BSAVA Manual of Canine and Feline Thoracic Imaging
second edition

Editors:

Tobias Schwarz
MA DrMedVet FRSB PGCAP FHEA DipECVDI DipACVR DVR FRCVS
Department of Veterinary Clinical Studies, Royal (Dick) School of Veterinary Studies,
The University of Edinburgh, Easter Bush Campus, Midlothian EH25 9RG

Peter Scrivani
DVM DipACVR
Department of Clinical Sciences, Cornell University College of Veterinary Medicine,
930 Campus Road, Box 36, Ithaca, NY 14853, USA

Published by:

British Small Animal Veterinary Association
Woodrow House, 1 Telford Way,
Waterwells Business Park, Quedgeley,
Gloucester GL2 2AB

A Company Limited by Guarantee in England
Registered Company No. 2837793
Registered as a Charity

ISBN: Print 978-1-910443-93-4 • Online 978-1-910443-94-1 • ePDF 978-1-913859-25-1 • EPUB 978-1-913859-26-8

The publishers, editors and contributors cannot take responsibility for information provided on dosages and methods of application of drugs mentioned or referred to in this publication. Details of this kind must be verified in each case by individual users from up to date literature published by the manufacturers or suppliers of those drugs. Veterinary surgeons are reminded that in each case they must follow all appropriate national legislation and regulations (for example, in the United Kingdom, the prescribing cascade) from time to time in force.

Save 15% off the digital version of this manual. By purchasing this print edition we are pleased to offer you a reduced price on online access at www.bsavalibrary.com
Enter offer code 15TI201 on checkout

Please note the discount only applies to a purchase of the full online version of the *BSAVA Manual of Canine and Feline Thoracic Imaging, 2nd edition* via **www.bsavalibrary.com**. The discount will be taken off the BSAVA member price or full price, depending on your member status. The discount code is for a single purchase of the online version and is for your personal use only. If you do not already have a login for the BSAVA website, you will need to register in order to make a purchase.

17348PUBS24

Printed in the UK by S&G Print Group, Merthyr Tydfil CF48 3TD

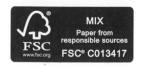

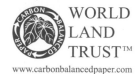

www.carbonbalancedpaper.com
CBP022977

Carbon Balancing is delivered by World Land Trust, an international conservation charity, who protects the world's most biologically important and threatened habitats acre by acre. Their Carbon Balanced Programme offsets emissions through the purchase and preservation of high conservation value forests.

Titles in the BSAVA Manuals series

Manual of Avian Practice: A Foundation Manual
Manual of Backyard Poultry Medicine and Surgery
Manual of Canine & Feline Abdominal Imaging
Manual of Canine & Feline Abdominal Surgery
Manual of Canine & Feline Advanced Veterinary Nursing
Manual of Canine & Feline Anaesthesia and Analgesia
Manual of Canine & Feline Behavioural Medicine
Manual of Canine & Feline Cardiorespiratory Medicine
Manual of Canine & Feline Clinical Pathology
Manual of Canine & Feline Dentistry and Oral Surgery
Manual of Canine & Feline Dermatology
Manual of Canine & Feline Emergency and Critical Care
Manual of Canine & Feline Endocrinology
Manual of Canine & Feline Endoscopy and Endosurgery
Manual of Canine & Feline Fracture Repair and Management
Manual of Canine & Feline Gastroenterology
Manual of Canine & Feline Haematology and Transfusion Medicine
Manual of Canine & Feline Head, Neck and Thoracic Surgery
Manual of Canine & Feline Musculoskeletal Disorders
Manual of Canine & Feline Musculoskeletal Imaging
Manual of Canine & Feline Nephrology and Urology
Manual of Canine & Feline Neurology
Manual of Canine & Feline Oncology
Manual of Canine & Feline Ophthalmology
Manual of Canine & Feline Radiography and Radiology: A Foundation Manual
*Manual of Canine & Feline Rehabilitation, Supportive and Palliative Care: Case Studies
    in Patient Management*
Manual of Canine & Feline Reproduction and Neonatology
*Manual of Canine & Feline Shelter Medicine: Principles of Health and Welfare in a
    Multi-animal Environment*
Manual of Canine & Feline Surgical Principles: A Foundation Manual
Manual of Canine & Feline Thoracic Imaging
Manual of Canine & Feline Ultrasonography
Manual of Canine & Feline Wound Management and Reconstruction
Manual of Canine Practice: A Foundation Manual
Manual of Exotic Pet and Wildlife Nursing
Manual of Exotic Pets: A Foundation Manual
Manual of Feline Practice: A Foundation Manual
Manual of Practical Animal Care
Manual of Practical Veterinary Nursing
Manual of Practical Veterinary Welfare
Manual of Psittacine Birds
Manual of Rabbit Medicine
Manual of Rabbit Surgery, Dentistry and Imaging
Manual of Raptors, Pigeons and Passerine Birds
Manual of Reptiles
Manual of Rodents and Ferrets
Manual of Small Animal Practice Management and Development
Manual of Wildlife Casualties

For further information on these and all BSAVA publications, please visit our website:
www.bsava.com

Contents

Contributors

Elizabeth Baines
MA VetMB DVR DipECVDI FHEA MRCVS
Willows Veterinary Centre and Referral Service,
Highlands Road, Solihull, West Midlands B90 4NH

Stacy Cooley
DVM DipACVR
Department of Clinical Sciences,
Carlson College of Veterinary Medicine,
Oregon State University, 700 SW 30th Street,
Corvallis, OR 97331-4801, USA

Joanna Dukes-McEwan
BVMS MVM PhD SFHEA DVC DipECVIM-CA(Cardiology) FRCVS
Cardiology Service, Small Animal Teaching Hospital,
Institute of Veterinary Science, University of Liverpool,
Leahurst Campus, Chester High Road,
Neston CH64 7TE

Anthony J. Fischetti
DVM MS DipACVR
Department of Diagnostic Imaging,
Schwarzman Animal Medical Center,
510 East 62nd Street, New York, NY 10065, USA

Mairi Frame
BVMS DVR DipECVDI FHEA MRCVS
Consultant in Veterinary Diagnostic Imaging
UK

Lorrie Gaschen
DVM PhD DrMedVet DipECVDI
School of Veterinary Medicine,
Louisiana State University, Baton Rouge,
Louisiana, LO 70803, USA

Karine Gendron
DVM DipECVDI DipACVR MRCVS
VetCT, Cambridge, UK

Alison King
BVMS MVM PhD DVR DipECVDI MRCVS
Vets Now Glasgow Hospital,
123–145 North Street, Glasgow G3 7DA

Ben van Klinken
MSc
SignalPET,
13101 Preston Road #110–313,
Dallas, TX 75240, USA

Tiziana Liuti
DVM PhD DipECVDI PGCAP FHEA FRSB FRCVS
Department of Veterinary Clinical Studies,
Royal (Dick) School of Veterinary Studies,
The University of Edinburgh, Easter Bush Campus,
Midlothian EH25 9RG

Maurizio Longo
DVM PhD Doctor Europaeus DipECVDI MRCVS
Antech Imaging Service,
University of Milan, Italy

Federica Morandi
DrMedVet MS DipACVR DipECVDI
Department of Small Animal Clinical Sciences,
The University of Tennessee,
Knoxville, TN 37996, USA

Ian Porter
DVM DipACVR
Department of Clinical Sciences,
Cornell University College of Veterinary Medicine,
930 Campus Road, Box 25, Ithaca, NY 14853, USA

Tobias Schwarz
MA DrMedVet FRSB PGCAP FHEA DipECVDI DipACVR DVR FRCVS
Department of Veterinary Clinical Studies,
Royal (Dick) School of Veterinary Studies,
The University of Edinburgh, Easter Bush Campus,
Midlothian EH25 9RG

Peter V. Scrivani
DVM DipACVR
Department of Clinical Sciences,
Cornell University College of Veterinary Medicine,
930 Campus Road, Box 36,
Ithaca, NY 14853, USA

Gabriela Seiler
DrMedVet DipECVDI DipACVR
Terry Companion Animal Veterinarian Medical Clinic,
College of Veterinary Medicine,
1052 William Moore Dr, Raleigh, NC 27606, USA

Neil Shaw
DVM DipACVIM
SignalPET,
13101 Preston Road #110–313,
Dallas, TX 75240, USA

Foreword

I feel honoured to write the Foreword for the *BSAVA Manual of Canine and Feline Thoracic Imaging, Second edition* edited by Tobias Schwarz and Peter Scrivani. This manual follows in the footsteps of the textbook *Thoracic Radiography: A text atlas of thoracic diseases of the dog and cat* published in 1984 by Peter Suter with contributions of Peter Lord. Peter Suter, who was Professor of Veterinary Radiology at the University of California, Davis and later Zurich University, sadly passed away in 2011. I still belong to the generation of radiologists having known Professor Peter F. Suter in person and his book was my bible for thoracic radiography during my residency. I regularly open this book to brush up my knowledge and find it still extremely valuable. I am very happy that many images from his book and in particular Peter Suter's spirit are found in the second edition of the *BSAVA Manual of Canine and Feline Thoracic Imaging*, showing that radiography is still work horse number one for thoracic imaging in dogs and cats.

This BSAVA Manual expands the classic radiographic knowledge by adding state-of-the-art modern imaging modalities and their interpretive principles. These modalities, such as ultrasonography and computed tomography, are used more and more by veterinarians throughout the world at all levels of veterinary care. By highlighting the relevance and limitations of these imaging modalities, we can achieve more accurate diagnoses and differentials for small animal patients with clinical signs of thoracic diseases.

The manual is structured into two major parts. The first part separately describes each modality used today in thoracic imaging. It provides information on when and how to use each modality and describes the modality-specific imaging anatomy. The second part is divided into all major thoracic body systems and describes normal and abnormal findings for each imaging modality. It gives very detailed interpretative principles and teaches the reader comprehensively about the abnormalities and their lists of differential diagnoses.

This manual serves veterinary students, small animal practitioners, trainees and specialists in diagnostic imaging alike as a modern comprehensive textbook and reference for small animal thoracic imaging. It should be ready at hand in the digital or physical bookshelf of every small animal radiology area.

Patrick R. Kircher
Prof.Dr.med.vet. PhD DipECVDI Executive MBA(UZH)
Vetsuisse Faculty Zürich

Preface

Thoracic radiography remains a challenge for many students and small animal practitioners alike. It is widely available in small animal practice, cost effective and requires only moderate skills to be performed well. Thoracic radiography is essential for the clinical work-up of most dogs and cats with cardiorespiratory signs. Often, it is used as an end-diagnostic tool, where treatment decisions are solely based on the radiographic interpretation. However, the thorax is arguably also the most difficult body area to interpret in radiography, due to the summation and constant motion of nearly all thoracic structures, the complexity of the functional aspects of the thoracic organs and the large degree of overlap of radiographic findings in physiological and pathological processes. Therefore, many clinicians and students are faced with the dilemma of having to interpret thoracic radiographs daily but finding it challenging to make their diagnoses with confidence. This manual is designed to aid novices and experienced veterinarians alike to give them a strong foundation to interpret canine and feline thoracic radiographs. In addition, the manual lays out when and how alternative imaging techniques are indicated to narrow down the differential list and to plan a therapeutic approach.

In 1984, Peter Suter published his textbook *Thoracic Radiography: A text atlas of thoracic diseases of the dog and cat*, the first ever comprehensive textbook on small animal thoracic radiology. It became the ultimate reference for students, small animal veterinarians and veterinary radiologists, but was soon out of print. The concept of the first edition of the *BSAVA Manual of Canine and Feline Thoracic Imaging*, published in 2008, was to bring a modern version of this book to the veterinary community and to include new thoracic imaging modalities. Peter Suter actively supported this effort and permitted many of his classic illustrations to be included in this manual. The first edition of the BSAVA Manual was a great success, but diagnostic imaging has evolved significantly over the last 16 years. There have been improvements in the diagnostic capabilities of all modalities allowing better and more specific diagnosis. Computed tomography is now commonly used as a first-line diagnostic tool for many patients with suspected thoracic diseases. Artificial intelligence has entered the arsenal of small animal thoracic imaging diagnostics. There are new concepts of thoracic image interpretation that need to be reflected in the interpretative process. Therefore, an update was urgently needed. In a world with exceeding technical improvements and expanding diagnostic modalities, it becomes even more important to have a strong and detailed foundation on thoracic anatomy, imaging anatomy, physiology and pathophysiology, something new co-editor Peter Scrivani is particularly dedicated to. For this second edition, we have put a lot of emphasis on these foundations and how they relate to specific imaging findings.

We are grateful to the many radiologists and other specialists from around the world who contributed to this manual by writing chapters, supplying images and providing feedback. Many thanks are also due to Victoria Johnson, co-editor of the first edition, for shaping the foundation of this manual in the second edition. Our aim was to ensure that the manual was as up-to-date, accurate and comprehensive as possible. The manual is organized into two sections: the first explaining the different imaging modalities and their recommended usage and the second illustrating the features of normalcy and disease of the main anatomical compartments of the thorax. We have emphasized the more common conditions and their diagnosis, but also provided the entire spectrum of thoracic diseases. High quality images of the interpretative principles and thoracic diseases are included in this manual.

We would like to extend our sincerest thanks to the publications team at BSAVA for their hard work and seemingly never-ending patience and all the authors for their time and expertise, and last but not least, all dogs and cats whose images were used in this manual. After all, dogs and cats are man's best friends!

Tobias Schwarz
Peter Scrivani
January 2024

Chapter 1

Basics of thoracic radiography and radiology

Ian Porter

Thoracic radiography is a cost-effective, non-invasive, readily available diagnostic and screening tool for thoracic and systemic disease in small animals that uses X-rays to create representative images of the internal form of an object. The procedure is relatively easy to perform but careful attention to technique is required to avoid degradation of image quality and optimize reduction of diagnostic uncertainty. In contrast to the ease of image acquisition, thoracic radiographic interpretation is challenging. Factors contributing to difficulty in thoracic radiographic interpretation include:

- Radiographs are planar images (two-dimensional representations of three-dimensional objects)
  - Lack of depth perception; commonly partially overcome by obtaining at least two orthogonal views
  - Object morphology depends on the direction of the radiographic view and the orientation of the X-ray beam; commonly mitigated by standardized patient positioning, routinely using a vertically oriented X-ray beam, and standardized hanging protocols for image orientation
- Anatomical depiction is primarily due to differential absorption of the X-ray beam, which produces shadows or silhouettes of objects in the image. Magnification, distortion, and geometric unsharpness also contribute to anatomical depiction. Phenomena associated with differential absorption of the X-ray beam include:
  - Contrast (the ability to distinguish separate objects based on opacity)
  - Positive and negative summation shadows (superimposition of structures)
  - Border effacement (lack of contrast between structures forming a novel silhouette)
- Patient variables
  - The wide range of normal anatomical and physiological variations
  - Fluid and gas redistribution according to gravity within hollow or tubular structures
- Wide overlapping spectrum of radiographic features of physiological and pathological processes
  - Similar imaging features in different diseases (lack of specificity)
  - Lack of morphological change until late in disease (lack of sensitivity).

Basics of radiography

X-rays are a form of ionizing radiation (electromagnetic energy), first discovered in 1895 by Wilhelm Röntgen who was able to produce a radiograph of a human hand. The discovery rapidly led to the development of clinical uses of radiography in medicine. Since that time, dramatic advancements have been made in the technology used to produce and detect X-rays, understanding of the hazards of ionizing radiation and the ability to maintain radiation exposure as low as reasonably achievable. Production of radiographs has progressed from photographic plates to film and, more recently, to digital radiography. The study of the effects of ionizing radiation on tissue has identified two types of adverse consequence. *Deterministic effects* are threshold dependent, meaning that there is no harmful effect below a certain level of exposure (threshold) to ionizing radiation; above the threshold, there is a predictable effect. Examples include radiation-induced cataracts and skin burns. Deterministic effects are infrequent in diagnostic imaging as the threshold for these effects is typically higher than the doses of radiation used in diagnostic procedures. In contrast, *stochastic effects* can occur at any exposure level. Exposure, however, does not equate to developing a harmful effect. The severity of the effect is not proportional to the exposure dose, but the risk for occurrence of effects is greater when the level of exposure is larger. Stochastic harmful effects of radiation exposure include carcinogenesis, teratogenesis, and mutagenesis. Because stochastic effects may occur with any level of exposure to ionizing radiation, it is important to limit unnecessary patient exposure and to follow strict radiation safety procedures to prevent unnecessary exposure of both staff and the public.

Digital radiography

Digital radiology has nearly replaced traditional film-based radiography and offers many advantages:

- Greater exposure latitude: a wide range of exposures can be used to produce a diagnostic image
- Post-processing: a choice of different density curves is available to examine relatively underexposed areas, such as the vertebral column, in the same detail as correctly exposed areas, such as the lung, in the same image

- Viewing digital images allows manipulations (e.g. magnification, window and level, pan) to maximize use of the available spatial and contrast resolutions obtained during image acquisition
- Digital images can be viewed remotely or digitally transferred for referral or interpretation
- Prior imaging studies can be rapidly retrieved for comparison
- A remote back-up database can be created.

Two types of digital radiography exist: computed radiography and direct radiography. As both rely on a traditional X-ray machine, often these technologies can be incorporated with existing X-ray equipment using different detectors.

Direct digital radiography

The flat panel detector is the most common type of digital radiography (DR) detector and there are two types:

- Direct detectors, where the incoming X-ray beam interacts with a photoconductor to liberate electrons that are collected and processed to create an electrical signal
- Indirect detectors, where an X-ray scintillator screen produces light that is collected and processed to create an electrical signal.

In both cases, the electrical signal is directly sent to the image processor and the resulting image is almost immediately displayed. Both wired and wireless systems are available, the latter offering more flexibility to position the plate for non-standard views, such as when using a horizontally oriented X-ray beam.

Computed radiography

A specialized cassette containing an imaging plate coated with a photostimulable phosphor (PSP) is used in computed radiography (CR) systems. When exposed to X-ray radiation, the PSP will immediately release a portion of the absorbed energy as light; the remaining energy becomes temporarily trapped in the PSP. To create the radiographic image, the plate is fed into a special reading device (Figure 1.1) where a laser scans the plate, releasing the stored energy in the form of luminescent light. The light is collected by a fibreoptic light guide and directed to a photomultiplier tube. The resulting electrical signal is proportional to the strength of the light released and becomes digitized to represent a pixel value for each specific location on the imaging plate. Once the plate is read, residual stored energy is released ('erased') by exposing it to a white light to prepare it for the next radiographic exposure. Compared with DR, the main disadvantage is that each cassette must be manually fed into the reader and the image reading process can take 1–2 minutes. This may create time limitations in a busy hospital, particularly if a single CR reader is supporting more than one radiology room. An advantage is that the plate is not tethered nor fixed to the imaging table and may be positioned more easily for non-standard views. CR cassettes are also very robust and relatively low in price. This allows purchase of multiple cassettes of different sizes, which facilitates a flexible workflow and redundancy of image capturing devices.

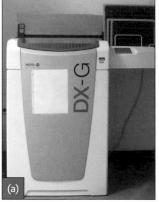
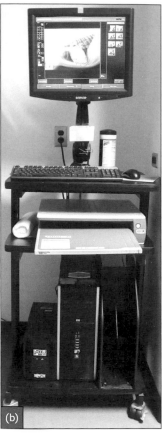

1.1 Computed radiography system including (a) a cassette reader and (b) digital workstation.

Thoracic radiography

Indications

Based on the patient's history and clinical findings, thoracic radiography is used to assess primary intrathoracic disease, thoracic involvement of systemic disease or both. There are many clinical indications for performing thoracic radiography (Figure 1.2). The goals of thoracic radiography may include reducing diagnostic uncertainty, determining the extent of an abnormality, planning treatment, or monitoring disease progression or response to treatment. In general, thoracic radiography:

- Identifies or confirms:
  - Presence of thoracic disease
  - Anatomical location of a disease within the thorax
  - Type of abnormality
  - Extent of abnormality
- Provides a definitive diagnosis or helps refine differential diagnoses
- Suggests additional procedures
- Documents the development/course of an abnormality.

• Coughing
• Dyspnoea
• Cardiovascular disease
• Suspected primary or metastatic neoplasia
• Regurgitation
• Thoracic body wall abnormalities
• Fever of unknown origin
• Planning an interventional procedure

1.2 Common indications for thoracic radiography.

Performing thoracic radiography

When deciding to perform thoracic radiography, it is important to consider the risks to the patient and the safety of those performing the study. For the patient, do the benefits outweigh the risks? What is the likelihood that the results may change the treatment plan? Is the patient stable enough to safely undergo the procedure? Should the patient first be stabilized, or could the procedure be modified based on the patient's clinical condition? If the benefits of performing the study do not outweigh the cost and risks, or if the results are unlikely to alter patient management, then the study should not be performed. When thoracic radiography is deemed necessary, it is important to consider how best to perform the examination by determining which views are needed and whether the patient should be sedated or manually restrained for positioning. In addition to acquiring well positioned and well exposed radiographs without motion, it is essential that radiographs be appropriately labelled with patient identification, date of the examination, patient side or recumbency, and veterinarian or clinic performing the examination. Care must be taken to minimize unnecessary exposure of personnel to ionizing radiation and prevent physical injury by fractious and aggressive patients.

Patient restraint and preparation

Animals presented for thoracic radiography are often afraid, in pain and/or dyspnoeic. With considerate handling and verbal reassurance, most patients can be restrained with a combination of positioning aids and sedation. Occasionally, manual restraint is necessary.

Chemical restraint

Sedation is highly recommended for thoracic radiography unless contraindicated by the clinical condition of the patient. Sedatives facilitate positioning by making the animal more amenable to handling. The level of sedation should depend upon the demeanour and general health of the animal. Quiet surroundings are essential for sedation to take effect, not only immediately after administration but during the radiographic procedure as well. If the animal is in pain, sedation will not occur unless analgesics are also administered.

Anaesthesia is not usually required for standard radiographic procedures; however, it may be required in difficult or painful patients. The clinical condition of the patient should be considered before performing general anaesthesia. Anaesthetic-induced atelectasis may hinder interpretation and therefore general anaesthesia is often not recommended unless necessary to ensure patient compliance. Repeated gentle inflation prior to obtaining radiographs, positive pressure ventilation, use of alveolar recruitment technique and use of different body positions may assist in preventing or resolving atelectasis.

Physical restraint and positioning aids

The following are commonly employed as positioning aids (Figures 1.3 and 1.4):

- Sandbags
- Troughs
- Foam wedges
- Ties and tape
- Gauze rolls

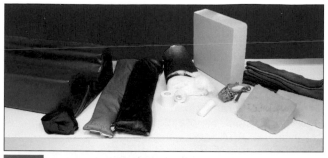

1.3 Commonly used aids for physical restraint.

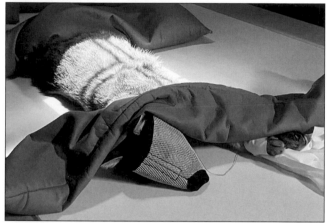

1.4 A sedated cat positioned for thoracic radiography using non-manual restraint devices (sandbags, tape and a cloth muzzle that covers the eyes).

- Cotton wool rolls
- Towels
- Muzzles.

Placing a dyspnoeic cat in a cardboard box can be a low-stress method to obtain a dorsoventral (DV) view.

Manual restraint

Holding a patient increases the risk of ionizing radiation exposure to the radiographer and, therefore, the use of manual restraint is often regulated by local laws. These laws differ from place to place and it is important to understand the laws governing veterinary radiology in the region where the veterinary hospital is located. In some jurisdictions (such as the UK), regulations prohibit routine manual restraint of animals during radiographic exposure and permit manual restraint (Figure 1.5) only when there is a strong clinical indication to do so (e.g. non-manual

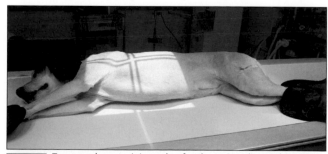

1.5 Two people restraining a dog for thoracic radiography. Using two people allows each person to remain as far from the primary beam and patient as possible. Manual restraint should only be performed when chemical and non-manual physical restraint are not possible or are ineffective.

physical restraint is not tolerated by the patient and chemical restraint is ineffective or contraindicated based on the patient's medical condition). In regions where regulations are more lenient, radiation protection (Figure 1.6) should remain a priority and be based on the principle of as low as reasonably achievable (ALARA).

ALARA refers to making every reasonable effort to maintain exposures to ionizing radiation as far below the legal dose limits as practical. The primary factors in achieving ALARA are distance, time and shielding. Distance is one of the most effective ways to reduce radiation dose; doubling the distance from the radiation source reduces exposure by a factor of four. Time is directly related to the number of exposures required. Time can be minimized by using sedation or anaesthesia for uncooperative patients, thereby reducing the number of exposures that require manual restraint and reducing the number of repeat exposures by facilitating proper patient positioning and minimizing patient motion. Shielding is provided in several ways, including shielding built in to radiation-producing equipment to prevent radiation leakage outside the primary beam, structural shielding within the facility that is designed to protect both radiation workers and the public (refer to local regulations), and personal protective equipment. Personal protective equipment includes lead-impregnated aprons, gloves, thyroid shields and radiation protective eyeglasses. Protective gloves and aprons are inadequate at protecting one from exposure to the primary X-ray beam because these items do not attenuate high-energy X-rays (Figure 1.7a). Personal protective equipment must be properly stored and regularly checked for physical damage such as cracks. It is important to recognize that substantial radiation exposure occurs outside the primary beam due to scatter and off-focus radiation (Figure 1.7b).

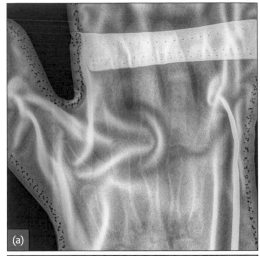

(a)

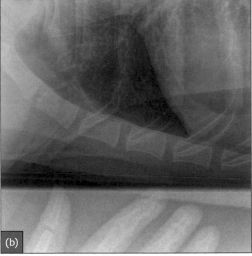

(b)

1.7 Radiographs of a human hand-and-wrist phantom. (a) The phantom is placed inside a 0.5 mm lead equivalent glove and exposed to the primary X-ray beam; the bones of the phantom are easily identified with the primary beam penetrating the lead glove and reaching the detector. (b) The phantom is placed beside a patient, over the detector but outside of the primary beam. Note the degree of exposure of the phantom due to scatter radiation.

- Manual restraint should be used only in exceptional circumstances and should not be permitted unless the X-ray machine is fitted with a light beam diaphragm
- The use of sedation or anaesthesia and positioning aids should always be considered before recourse to manual restraint
- Only those who are absolutely required to perform the study should be allowed in the room during the radiographic exposure
- A maximal distance from the primary beam should be maintained
- Two people may be required so that each is as far away from the primary beam as possible (see Figure 1.5)
- Personal dosimetry devices must be used
- Personal protection such as lead aprons, gloves, thyroid protectors and lead-impregnated glasses must be worn
- People who are pregnant or under the age of 18 should not be present in the room during the radiographic exposure

1.6 Essential steps in radiation safety.

Technique

Collimation

Collimators are used to regulate the size and shape of the X-ray beam (field of view). A light source placed inside the collimator will show the centre and exact size of the X-ray field; the field of view should be limited to only the required anatomy. Careful centring allows accurate collimation. Collimation of the X-ray beam to the area of the body under investigation has two important functions:

- Limit unnecessary radiation exposure to the patient
- Reduce excessive scatter radiation that will reduce radiographic contrast.

Scatter radiation is radiation that spreads out from the primary X-ray beam because of interactions with the object examined. Scatter radiation is minimized by including only the necessary parts of the body in the primary X-ray beam. Frequently, this is achieved by collimating the primary beam such that the field of view is as small as needed. Scatter radiation, however, is maximized when the examined object is 30 x 30 cm. Above this point, collimation does not further reduce scatter radiation and only reduces patient exposure and delineates the extent of the primary X-ray beam. Room air surrounding the object has a negligible contribution to scatter.

Grids

Grids improve radiographic contrast by absorbing scatter radiation. In doing so they also absorb part of the primary beam, requiring an increase in radiographic exposure. Regions of anatomy thicker than 10 cm should be radiographed using a grid. In regions less than 10 cm thick, scatter is insufficient to result in substantial image degradation; avoiding a grid in these cases will allow the use of lower exposure factors and prevent any possible grid-related artefacts (Figure 1.8). A moving (Potter–Bucky)

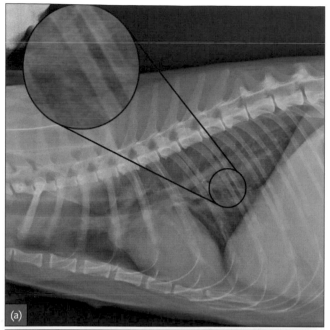

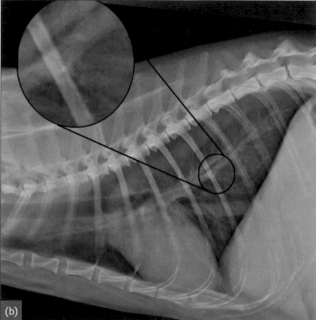

1.8 Lateral thoracic radiographs of a cat acquired with (a) a stationary grid and (b) tabletop (without the use of a grid). In the magnified inserts, notice the prominent parallel grid lines displayed across the image in (a).

grid will reduce the appearance of grid lines on the radiograph. It is important to be aware of other possible artefacts such as grid cut-off. Grid cut-off is excessive absorption of radiation by the grid due to technical causes, including an upside down (focused) grid, decentring of the grid relative to the primary beam, incorrect focus-to-grid distance and an off-level grid (the grid not being perpendicular to the primary beam).

Exposure

An exposure chart guides selection of the kilovoltage peak (kVp) potential across the X-ray tube and the mAs, which is the product of the X-ray tube current in milliamperes (mA) and length of exposure in seconds (s), based on body region and tissue thickness in centimetres. The kVp determines mainly the photon energy spectrum (the quality of

the X-ray beam) and the mAs dictates the number of photons emitted (the quantity of X-ray photons in the beam). Together, the kVp and mAs determine the intensity of the X-ray beam. Radiographic contrast (or contrast resolution) refers to the difference in opacity (shade of grey) between different structures in the image. When a lower kVp technique is used, more of the X-ray beam is absorbed proportional to the cubed atomic number of the exposed tissue (photoelectric effect) and less is absorbed proportionally to the physical density of the tissue or scattered (Compton effect). The result is a high-contrast radiograph with fewer shades of grey (i.e. objects are mostly black or white). When a higher kVp technique is used, the opposite is true; more of the X-ray beam is linearly absorbed or scattered (Compton effect) and less is exponentially absorbed (photoelectric effect), resulting in a low-contrast radiograph with many shades of grey. In thoracic radiography, a high kVp is used because a low-contrast image with a wide range of tones of grey is desired to enable better evaluation of lung detail. In addition, when the higher kVp setting is used, the mAs is reduced to produce the correct radiographic exposure; this is important in reducing motion artefacts since the reduction in mAs is mostly accomplished by reducing the duration of the exposure (Figure 1.9).

The ideal radiographic technique for the thorax is:

* High kVp
* Low mAs (specifically, short exposure time).

Timing: inspiration *versus* expiration

In almost all cases, exposure should occur at the end of the inspiratory phase, when the lungs are fully expanded. Radiographs acquired at the end of expiration show reduced lung size and pulmonary opacification that may mimic lung disease. End-expiratory radiographs are useful in certain situations, for example when evaluated together with the inspiratory view to detect dynamic changes in the lung (e.g. air-trapping, identification of pulmonary fibrosis) or trachea and in diagnosis of small volume pneumothorax. It is important to understand that lungs do not

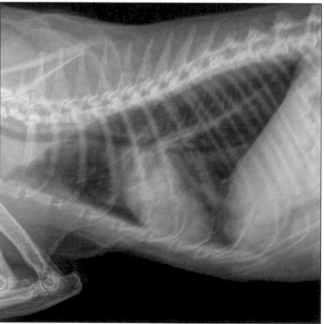

1.9 Right lateral thoracic radiograph of a cat demonstrating patient motion artefact.

appear darker (less opaque) on inspiratory radiographs because they contain more air, which does not attenuate X-rays, but because they contain less blood and soft tissue structures are spaced further apart. Under the increased inspiratory lung pressure, the heart and pulmonary vessels are compressed and some of the blood is moved out of the thorax. Soft tissue structures of the lungs are spaced further apart with increased air volume. This leads to less fluid and soft tissue in the thorax that would otherwise attenuate X-rays.

Standard radiographic views

Radiographs are named by the entrance and exit points of the projected X-ray beam through the patient. For example, a 'ventrodorsal' (VD) view indicates that the beam entered the ventral aspect of the patient and exited the dorsal aspect of the patient. By convention, there is an exception to this rule whereby lateral radiographs are commonly shortened to indicate the side of the patient closest to the detector. For example, a 'right–left lateral radiograph' may be reduced to 'left lateral radiograph'. In small animals, it is assumed that a vertically oriented X-ray beam is used unless specified otherwise. Therefore, the name of the radiographic view also indicates patient recumbency. Because the X-ray tube is usually suspended above the patient, a ventrodorsal view is made with the patient in dorsal recumbency (i.e. the back being against the table or detector). A right–left lateral view (a left lateral radiograph) indicates that the patient is in left lateral recumbency.

Before discussing differences between views, it is important to understand three concepts:

- Pulmonary atelectasis
- Gravity-dependent redistribution
- Image magnification and penumbra (Figure 1.10)

These concepts are important in understanding the differences between views and why abnormalities might not be detected if the appropriate views are not acquired (Figure 1.11).

Atelectasis refers to collapse or incomplete expansion of the pulmonary parenchyma, for which there are many causes (see Chapter 12). In recumbent patients, the 'down' (gravity-dependent) regions of the lung are most susceptible to atelectasis due to the lung's inherent elasticity (it tends to collapse under the weight of the overlying lung and viscera including the heart) and due to cranial displacement of the diaphragm because of gravity on the abdominal viscera. While some degree of gravity-dependent atelectasis is common, the severity may be exacerbated in patients who are deeply sedated, in patients under general anaesthesia and on supplemental oxygen where there is less stimulus for deep inspiration, in patients who are obese and have substantial intrathoracic fat accumulations, and in patients who have been in unchanged recumbency for prolonged periods of time. Opacification of atelectatic regions of lung can vary from minimal to substantial, depending on the volume of atelectatic lung and the degree of hypoxic pulmonary vasoconstriction in that lung. When opacification occurs, it may mimic the appearance of pathology (e.g. pneumonia) or mask abnormalities within the lung (e.g. nodules).

Gravity-dependent redistribution affects gas and fluid within the pleural cavity, cavitary lesions, and hollow viscera such as the oesophagus. Repositioning the patient can cause a redistribution of fluid and gas that may help in the diagnosis of an abnormality (for example, a horizontal beam view may detect a fluid–gas interface within a pulmonary abscess) or help redistribute fluid to aid in seeing the anatomy (for example, when pleural fluid is present).

Image magnification is defined as the size of an object in an image divided by the actual object size. Penumbra is a loss of sharpness around the margins of an object and occurs because the focal spot of the anode in the X-ray tube has a finite dimension rather than being a point source.

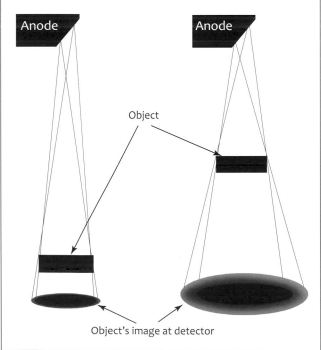

1.10 Magnification and penumbra. The objects on the left and right are equal in size. The object on the right is farther away from the detector than the object on the left; the resulting image of the object on the right is magnified and has penumbra (unsharpness) around its margin.

- It is easier to detect lung lesions and evaluate normal lung anatomy in the non-gravity-dependent lung (lateral views) or lung region (DV or VD views)
- In the gravity-dependent region of the lung, increased pulmonary opacification due to atelectasis may silhouette with pulmonary abnormalities resulting in false-negative diagnoses or reduced diagnostic confidence
- Although the non-dependent lung is easier to evaluate on lateral views, the dependent lung can also be seen and summates with the non-dependent lung
- Pathology in the non-dependent lung will be magnified and have penumbra (unsharpness) but the improved contrast that occurs between well inflated non-dependent lungs and soft tissue pulmonary abnormalities more than compensates for having penumbra
- The thoracic body wall located closest to the detector is easier to evaluate because magnification and penumbra are minimized
- When pleural fluid is present and the patient is in ventral recumbency, the fluid will pool in the narrower ventral portion of the thoracic cavity that also contains the heart. Consequently, the fluid will be deeper and attenuate X-rays to the same extent as the heart, producing border effacement of the cardiac silhouette on the DV view (Figure 1.12a). When the patient is positioned for a VD radiograph, the fluid will pool dorsally over a wider area and cause retraction of the caudodorsal margins of the lungs from the body wall (Figure 1.12b). When a small volume of pleural fluid is present, it will usually be more easily detected in a VD radiograph than in a DV radiograph
- A DV rather than a VD view is preferred for patients in respiratory distress

1.11 Important considerations in selecting and interpreting radiographic views.

Image magnification and unsharpness due to penumbra are minimized when the focal spot is small and the object of interest is closest to the detector, and increase with increasing distance of the object from the detector. Sufficient distance between the X-ray source and object also may be important when using a horizontal beam.

A routine radiographic examination of the thorax includes three views: both lateral views and at least one ventrodorsal or dorsoventral view. In some cases, acquisition of both DV and VD views may provide additional information (Figure 1.12). Historically, references have stated the minimal standard of routine thoracic radiography is to obtain at least two orthogonal views, when possible. With the adoption of digital radiography, which has eliminated the cost of expendable inputs such as film and has resulted in rapid image processing (particularly with DR systems), many recommend routinely obtaining three views. In some cases, based on the clinical condition of the patient, the study may need to be abbreviated by eliminating views that will cause unnecessary risk or stress to the patient, though it is important to realize that elimination of views may result

in loss of information and the potential for abnormalities to go undetected. If an examination is abbreviated, then the views that are most likely to yield a diagnosis should be acquired. For example, if there is concern for aspiration pneumonia, which occurs most commonly in the right middle lung lobe, then a left lateral view (to best evaluate the right middle and cranial lung lobes) and a VD view (to best evaluate the cranioventral lung field) may be prioritized. For cardiac conditions, the heart will be in a more consistent position on a right lateral view due to the cardiac notch of the lungs being located on the right side, whereas a DV view will better evaluate the caudodorsal lung field and pulmonary blood vessels while creating less magnification of the cardiac silhouette. For a metastasis check, both lateral views and a DV view are recommended when possible. Additional, non-routine views are described below (see 'Supplementary views'). It is important to understand how and why these should be performed.

Technique for standard views
Lateral views

1. Position the patient in right or left lateral recumbency.
2. Place a sandbag over the neck with the sand distributed to either end (so as not to compress the airway and blood vessels).
3. Extend the thoracic limbs forward and secure with sandbags or ties to avoid superimposition of the limbs over the cranial thorax.
4. Position a sandbag over the hindquarters or wrapped around the pelvic limbs. Gently extend the head and neck to avoid positional variation of the trachea.
5. The sternum and vertebrae should be level with each other; a foam positioning wedge under the sternum and/or back may be required depending on patient conformation (Figure 1.13).
6. Centre the X-ray beam at the caudal aspect of the scapula and two-thirds of this distance ventrally over the thorax (Figure 1.14). Collimation should include the thoracic inlet and whole diaphragm (including part of the liver).

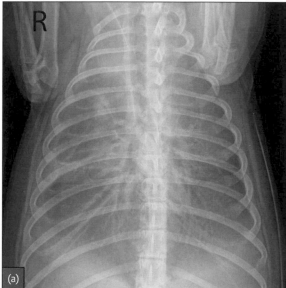

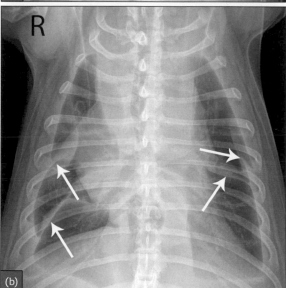

1.12 (a) DV and (b) VD thoracic radiographs of a dog with pleural fluid. Notice the redistribution of fluid between views with border effacement of the cardiac silhouette on the DV radiograph and the retraction of the dorsal aspect of the lungs from the lateral thoracic body walls with wide interlobar fissures (arrowed) on the VD view.

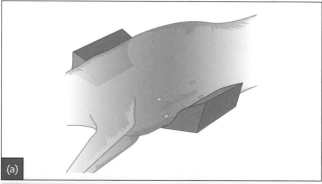

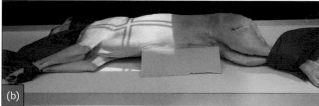

1.13 Patient positioning for a right lateral thoracic radiograph. (a) In some patients, foam wedges may be needed to comfortably level the patient both dorsally and ventrally. (b) The patient is positioned and restrained in right lateral recumbency using sandbags for physical restraint and a foam wedge to level the sternum and vertebral column.

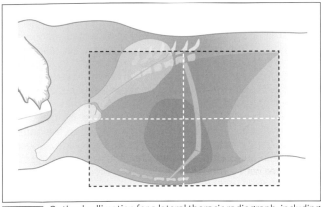

1.14 Optimal collimation for a lateral thoracic radiograph, including centring of the X-ray beam.

7. Include a left or right marker in the collimated area, usually the axillary region, to indicate the recumbency of the patient.
8. In almost all instances, radiographic exposure should be made on full inspiration.

Dorsoventral and ventrodorsal views

DV view:

1. Position the animal in ventral recumbency with elbows to either side of the thorax and the pelvic limbs flexed, resulting in a crouching position.

2. It may be helpful to support the paws of the pelvic limb with sandbags to avoid slipping.
3. Some patients may be more comfortable when placed in a trough or when supported by a foam block under the sternum (Figure 1.15).
4. Ensure that the animal is straight with sternum and vertebrae summating.
5. Gently extend the neck and, if necessary, rest it on a foam block.
6. Place a sandbag across the neck, taking care not to compromise the airway.
7. Centre the beam on the vertebral column, immediately caudal to the scapulae.
8. Collimate to include the thoracic inlet, diaphragm and cranial abdomen, and the lateral aspects of the thorax.
9. Include a right or left marker in the collimated area, usually in the axillary region, to indicate the patient's right or left side.

VD view:

1. Place the animal in dorsal recumbency in a trough or bean bag.
2. Pull the thoracic limbs forward and fix them in position with sandbags (Figure 1.16); alternatively, ties or tape may be used to secure the limbs.
3. The vertebrae and sternum should summate.
4. Centre the beam on the centre of the sternum.
5. Collimation and labelling are as described for the DV view.

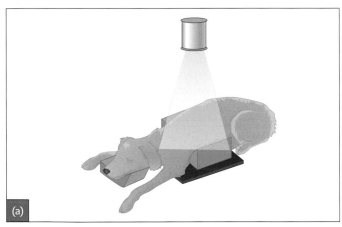

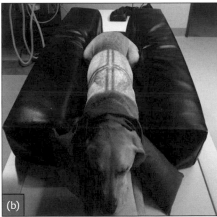

1.15 Patient positioning for a DV thoracic radiograph using (a) foam wedges and (b) a trough. These positioning aids help maintain the proper position while keeping the patient comfortable.

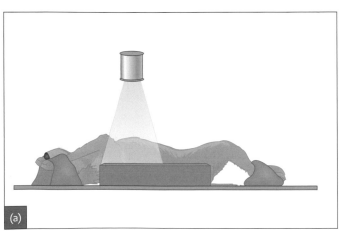

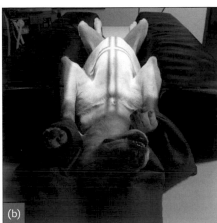

1.16 (a, b) Patient positioning for a VD thoracic radiograph using a trough and sandbags.

Supplementary views

DV or VD (decubitus/horizontal) view

This view may improve sensitivity in detection of a small pneumothorax or small volumes of pleural fluid. Consideration must be given to radiation safety; the X-ray beam must only be directed at suitable equipment (e.g. lead-backed cassettes) or a suitable barrier or wall that provides sufficient shielding.

The technique is as follows (Figure 1.17):

1. The patient may be placed in left or right lateral recumbency. The decision will depend on the indication for obtaining this view.

2. Direct the X-ray beam horizontally by turning the X-ray tube head through 90 degrees.
3. Position the cassette against the back or sternum. The use of a cassette holder is recommended; if unavailable, the cassette may need to be supported by sandbags to remain upright.
4. It is important to maintain the usual film/detector–focus distance (FFD).
5. If a grid is used, the tube head should be aligned carefully with respect to the grid to avoid grid cut-off.
6. Include a right or left marker in the collimated area to indicate the patient's right or left side. A positional marker with a moveable bead may be used to show the direction of gravity and patient recumbency.

Left–right lateral (standing/horizontal) or right–left lateral (standing/horizontal) view

Either view may be used in animals with severe respiratory compromise that cannot be positioned in lateral recumbency to obtain a standard lateral view. These views are useful for the detection of pneumothorax, pleural fluid and gas–fluid interfaces of cysts or abscesses. An example of a gas–fluid interface is provided in Figure 1.18. A similar view can be achieved with the animal in ventral recumbency or in a sitting position. It may be easier to extend the thoracic limbs adequately in ventral recumbency than in a standing position. These views are less sensitive for the detection of small volumes of pleural fluid when compared with the decubitus view.

The technique is as follows (Figure 1.19):

1. Position the cassette in a cassette holder against the thoracic body wall (costal region).
2. Rotate the tube head 90 degrees and centre and collimate as for a lateral recumbent view.

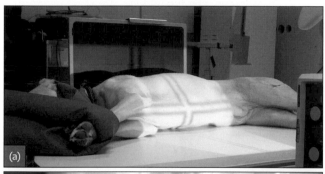

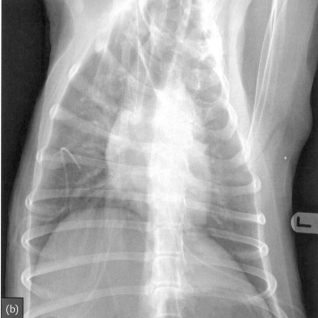

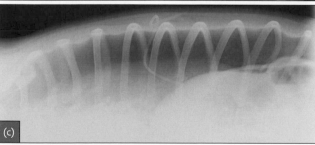

1.17 (a) Patient positioning for a VD (right decubitus/horizontal) thoracic radiograph. Note that collimation is insufficient; the X-ray beam should be collimated to only include the required region of anatomy and never extend beyond the margins of the detector. (b) DV thoracic radiograph of a dog with idiopathic pneumothorax that was drained. It is difficult to ascertain whether residual pleural gas is present or not. (c) VD (left decubitus/horizontal) thoracic radiograph of the same dog as in (b) demonstrating the presence of a large volume of right-sided pleural gas.

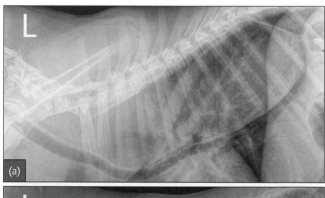

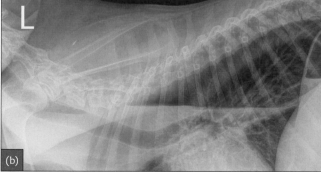

1.18 (a) Left–right lateral thoracic radiograph and (b) left–right lateral (standing/horizontal) thoracic radiograph of a 5-year-old German Shepherd Dog with megaoesophagus. Compare the distribution of air and fluid within the oesophageal lumen between the views. A distinct gas–fluid interface is only detected on the horizontal beam view.

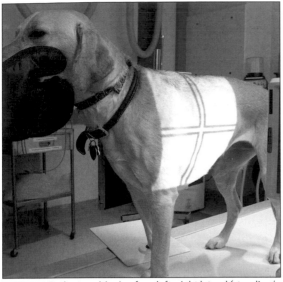

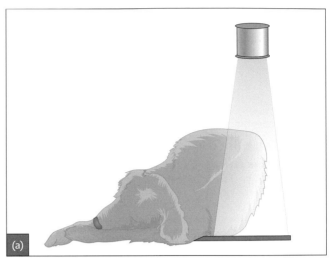

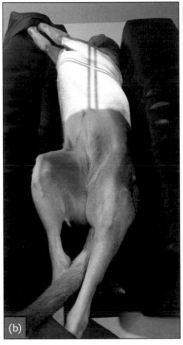

1.19 Patient positioning for a left–right lateral (standing/horizontal) thoracic radiograph.

1.21 Patient positioning for (a) an oblique DV thoracic radiograph and (b) an oblique VD thoracic radiograph.

3. Like the VD (decubitus/horizontal) view, careful attention to radiation safety, FFD and grid alignment is necessary.
4. Include a left or right marker to indicate the side of the patient closest to the detector. A positional marker with a moveable bead may be used to show the direction of gravity.

Lesion-oriented oblique view

This view is indicated for the assessment of abnormalities of the thoracic body wall (Figure 1.20) and for the demonstration of the oesophagus, avoiding its superimposition with the vertebral column.

The technique is similar to that for obtaining a DV or VD radiograph, except that the patient is rotated so that the abnormality is projected tangentially to the X-ray beam (Figure 1.21); the degree of obliquity depends on the location of the abnormality. The exposure factors may need to be lower than those for the standard DV or VD view.

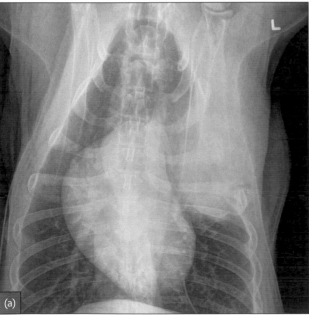

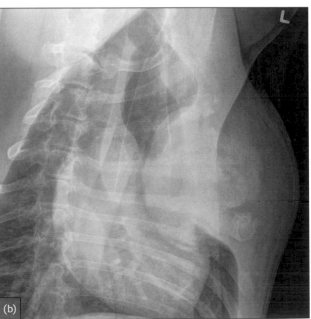

1.20 (a) VD and (b) lesion-oriented oblique VD thoracic radiographs of a dog with a mass arising from the left fourth rib. Notice how the oblique VD radiograph highlights the osseous portion of the mass.

VD 'humanoid' view (VD with the thoracic limbs retracted caudally)

This view is indicated for the assessment of abnormalities in the cranial thorax as it eliminates superimposition of the scapulae. The technique is similar to that for a VD view, except the thoracic limbs are retracted caudally, to lie adjacent to the body wall, and are secured with tape or sandbags (Figure 1.22).

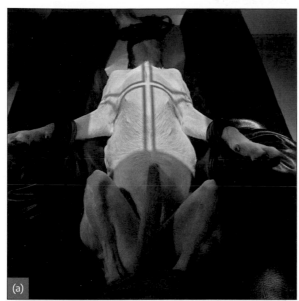

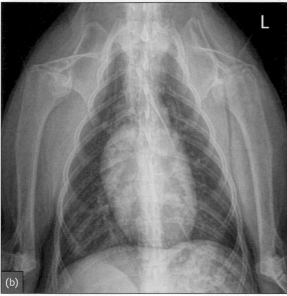

1.22 (a) Patient positioning for the 'humanoid' view. (b) The resulting radiograph demonstrating the displacement of the scapulae from the cranial aspect of the thorax.

Fluoroscopy and dynamic digital radiography

Fluoroscopy is an imaging modality that allows real-time viewing of images created by detection of X-ray transmission through the patient. Current systems fall into one of two categories based on their detector type:

- Conventional fluorescent screen and image intensifier-based systems

- Digital flat panel detectors, which do not use a fluorescent screen and hence, technically, are not fluoroscopy devices. These systems are more appropriately called dynamic digital radiography (DDR) units.

Flat panel detectors offer several advantages including more compact equipment size, lower doses of radiation to the patient, wider dynamic range and absence of geometric image deformation. Some of the newest systems offer a gantry that can acquire images while rapidly rotating 180 degrees around the patient, producing a three-dimensional acquisition, in a manner akin to computed tomography (CT). Most fluoroscopic and DDR systems offer a pulsed acquisition, where the generator produces a series of short-duration X-ray pulses (3–10 milliseconds) at a rate of about 3–30 pulses/second (frames per second). The short pulses and high frame rates can produce excellent temporal resolution. In procedures where high temporal resolution is not required, the frame rate should be reduced to minimize radiation exposure to the patient and operator. When compared with radiography, the dynamic component of fluoroscopy adds valuable information to the thoracic examination, particularly in the assessment of functional abnormalities and in rapidly performing image-guided interventions.

Indications

- Dysphagia (e.g. pharyngeal or cricopharyngeal dysfunction).
- Oesophageal disorders (e.g. strictures, foreign body, dysmotility).
- Tracheal collapse.
- Tracheal stent placement.
- Sliding hernias (e.g. hiatal, lung).
- Evaluation of diaphragmatic paralysis.
- Angiocardiography and therapeutic procedures (e.g. balloon valvuloplasty).
- Biopsy guidance (e.g. lung biopsy).

Safety

Personnel are often required to remain in the room for procedures because anaesthesia is contraindicated for most functional examinations and interventions. All personnel in the room during the procedure are required to use personal protective equipment (e.g. lead apron, thyroid guard, gloves, glasses, curtain or barrier) and dosimeters. In addition, the following precautions should be followed:

- Permit only those people necessary for the procedure to be in the room
- Limit the duration of the radiographic exposure and the imaging frame rate as much as possible
- Collimate the field of view and ensure personnel remain outside the primary X-ray beam
- Avoid manual restraint when possible (i.e. use chemical restraint, sandbags or tape, place animal in a box)
- Only perform when clinically indicated.

Contrast radiography

The most common applications of contrast radiography in the thorax include angiography and oesophagography. Angiographic studies are typically performed in a referral setting. Oesophagography may be performed in both private and referral practice.

Contrast media

The two main types of contrast media used in thoracic radiography are barium sulphate and iodine. Both have a high atomic number relative to tissues, making them much more efficient at absorbing the X-ray beam. Multiple formulations are available for both barium- and iodine-based contrast agents; understanding the properties and risks associated with each is important.

Barium sulphate is inexpensive and commonly used for digestive tract contrast studies. It provides superior mucosal detail in the oesophagus compared with iodinated media. It is water insoluble, not absorbed from the digestive tract, and available in the form of liquid suspension or paste. Hard water will cause the liquid suspension to precipitate. Leakage of barium sulphate into the mediastinum (or peritoneal cavity) can cause morbidity, due to mediastinitis (or peritonitis) with secondary fibrosis and granuloma formation, and potentially mortality. Barium sulphate within the digestive tract during an endoscopic procedure will inhibit examination of the anatomy and may cause equipment damage or malfunction (e.g. plugging of the biopsy channel). If barium in the liquid suspension form is aspirated into the airway or lung, then the consequences are usually negligible when the aspirated volume is small; when larger volumes are aspirated, rare consequences include pneumonia and granulomatous reactions. If aspirated barium reaches the alveoli, it may persist there with permanent detection on radiographs. It may also be phagocytized by macrophages and migrate to regional lymph nodes, where it may persist. The paste form is viscous and poses a greater risk for asphyxiation when aspirated; it should not be used if there is concern for aspiration. If oesophageal rupture or a bronchoesophageal fistula is suspected, then barium sulphate should be avoided.

Iodine-based contrast media are divided into two main classes: ionic (hyperosmolar) and non-ionic (low osmolar or iso-osmolar).

- Ionic iodinated contrast media (e.g. diatrizoate meglumine and diatrizoate sodium solution, Gastrografin®) administered orally will result in interstitial fluid being drawn into the lumen of the gastrointestinal tract and therefore should not be administered orally to hypovolaemic patients as hypovolaemic shock may result. If aspirated, ionic contrast media may cause severe pulmonary oedema and they are therefore contraindicated in patients at risk for aspiration, including those with bronchoesophageal fistula.
- Non-ionic iodinated contrast media (e.g. iohexol, Omnipaque®) have far fewer side effects. Non-ionic contrast media are indicated in cases where a digestive tract perforation or bronchoesophageal fistula is suspected, or when there is concern for aspiration.

Oesophagography

The oesophagus is not normally visible on survey radiographs, although it can be seen when its lumen is distended with air, fluid, food or foreign material. Orally administered contrast agents allow evaluation of the oesophagus; however, consideration must be given to the most appropriate imaging modality (radiography versus fluoroscopy), type and formulation of contrast media and to the risks of the procedure. If a functional disorder is suspected, fluoroscopy is generally required to evaluate the dynamic changes that occur during swallowing (e.g. cricopharyngeal achalasia). A static radiographic study may be sufficient to detect structural abnormalities (e.g. foreign body) or show the location of the oesophagus. In either case, care must be taken to minimize the risk of aspiration, particularly when a swallowing disorder is suspected.

Indications for oesophagography

- Oesophageal foreign body.
- Oesophageal mural mass.
- Megaoesophagus.
- Oesophageal stricture, vascular ring anomaly.
- Oesophageal perforation.
- Oesophagitis.
- Oesophageal diverticulum.
- Tracheoesophageal fistula.
- Dysphagia.
- Mediastinal mass.
- Hiatal hernia or gastro-oesophageal reflux.

Technique: static positive contrast oesophagography

1. Sedation should be avoided.
2. Prepare a mixture of 10 ml barium sulphate suspension with soft food or dry kibble.
   - Substitute barium sulphate suspension with a 50:50 mixture of non-ionic iodinated contrast medium with water or broth if there is concern for gastrointestinal perforation, aspiration or bronchoesophageal fistula, or if endoscopy is to follow.
3. Obtain orthogonal survey radiographs of the neck and thorax.
4. In right lateral recumbency, orally administer 60% weight-to-volume barium sulphate suspension (use barium paste if a foreign body or mural mass is present as it will adhere better to the surface, or a 50:50 mixture of non-ionic iodinated contrast medium if there is concern for digestive tract perforation, the risk of aspiration is deemed to be high, a bronchoesophageal fistula is suspected or endoscopy is to follow). If there is concern for gastro-oesophageal reflux or a sliding hiatal hernia, left lateral recumbency may be more sensitive.
   - Cat: 5–7 ml.
   - Small-to-medium dog: 15 ml.
   - Large dog: 20–30 ml.
5. Immediately obtain lateral and VD radiographs of the neck and thorax. Note, a VD view taken with the beam angled 15–30 degrees from left ventral to right dorsal might be required to evaluate the oesophagus due to its midline location and summation with the vertebral column.
6. If there is insufficient contrast material, repeat the procedure.

If no abnormality is detected, proceed to administer the pre-prepared contrast-soaked food. Evaluation with contrast-soaked food is useful to detect partial obstructions (e.g. oesophageal stricture) that allow liquid to pass normally. Do not proceed if a perforation is suspected. The ingested food should not be mistaken for filling defects or mucosal irregularity.

7. In right lateral recumbency, offer or place food into the patient's mouth.
8. Immediately obtain lateral and VD radiographs of the neck and thorax. It may be necessary to use an oblique VD view (as above).
9. If there is insufficient food, then repeat the procedure.

Dynamic oesophagography is performed using fluoroscopy. The technique is beyond the scope of this chapter. Standardized procedures have been reported (Harris, 2017); however, it is important to note that there is substantial variation in how different institutions perform this procedure (e.g. right lateral *versus* standing, bolus size and consistency). These variables may affect quantitively measured outcomes of the procedure (Pollard, 2019).

Variations in radiographic anatomy

Considerable variation exists in the normal radiographic appearance of the thorax, especially in the dog. Recognizing normal anatomical variation and being able to differentiate it from pathological conditions is essential. These variations are introduced below and described in more detail in Chapters 8–12.

Breed

This has little influence on the normal appearance of a feline radiograph, but considerable impact on the evaluation of canine thoracic radiographs (Figure 1.23). Three main canine body types should be recognized:

- Deep, narrow-chested conformation (e.g. Afghan Hound, Irish Setter, Greyhound)
- Intermediate thoracic conformation (e.g. German Shepherd Dog, Boxer, Golden Retriever, Standard Poodle)
- Wide, shallow conformation (e.g. Boston Terrier, Bulldog).

These conformational variations have importance in the evaluation of structures such as the mediastinum and cardiac silhouette (see Chapters 8–12). Additional factors to consider are breed-related vertebral abnormalities (e.g. wedge, butterfly) that can lead to kyphosis, scoliosis or lordosis. Sternal abnormalities (such as pectus excavatum) will also influence the radiographic appearance of the thorax. Alterations in the vertebral or sternal curvature may result in the view of normal soft tissue structures over the lung fields. Chondrodystrophic breeds (especially the Basset Hound) often have unusual costal cartilages and costochondral junctions, which may appear nodule-like and create confusing shadows that summate with the lungs.

Age

In young animals, the thymus may be detected in the cranial and ventral mediastina (Figure 1.24); it reaches a maximum size at about 4 months and then progressively undergoes involution until it is no longer radiographically visible (usually not seen after the age of 6 months). Depending on the age of the animal, open physes may be observed in the skeleton. Many old dogs have varying degrees of spondylosis deformans, degenerative sternal changes, mineralized costochondral junctions, bronchial walls, tracheal rings and pulmonary osteomas. Mildly thick pleurae may occasionally be detected in older animals. Older cats may have varying degrees of spondylosis deformans and a tortuous and apparently elongated aorta, which is often accompanied by a more 'horizontal' orientation of the cardiac silhouette, often with increased sternal contact (Figure 1.25). Fragmented costal cartilages are seen as a normal variation in some older cats.

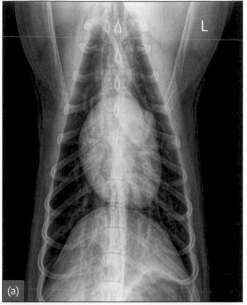

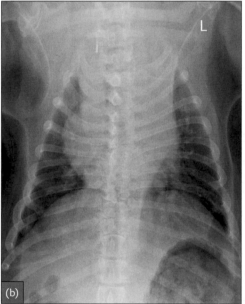

1.23 Normal DV thoracic radiographs of (a) an 8-year-old neutered Greyhound bitch with a deep narrow-chested conformation and (b) a 7-year-old male Bulldog with a wide shallow-chested conformation, breed-related vertebral abnormalities, and a wide cranial mediastinum due to fat accumulation.

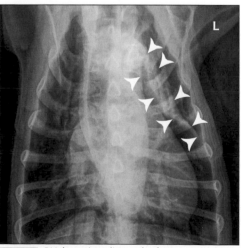

1.24 DV thoracic radiograph of a 4-month-old German Shepherd Dog bitch with a visible thymus (arrowheads).

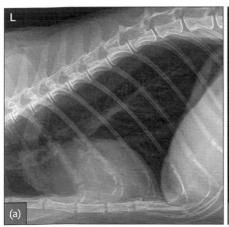
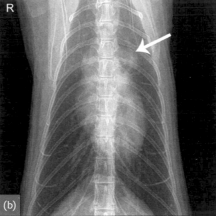
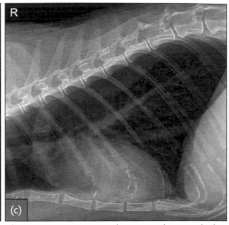

1.25 (a–c) Three orthogonal thoracic radiographs of a 15-year-old Domestic Shorthaired cat. Note the aorta is tortuous and appears elongated. The long axis of the heart is more parallel to the sternum with increased sternal contact. These findings are common age-related changes of minor consequence. (b) On the VD view, the tortuous aorta (arrowed) should not be mistaken for a mass. L = left; R = right.

Sex

Females often have prominent nipples and skin folds (especially pregnant or older post-parturient bitches); these can be confused with pulmonary nodules when they summate with the lungs.

Body condition

Obesity influences the interpretation of many thoracic structures. Large amounts of fat will alter the appearance of the cardiac silhouette (mimicking cardiomegaly) and widen the cranial mediastinum, and can create an overall increase in the opacity of the lungs (e.g. due to inability to fully expand the lungs secondary to intrathoracic fat accumulation, and summation of intrathoracic and body wall fat with the lungs). Exposure factors may need to be increased for thoracic radiography in obese animals. Interpretation of radiographs of overweight patients may be challenging (see Figure 1.37). Emaciated animals will appear to have hyperlucent lungs and exposure factors may need to be reduced in these animals to create a diagnostic radiograph. Vascular structures in the cranial mediastinum may be detected in a thin animal (Figure 1.26), especially in narrow-chested breeds. Severe emaciation can result in microcardia, seen as a small cardiac silhouette.

Respiratory phase

It is important to recognize the differences between radiographs obtained at full inspiration and those obtained during expiration. Figure 1.27 outlines the major differences, and these are demonstrated in Figure 1.28.

Cardiac cycle

The influence of cardiac motion on a radiograph varies. Generally, the edges of the cardiac silhouette should appear slightly hazy due to the presence of cardiac motion during the radiographic exposure, and a sharply marginated, enlarged cardiac silhouette should alert the clinician to the possibility of pericardial fluid. The changes between systole and diastole are best seen in large dogs, on DV or VD views and with short exposure times (Figure 1.29). Near end-systole, the ventricular area is small,

and the atria are well rounded and bulging out. At end-diastole, the ventricles are larger and rounder and the atria are less conspicuous. The pulmonic trunk varies a great deal during the cardiac cycle and will appear more prominent during systole.

Body position

There are inherent differences between left and right lateral views and between DV and VD views. It is often possible to identify which view has been obtained based on the appearance of certain anatomical structures; however, this is not always the case. The principles are shown in Figures 1.30 to 1.33. The differences are more pronounced in larger dogs than in small dogs and cats.

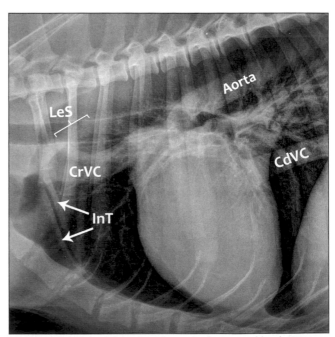

1.26 Right lateral thoracic radiograph of a 4-year-old male German Shepherd Dog with minimal fat accumulation in the cranial mediastinum and increased visibility of the left subclavian artery (LeS), cranial vena cava (CrVC) and internal thoracic arteries/veins (InT). CdVC = caudal vena cava.

Radiographic features	Inspiration	Expiration
Overall pulmonary opacity	• Opacity decreased • Good contrast to vascular structures, bronchial walls and heart	• Opacity increased • Poor contrast to vascular and bronchial walls; bronchial lumen may be seen
Lateral radiograph		
Cranioventral thorax	• Opacity decreased • Slight separation of right ventricular margin from sternum	• Opacity increased • Extended contact between right ventricular margin and sternum
Caudodorsal thorax	• Lumbodiaphragmatic recess located around T12 and open • Distances from vertebrae to carina and from lumbodiaphragmatic recess to CdVC are increased	• Lumbodiaphragmatic recess located around T11 and closed • Distances from vertebrae to carina and from lumbodiaphragmatic recess to CdVC are diminished
'Postcardiac triangle' between caudal cardiac border, ventral diaphragm and CdVC (accessory lobe area)	• Minimal or no contact between cardiac silhouette and diaphragm • Horizontal position of CdVC • Less opaque, large accessory lobe area • Flattened diaphragm	• Cardiac border and diaphragm contact or intersect • Caudally ascending position of CdVC • More opaque, small accessory lobe area • Rounded diaphragm
Relative and absolute cardiac size (cardiothoracic ratio)	• Diminished (i.e. small cardiac size with respect to thoracic size)	• Increased (i.e. larger cardiac size with respect to thoracic size)
Dorsoventral radiograph		
Changes of caudal thorax (the appearance of the cranial aspect of the thorax changes less with respiration)	• Widened and lengthened • Diaphragmatic cupula approximately at T8–T10 • Open costodiaphragmatic recesses	• Narrowed and shortened • Diaphragmatic cupula approximately at T7–T8 • Narrowed costodiaphragmatic recesses
Cardiac size	• Relatively and absolutely smaller than on expiration	• Relatively and absolutely larger than on inspiration

1.27 Radiographic features of inspiration and expiration in dogs. The lumbodiaphragmatic recess is the angular region between the diaphragm and the thoracolumbar vertebral column on a lateral radiograph. The costodiaphragmatic recess is the angular region between the diaphragm and the ribs on DV and VD radiographs. CdVC = caudal vena cava; T7–T12 = seventh–twelfth thoracic vertebrae.
(Adapted from Suter, 1984)

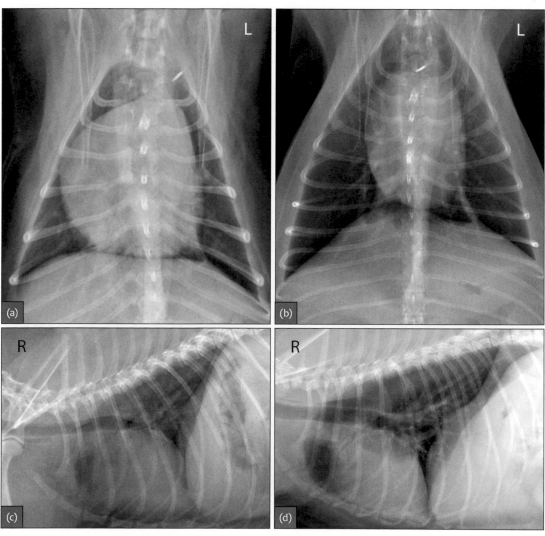

1.28 Normal (a, b) VD and (c, d) right lateral thoracic radiographs of a 6-year-old Border Collie bitch acquired during (a, c) expiration and (b, d) inspiration.

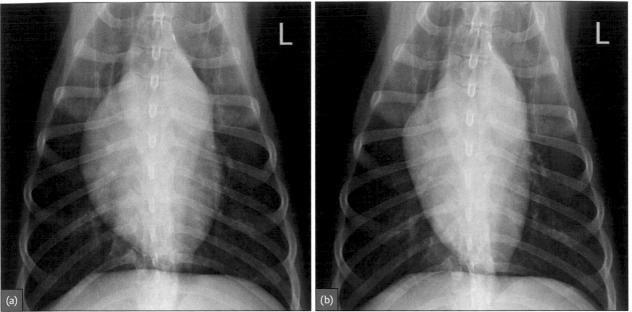

1.29 Sequential VD thoracic radiographs of a 14-year-old English Setter acquired during (a) diastole and (b) systole. Compare the size and shape of the cardiac silhouette.

Structure	Right lateral	Left lateral
Diaphragm	The crura appear parallel	The crura appear Y-shaped
Gastric lumen gas	Gas in the fundus, seen dorsally and caudal to the left diaphragmatic crus	Gas is present ventrally within the pyloric antrum and canal
Caudal vena cava	Merges with the most cranial crus (right crus)	Extends caudal to the most cranial crus (left crus) and merges with the more caudal crus (right crus)
Lung	Left lung is seen better	Right lung is seen better
Cardiac silhouette	More oval or egg-shaped	More rounded. The apex may be displaced slightly dorsally from the sternum
Cranial lobar pulmonary arteries and veins	Vessels overlap more frequently making it harder to distinguish left from right cranial lobar blood vessels	Easier to distinguish left from right cranial lobar blood vessels
Cranial sternal lymph nodes	May be seen as a normal finding on this view, with a mean length of 30 mm	Seen less frequently

1.30 Differences between left and right lateral recumbent thoracic radiographs.

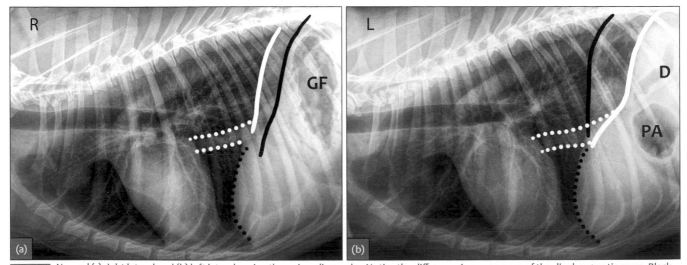

1.31 Normal (a) right lateral and (b) left lateral canine thoracic radiographs. Notice the difference in appearance of the diaphragmatic crura. Black line = left crus; black dotted line = diaphragmatic cupula; D = duodenum; GF = gastric fundus; PA = pyloric antrum; white line = right crus; white dotted line = caudal vena cava.

Structure	Ventrodorsal	Dorsoventral
Diaphragm	Crura summate with the cupula giving a three-humped appearance	A single smooth curve of the cupula is seen
Gastric lumen gas	Gas present in the body (centrally) or the pyloric antrum and canal (seen on the right side)	Gas present in the fundus (seen on the left side)
Major blood vessels	Changes in size tend to be more conspicuous. Also, a greater length of the caudal vena cava than on the DV view	Changes in size are not seen as easily
Lungs	Accessory lobe seen better as heart moves more cranially. In general, cranioventral lung field is seen best	Accessory lobe less aerated due to cranial displacement of the midportion of the diaphragm. In general, caudodorsal lung field is seen best
Caudal lobar pulmonary arteries and veins	Not seen as easily as on the DV view	Seen more easily due to the well inflated surrounding lungs and the effect of magnification
Cardiac silhouette	Elongated. Pulmonic trunk may appear bulging as a normal variation	More oval due to a more upright position

1.32 Differences between VD and DV thoracic radiographs.

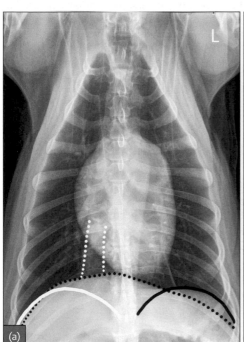 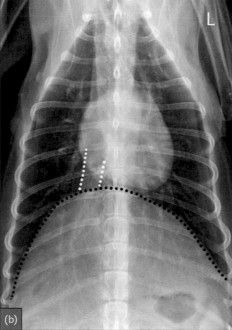

1.33 Normal (a) VD and (b) DV canine thoracic radiographs. Notice the difference in cardiac size and shape due to magnification and view, and the appearance of the diaphragmatic crura. (b) The pulmonary blood vessels in the caudodorsal lung field extend caudal to the dotted diaphragmatic line and form a positive summation shadow with the liver. Black line = left crus; black dotted line = diapragmatic cupula; white line = right crus; white dotted line = caudal vena cava.

Essential principles of interpretation

As previously noted, a radiograph is a planar image. The image comprises a grid of pixels and each pixel has a grayscale value which represents the amount of X-ray beam absorption that occurred along a straight path from the X-ray source to the detector. Because the amount of X-ray absorption is a summation of all structures along the path, there is a loss of depth perception: it is impossible to determine whether the object that caused the most absorption of the X-ray beam was near to or far from the detector. The impact of the loss of depth perception in the image can be partially mitigated by obtaining different radiographic views. This is commonly accomplished by obtaining at least two orthogonal views (views acquired at a 90-degree angle to each other; see Figure 1.36).

Radiographic opacities

Radiopacity refers to the grayscale appearance of tissues and organs in the radiograph and denotes the ability of X-rays to pass through structures. Radiopacity is a result of differential attenuation of the X-ray beam and depends on the composition (effective atomic number), density and size of the tissue or organ. Structures that allow greater transmission of X-rays will appear darker (less opaque) and structures that attenuate more X-rays will appear whiter (more opaque). On radiographs, five categories of opacity are recognized (from least to most opaque):

- Air
- Fat
- Water/soft tissue
- Bone/mineral
- Metal.

The ability to differentiate tissues and organs based on differences in opacity (signal intensity) is called contrast resolution. Compared with CT and magnetic resonance imaging (MRI), the contrast resolution of radiographs is somewhat limited.

The radiographic opacity of a tissue or region is evaluated relative to the opacity of other tissues and organs within the same image and assumes that adjacent tissues have similar thickness. As tissue in one region becomes thicker relative to another region, the radiographic opacity may be different to that expected based on the tissue composition because the attenuation of the X-ray beam increases as thickness increases. For example, a body wall lipoma may appear to have a soft tissue opacity relative to the adjacent body wall fat, due to the greater thickness in the region of the lipoma, even though both are composed of fat.

In a radiograph, tissues and organs may form a shadow or silhouette that represents the gross appearance of that structure (e.g. cardiac silhouette). However, some structures may not be normally visible on radiograph or may have an unexpected appearance for several reasons. Two phenomena associated with differential attenuation of the X-ray beam that may produce unexpected appearances are summation shadows and border effacement.

Summation shadows

The presence of two or more structures within the path of the X-ray beam may create an opacity that does not represent an anatomical structure within the object or patient. These opacities are referred to as summation shadows. Summation shadows can be positive (more opaque) or negative (less opaque). Positive summation shadows occur when the X-ray beam is attenuated more than expected (e.g. summation of two or more structures may create a distinct, more opaque shadow). Negative summation shadows occur when the X-ray beam is attenuated less than expected. Negative summation is usually due to gas or fat in the path of the X-ray beam or examination of a thinner area.

Border effacement (silhouette sign)

If adjacent portions of the X-ray beam are attenuated to the same degree, then it is impossible to differentiate the border of structures along that path. This phenomenon may create an unexpected shadow that is a novel silhouette on the radiograph. This disappearance of individual silhouettes is called border effacement. Note that because planar images lack depth perception, objects do not have to be at the same distance from the cassette to appear adjacent in the image and produce border effacement. In practice, border effacement only occurs with fluid and soft tissue structures. Some common examples include:

- The heart surrounded by pleural fluid
- Pulmonary blood vessels surrounded by consolidated lung.

Röntgen signs (named after Wilhelm Conrad Röntgen, who discovered X-rays)

When structures are evaluated radiographically, consideration should be given to the following characteristics:

- Size
- Shape
- Opacity
- Location

- Number
- Architecture
- Function.

Alterations in these characteristics are Röntgen signs. In most instances, the presence of a sign indicates the presence of an abnormal state and the absence of a sign indicates normal condition (there are some exceptions). The signs associated with function are only applicable in specific situations such as a contrast study or a dynamic fluoroscopic study.

Mass and mass effect

Inflammatory, neoplastic and degenerative diseases can alter the size (e.g. fluid infiltration, focal fluid accumulation, vascular congestion, cellular infiltration or hypertrophy), shape and opacity (e.g. when gas is replaced by fluid) of normal structures. Many of these conditions also may result in the development of lesions that are mass-like (circumscribed) or infiltrative (non-circumscribed). These masses are generally recognized because of a change in opacity, displacement/compression of adjacent structures or both. When a discrete mass is not identified, then the effect of the mass causing displacement or compression of adjacent structures may be observed. This *mass effect* is an essential diagnostic tool that allows recognition of a potential mass as well as its position, extent and origin.

Approach to evaluation of the thoracic radiograph

Before beginning evaluation of a thoracic radiographic study, it is important to have an accurate clinical history and to understand the reason the study was performed. Once that information is obtained, the following should be considered:

- Is the study correctly labelled, including patient name or ID, date, clinic name, client name and positional markers?
- Are the views provided adequate to answer the clinical question? Is the relevant anatomy included and were all appropriate views obtained?
- Is the radiographic technique correct? It is important to be able to recognize good technique, including correct exposure (Figure 1.34) and proper patient positioning. It is also important to recognize common artefacts, which may be helpful or harmful to the interpretation. Radiographic artefacts may be system specific (Figure 1.35). The full range of radiographic artefacts is beyond the scope of this chapter and excellent resources are available elsewhere (e.g. Drost *et al.*, 2008; Jiménez *et al.*, 2008; Jiménez *et al.*, 2009; Walz-Flannigan, 2018)
- Are prior studies of the patient available for comparison?

Once it is determined that the clinical information provided is sufficient and accurate, and that the study technique is appropriate, a *systematic approach* should be applied for evaluation of the images. This approach may be performed before or after evaluation of the most salient abnormalities. The approach will vary by reader; however, the goal remains the same: a complete and thorough evaluation of the images. Approaches may include:

- An *organ approach* where the observer makes a conscious effort to evaluate every organ on the images in the same order each time
- An *area approach* where the observer evaluates the images by starting centrally and working towards the periphery or vice versa (or cranially to caudally, etc.).

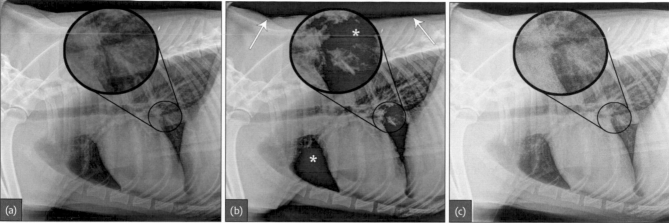

1.34 Lateral thoracic radiographs of a dog acquired on a DR system demonstrating (a) correct exposure, (b) overexposure, and (c) underexposure. (b) Arrows indicate regions of the thoracic body wall where saturation artefacts have occurred (in saturation, information is lost or 'clipped' from an image when an exposure exceeds the dynamic range of the image-processing algorithm and/or the image detector); * indicates regions where overexposure has occurred to a degree where the calibration mask of the system is visible (seen as linear 'plank-like' lines, sometimes referred to a planking artefact). (c) The image is 'grainy' or 'has noise' due to insufficient radiation reaching the detector (quantum mottle).

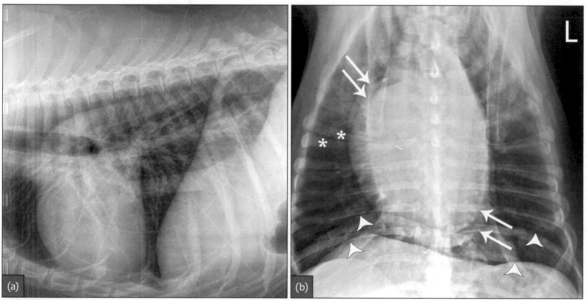

1.35 (a) Lateral and (b) VD thoracic radiographs of a dog obtained using a CR system. (a) The radiograph was obtained with the CR detector cassette upside down. Notice the circles and radiating lines summating with the thorax. (b) The radiograph demostrates a double exposure. Notice the double images of the cardiac silhouette (arrowed), diaphragm (arrowheads), and ribs (* = duplicate images of the same rib).

Regardless of the order of approach, it is always important to:

- Maximize the use of available spatial and contrast resolution by using the zoom and window/level features
- View multiple radiographs simultaneously (especially orthogonal views) to accurately localize and fully characterize any abnormality (Figure 1.36)
- Consider how factors such as anatomical variation and positioning may influence interpretation (Figures 1.37 and 1.38):
  - Breed and conformation
  - Age
  - Body condition
  - Phase of respiration (and whether it changes between views)
  - Patient position.

During the evaluation it may become obvious that additional clinical information or additional views are necessary as part of the study (see Figures 1.37 and 1.39). If this information is unattainable, then the limitations need to be factored into the final interpretation. A more detailed description of interpretation is provided in Chapter 7.

As discussed in the introduction to this chapter, thoracic radiographic interpretation is challenging. As a result, errors are inevitable. Errors may occur for many reasons, and it is important to be aware of common types and try to avoid them. Some of the more common errors include:

- Under-reading: an abnormality is seen but is not reported or is interpreted as normal
- Over-reading: normal anatomy is interpreted as abnormal, or too much importance is assigned to findings, especially incidental findings of minor consequence
- Satisfaction of search: after finding a first abnormality, the reader fails to continue to look for additional abnormalities
- Faulty reasoning: abnormalities are detected but attributed to the wrong cause
- Failure to detect abnormalities outside the region of interest (but visible in the images)

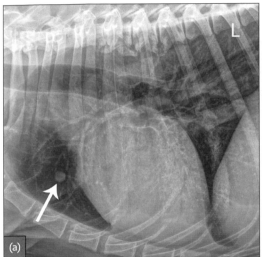

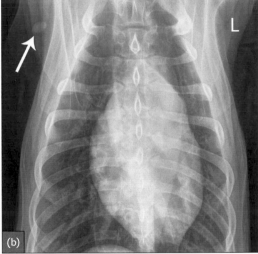

1.36 (a) Left lateral and (b) VD thoracic radiographs of an 11-year-old male Flat Coated Retriever. Radiography was performed to test for thoracic metastasis. (a) There is concern for a pulmonary nodule *versus* a positive summation shadow (arrowed). (b) On the orthogonal view, the nodule is confirmed to be a superficial nodule on the body wall (arrowed), not a lung nodule.

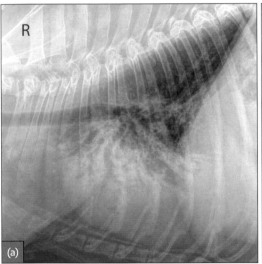

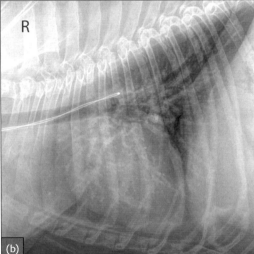

1.37 Right lateral thoracic radiographs of an obese Boston Terrier under general anaesthesia. (a) Image acquired after a period of lateral recumbency. The findings are highly concerning for cranioventral lung consolidation due to a disease such as aspiration pneumonia. (b) Image obtained approximately 10 minutes later after temporarily repositioning the patient and improving ventilation. Resolution of pulmonary opacification and improved lung expansion confirmed the finding was due to atelectasis.

- Satisfaction of report: uncritical reliance on the conclusion of a prior report leads to perpetuation of error through consecutive studies
- Failure to consult prior imaging studies
- Reliance on inaccurate or incomplete clinical history.

Unconscious bias may predispose the reader to error. Some of the more common examples of bias include:

- Anchoring bias: the reader fixes on an early impression and fails to adapt or change their opinion as subsequent information is obtained
- Framing bias: the reader is unduly influenced by the way the clinical question is framed
- Availability bias: tendency to suggest diagnosis that readily comes to mind
- Confirmation bias: tendency to seek evidence to support a diagnostic hypothesis that is already made and ignore evidence that would refute that hypothesis.

Techniques such as interpreting the study before reviewing the clinical history and subsequently reinterpreting the study while considering the clinical information may help reduce bias in image interpretation. When uncertain of a diagnosis in an unusual case, consulting a colleague is often helpful as they may raise different differential diagnoses or have prior experience with a similar case. Re-evaluating the study after some time has passed may also be beneficial.

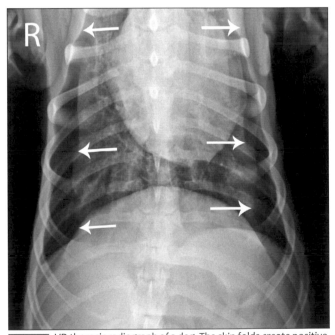

1.38 VD thoracic radiograph of a dog. The skin folds create positive summation shadows with the lungs (arrowed). The less opaque regions lateral to the skin folds should not be confused with a pneumothorax. An easy way to identify skin folds is that they often extend across the body wall or beyond the margin of the thorax (pneumothorax does not).

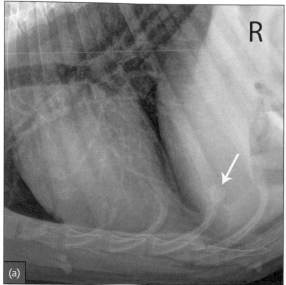
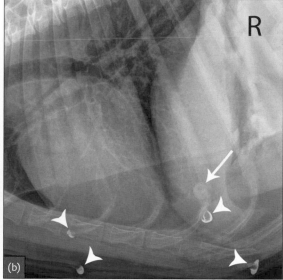

1.39 Lateral thoracic radiographs of a 10-year-old Staffordshire Bull Terrier bitch diagnosed with mammary carcinoma. Radiography was performed to test for thoracic metastasis. (a) On the initial radiograph, a soft tissue nodule was observed (arrowed) that might be a pulmonary nodule, body wall nodule or nipple. No body wall nodule was palpated. (b) After application of barium paste topically to the nipples, the nodule (arrowed) is distinct from the nipples (arrowheads), supporting a diagnosis of a pulmonary nodule.

References and further reading

Brady AP (2017) Error and discrepancy in radiology: inevitable or avoidable? *Insights into Imaging* **8**, 171–182

Bushberg JT, Seibert JA, Leidholdt EM and Boone JM (2011) *The Essential Physics of Medical Imaging, 3rd edn.* Lippincott Williams & Wilkins, Philadelphia

Curry TS, Dowdey JE and Murray RC Jr (1990) *Christensen's Physics of Diagnostic Radiology, 4th edn.* Lippincott Williams & Wilkins, Philadelphia

Drost WT, Reese DJ and Hornof WJ (2008) Digital radiography artifacts. *Veterinary Radiology & Ultrasound* **49**, S48–S56

Gaschen L (2018) Canine and feline esophagus. In: *Textbook of Veterinary Diagnostic Radiology, 7th edn*, ed. DE Thrall and WR Windmer, pp. 596–617. Elsevier, St. Louis

Harris RA, Grobman ME, Allen MJ *et al.* (2017) Standardization of a videofluoroscopic swallow study protocol to investigate dysphagia in dogs. *Journal of Veterinary Internal Medicine* **31**, 383–393

Jiménez DA and Armbrust LJ (2009) Digital radiographic artifacts. *Veterinary Clinics of North America: Small Animal Practice* **39**, 689–709

Jiménez DA, Armbrust LJ, O'Brien RT and Biller DS (2008) Artifacts in digital radiography. *Veterinary Radiology & Ultrasound* **49**, 321–332

Lynch KC, Oliveira CR, Matheson JS, Mitchell MA and O'Brien RT (2012) Detection of pneumothorax and pleural effusion with horizontal beam radiography. *Veterinary Radiology & Ultrasound* **53**, 38–43

Muhlbauer MC and Kneller SK (2013) *Radiography of the Dog and Cat: Guide to Making and Interpreting Radiographs.* John Wiley & Sons Inc., Ames

Nickoloff EL (2011) AAPM/RSNA Physics tutorial for residents: flat panel fluoroscopic systems. *RadioGraphics* **31**, 591–602

Owen M (2018) Radiographic, computed tomography, and magnetic resonance contrast media. In: *Textbook of Veterinary Diagnostic Radiology, 7th edn*, ed. DE Thrall and WR Windmer, pp. 96–109. Elsevier, St. Louis

Pollard RE (2019) Videofluoroscopic evaluation of the pharynx and upper esophageal sphincter in the dog: a systematic review of the literature. *Frontiers in Veterinary Science* **6**, 177

Robertson ID and Thrall DE (2018) Digital radiographic imaging. In: *Textbook of Veterinary Diagnostic Radiology, 7th edn*, ed. DE Thrall and WR Windmer, pp. 23–38. Elsevier, St. Louis

Rudorf H, Taeymans O and Johnson V (2008) Basics of thoracic radiography and radiology. In: *BSAVA Manual of Canine and Feline Thoracic Imaging, 1st edn*, ed. T Schwarz and V Johnson, pp. 1–19. BSAVA Publications, Gloucester

Suter PF (1984) Principles of radiographic examination and radiographic interpretation. In: *Thoracic Radiography: A Text Atlas of Thoracic Diseases of the Dog and Cat*, ed. PF Suter and PF Lord, pp. 1–77. Peter F. Suter, Wettswil

Thrall DE (2018a) Introduction to radiographic interpretation. In: *Textbook of Veterinary Diagnostic Radiology, 7th edn*, ed. DE Thrall and WR Windmer, pp. 110–122. Elsevier, St. Louis

Thrall DE (2018b) Principles of radiographic interpretation of the thorax. In: *Textbook of Veterinary Diagnostic Radiology, 7th edn*, ed. DE Thrall and WR Windmer, pp. 568–582. Elsevier, St. Louis

Thrall DE and Windmer WR (2018) Radiation protection and physics of diagnostic imaging. In: *Textbook of Veterinary Diagnostic Radiology, 7th edn*, ed. DE Thrall and WR Windmer, pp. 2–22. Elsevier, St. Louis

Wallack ST (2003) Static barium esophagram. In: *The Handbook of Veterinary Contrast Radiography*, pp. 45–53. San Diego Veterinary Imaging, Solana Beach

Walz-Flannigan AI, Brossoit KJ, Magnuson DJ and Schueler BA (2018) Pictorial review of digital radiography artifacts. *RadioGraphics* **38**, 833–846

Chapter 2

Basics of thoracic ultrasonography

Gabriela Seiler, Joanna Dukes-McEwan and Lorrie Gaschen

General thoracic ultrasonography

Indications

Non-cardiac thoracic ultrasonography has established itself in veterinary medicine as complementary to thoracic radiography in many cases. Due to reflection of the ultrasound beam at soft tissue–gas interfaces, such as the lung surface, ultrasound evaluation is limited to structures or lesions that are not surrounded by air. A complete set of thoracic radiographs should always be acquired initially to get an overview of possible thoracic pathology and to determine areas of interest that can be addressed with ultrasonography. In trauma patients, point-of-care ultrasound examinations, such as thoracic focused assessment with sonography for trauma (tFAST) protocols, have proved to be useful methods to rapidly assess binary variables such as presence or absence of pleural and pericardial effusion and pneumothorax. Point-of-care thoracic ultrasonography may also aid in detecting pulmonary changes which, in conjunction with left atrial enlargement, can be a sign of congestive heart failure. Protocols for these point-of-care examinations have been published, but the general principles of thoracic imaging described below apply. Non-cardiac thoracic ultrasonography is also used for more comprehensive examination of thoracic pathology together with other imaging methods such as thoracic radiography. Finally, thoracic ultrasonography is frequently used to sample thoracic lesions detected with other imaging modalities such as radiography or computed tomography (CT).

Indications for thoracic ultrasonography include:

- Pleural effusion obscuring thoracic or mediastinal contents
- Pleural thickening or pleural masses
- Mediastinal widening with suspicion of a mediastinal mass
- Lung consolidation or nodules
- Thoracic wall lesions
- Suspicion of diaphragmatic hernia
- Suspicion of lung lobe torsion
- Diagnostic fine-needle aspiration or biopsy
- Therapeutic pleural fluid removal.

Restraint and patient preparation

Patients are routinely prepared by clipping the hair coat in the region of interest, cleaning the skin with alcohol and applying coupling gel. Wetting the haircoat with alcohol without clipping may provide sufficient access and image quality in some areas such as the cranial mediastinum through the axillary region. For fine-needle aspiration and biopsy procedures, aseptic preparation of the skin is required.

Most patients can be examined awake with minimal restraint, in lateral or dorsal recumbency. Dyspnoeic patients should be examined in the position they tolerate best, in ventral recumbency or standing. In the absence of, or with minimal, pleural effusion, scanning from the dependent side may be essential to evaluate the heart, mediastinum, pleural surface and pulmonary lesions. Sedation is generally recommended for any sampling procedures. General anaesthesia is recommended if biopsy specimens are taken of any thoracic structures, particularly the lung, in order to control respiratory movement.

Coagulation profiles should also be obtained prior to ultrasound-guided biopsy. These are generally not required for fine-needle aspiration techniques unless there is a clinical suspicion of a coagulopathy.

Technique

A non-cardiac thoracic ultrasound examination is often targeted to an area of interest identified on survey radiographs, for example the cranial mediastinum; however, it is recommended to use multiple access windows both dorsally and ventrally on both sides to get an overview of pleural and peripheral pulmonary pathology. Depending on the location of the suspected lesion (mediastinum, thoracic wall, pulmonary parenchyma), different windows must be used. These may be intercostal, parasternal, subcostal, transhepatic or via the thoracic inlet (see 'Examination method', below).

Equipment

- Small footprint transducer (sector, microconvex) for deeper structures such as mediastinum.
- Linear array transducer for superficial structures such as the pleural surface, particularly in smaller patients.
- Transducer frequency should be as high as possible but with adequate depth penetration:
  - Small dogs, cats: 7.5–15 MHz
  - Large-breed dogs may require lower frequency for adequate penetration: 3.5–7.5 MHz.

Examination method

Using each intercostal space as a scan window, the thorax is examined in a longitudinal and transverse image plane, following the intercostal spaces as far dorsally as the aerated lungs allow. The caudal and cranial mediastinum can be evaluated with a subxiphoid and thoracic inlet view, respectively. Both sides of the thorax are routinely examined. The structures described below are identified.

Body wall, pleural and lung surface: The body wall is characterized by alternating layers of hypo- and hyperechoic tissue, representing layers of skin, subcutaneous fat and muscle. Normal ribs are seen as round (in short axis) or linear (in long axis) structures with a distal acoustic shadowing (Figure 2.1). The surface of the ribs is smooth and hyperechoic; any interruption of the cortex is a sign of either rib fracture or an aggressive lesion with lysis. The body wall is best examined using a linear transducer (Figures 2.1 and 2.2).

The two layers of the pleura are not visible as separate structures unless thickened. The visceral pleura and lung surface are recognizable as a bright hyperechoic, smooth and continuous line. The hyperechogenicity is caused by the soft tissue–gas interface at the lung surface, resulting in strong reflection of the ultrasound beam (Figure 2.2). It is important to observe the motion of the lung surface during the respiratory cycle. If the pleural space is normal, the lung surface can be seen gliding back and forth along the thoracic wall during inspiration and expiration. This motion is sometimes called a 'glide sign'. If this motion is absent, pneumothorax should be suspected. If the lung is normally aerated, almost all the ultrasound waves are reflected on the surface and the ultrasound beam is not able to penetrate the deeper portions of the lung. It is important to recognize this limitation of ultrasonography; a normal lung surface does not mean there are no lesions deeper within the lung. A normal lung surface creates reverberation artefacts, which present as multiple linear echoes deep and parallel to the lung surface (Figure 2.2). The intensity of these parallel lines decreases with increasing depth. The reverberation artefact, also called A-lines in thoracic imaging, is caused by multiple reflections between the highly reflective lung surface and the transducer–skin interface.

Interruption of the normal reverberation artefact or A-lines, and the presence of a column of densely spaced, small linear artefacts (comet tail artefacts or B-lines) (Figure 2.3) that arise from the pleural surface and extend to the deep edge of the ultrasound image, are a sign of abnormally aerated lung. B-lines move in concert with the lung surface and do not decrease in intensity as they reach deeper portions of the image. They are thought to be caused by ultrasound waves reverberating within a fluid-filled lesion surrounded by air and are a non-specific finding that can be seen with interstitial lung pathology such as cardiogenic or non-cardiogenic oedema, lung contusions, fibrosis, inflammation or diffuse neoplasia. Larger consolidations that would present radiographically as alveolar-type disease present as hypoechoic areas of lung tissue without, or with only focal pockets of, residual gas (Figure 2.4). Peripherally located nodules and masses are recognized by their rounded, well demarcated shape, unless they are surrounded by haemorrhage and inflammation, in which case they may have a more irregular and poorly delineated shape (Figure 2.5). Observation of the

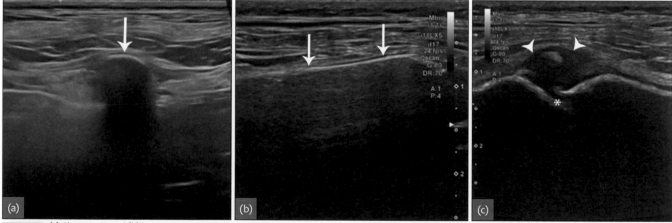

2.1 (a) Short-axis and (b) long-axis images of a normal canine rib, compared with (c) a long-axis image of a chronic rib fracture. Note the smooth hyperechoic surface of the normal rib (arrowed) whereas the fractured rib has an interrupted cortex (✳) surrounded by hypoechoic callus (arrowheads). The body wall is characterized by alternating hyperechoic and hypoechoic layers.

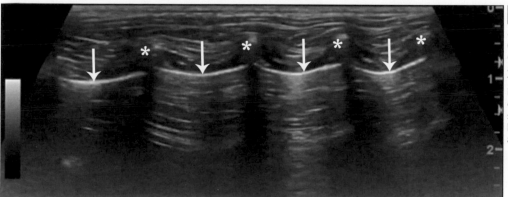

2.2 Longitudinal image of a normal feline thorax using a linear array transducer. The ribs (✳, displayed in short axis) cast a distal shadow. Note the striated appearance of the thoracic wall. The lung surface is a smooth, hyperechoic line (arrowed). Multiple echogenic lines parallel to the lung surface extending distal to the lung surface represent reverberation artefacts or A-lines.

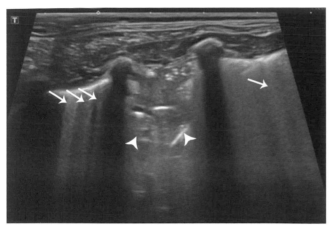

2.3 Comet tail or B-line artefacts originating from the lung surface (arrowed) of a dog with suppurative inflammation of the lungs. Centrally, there is an area of lung consolidation present (arrowheads).

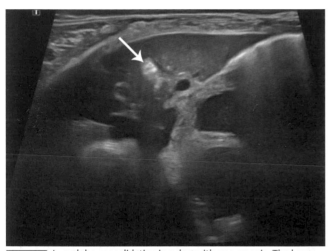

2.4 Lung lobe consolidation in a dog with pneumonia. The lung lobe has a 'hepatized' appearance with a central residual gas pocket (arrowed).

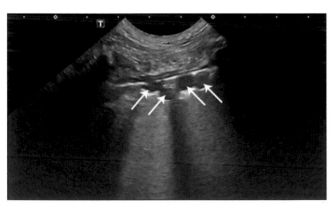

2.5 Multiple hypoechoic nodules along the lung surface (arrowed) of a Maltese with metastatic carcinoma.

respiratory movement and appearance of gas within a lesion allows differentiation between lesions of pulmonary and extrapulmonary origin.

Mediastinum: Ultrasound examination of the mediastinum is usually limited to the ventral aspect as the dorsal mediastinum is normally surrounded by aerated lung. The caudal mediastinum is very thin, accommodating the caudal vena cava, oesophagus and accessory lung lobe and, in overweight animals, some fat. These structures are best seen close to the diaphragm using a subxiphoidal or subcostal approach with the liver as the acoustic window. The most dorsal part of the caudal mediastinum containing the aorta and azygos vein is usually not accessible ultrasonographically. Normal lung aeration often obscures caudal mediastinal structures and can cause a mirror image artefact (Figure 2.6). Caudal mediastinal structures are best seen in the presence of pleural space pathology such as pleural effusion (Figure 2.7). If pleural effusion is present, the caudoventral mediastinum may be visible as a thin undulating hyperechoic structure.

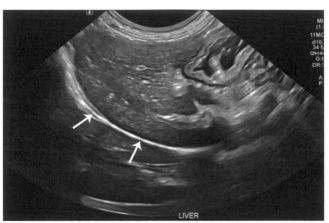

2.6 Subxiphoidal long-axis view of the diaphragm and caudal mediastinum in a cat without thoracic disease. The diaphragm is represented by a curvilinear hyperechoic line (arrowed). The tissue cranial to the diaphragm represents a mirror image artefact and not mediastinal pathology; note the symmetry of the structures within this tissue with the liver.

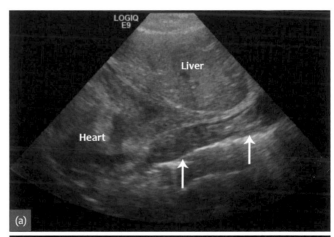

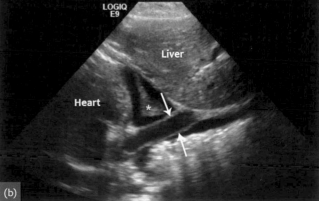

2.7 Longitudinal images of the caudal mediastinum of a cat using a subcostal approach. (a) The caudal thoracic oesophagus and gastro-oesophageal junction are visible (arrowed). (b) The caudal vena cava (arrowed) is surrounded by pleural effusion. A portion of the consolidated accessory lung lobe (*) is surrounded by fluid as well. Histopathology of the accessory lung lobe and cytology of pleural fluid were consistent with carcinoma.

The cranial mediastinum is best examined using a parasternal intercostal window. A thoracic inlet view may be beneficial in patients with very cranially located lesions. In this view, the trachea is easy to identify based on the structure of the cartilage rings, which give the trachea a rippled surface, and the air column within the trachea, which produces reverberation artefacts. The jugular veins are easily compressed and are bilateral tubular anechoic structures close to the skin surface, whereas the common carotid arteries are round anechoic slightly pulsating structures (Figure 2.8). If an intercostal approach is chosen, it is important to pull the thoracic limb as far cranially as possible to access the cranial intercostal spaces. The transducer is placed just dorsal to the sternum and cranial to the heart.

In the presence of pleural effusion, the ventral portion of the cranial mediastinum is a thin strip of echogenic tissue, depending on the amount of mediastinal fat, and can be examined quite easily for presence of lymphadenopathy or other masses (Figure 2.9). The cranial vena cava, if visible, is a good landmark to identify the surrounding mediastinum and should be examined for evidence of thrombosis in animals with pleural effusion (Figure 2.10).

Normal sternal or mediastinal lymph nodes are not differentiated from the surrounding mediastinal fat but present as hypoechoic rounded retrosternal structures when enlarged (Figure 2.11). Mediastinal fat is fairly uniform and can be recognized by its coarse structure, poor margination and poor transmission of the ultrasound beam. Occasional vascular structures may be seen extending through the cranial mediastinal fat (Figure 2.12). Especially in brachycephalic breeds and obese animals, a large amount of fat can be observed in the mediastinum and should not be confused with a mediastinal mass. Most mediastinal masses or abnormal lymph nodes are hypoechoic or sometimes heterogeneous, well defined and rounded (see Figure 2.11). In young animals, thymic tissue is present cranial to the heart, best seen from the left side. It has a granular, homogeneous texture and contains a large number of blood vessels.

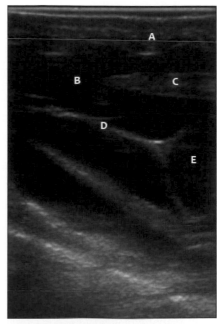

2.9 Longitudinal parasternal view of the cranial thorax of a cat with pleural effusion. The entire width of the cranial thorax is visible: the thoracic wall (A), pleural space with anechoic effusion (B), collapsed cranial lung lobes (C), cranial mediastinum (D), which is very thin without evidence of lymphadenopathy or fat, and the heart (E).

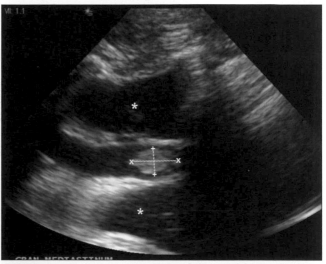

2.10 Longitudinal parasternal view of the cranial thorax of a cat with bilateral chylous pleural effusion (∗) and thrombosis of the cranial vena cava (indicated by calipers).

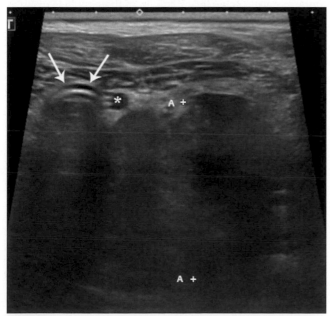

2.8 Transverse view of the thoracic inlet in a dog with ectopic thyroid carcinoma (indicated by calipers). The trachea is a curvilinear structure with distal reverberation artefact (arrowed). The adjacent round hypoechoic structure is the common carotid artery (∗).

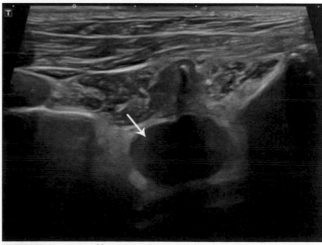

2.11 Parasternal long-axis view immediately dorsal to the sternum in a Labrador Retriever with acute myeloid leukaemia. The sternal lymph node is enlarged, rounded and hypoechoic (arrowed).

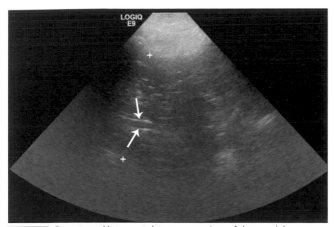

2.12 Parasternal intercostal transverse view of the cranial mediastinum in an obese dog. The mediastinum is wide due to fat deposition (indicated by calipers). The fat is hypoechoic with a coarse structure. A vessel is visible centrally (arrowed).

Diaphragm: The diaphragm is normally not seen as a separate structure; the highly reflective hyperechoic lung interface blends in with it. The diaphragm is only seen in its full thickness in cases of pleural and peritoneal effusion (Figure 2.13). A normal diaphragm has a smooth, curvilinear, continuous surface. Examination is best performed with a subcostal approach, placing the transducer just caudal to the rib cage and examining the diaphragm in sagittal, dorsal and transverse planes. Evaluation of diaphragmatic motion using M-mode has been described in dogs. In the presence of pleural effusion, the cranial surface of the diaphragm may also be evaluated using an intercostal window. Care should be taken not to confuse consolidated lung tissue or pericardial fat with herniated abdominal organs; an ultrasound examination of the cranial abdominal organs usually helps to determine the origin of abnormal intrathoracic tissue.

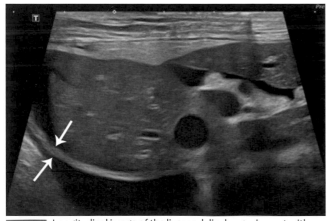

2.13 Longitudinal image of the liver and diaphragm in a cat with bicavitary effusion. The diaphragm is outlined by peritoneal and pleural effusion (arrowed).

Fine-needle aspiration and biopsy
Fine-needle aspiration

Fine-needle aspiration of thoracic structures generally requires sedation although samples of pleural effusion can usually be obtained from cooperative awake patients. A local anaesthetic may be helpful to alleviate patient discomfort. Most thoracic aspiration can be performed using 22 G needles. Highly cellular and viscous pleural effusion may require use of a larger needle. Intravenous or butterfly catheters or any other type of needle can be used depending on the ultrasonographer's preference and comfort. For therapeutic drainage of pleural effusion an extension set with a three-way stopcock is necessary. Ultrasound-guided drainage of pleural effusion is advantageous especially in patients with chronic or loculated effusion where exact needle placement is pivotal to successfully removing most of the effusion. To obtain pleural fluid, the largest, least septated fluid pocket cranial or caudal to the heart is identified and the position of the needle or catheter is continuously observed during the procedure, to allow placement to be adjusted if needed. For example, the needle should be retracted if the lung surface, fat or fibrin strands approach the needle in order to avoid laceration of lung tissue or obstruction of the needle.

Fine-needle aspiration of solid thoracic lesions such as mediastinal, pulmonary and thoracic wall masses should only be performed by an ultrasonographer experienced with ultrasound-guided fine-needle aspiration. For all lesions, an acoustic window for a safe approach to the lesion must be identified. If needle placement has to be close to a rib, the cranial aspect of a rib should be selected in order to avoid intercostal vasculature. Doppler ultrasonography should be used to identify large vessels in the path of the lesion or within the lesion. Fine-needle aspiration of lung masses can only be performed if the lesion is superficial and not covered by more than 1–2 cm of aerated lung tissue. It is essential in these cases to localize the mass on survey radiographs before starting the procedure. A thin layer of air-filled lung tissue can be reduced by keeping the animal in lateral recumbency with the affected side down for 5–10 minutes. Atelectasis of the lung tissue is usually sufficient to see and sample the lesion either from the dependent or the non-dependent side, as the lung stays atelectatic for a few minutes. Hyperventilation of the intubated patient is helpful to temporarily halt respiratory motion when aspirating lung lesions. In heavily sedated patients, the needle should be placed in the thoracic wall, ensuring visibility of the entire needle path, and advanced into the lesion during the expiratory pause to obtain a sample quickly and carefully (Figure 2.14). Risk of lung laceration increases with the time the needle remains in the thoracic cavity, especially if the tip of the needle is close to the lung surface. The thoracic cavity should be examined after each procedure for the presence of haemorrhage and pneumothorax.

Biopsy

Biopsies of mass lesions should always be performed under general anaesthesia; this is particularly important for lung lesions where it is essential to control respiratory motion. A coagulation profile should be checked prior to

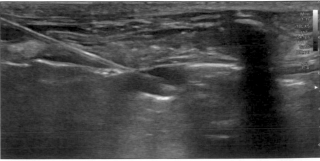

2.14 Fine-needle aspiration of a pulmonary nodule using a 22 G needle. The needle (seen on the left side of the image) is inserted through the body wall and into the pulmonary nodule.

the procedure. A 14–18 G automated or semiautomatic biopsy device is most commonly used. The skin is aseptically prepared and a small incision is made with a scalpel blade. The depth of the lesion should be measured and the length of the biopsy throw adjusted. Colour Doppler ultrasonography is useful to make sure no large vessels are in the biopsy path. The thoracic cavity should be checked for the presence of haemorrhage or pneumothorax after the procedure.

Complications

Pneumothorax can occur, more commonly after biopsy but also after fine-needle aspiration of pulmonary lesions. Presence of free pleural air is easily recognized during or immediately after the procedure if the lesion suddenly disappears and a broad hyperechoic layer appears directly underneath the thoracic wall with distal reverberation artefacts but no gliding motion along the thoracic wall. The extent of the pneumothorax and lung collapse is best assessed radiographically. Even though pneumothorax is a rare complication, equipment to perform a therapeutic thoracocentesis should always be available during aspiration or biopsy techniques. Haemorrhage is an uncommon complication of thoracic interventional procedures and is usually minimal and self-limiting in patients with normal platelet count and coagulation profile. Intervention is only required occasionally.

Echocardiography

Indications

Echocardiography (cardiac ultrasonography) has revolutionized the non-invasive assessment of cardiac disease. The ability of ultrasonography to discriminate between soft tissue (myocardium) and fluid (the blood pool) permits easy assessment of:

- The structure, size and relative proportions of the specific heart chambers and walls
- Heart valves
- Great vessels
- Cardiac function (particularly systolic function)
- The presence of a pericardial or pleural effusion.

It should be appreciated that echocardiography is complementary to thoracic radiography. Both techniques are essential in the investigation of a cardiac patient, particularly in conditions associated with left-sided volume overload, as radiographs demonstrate the haemodynamic significance of this on the pulmonary vasculature and lungs.

- Quantitative echocardiography allows standard assessment of chamber size or wall measurements, which can be compared with reference values for the species, breed or size of animal where these data are available. Measurements can be carried out on both two-dimensional (2D) and M-mode images.
- Doppler echocardiography demonstrates the direction, velocity and character of flow within the heart and great vessels. It is indicated for the identification of the cause of a heart murmur detected clinically, and for assessing its clinical significance.
- A complete systematic 2D, M-mode and Doppler echocardiographic examination will enable a diagnosis

to be made and assessment of the severity of most acquired or congenital heart diseases in animals, without resorting to invasive procedures such as cardiac catheterization and angiocardiography.

Information required from echocardiography

The clinician or echocardiographer may have different priorities for a given patient or presentation.

- Emergency ultrasonography – point-of-care ultrasonography (e.g. tFAST examination) is especially important for a patient presenting with potentially life-threatening clinical signs such as dyspnoea. Pleural effusion can be rapidly identified or excluded. If the dyspnoea is due to cardiogenic pulmonary oedema, the left atrium is normally dilated. Lung B-lines reflect a pulmonary infiltrate, which could be cardiogenic pulmonary oedema.
- A comprehensive Doppler echocardiographic examination, including 2D, M-mode, colour flow, spectral Doppler and tissue Doppler studies, is required to complete a systematic assessment of patients with acquired and congenital heart disease and fully examine chamber size, function and valves.
- Goal-focused echocardiography may be part of a follow-up examination (e.g. to assess left atrial size or left-sided filling pressures following treatment, or to assess for recurrence of pleural or pericardial effusion following thoracocentesis or pericardiocentesis). In some cases, it is performed to identify the phase of disease (e.g. in breeds with a systolic left apical heart murmur suspected of having preclinical myxomatous mitral valve disease (MMVD) to assess left atrial and left ventricular size in order to differentiate between Stage B1 and Stage B2 MMVD and decide whether treatment is indicated; or in cats with an asymptomatic heart murmur to assess left atrial size and, if the left atrium is dilated, determine the risk of events associated with myocardial disease).

Restraint and patient preparation

Animals with life-threatening pulmonary oedema or arrhythmias should always be stabilized prior to a full echocardiographic examination. Dyspnoeic cats should never be restrained in lateral recumbency. Treatment and stabilization over 24–48 hours may be required before a full echocardiographic assessment can be made, once the patient is breathing normally. As ultrasonography is exquisitely sensitive at detecting fluid, rapid thoracic imaging of a dyspnoeic animal (in ventral recumbency) identifies pleural effusion, which can then be drained, or B-lines with left atrial dilatation, which prompts treatment of left-sided congestive heart failure (L-CHF).

The fur is clipped from the left and right sides of the thorax, over the area of the palpable cardiac impulse. If the subcostal view is to be utilized, a small square caudal to the xiphisternum should also be clipped. In fine-coated animals, clipping may not be essential but facilitates more rapid attainment of good quality ultrasound images. Acoustic coupling gel is generously applied.

Animals are gently restrained in lateral recumbency (right then left). Care should be taken to avoid causing stress through over-restraint, especially in cats (they may need more than one handler restraining them). The distal fore- and hindlimbs should be held by the handler(s) to prevent the patient rising from the table, thus allowing the operator to keep equipment and transducers safe from damage. The animal should be comfortable and on bedding material; they may actually fall asleep in quiet, calm conditions.

Chemical restraint is not normally required. As sedative drugs may influence heart rate, contractility, wall thickness and flow velocities, they are best avoided. However, it is appreciated that they may be indicated in uncooperative or very stressed patients. Similar drugs and dose rates are used in cardiac patients and for radiographic positioning:

- Suggested sedation for dogs with heart disease: intravascular or intramuscular injection of butorphanol (0.3 mg/kg). This can be topped up with alfaxalone to effect to achieve the required level of sedation
- Suggested sedation for cats with heart disease: initially calm cats should be given intramuscular or intravenous butorphanol (0.2–0.3 mg/kg). If a cat is extremely uncooperative, various agents can be used in addition to give the desired level of sedation. These include one of the following options:
  - Alfaxalone i.v. to effect (e.g. 1–2 mg/kg bolus initially) (can also use 2–3 mg/kg i.m.)
  - If the cat is known or presumed to have hypertrophic obstructive cardiomyopathy, low dose medetomidine can reduce the severity of any dynamic left ventricular outflow tract obstruction (e.g. 5 μg/kg i.m. or i.v.)
  - Less common: an intramuscular injection of midazolam (0.2 mg/kg) and ketamine (5 mg/kg) can be given in the same syringe. (Ketamine will increase heart rate, making assessment of diastolic function difficult, and wall thickness may be artefactually increased.)

In a cat known to be stressed during examination, owner-administered oral gabapentin (50 or 100 mg per cat; 10–20 mg/kg orally) or trazodone (50 mg per cat; 5–10 mg/kg orally) about 1–2 hours before echocardiography can make the animal less stressed and therefore more amenable to undergoing an echocardiographic examination.

Electrocardiographic electrodes need to be applied. This is important to time cardiac events. However, it is appreciated that some cats may not accept electrode placement. As a complete study takes a minimum of 30 minutes, it is preferable to use adhesive electrodes (on the main pads of the paws) rather than crocodile clips on the skin. Normally, a lead II is obtained to optimize complex size and recognition, with electrodes on the right forelimb and the left hindlimb and the earth lead positioned wherever else is convenient (e.g. right hindlimb).

The right-sided views are used for 2D and M-mode images and measurements. Image quality is good as the heart is perpendicular to the ultrasound beam. For the right-handed operator, the animal remains in this position for the subcostal view.

The animal is turned over, still with sternum towards the operator, for the left-sided views. These give a 'vertical' heart, so image quality is less good, as structures other than the heart base are parallel to the ultrasound beam. However, alignment with intracardiac flow is optimized, facilitating Doppler studies. Access over several rib spaces (third to sixth) is required for all standard left-sided views; the animal may need to be repositioned during the course of the study, to permit access for all views.

Technique

The conventional standard display of images is that right-sided and basilar structures are displayed to the right of the screen (with a single exception: the left apical four-chamber view, which is displayed like a dorsoventral (DV) radiograph, with left to the right side of the screen). To achieve this with the operator's thumb on the transducer thumb-mark near the animal's sternum, the left–right image reverse facility of the ultrasound machine may be required.

2D (also known as B-mode) images represent a 'slice' through a complex, three-dimensional (3D) structure. Cardiac anatomy must be thoroughly appreciated to acquire and interpret these views; a model of the heart adjacent to the ultrasound machine can facilitate this. Most of the anatomy is appreciated from these 2D views. The standard 2D views are also essential:

- To position the M-mode cursor for M-mode studies
- For colour flow interrogation of the heart valves, septa and great vessels
- To position the spectral Doppler cursor (for pulsed wave (PW) or continuous wave (CW) Doppler) to record blood flow direction, velocity and character.

In general, the right parasternal (RPS) views are used to assess the anatomy and for M-mode studies. The left apical and left parasternal (LPS) views are used for Doppler studies. 2D images are described as being long-axis or short-axis, depending on whether the ventricular axis or aorta is being displayed in longitudinal or cross-sectional planes, respectively.

Equipment

A sector transducer (phased array) is required to image the heart through windows between the lung lobes and the ribs. A linear transducer or a curvilinear transducer with a large footprint is not appropriate, as it would not permit acquisition of images acquired by rotation or angulation.

A range of transducers, offering various frequencies, is normally required to scan veterinary patients:

- Cats and very small dogs require a 7.5–12 MHz transducer
- Medium-sized dogs require a 5.0–7.5 MHz transducer
- Giant breeds of dog require a 2.5–4.0 MHz transducer
- The highest frequency transducer offering appropriate penetration should be selected to optimize image resolution
- Note that most modern transducers can have the frequency adjusted within the prescribed range
- For Doppler studies, a lower frequency transducer may be required than that for optimal ultrasound imaging; transducers may need to be changed during the study.

A purpose-designed echocardiography table should be used, with a hole or a wedge over which the animal lies in lateral recumbency. Images are acquired through the dependent chest wall. The hypostatic effects on the dependent lung minimize air interference on the cardiac images.

Cardiac software is required on the ultrasound machine. Machine settings ('knobology') will depend on the manufacturer, but in general, fast frame rates and low persistence are required for echocardiography. Some other general tips include:

- Use a sector angle appropriate for the view you want to obtain. It can be narrowed down to a particular region of interest (which improves frame rate)

- Optimize image depth for the size of heart, so the entire heart almost fills the depth of the image
- Consider harmonic (octave) imaging. Mainly useful for obese or large patients. The reflected ultrasound beam is received at double the frequency of the transmitted ultrasound beam, so image quality is better with fewer artefacts such as reverberation. Harmonic frequencies rapidly attenuate, so there is an optimal depth for their use (4–8 cm). Harmonic imaging can make heart valves appear thicker, but this is rarely a problem with modern machines
- Adjust focus. Multiple focal zones may be selectable on many machines. For animals, only one is required; position within the middle of the left ventricle (LV)
- Set the gain so that the blood pool is black and greyscale is ideal for the myocardium
- Set time gain compensation (TGC) to correct for attenuation of the ultrasound beam in the far field. Aim for uniform greyscale of the ventricular myocardium throughout the depth of the image. In cardiology the TGC sliders are often almost vertical; however, some transducers allow gain in the far field allowing for ultrasound beam attenuation at depth with high-frequency transducers.
- Set reject low if soft echoes such as spontaneous echo-contrast need to be visualized.

A simultaneous electrocardiogram (ECG) should be recorded with the images. Accurate measurement depends on defining phases of diastole or systole. Generally, end-diastolic measurements are taken at the start of the QRS complex. End-systolic measurements are usually taken when the LV cavity is smallest (or at the end of the ECG T wave).

Standard 2D (B-mode) views of the heart

Acquisition of the standard RPS views is described and illustrated in Figure 2.15; the subcostal view is also shown. The corresponding observations, measurements and calculations are also indicated in Figure 2.15. Acquisition of the standard left apical and LPS views is described and illustrated in Figure 2.16.

M-mode echocardiography

M-mode measurements are one-dimensional (1D). The images are motion–time graphs. Temporal resolution is very high (in contrast to 2D and spectral Doppler images). The M-mode cursor can be accurately positioned on the 2D image.

M-mode measurements need to be carefully and consistently acquired for them to be useful in patient follow-up or in comparison with reference values for the species, breed and weight, where these data are available. Acquisition of M-mode images and methods of measurement are detailed in Figure 2.17.

With modern echocardiographic equipment and high frame rates for 2D echocardiography, the role of M-mode in cardiac evaluation has been dismissed by some cardiologists. However, it can give useful additional information to 2D imaging, especially when superior temporal resolution is required.

On some machines, 'anatomical M-mode' is available. An M-mode cursor can be placed on an acquired 2D image to generate an M-mode image. However, this will only have a similar temporal resolution to 2D and its main use is if the M-mode study was forgotten at the time of image acquisition.

M-mode reference values: Breed-specific reference values should be consulted whenever they are available. Where they are not available, weight-based reference ranges can be used. These have been generated by allometric scaling to bodyweight. The indices of each measured M-mode variable in diastole and systole are generated by dividing by approximately the cube root of the bodyweight in kg (but the actual exponent varies); these have recently been updated from the original allometric scaling publication (Cornell *et al.*, 2004; Esser *et al.*, 2020). Note that sighthound breeds are different from other canine breeds.

Since cats are relatively uniform in breed and size (compared with the canine population), standard feline reference values can be consulted for most cats; breed- and weight-specific values should be compared for extremes of size and breed (Häggström *et al.*, 2016).

Doppler echocardiography

J. Christian Doppler originally defined the Doppler principle. This states that there is an apparent change in transmitted frequency, reflected back to the source off a target, which occurs as a result of the movement of the source or the target. This phenomenon is readily appreciated as a police car with siren noise approaches then passes an observer; the sound is of higher frequency as it approaches, and lower frequency as it moves away from, the observer. There are several practical applications, not least important of which is Doppler echocardiography.

In Doppler echocardiography, a pulse of sound is emitted from the transducer and reflected off moving targets within the heart, the red blood cells (RBCs). The apparent shift in frequency of the sound reflected back to the transducer, termed the Doppler shift, is proportional to the velocity of the RBCs (accounting for their speed and direction of movement). The software of a Doppler echocardiography machine converts this Doppler shift into an audible signal and a visual display and calculates the velocity of the RBCs. The flow through each valve varies during the cardiac cycle; these events can be plotted against time (with a simultaneously recorded ECG). This gives the spectral Doppler trace, a velocity–time graph.

In PW Doppler, a sample volume may be positioned within the area of interest. A pulse of ultrasound waves is emitted by the crystal in the transducer and is reflected back to the transducer before another pulse is transmitted. Only the RBCs in the area of interest are assessed. Because of the time required for sampling in this way, only low velocities can be measured. According to Nyquist's theorem, the maximum velocity of flow that can be measured using PW Doppler must produce a Doppler shift no higher than half the pulse repetition frequency (PRF). If blood is moving at a velocity exceeding the Nyquist limit of the machine settings (the Doppler shift exceeds half the PRF), it is shown 'wrapped around' in the opposite direction; this is called aliasing. Aliasing, thus, results in directional ambiguity.

PW Doppler gives information about flow velocity and direction of flow (towards the observer is displayed above the baseline, away is displayed below the baseline of the spectral trace). Character of flow is also illustrated with PW Doppler. Laminar flow, due to RBCs moving in 'sheets', uniformly accelerating and decelerating, is indicated by a clean 'envelope' (see Figure 2.18). Turbulent flow tends to occur at higher velocities, with whorls and eddies of flow, giving a filled in, less tidy signal on PW spectra. PW Doppler may be limited by the depth of image being interrogated.

Right parasternal long-axis four-chamber view

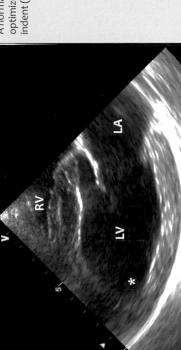

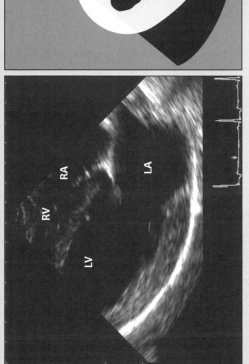

A normal Greyhound.

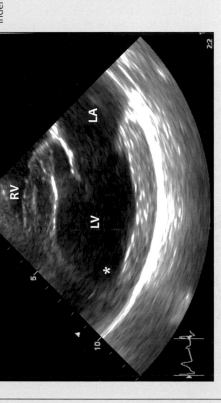

A normal Great Dane. LV length and area are optimized. The LV apex can be seen as an indent (∗).

Acquisition of the view

- Operator thumb on thumb-mark of transducer
- Position transducer over where cardiac impulse is easily palpable
- Beam is directed approximately parallel to the ribs, towards the caudodorsal scapula
- Transducer perpendicular to the thoracic wall
- Slide up the intercostal space for a 'horizontal' heart (important before acquiring M-mode), or slide down towards the sternum for a 'tipped' view (useful for colour flow screening)
- When determining LV shape and geometry, aim to optimize LV length and area. The transducer (and ultrasound beam) is directed more caudosternally (i.e. towards the LV apex)
- Optimize the LA. Assess its size and shape. A normal LA is almost square in systole. The IAS flares to the right and the chamber looks more rounded when enlarged
- Dorsal to the LA, image the PVe and RPA (in cross-section) and compare the diameters of these. A more dilated PVe suggests actual or imminent L-CHF. A more dilated RPA may be seen in pulmonary hypertension
- Assess MV and check for prolapse
- Colour flow Doppler; check MV and TV
- To image more of the right heart, the transducer may need to be moved one rib space cranially and a tipped view optimizes the right heart
- Check the IAS (anatomy and with colour flow Doppler)

Observations, measurements and calculations

- Optimize LV length and area. 2D methods (e.g. Simpson's rule; see Figure 2.19) can be used to trace the endocardial border of the LV (closing at the level of the mitral annulus) to determine LV volumes in diastole and systole
- An indication of whether the LV is rounded, such as in remodelling with disease, can be shown by calculating the *index of sphericity*. This is the ratio of LV diastolic length over 'width' (at chordal level, or use the M-mode dimension). Note: there are breed/conformational differences in this, and it is not sensitive or specific (e.g. for diagnosis of DCM)
- In cats, regions of focal hypertrophy may be recognized (in HCM). These segments should be measured in diastole; a measurement of ≥6 mm defines LV hypertrophy in the adult cat
- Size of the LA can be measured, at end of systole (frame before MV opens), by measuring the maximal width of the LA, parallel to the mitral annulus. This LA max can be compared with aortic annulus diameter (normal ratio <2.5) or can be indexed for bodyweight
- Assess the MV for the presence of prolapse or flail (associated with MMVD and ruptured chordae tendinae, respectively)

2.15 Right parasternal (RPS) and subcostal views. amv = anterior mitral valve leaflet; Ao = aorta; AoV = aortic valve; APM = anterior papillary muscle; CdVC = caudal vena cava; CW = continuous wave; DCM = dilated cardiomyopathy; HCM = hypertrophic cardiomyopathy; IAS = interatrial septum; IVS = interventricular septum; LA = left atrium; LAA = left atrial appendage; L-CHF = left-sided congestive heart failure; LPA = left pulmonary artery; LV = left ventricle; LVFW = left ventricular free wall; LVOT = left ventricular outflow tract; MMVD = myxomatous mitral valve disease; MPA = main pulmonary artery (pulmonic trunk); MV = mitral valve; pmv = posterior mitral valve leaflet; PPM = posterior papillary muscle; PVe = pulmonary vein; PW = pulsed wave; RA = right atrium; R-CHF = right-sided congestive heart failure; RPA = right pulmonary artery; RV = right ventricle; RVOT = right ventricular outflow tract; TV = tricuspid valve; VSD = ventricular septal defect. (continues)

(Line diagrams adapted and reproduced from Boon (1998) with permission from the publisher)

Right parasternal long-axis four-chamber view continued

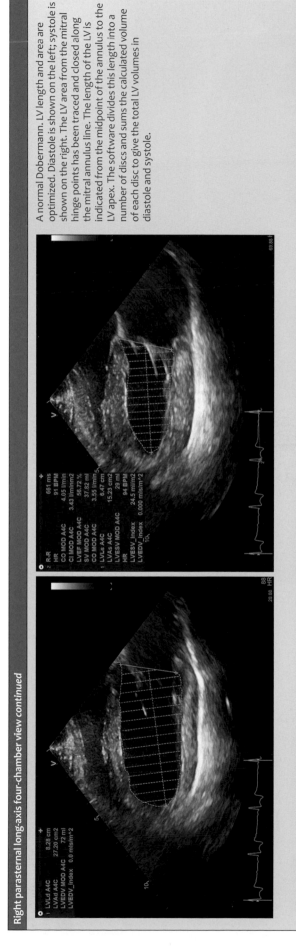

A normal Dobermann. LV length and area are optimized. Diastole is shown on the left; systole is shown on the right. The LV area from the mitral hinge points has been traced and closed along the mitral annulus line. The length of the LV is indicated from the midpoint of the annulus to the LV apex. The software divides this length into a number of discs and sums the calculated volume of each disc to give the total LV volumes in diastole and systole.

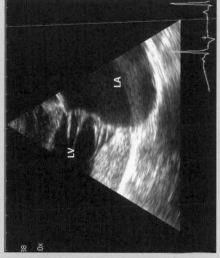

A Collie cross with MMVD. In systole, parts of the valve 'balloon' on the left atrial side of the mitral annulus line (mitral prolapse). This is an abnormal finding.

LA dilatation in a Great Dane with DCM (early systolic frame). The LA looks more rounded and the IAS is flared towards the right.

A normal Great Dane. This view can be used to assess the structures dorsal to the LA. The PVe enters the LA parallel to the septum and the RPA branch is seen dorsal to the LA. The diameter of the PVe and RPA should be compared and should be similar to one another.

See also Figure 2.22

2.15 (continued) Right parasternal (RPS) and subcostal views. amv = anterior mitral valve leaflet; Ao = aorta; AoV = aortic valve; APM = anterior papillary muscle; CdVC = caudal vena cava; CW = continuous wave; DCM = dilated cardiomyopathy; HCM = hypertrophic cardiomyopathy; IAS = interatrial septum; IVS = interventricular septum; LA = left atrium; LAA = left atrial appendage; L-CHF = left-sided congestive heart failure; LPA = left pulmonary artery; LV = left ventricle; LVFW = left ventricular free wall; LVOT = left ventricular outflow tract; MMVD = myxomatous mitral valve disease; MPA = main pulmonary artery (pulmonic trunk); MV = mitral valve; pmv = posterior mitral valve leaflet; PPM = posterior papillary muscle; PV = pulmonic valve; PVe = pulmonary vein; PW = pulsed wave; RA = right atrium; R-CHF = right-sided congestive heart failure; RPA = right pulmonary artery; RV = right ventricle; RVOT = right ventricular outflow tract; TV = tricuspid valve; VSD = ventricular septal defect. (continues)

(Line diagrams adapted and reproduced from Boon (1998) with permission from the publisher)

Right parasternal long-axis five-chamber view

Acquisition of the view

- From the four-chamber view, rotate the thumb about 10 degrees towards the animal's rump (anticlockwise) and angle cranially
- The long-axis view of the Ao ('chamber 5') should be clear
- Check LVOT and Ao for turbulence or aortic insufficiency using colour flow Doppler

Observations, measurements and calculations

- The aortic annulus diameter can be measured between the open aortic valves
- The basal septum in cats with primary or secondary myocardial disease, or in aged cats, may be prominent or grossly hypertrophied: measure diastolic wall thickness of this region, parallel to the endocardium
- Examine the subvalvular region, the aortic valves and the ascending aortic arch
- Exclude VSDs in membranous part of septum (but note that small VSDs may not be imaged without colour flow Doppler)

See also Chapter 9

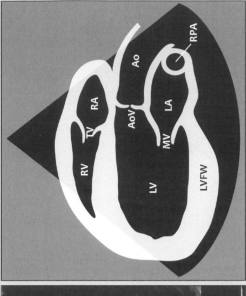

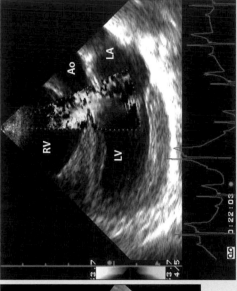

A normal Greyhound, including the ascending Ao. The LAA or LA may be seen.

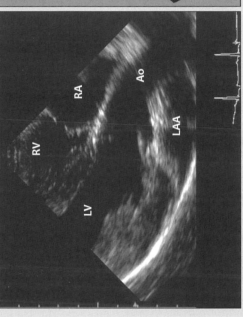

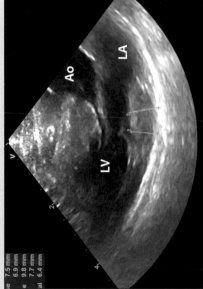

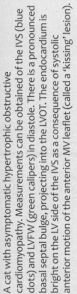

A cat with asymptomatic hypertrophic obstructive cardiomyopathy. Measurements can be obtained of the IVS (blue dots) and LVFW (green calipers) in diastole. There is a pronounced basal septal bulge, projecting into the LVOT. The endocardium is bright on the LV side of the IVS as a consequence of systolic anterior motion of the anterior MV leaflet (called a 'kissing' lesion).

A Shetland Sheepdog, with colour flow Doppler over the base of the IVS. Turbulent flow from the LVOT into the RV in systole supports the presence of a VSD.

2.15 (continued) Right parasternal (RPS) and subcostal views. amv = anterior mitral valve leaflet; Ao = aorta; AoV = aortic valve; APM = anterior papillary muscle; CdVC = caudal vena cava; CW = continuous wave; DCM = dilated cardiomyopathy; HCM = hypertrophic cardiomyopathy; IAS = interatrial septum; IVS = interventricular septum; LA = left atrium; LAA = left atrial appendage; L-CHF = left-sided congestive heart failure; LPA = left pulmonary artery; LV = left ventricle; LVFW = left ventricular free wall; LVOT = left ventricular outflow tract; MMVD = myxomatous mitral valve disease; MPA = main pulmonary artery (pulmonic trunk); MV = mitral valve; pmv = posterior mitral valve leaflet; PPM = posterior papillary muscle; PV = pulmonic valve; PVe = pulmonary vein; PW = pulsed wave; RA = right atrium; R-CHF = right-sided congestive heart failure; RPA = right pulmonary artery; RV = right ventricle; RVOT = right ventricular outflow tract; TV = tricuspid valve; VSD = ventricular septal defect. (continues)

(Line diagrams adapted and reproduced from Boon (1998) with permission from the publisher)

Right parasternal short-axis view

Acquisition of the view

- From the four-chamber view, with the heart as horizontal as possible, rotate the transducer 90 degrees anticlockwise, towards the rump
- The LV is displayed in cross-section, with the RV wrapped around the septum in a crescent shape
- Check the LV is rounded as normal. The septum may be flattened if RV pressure is increased (e.g. in pulmonic stenosis)
- Slide or angle up the intercostal space to image at level of apex, level of papillary muscles and level of chordae tendinae. Aim for the LV to be symmetrical. The M-mode cursor can be positioned to bisect the LV cavity at the chordal level
- Note that, during angling up from apex to base, as the heart is twisted, slightly more rotation is required towards the heart base
- Slide or angle more dorsally to record the 'fish-mouth' view of the MV, ensuring both anterior and posterior leaflets are imaged. Mitral M-mode studies can be positioned from this view
- With slightly more rotation, and cranial angulation, the short-axis view of the Ao, central within the heart, is obtained, at aortic valve level (Mercedes Benz sign). As well as including aortic valve leaflets, optimize the LA with LAA

Observations, measurements and calculations

- From RPS short-axis view at the level of chordae tendinae or papillary muscles, check normal relationship of LV and RV and whether there is any septal flattening suggesting increased RV pressure
- In cats, can accurately measure the wall thickness in diastole to diagnose hypertrophy (≥6 mm). 2D measurements may be preferable for the LV in cats with papillary muscles or false tendons interfering with M-mode imaging, making it difficult to assess endocardial boundaries of the walls
- Can make subjective assessment of papillary muscle hypertrophy (common in feline HCM)
- M-mode LV at chordae tendinae level
- Assess the MV leaflets
- Use to position the M-mode cursor for mitral M-mode

From RPS short-axis view, at the level of aortic valves and LA:

- From an early diastolic frame (frame following closure of aortic valve leaflets) measure the diameter of the Ao at valve level, and measure the left atrial size in the same direction (avoiding ending measurement within PVe). The normal ratio of LA:Ao is <1.6
- Can also record M-mode of Ao (measured in diastole) to LA (measured in systole). M-mode is useful to assess aortic root motion and aortic valve opening, but it is not reliable at left atrial size in dogs

See also Chapter 9

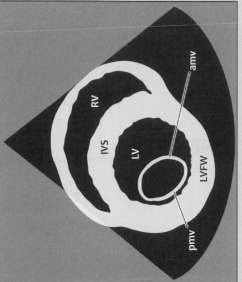

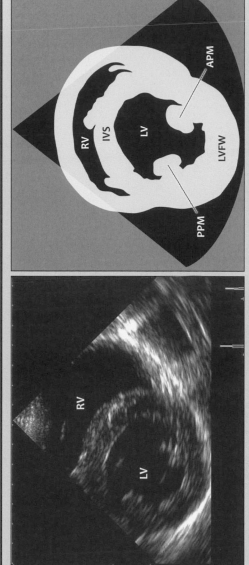

Left and right ventricles at the level of the chordae tendinae in a normal Greyhound.

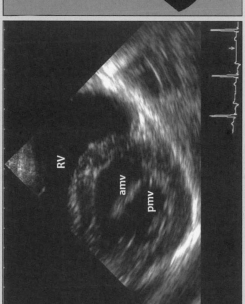

LV at MV level in a normal Greyhound.

2.15 (continued) Right parasternal (RPS) and subcostal views. amv = anterior mitral valve leaflet; Ao = aorta; AoV = aortic valve; APM = anterior papillary muscle; CdVC = caudal vena cava; CW = continuous wave; DCM = dilated cardiomyopathy; HCM = hypertrophic cardiomyopathy; IAS = interatrial septum; IVS = interventricular septum; LA = left atrium; LAA = left atrial appendage; L-CHF = left-sided congestive heart failure; LPA = left pulmonary artery; LV = left ventricle; LVFW = left ventricular free wall; LVOT = left ventricular outflow tract; MMVD = myxomatous mitral valve disease; MPA = main pulmonary artery (pulmonic trunk); MV = mitral valve; pmv = posterior mitral valve leaflet; PPM = posterior papillary muscle; PV = pulmonic valve; PVe = pulmonary vein; PW = pulsed wave; RA = right atrium; R-CHF = right-sided congestive heart failure; RPA = right pulmonary artery; RV = right ventricle; RVOT = right ventricular outflow tract; TV = tricuspid valve; VSD = ventricular septal defect. (continues)

(Line diagrams adapted and reproduced from Boon (1998) with permission from the publisher)

Right parasternal short-axis view *continued*

AoV level: when clearly seen, the aortic valves form a 'Mercedes Benz' sign.

Left atrial enlargement, shown by ratio of the diastolic short-axis dimension of the LA, indexed to the aortic diameter in diastole. (a) A dog with advanced MMVD. AoV level, showing measurement in diastole of the aortic diameter (measurement 1) and the left atrial diameter, along the same plane (measurement 2). The ratio in this dog was 57.7:16.2 (3.56; normal <1.6). (b) A cat with severe congestive heart failure due to end-stage HCM. AoV level, showing measurement in diastole of the aortic diameter (measurement 1) and the left atrial diameter, along the same plane (measurement 2). The ratio in this cat was 22.1:9.7 (2.28).

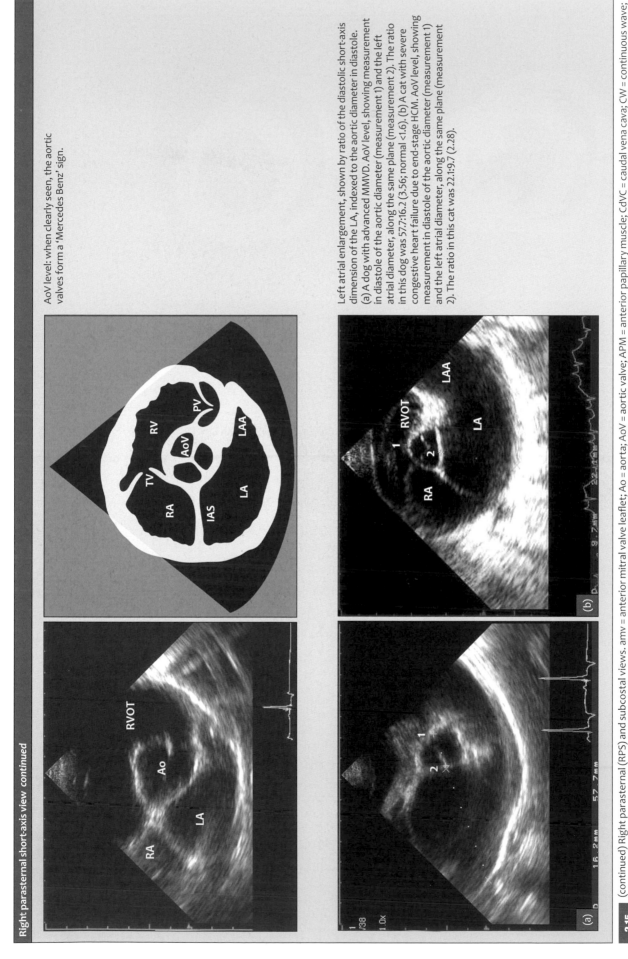

2.15 (continued) Right parasternal (RPS) and subcostal views. amv = anterior mitral valve leaflet; Ao = aorta; AoV = aortic valve; APM = anterior papillary muscle; CdVC = caudal vena cava; CW = continuous wave; DCM = dilated cardiomyopathy; HCM = hypertrophic cardiomyopathy; IAS = interatrial septum; IVS = interventricular septum; LA = left atrium; LAA = left atrial appendage; L-CHF = left-sided congestive heart failure; LPA = left pulmonary artery; LV = left ventricle; LVFW = left ventricular free wall; LVOT = left ventricular outflow tract; MMVD = myxomatous mitral valve disease; MPA = main pulmonary artery (pulmonic trunk); MV = mitral valve; pmv = posterior mitral valve leaflet; PPM = posterior papillary muscle; PV = pulmonic valve; PVe = pulmonary vein; PW = pulsed wave; RA = right atrium; R-CHF = right-sided congestive heart failure; RPA = right pulmonary artery; RV = right ventricle; RVOT = right ventricular outflow tract; TV = tricuspid valve; VSD = ventricular septal defect. (continues)
(Line diagrams adapted and reproduced from Boon (1998) with permission from the publisher) ▲

Right parasternal cranial long-axis view of aorta

Acquisition of the view

- From short-axis Ao, rotate back clockwise until the Ao is seen in long axis
- Alternatively, move a rib space cranial from the RPS five-chamber view

Observations, measurements and calculations

- Can assess aortic valves and subvalvular region, and whether there is any post-stenotic dilatation of the aortic arch
- Measure aortic diameter (systole; aortic annulus and valve level) to enable calculation of LA max:Ao long-axis systolic ratio or cross-sectional area and forward stroke volume)

View optimizing the proximal Ao and aortic annulus. The aortic annulus diameter is measured during systole (between the hinge points of the open AoV leaflets) (arrowed).

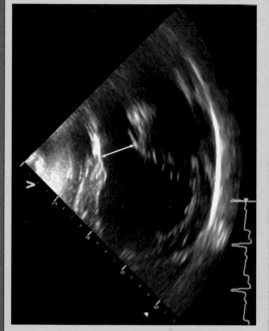

Right parasternal cranial short-axis view

Acquisition of the view

- From a cranial view of the long-axis Ao, angle the transducer dorsally. The Ao will become short-axis, and a long-axis view of the RVOT and pulmonic valves is acquired
- Fan slightly more dorsally and cranially to optimize the pulmonic trunk and bifurcation of the left and right pulmonary arteries
- Use colour flow Doppler for the pulmonic valves and pulmonic trunk

Observations, measurements and calculations

- From RPS cranial short-axis view, optimized for pulmonic trunk, can assess pulmonic valves and pulmonic trunk
- Can measure MPA diameter, at valve level, in systole
- The MPA should be equal in diameter or less wide than the Ao. Increased diameter, with normal pulmonic valves, may suggest pulmonary hypertension
- This view is used for Doppler assessment of the pulmonic valves, pulmonary outflow and pulmonic insufficiency

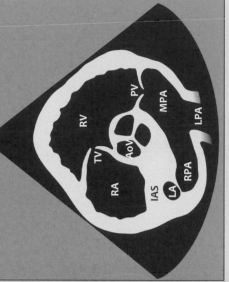

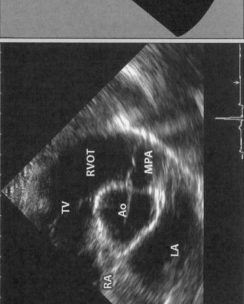

AoV level, optimized for PV and proximal MPA in a normal Greyhound.

2.15 (continued) Right parasternal (RPS) and subcostal views. amv = anterior mitral valve leaflet; Ao = aorta; AoV = aortic valve; APM = anterior papillary muscle; CdVC = caudal vena cava; CW = continuous wave; DCM = dilated cardiomyopathy; HCM = hypertrophic cardiomyopathy; IAS = interatrial septum; IVS = interventricular septum; LA = left atrium; LAA = left atrial appendage; L-CHF = left-sided congestive heart failure; LPA = left pulmonary artery; LV = left ventricle; LVFW = left ventricular free wall; LVOT = left ventricular outflow tract; MMVD = myxomatous mitral valve disease; MPA = main pulmonary artery (pulmonic trunk); MV = mitral valve; pmv = posterior mitral valve leaflet; PPM = posterior papillary muscle; PV = pulmonic valve; PVe = pulmonary vein; PW = pulsed wave; RA = right atrium; R-CHF = right-sided congestive heart failure; RPA = right pulmonary artery; RV = right ventricle; RVOT = right ventricular outflow tract; TV = tricuspid valve; VSD = ventricular septal defect. (continues)
(Line diagrams adapted and reproduced from Boon (1998) with permission from the publisher)

Subcostal view

Acquisition of the view

- Position transducer caudal to the xiphisternum, angling cranially. The thumb is ventral, towards the operator. The depth of field needs to be increased for imaging the heart and ascending Ao, beyond the liver and diaphragm. The transducer may need to be pushed into the cranial abdomen (which is not comfortable for most dogs). Slight rotation of the transducer results in opening up the Ao. The CW cursor can be used to position for aortic outflow peak velocity
- This view is also useful to assess for evidence of R-CHF: ascites, hepatic venous congestion, dilatation of the CdVC

Observations, measurements and calculations

- This view is as parallel as possible to the aortic outflow. The Ao is central within the thorax and imaging from the midline optimizes alignment
- Spectral Doppler is used to record peak aortic velocity. In most dogs, peak aortic velocities are obtained from this view
- Note that a low frequency transducer is required for the depth of penetration, and CW Doppler may be required rather than PW to obtain a signal at this depth
- Confirms actual or imminent R-CHF

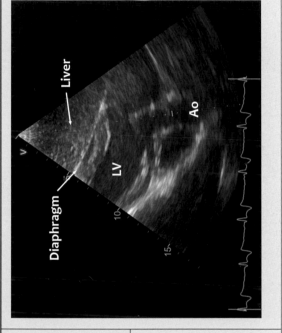

A normal Dobermann. This view is transhepatic and transdiaphragmatic and allows good alignment with aortic outflow because the ascending Ao is very central in the thorax. This permits accurate recording of peak aortic velocities. Due to the depth of the image in large dogs, CW Doppler may be required. The hepatic veins and CdVC can also be assessed.

2.15 (continued) Right parasternal (RPS) and subcostal views. amv = anterior mitral valve leaflet; Ao = aorta; AoV = aortic valve; APM = anterior papillary muscle; CdVC = caudal vena cava; CW = continuous wave; DCM = dilated cardiomyopathy; HCM = hypertrophic cardiomyopathy; IAS = interatrial septum; IVS = interventricular septum; LA = left atrium; LAA = left atrial appendage; L-CHF = left-sided congestive heart failure; LPA = left pulmonary artery; LV = left ventricle; LVFW = left ventricular free wall; LVOT = left ventricular outflow tract; MMVD = myxomatous mitral valve disease; MPA = main pulmonary artery (pulmonic trunk); MV = mitral valve; pmv = posterior mitral valve leaflet; PPM = posterior papillary muscle; PV = pulmonic valve; PVe = pulmonary vein; PW = pulsed wave; RA = right atrium; R-CHF = right-sided congestive heart failure; RPA = right pulmonary artery; RV = right ventricle; RVOT = right ventricular outflow tract; TV = tricuspid valve; VSD = ventricular septal defect. (Line diagrams adapted and reproduced from Boon (1998) with permission from the publisher)

Left apical four-chamber view

Acquisition of the view

- Feel for the cardiac apex
- Position transducer at the cardiac apex, with thumb about 30–45 degrees to the intercostal space, towards the head at the cardiac apex, angling dorsally
- The transducer is almost parallel to the thoracic wall
- To include the apex, move nearer the sternum, and possibly more caudally, to optimize LV length. Aim for a 'vertical' heart
- Note: in all but very deep, narrow-chested breeds, the anatomical LV apex is not included as it is more diaphragmatically directed
- This view is used for mitral Doppler studies
- To include more right heart, move one or two rib spaces cranially (e.g. to record TV studies)

Observations, measurements and calculations

- May be used to assess LV length and volume (but apex not included) (RPS long-axis four-chamber view more likely to optimize LV length and area in most dogs)
- Colour flow Doppler interrogation of the MV and TV
- Spectral Doppler assessment of mitral and tricuspid flow, mitral and tricuspid regurgitation
- When RV optimized, can determine right ventricular area in diastole and systole, and FAC. FAC = (diastolic area – systolic area)/ diastolic area. See also Figure 2.23
- Position M-mode cursor for mitral (septal and lateral) or tricuspid annular plane systolic excursion; cursor must be parallel to each wall in turn
- Use for recording PW Doppler of pulmonary venous flow
- Use for calculation of mitral early flow propagation (Vp) with colour M-mode
- Use of PW-TDI studies of myocardial motion of longitudinal fibres at the mitral annulus (septal and lateral) and tricuspid annulus. Cursor must be parallel to each wall in turn

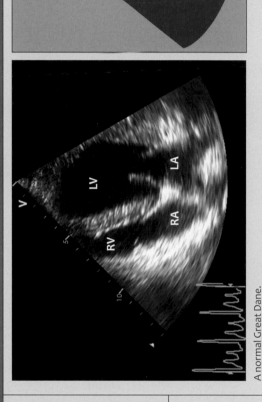

A normal Great Dane.

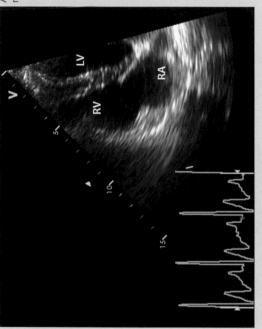

A normal Great Dane. View optimizing the right heart.

2.16 The left apical and parasternal views. Ao = aorta; AoV = aortic valve; CW = continuous wave; FAC = fractional area change; HOCM = hypertrophic obstructive cardiomyopathy; IAS = interatrial septum; IVS = interventricular septum; LA = left atrium; LAA = left atrial appendage; LPA = left pulmonary artery; L-CHF = left-sided congestive heart failure; LV = left ventricle; LVFW = left ventricular free wall; LVOT = left ventricular outflow tract; MAPSE = mitral annulus plane systolic excursion; MPA = main pulmonary artery (pulmonic trunk); MV = mitral valve; PDA = patent ductus arteriosus; PV = pulmonic valve; PW = pulsed wave; PW-TDI = pulsed wave tissue Doppler imaging; RA = right atrium; RPA = right pulmonary artery; RPS = right parasternal; RV = right ventricle; RVOT = right ventricular outflow tract; TAPSE = tricuspid annulus plane systolic excursion; TV = tricuspid valve; Vp = left ventricular early flow propagation velocity. (continues)

(Line diagrams adapted and reproduced from Boon (1998) with permission from the publisher)

Left apical four-chamber view continued

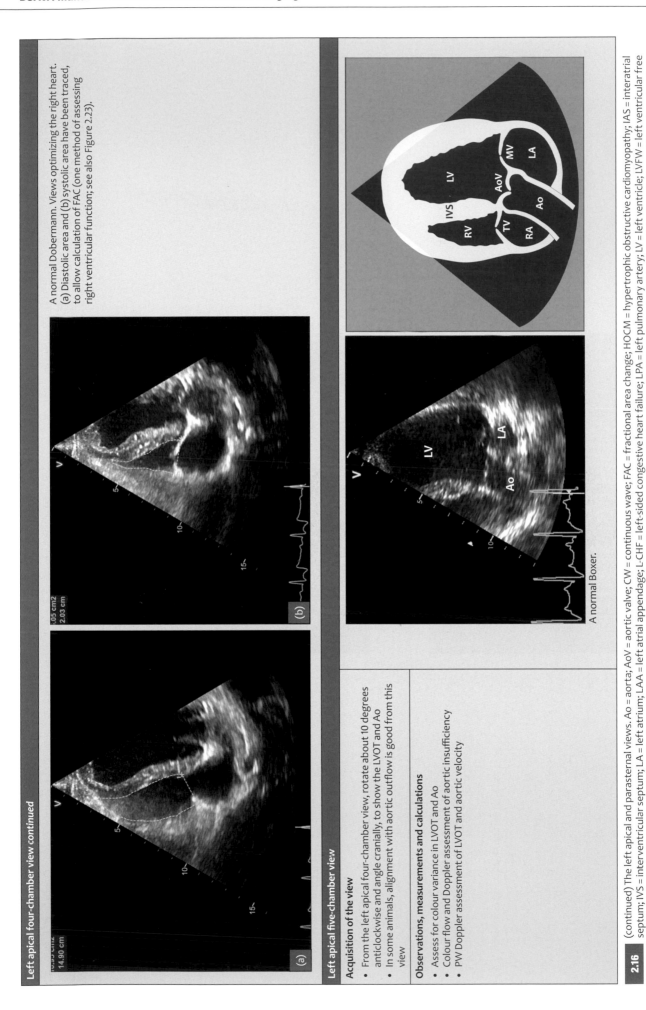

A normal Dobermann. Views optimizing the right heart. (a) Diastolic area and (b) systolic area have been traced, to allow calculation of FAC (one method of assessing right ventricular function; see also Figure 2.23).

(a)

(b)

105 cm2
2.03 cm

14.90 cm

Left apical five-chamber view

Acquisition of the view

- From the left apical four-chamber view, rotate about 10 degrees anticlockwise and angle cranially, to show the LVOT and Ao
- In some animals, alignment with aortic outflow is good from this view

Observations, measurements and calculations

- Assess for colour variance in LVOT and Ao
- Colour flow and Doppler assessment of aortic insufficiency
- PW Doppler assessment of LVOT and aortic velocity

A normal Boxer.

2.16 (continued) The left apical and parasternal views. Ao = aorta; AoV = aortic valve; CW = continuous wave; FAC = fractional area change; HOCM = hypertrophic obstructive cardiomyopathy; IAS = interatrial septum; IVS = interventricular septum; LA = left atrium; LAA = left atrial appendage; L-CHF = left-sided congestive heart failure; LPA = left pulmonary artery; LV = left ventricle; LVFW = left ventricular free wall; LVOT = left ventricular outflow tract; MAPSE = mitral annulus plane systolic excursion; MPA = main pulmonary artery (pulmonic trunk); MV = mitral valve; PDA = patent ductus arteriosus; PV = pulmonic valve; PW = pulsed wave; PW-TD = pulsed wave tissue Doppler imaging; RA = right atrium; RPA = right pulmonary artery; RPS = right parasternal; RV = right ventricle; RVOT = right ventricular outflow tract; TAPSE = tricuspid annulus plane systolic excursion; TV = tricuspid valve; Vp = left ventricular early flow propagation velocity. (continues)

(Line diagrams adapted and reproduced from Boon (1998) with permission from the publisher)

Left apical two-chamber view

Acquisition of the view

- From the left apical four-chamber view, as far caudally as possible, rotate 90 degrees for the two-chamber view (LA and LV)
- Includes the LAA – but to fully assess this, the transducer must be moved much further cranially and dorsally up the intercostal space

Observations, measurements and calculations

- Orthogonal long-axis view; used for more accurate assessment of LV length and volumes (e.g. full Simpson's rule; see Figure 2.19)
- Sometimes used to assess mitral inflow or regurgitation (e.g. eccentric jets)
- Can record MAPSE or PW-TDI velocities at orthogonal points to those recorded in the four-chamber view. Rarely indicated (unless investigating asynchronous wall motion)

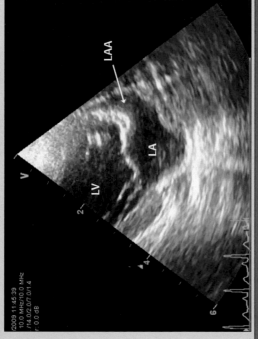

View showing the LV and LA with its appendage (LAA).

Left apical three-chamber view

Acquisition of the view

- From the apical two-chamber view, angle cranially until the LVOT and Ao are apparent
- Sometimes, good alignment with aortic outflow is possible here

Observations, measurements and calculations

- Assess colour variance of LVOT and Ao
- Colour flow and Doppler assessment of aortic insufficiency
- PW Doppler assessment of LVOT and aortic velocity, to indicate whether there is a step-up in velocity and/or to record peak aortic velocity

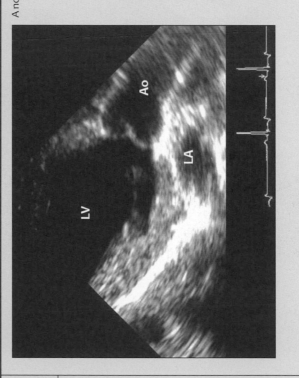

A normal Greyhound.

2.16 (continued) The left apical and parasternal views. Ao = aorta; AoV = aortic valve; CW = continuous wave; FAC = fractional area change; HOCM = hypertrophic obstructive cardiomyopathy; IAS = interatrial septum; IVS = interventricular septum; LA = left atrium; LAA = left atrial appendage; L-CHF = left-sided congestive heart failure; LPA = left pulmonary artery; LV = left ventricle; LVFW = left ventricular free wall; LVOT = left ventricular outflow tract; MAPSE = mitral annulus plane systolic excursion; MPA = main pulmonary artery (pulmonic trunk); MV = mitral valve; PDA = patent ductus arteriosus; PV = pulmonic valve; PW = pulsed wave; PW-TDI = pulsed wave tissue Doppler imaging; RA = right atrium; RPA = right pulmonary artery; RPS = right parasternal; RV = right ventricle; RVOT = right ventricular outflow tract; TAPSE = tricuspid annulus plane systolic excursion; TV = tricuspid valve; Vp = left ventricular early flow propagation velocity. (continues)

(Line diagrams adapted and reproduced from Boon (1998) with permission from the publisher)

Left cranial parasternal long-axis view of the aorta

Acquisition of the view

- Moving 1–2 rib spaces cranially from the apical views, the ascending aortic arch can be assessed

Observations, measurements and calculations

- Used to assess for post-stenotic dilation in aortic stenosis
- Search for periaortic masses
- Used to measure aortic annulus diameter (during systole, between the open aortic valve leaflets, at their hinge point) to calculate forward stroke volume

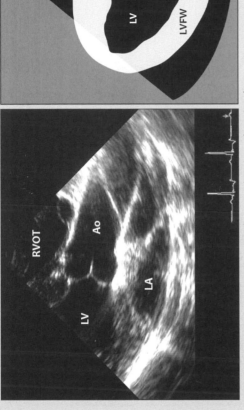

A normal Greyhound. View optimizing the ascending Ao and aortic valves.

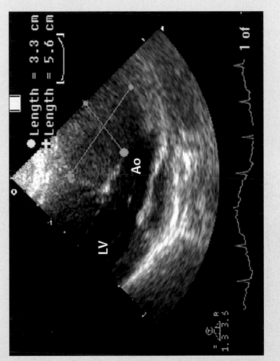

A Boxer with a periaortic mass, presumed to be a chemodectoma. See also Chapter 9.

2.16 (continued) The left apical and parasternal views. Ao = aorta; AoV = aortic valve; CW = continuous wave; FAC = fractional area change; HOCM = hypertrophic obstructive cardiomyopathy; IAS = interatrial septum; IVS = interventricular septum; LA = left atrium; LAA = left atrial appendage; L-CHF = left-sided congestive heart failure; LPA = left pulmonary artery; LV = left ventricle; LVFW = left ventricular free wall; LVOT = left ventricular outflow tract; MAPSE = mitral annulus plane systolic excursion; MPA = main pulmonary artery (pulmonic trunk); MV = mitral valve; PDA = patent ductus arteriosus; PV = pulmonic valve; PW = pulsed wave; PW-TDI = pulsed wave tissue Doppler imaging; RA = right atrium; RPA = right pulmonary artery; RPS = right parasternal; RV = right ventricle; RVOT = right ventricular outflow tract; TAPSE = tricuspid annulus plane systolic excursion; TV = tricuspid valve; Vp = left ventricular early flow propagation velocity. (continues)

(Line diagrams adapted and reproduced from Boon (1998) with permission from the publisher)

Left cranial parasternal short-axis view optimizing the pulmonic trunk

Acquisition of the view

- From the long-axis Ao, angle dorsally (almost parallel with the thoracic wall) and slightly cranially; the Ao will become short-axis and the pulmonic trunk should be imaged
- To optimize alignment with the pulmonic trunk, the transducer may need to be moved into another rib space cranially
- This view can also be used to image the ductus of a PDA

Observations, measurements and calculations

- Used to align with transpulmonic flow, for colour flow and spectral Doppler assessment of pulmonary flow (e.g. assessment of pulmonic stenosis)
- Used to screen for PDA and align with PDA flow (colour flow and CW Doppler)

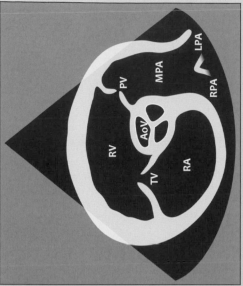

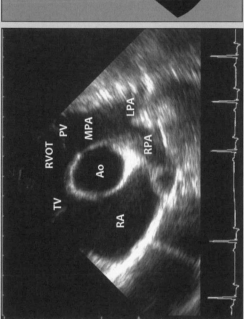

A normal Greyhound. View optimizing for the MPA and bifurcation into RPA and LPA.

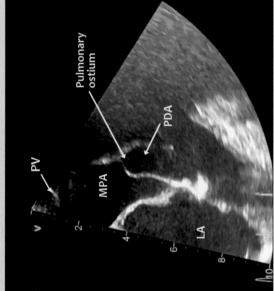

PDA in a Cocker Spaniel cross, which presented in L-CHF. View optimizing the MPA and the PDA as it enters the MPA. The pulmonary ostium (narrowest point of the ductus) is shown.

2.16 (continued) The left apical and parasternal views. Ao = aorta; AoV = aortic valve; CW = continuous wave; FAC = fractional area change; HOCM = hypertrophic obstructive cardiomyopathy; IAS = interatrial septum; IVS = interventricular septum; LA = left atrium; LAA = left atrial appendage; L-CHF = left-sided congestive heart failure; LPA = left pulmonary artery; LV = left ventricle; LVFW = left ventricular free wall; LVOT = left ventricular outflow tract; MAPSE = mitral annulus plane systolic excursion; MPA = main pulmonary artery (pulmonic trunk); MV = mitral valve; PDA = patent ductus arteriosus; PV = pulmonic valve; PW = pulsed wave; PW-TDI = pulsed wave tissue Doppler imaging; RA = right atrium; RPA = right pulmonary artery; RPS = right parasternal; RV = right ventricle; RVOT = right ventricular outflow tract; TAPSE = tricuspid annulus plane systolic excursion; TV = tricuspid valve; Vp = left ventricular early flow propagation velocity. (continues)

(Line diagrams adapted and reproduced from Boon (1998) with permission from the publisher)

Left cranial parasternal short-axis view (left atrial appendage)

Acquisition of the view

- Important to assess in cats, to establish risk for thromboembolic complications (see also Chapter 9)
- The LAA is slightly cranial to the pulmonary artery, and is usually easy to identify if dilated. Some rotation (clockwise) may be required as well as cranial angulation (see the two-chamber view)

Observations, measurements and calculations

- Assess for presence of LAA thrombus or spontaneous echocontrast
- LAA flow assessment. With PW spectral Doppler, sample volume at the junction between LAA and body of LA, can record LAA flow velocity

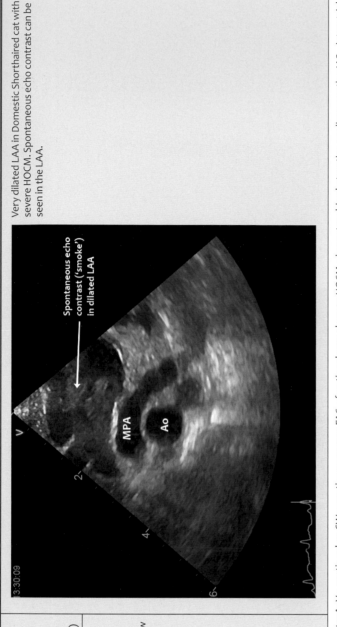

Spontaneous echo contrast ('smoke') in dilated LAA

MPA

Ao

Very dilated LAA in Domestic Shorthaired cat with severe HOCM. Spontaneous echo contrast can be seen in the LAA.

2.16 (continued) The left apical and parasternal views. Ao = aorta; AoV = aortic valve; CW = continuous wave; FAC = fractional area change; HOCM = hypertrophic obstructive cardiomyopathy; IAS = interatrial septum; IVS = interventricular septum; LA = left atrium; LAA = left atrial appendage; LPA = left pulmonary artery; LV = left ventricle; LVFW = left ventricular free wall; LVOT = left ventricular outflow tract; MAPSE = mitral annulus plane systolic excursion; MPA = main pulmonary artery (pulmonic trunk); MV = mitral valve; PDA = patent ductus arteriosus; PV = pulmonic valve; PW = pulsed wave; PW-TDI = pulsed wave tissue Doppler imaging; RA = right atrium; RPA = right pulmonary artery; RPS = right parasternal; RV = right ventricle; RVOT = right ventricular outflow tract; TAPSE = tricuspid annulus plane systolic excursion; TV = tricuspid valve; Vp = left ventricular early flow propagation velocity.
(Line diagrams adapted and reproduced from Boon (1998) with permission from the publisher)

Left ventricular M-mode (chordae tendinae level)

Acquisition of the image

- Make sure the RPS long-axis four-chamber view is as 'horizontal' as possible, with the M-mode cursor transecting chordae tendinae of both mitral valve leaflets. The cursor should be perpendicular to the endocardium of both the septum and the free wall
- Change to short-axis view, and ensure the M-mode cursor bisects a symmetrical LV cavity
- Record M-mode trace, ensuring endocardium of both sides of the septum and the LVFW can be seen. Make sure papillary muscles are not transected. It is acceptable to see chordae within the LV cavity

Measurements and calculations

- From still images, the standard LV measurements can be obtained
- An ECG is essential for accurate M-mode measurements. End-diastolic measurements are made at the start of the QRS complex; systolic measurements are made at the nadir of septal motion or the smallest LV dimension
- In obtaining measurements, use the 'leading edge to leading edge' technique; i.e. the endocardium nearest the transducer is included but far endocardium is excluded. This ensures effects of gain and endocardial brightness do not influence measurements
- **Measurements:**
  - IVS in diastole and systole (IVSd, IVSs), LVID in diastole and systole (LVIDd, LVIDs)
  - LVFW wall in diastole and systole (LVFWd, LVFWs)
  - RV may be measured in diastole (RVd)
- **Calculation:** FS(%) = [[LVIDd - LVIDs]/LVIDd] × 100

Positioning of the M-mode cursor to bisect the LV cavity (right). Everything along this cursor line is plotted against time to give the M-mode image (left).

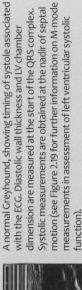

A normal Greyhound, showing timing of systole associated with the ECG. Diastolic wall thickness and LV chamber dimension are measured at the start of the QRS complex. Systolic measurements are obtained at the nadir of septal motion (see Figure 2.19 for further information on M-mode measurements in assessment of left ventricular systolic function).

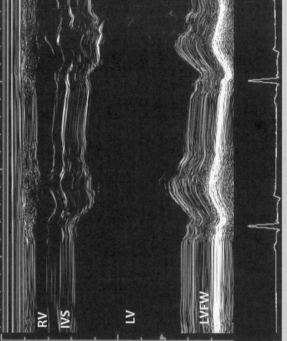

2.17 M-mode views, measurements and calculations. amv = anterior mitral valve leaflet; Ao = aorta; AoR = aortic regurgitation; DCM = dilated cardiomyopathy; ECG = electrocardiogram; EPSS = mitral valve E point to septal separation; ET = left ventricular ejection time; FS = fractional shortening; HCM = hypertrophic cardiomyopathy; HOCM = hypertrophic obstructive cardiomyopathy; IVS (with d or s) = interventricular septum (in diastole or systole); LA = left atrium; LAA = left atrial appendage; LPA = left pulmonary artery; LV = left ventricle; LVFW (with d or s) = left ventricular free wall (in diastole or systole); LVID (with d or s) = left ventricular internal diameter (in diastole or systole); LVOT = left ventricular outflow tract; MA = mitral annulus; MAPSE = mitral annulus plane systolic excursion; PEP = pre-ejection period; pmv = posterior mitral valve leaflet; RA = right atrium; RPA = right pulmonary artery; RPS = right parasternal; RV = right ventricle; RVFW = right ventricular free wall; SAM = systolic anterior motion; TAPSE = tricuspid annulus plane systolic excursion. (continues)

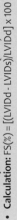

Mitral valve M-mode

Acquisition of the image

- From the fish-mouth view of the mitral valve, position the M-mode cursor so it transects both leaflets in a symmetrical LV cavity
- Change to M-mode and record the excursions of the anterior and posterior leaflets with time
- In an animal in sinus rhythm, the valve opens twice: once in early diastole (E peak or E point of the anterior leaflet), with partial closure during diastasis, then a late diastolic peak following the P wave of the ECG, corresponding to atrial emptying (A peak)
- The posterior leaflet should move to a lesser magnitude in the opposite direction, towards the LVFW
- Both leaflets are closed together in systole and course slightly anteriorly, towards the septum

Measurements and calculations

- Measurements include the EPSS. This may increase when the LV is rounded, or with reduced stroke volume (e.g. in DCM; see also Chapter 9). This distance should be less than 7 mm in a dog of any breed
- Due to the high temporal resolution of M-mode, the presence of SAM of the amv can be best appreciated and documented on this view (e.g. cats with HOCM; see also Chapter 9)
- Diastolic flutter of the amv can be seen associated with significant AoR
- Abnormal MV movement, with the posterior leaflet failing to move in the opposite direction of the anterior leaflet, can be documented in mitral stenosis (e.g. mitral dysplasia in bull terriers)

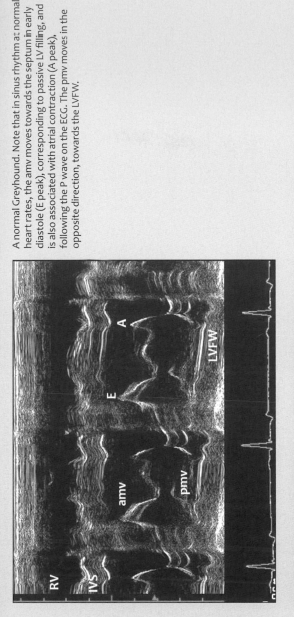

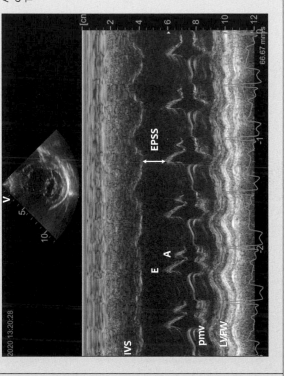

A normal Greyhound. Note that in sinus rhythm: normal heart rates, the amv moves towards the septum in early diastole (E peak), corresponding to passive LV filling, and is also associated with atrial contraction (A peak), following the P wave on the ECG. The pmv moves in the opposite direction, towards the LVFW.

A Labrador Retriever with DCM associated with taurine deficiency (partly reversible with supplementation). There is a large EPSS.

2.17 (continued) M-mode views, measurements and calculations. amv = anterior mitral valve leaflet; Ao = aorta; AoR = aortic regurgitation; DCM = dilated cardiomyopathy; ECG = electrocardiogram; EPSS = mitral valve E point to septal separation; ET = left ventricular ejection time; FS = fractional shortening; HCM = hypertrophic cardiomyopathy; HOCM = hypertrophic obstructive cardiomyopathy; IVS (with d or s) = interventricular septum (in diastole or systole); LA = left atrium; LAA = left atrial appendage; LPA = left pulmonary artery; LV = left ventricle; LVFW (with d or s) = left ventricular free wall (in diastole or systole); LVID (with d or s) = left ventricular internal diameter (in diastole or systole); LVOT = left ventricular outflow tract; MA = mitral annulus; MAPSE = mitral annulus plane systolic excursion; PEP = pre-ejection period; pmv = posterior mitral valve leaflet; RA = right atrium; RPA = right pulmonary artery; RPS = right parasternal; RV = right ventricle; RVFW = right ventricular free wall; SAM = systolic anterior motion; TAPSE = tricuspid annulus plane systolic excursion. (continues)

Mitral valve M-mode continued

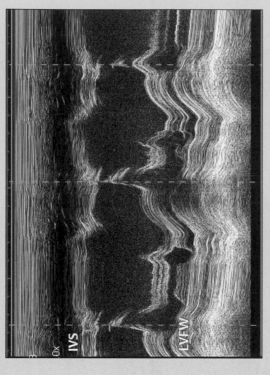

A Domestic Shorthaired cat with severe HOCM (asymmetrical, predominantly septal hypertrophy). The amv can be seen to open towards the IVS during systole (arrowed) as well as opening normally during diastole. This SAM of the amv is typical of HOCM (see also Chapter 9).

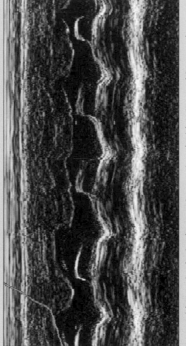

A German Shepherd Dog with severe AoR associated with subaortic stenosis. Mitral valve leaflets were thickened due to concurrent mitral dysplasia. Note the diastolic flutter of the amv; a consequence of the aortic regurgitant jet affecting this leaflet in diastole.

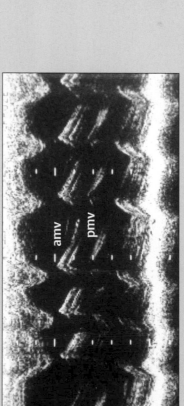

A Bull Terrier with congenital mitral stenosis as part of mitral dysplasia. This dog had severe left atrial enlargement and atrial fibrillation, which meant that there was no A peak of anterior mitral motion. Note that the posterior leaflet is not moving in the opposite direction but tends to be dragged in the same direction as the anterior leaflet (see also Chapter 9).

A cat with acquired mitral stenosis associated with HCM. In this case, the posterior leaflet appears immobile.

2.17 (continued) M-mode views, measurements and calculations. amv = anterior mitral valve leaflet; Ao = aorta; AoR = aortic regurgitation; DCM = dilated cardiomyopathy; ECG = electrocardiogram; EPSS = mitral valve E point to septal separation; ET = left ventricular ejection time; FS = fractional shortening; HCM = hypertrophic cardiomyopathy; HOCM = hypertrophic obstructive cardiomyopathy; IVS (with d or s) = interventricular septum (in diastole or systole); LA = left atrium; LAA = left atrial appendage; LPA = left pulmonary artery; LV = left ventricle; LVFW (with d or s) = left ventricular free wall (in diastole or systole); LVID (with d or s) = left ventricular internal diameter (in diastole or systole); LVOT = left ventricular outflow tract; MA = mitral annulus; MAPSE = mitral annulus plane systolic excursion; PEP = pre-ejection period; pmv = posterior mitral valve leaflet; RA = right atrium; RPA = right pulmonary artery; RPS = right parasternal; RV = right ventricle; RVFW = right ventricular free wall; SAM = systolic anterior motion; TAPSE = tricuspid annulus plane systolic excursion. (continues)

M-mode at aortic valve level

Acquisition of the image

- From the cranial short-axis view of the aortic valve leaflets, position M-mode cursor through the centre of the Ao and the LA/LAA
- Try to record the aortic valve leaflets throughout the cardiac cycle (normally, only one is recorded in dogs)

Measurements and calculations

- Assess aortic root excursion in systole. In conditions of poor systolic function (e.g. DCM), the aortic root remains 'flat' during systole
- **Measurements:**
  - Aortic diameter (diastole: start of QRS on ECG)
  - LA (systole: maximal width)
- **Calculation:**
  - M-mode LA:Ao ratio
  (Note: it is difficult to consistently transect the same portion of the LA and LAA in different individuals, so 2D methods of assessing LA size are now preferred)
- Assess aortic valve movement. Notched systolic movement with mid-systolic closure may be seen in patients with dynamic LVOT obstruction
- Systolic time intervals:
  - Measure the PEP from the start of the QRS complex to opening of aortic valve
  - Measure the ET as the duration of aortic valve opening
  - The PEP:ET ratio is a sensitive indicator of systolic function. Normal ratio is 0.25–0.40

A normal Greyhound. Note that the aortic root (Ao) moves anteriorly (cranially; upwards) during systole. The aortic valves transcribe a 'box' shape during systole. To calculate the LA:Ao ratio, the aortic root diameter is measured in end-diastole (start of QRS complex; measurement 1) and the maximum left atrial dimension is measured during systole (measurement 2).

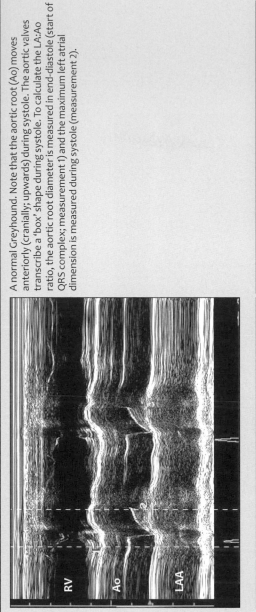

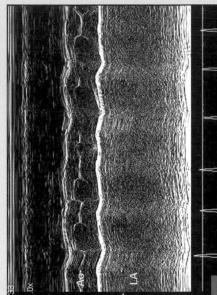

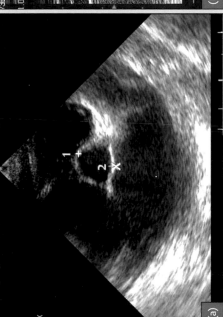

A cat with a non-specific cardiomyopathy with severe left atrial enlargement and systolic dysfunction. The cat was also in atrial fibrillation. (a) Cranial short-axis view of the aortic root and LA, indicating the 2D measurements. The M-mode cursor was positioned on this image: the aortic root and left atrial measurements are in a slightly different plane than the 2D measurements. (b) M-mode view of the aortic root (Ao) and the LA. This view also confirms the severe left atrial enlargement. Note also that the aortic root is 'flat' with minimal anterior excursion, providing additional evidence of the impaired systolic function. The atrial fibrillation is resulting in variable opening of the aortic valves and there is premature closure of the aortic valves during systole (the valves no longer transcribe a rectangular box). This finding is common in cases of impaired systolic function.

2.17 (continued) M-mode views, measurements and calculations. amv = anterior mitral valve leaflet; Ao = aorta; AoR = aortic regurgitation; DCM = dilated cardiomyopathy; ECG = electrocardiogram; EPSS = mitral valve E point to septal separation; ET = left ventricular ejection time; FS = fractional shortening; HCM = hypertrophic cardiomyopathy; HOCM = hypertrophic obstructive cardiomyopathy; IVS (with d or s) = interventricular septum (in diastole or systole); LA = left atrium; LAA = left atrial appendage; LPA = left pulmonary artery; LV = left ventricle; LVFW (with d or s) = left ventricular free wall (in diastole or systole); LVID (with d or s) = left ventricular internal diameter (in diastole or systole); LVOT = left ventricular outflow tract; MA = mitral annulus; MAPSE = mitral annulus plane systolic excursion; PEP = pre-ejection period; pmv = posterior mitral valve leaflet; RA = right atrium; RPA = right pulmonary artery; RPS = right parasternal; RV = right ventricle; RVFW = right ventricular free wall; SAM = systolic anterior motion; TAPSE = tricuspid annulus plane systolic excursion. (continues)

M-mode at aortic valve level continued

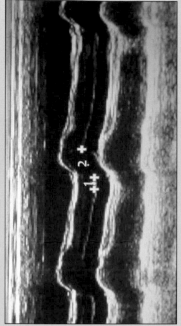

A Jack Russell Terrier with dynamic LVOT obstruction associated with SAM. The aortic valve movement is abnormal in this case, showing premature closure then slight opening again (arrowed) (systolic notching or 'double-diamond' appearance). This is typical of dynamic LVOT obstruction, such as in HOCM. The excellent temporal resolution offered by M-mode facilitates identification of these very brief events during systole.

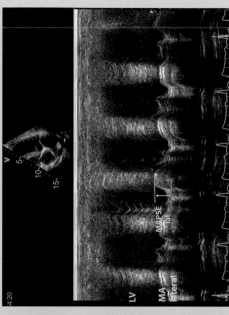

A Great Dane. This view shows measurement of the systolic time intervals: PEP and ET. The PEP is measured from the start of the QRS complex to the opening of the aortic valves (measurement 1) (here 80 ms). The ET is the duration that the aortic valves open for (measurement 2) (here 195 ms). Both parameters are heart rate dependent. However, the PEP:ET ratio is relatively heart rate independent and is an indicator of systolic function. In this dog, the PEP:ET ratio was 0.41 (slightly higher than the reference values of 0.25–0.40).

Mitral annular plane systolic excursion (also known as mitral annulus motion)

Acquisition of the image

- From the left apical four-chamber view (or the orthogonal two-chamber view), position the M-mode cursor so it is parallel to the wall under interrogation and perpendicular to the mitral annulus
- For the left apical four-chamber view, both the septal and lateral annulus can be recorded
- Record M-mode of MAPSE
- As longitudinal fibres contract, the annulus moves towards the apex during systole

Measurements and calculations

- Measure the magnitude of MAPSE for each wall, from end-diastole to systole
- This corresponds to longitudinal fibre shortening and apicobasilar contractility
- Regional wall motion abnormalities (dyssynchronous contraction) may result in discordant readings from the two or four sampling points around the mitral annulus. See also Figure 2.19

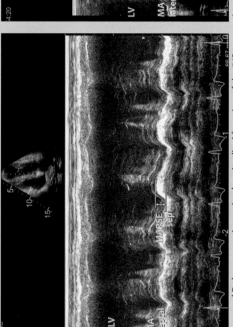

A normal Dobermann. Assessing longitudinal function of the IVS. MAPSE magnitude measured as shown.

A normal Dobermann. Assessing longitudinal function of the LVFW. MAPSE magnitude measured as shown.

2.17 (continued) M-mode views, measurements and calculations. amv = anterior mitral valve leaflet; Ao = aorta; AoR = aortic regurgitation; DCM = dilated cardiomyopathy; ECG = electrocardiogram; EPSS = mitral valve E point to septal separation; ET = left ventricular ejection time; FS = fractional shortening; HCM = hypertrophic cardiomyopathy; HOCM = hypertrophic obstructive cardiomyopathy; IVS (with d or s) = interventricular septum (in diastole or systole); LA = left atrium; LAA = left atrial appendage; LPA = left pulmonary artery; LV = left ventricle; LVFW (with d or s) = left ventricular free wall (in diastole or systole); LVID (with d or s) = left ventricular internal diameter (in diastole or systole); LVOT = left ventricular outflow tract; MA = mitral annulus; MAPSE = mitral annulus plane systolic excursion; PEP = pre-ejection period; pmv = posterior mitral valve leaflet; RA = right atrium; RPA = right pulmonary artery; RPS = right parasternal; RV = right ventricle; RVFW = right ventricular free wall; SAM = systolic anterior motion; TAPSE = tricuspid annulus plane systolic excursion. (continues)

Tricuspid annular plane systolic excursion

Acquisition of the image

- In the normal RV, right ventricular systolic function mainly depends on contraction of the longitudinal fibres
- From a left apical four-chamber view which optimizes the right heart, position the M-mode cursor so it is parallel to the RVFW, and the movement of the tricuspid annulus is perpendicular to the cursor
- Record M-mode of TAPSE

Measurements and calculations

- Measure the magnitude of TAPSE, from end-diastole to systole
- This corresponds to longitudinal fibre shortening and right ventricular systolic function
- See also Figure 2.23

4 TAPSE	1.85 cm
3 TAPSE	1.46 cm
2 TAPSE	1.95 cm
1 TAPSE	2.06 cm

A normal Dobermann. Assessing longitudinal function of the RVFW. TAPSE magnitude measured as shown.

2.17 (continued) M-mode views, measurements and calculations. amv = anterior mitral valve leaflet; Ao = aorta; AoR = aortic regurgitation; DCM = dilated cardiomyopathy; ECG = electrocardiogram; EPSS = mitral valve E point to septal separation; ET = left ventricular ejection time; FS = fractional shortening; HCM = hypertrophic cardiomyopathy; HOCM = hypertrophic obstructive cardiomyopathy; IVS (with d or s) = interventricular septum (in diastole or systole); LA = left atrium; LAA = left atrial appendage; LPA = left pulmonary artery; LV = left ventricle; LVFW (with d or s) = left ventricular free wall (in diastole or systole); LVID (with d or s) = left ventricular internal diameter (in diastole or systole); LVOT = left ventricular outflow tract; MA = mitral annulus; MAPSE = mitral annulus plane systolic excursion; PEP = pre-ejection period; pmv = posterior mitral valve leaflet; RA = right atrium; RPA = right pulmonary artery; RPS = right parasternal; RV = right ventricle; RVFW = right ventricular free wall; SAM = systolic anterior motion; TAPSE = tricuspid annulus plane systolic excursion.

High pulse repetition frequency (HPRF) spectral Doppler describes additional sample volumes along the cursor line, as well as the region of interest at a particular valve. The transducer does not wait for a pulse of ultrasound waves to be reflected back prior to transmitting another pulse; this allows much higher velocities to be assessed and displayed in a spectrum by the machine without aliasing. It also allows sampling of velocities from regions at greater depth. It is presumed the region of interest is being predominantly sampled, but it is important to exclude significant impact due to sampling of flow by the other sample volumes (e.g. when trying to record pulmonary venous flow (PVF) from a left apical view, it is possible that transmitral flow is also being sampled).

CW Doppler echocardiography also produces a spectral display. Ultrasound waves are continuously emitted from, and received back by, the transducer; the frequency shift is converted by the machine into a spectral signal that is not limited by aliasing, so very high velocities can be measured. Sampling is not specific to one region of interest; it is all along the cursor line. Most modern machines allow positioning of the CW cursor on a 2D image to ensure correct alignment with flow (steerable CW). CW Doppler is required for recording the velocity of mitral regurgitant jets or very high velocities in aortic or pulmonic stenosis. CW Doppler may also be required if assessment of flow at depth is required, for example aortic flow from a subcostal view in a large or giant-breed dog.

If spectral Doppler signals are weak (or have low signal:noise ratio), reducing the frequency of the transducer (with steerable frequencies) or changing to a lower frequency transducer will improve spectral Doppler signals (PW or CW).

When measuring velocities from spectral Doppler traces, the peak at the brightest line of the spectral signal (modal velocity) should be measured. With turbulent flow (e.g. in aortic stenosis), there may be some faint apparently higher velocity signals (these appear like a beard on a chin: measure the end of the chin, not the end of the beard).

Colour flow: This is a specialized form of PW Doppler echocardiography. Within a sector, which can be directed over the area of interest within a 2D image, there is a large number of 'sample volumes' or pixels, which are individually colour-coded according to direction and character of flow (see Figure 2.18).

On most ultrasound machines blood moving towards the transducer is colour-coded red and blood moving away from the transducer is colour-coded blue – the BART map (blue away, red towards). Different colour shades are usually provided to give an impression of flow velocity (the higher the velocity, the brighter the hue). Again, the Nyquist limit can be exceeded and fast blood moving away from the transducer may have a normal blue outline but an aliased core of red. The Nyquist limit is normally set as high as possible (e.g. at least 80 cm/s) to avoid colour aliasing of normal cardiac flow.

Most colour flow Doppler echocardiography machines have maps to indicate colour variance or turbulent flow; these are usually colour-coded green/yellow and have a 'speckled' or 'mosaic' appearance, e.g. such as may be seen in a mitral regurgitant jet.

Colour flow Doppler can rapidly screen for abnormal flow, such as a ventricular septal defect (VSD): the left-to-right shunting causes a turbulent jet to cross into the right ventricle (RV), usually just below the tricuspid valve. Imaging of this jet allows placement of a PW or steerable

CW cursor over it to obtain a spectral signal, so that velocity may be accurately measured. Colour flow Doppler echocardiography may therefore be considered as a form of non-invasive angiography.

Importance of being aligned with flow: All Doppler echocardiography is dependent on positioning. It is very important for the cursor to be as parallel to blood flow as possible (it must be within 20 degrees). The reason for this can be understood from the Doppler equation.

The Doppler equation

$$f_2 = \frac{2f_0}{c} \, v \, \text{Cos}\theta$$

Where f_2 = reflected frequency
f_0 = transmitted frequency
v = maximal velocity
c = velocity of ultrasound waves in blood
θ = angle between ultrasound beam and direction of blood flow.

Rearranging the equation:

$$v = \frac{c}{2f_0 \, \text{Cos}\theta} \, f_2$$

As every attempt to be parallel to flow is made, θ is 0 degrees and the cosine of this is 1.
(θ must be <20 degrees for the angle factor to be ignored).
This allows the equation to be modified to:

$$v = \frac{c}{2f_0} \, f_2$$

As $\frac{c}{2}$ is constant

$$v \propto \frac{f_2}{f_0}$$

i.e. the velocity of RBCs is proportional to the frequency shift between reflected and transmitted ultrasound waves.

It is very important to attempt to obtain as perfect spectral Doppler signals as possible, and to record maximal velocities, as these will represent best parallel alignment with flow. This may involve interrogating a valve from several different positions (e.g. aortic velocity in aortic stenosis from left apical and subcostal views; assessing pulmonary flow from both RPS and LPS cranial windows). The use of any angle correction facility on the machine is considered bad practice in cardiology. Despite apparent alignment in 2D, it may not be correct in the third dimension (e.g. if the structure is going 'into or out of' the screen). Much of the learning curve in Doppler echocardiography is spent perfecting alignment with intracardiac flows. The Doppler sound can be useful – the volume should be turned up provided patients tolerate it. With laminar flow, the sound with good alignment is usually musical. Lack of alignment or turbulent flow results in a harsh sound.

Modified Bernoulli equation – non-invasive Doppler-derived pressure gradients: An estimate of pressure gradient (PG) across a valve can be determined from the peak velocity of flow through that valve using the modified Bernoulli equation. Thus, the severity of pulmonic or aortic stenosis can be assessed non-invasively, without selective cardiac catherization.

Modified Bernoulli equation

$$PG \approx 4v^2$$

Where   PG = pressure gradient (mmHg)
           v = maximal velocity (m/s)

Where the pressure of one chamber is known or assumed, the modified Bernoulli equation can be used to estimate pressure of the other side of a valve. For example, in aortic stenosis, if systolic blood pressure is recorded as 120 mmHg, and the PG derived from Doppler studies is 80 mmHg, then the LV systolic pressure must be 200 mmHg.

In the absence of pulmonic stenosis, and the presence of tricuspid regurgitation and pulmonic regurgitation jets from which good quality spectral Doppler signals can be recorded, both systolic and diastolic pressure in the pulmonic trunk (main pulmonary artery) can be determined using the modified Bernoulli equation.

Practicalities of a complete Doppler study: Figure 2.18 gives the techniques for acquiring spectral Doppler studies from each heart valve, and the measurements that may be obtained. The cursor and sample volumes are positioned based on the 2D and colour flow Doppler images. Listening to the Doppler sound as well as examining spectral Doppler traces can help with optimization of alignment with flow and with discrimination between laminar and turbulent flow.

Other tips include:

* Setting an appropriate baseline and velocity scale for the spectral Doppler to be obtained; spectra should be displayed as optimally as possible
* Using fast sweep speed especially if durations are to be measured
* For low-velocity signals, making sure the wall filter (low-velocity reject) is minimal, so that spectra can be seen and intersect with the baseline. This can be increased if high velocities are to be assessed
* For weak spectral Doppler signals, having the gain turned high and then reducing it once the spectra have been optimized. The Doppler gain setting should be sufficient to allow some background shading. If signals remain weak, change to a lower frequency
* Setting colour Doppler gain by turning up the gain to see some colour speckle on the 2D image, not associated with flow, and then reducing again until this is no longer seen.

Assessing cardiac function

In simplest terms, cardiac function can be divided into:

* Systolic function
* Diastolic function.

Doppler echocardiography can give a non-invasive method of assessing these, but it is important to be aware of the limitations of each technique. These traditionally concentrate on the left heart, but there has been recent interest in assessing right ventricular function as well.

Assessment of left ventricular systolic function

Figure 2.19 details the M-mode, 2D and Doppler methods of assessing systolic function, with advantages and limitations of each technique. To make an overall assessment of systolic function, an integrated approach is required, rather than relying on one single method.

Assessment of left ventricular diastolic function

The study of diastolic function ('diastology') requires recognition of the phases of diastole:

1. Isovolumic relaxation phase.
2. Early rapid filling of the LV (depending on LV active relaxation).
3. Diastasis.
4. Late LV filling, corresponding to left atrial contraction (following P wave of the ECG).

Most of the echocardiographically derived parameters of diastolic function will be preload and heart rate sensitive. Elevated filling pressures (L-CHF) or tachycardia may confound the interpretation of diastolic function.

PW Doppler assessment of diastolic function from isovolumic relaxation time (IVRT), mitral inflow and PVF is shown in Figure 2.20. Additional parameters of diastolic function can be derived from mitral regurgitant jets ($-^{dP}/_{dt}$) and the velocity of propagation of left ventricular inflow towards the LV apex (Vp) and are also detailed in Figure 2.20.

Index of myocardial performance

The index of myocardial performance (IMP, also known as the Tei index), an index of combined systolic and diastolic function, has been proposed (Figure 2.20).

Pulsed wave tissue Doppler imaging

Pulsed wave tissue Doppler imaging (PW-TDI) is used to assess myocardial function. PW-TDI utilizes settings that ignore the high-velocity, low-amplitude signals of the blood pool and record the low-velocity, high-amplitude signals of myocardial motion. The basic limitations of Doppler apply; only fibres parallel with the ultrasound beam will have myocardial velocities accurately recorded. Furthermore, velocities may be influenced by translational movement of the heart within the thorax. There are various applications of tissue Doppler. PW-TDI signals of the longitudinal fibres of the LV myocardium are relatively easy to acquire and interpret for clinical echocardiography (Figure 2.21).

Assessment of left-sided filling pressures

Most acquired cardiac disease in dogs and cats leads initially or predominantly to L-CHF. Thoracic radiographs are still considered to be the 'gold standard' to confirm the presence of cardiogenic pulmonary oedema. However, a number of subjective findings and ratios calculated from Doppler echocardiographic variables can indicate actual or imminent L-CHF. The 2D assessments include left atrial dilatation, with bowing (rather than just flaring) of the interatrial septum and dilated pulmonary veins entering the left atrium. Suggested assessment are shown in Figure 2.22. Not all of these have been validated in naturally occurring disease but they are still clinically useful.

Assessment of right ventricular systolic function

Because of its complex geometry with two components – the inflow and outflow parts – assessment of RV volume or function is difficult. In the normal RV, the systolic function depends mainly on contraction of the longitudinal fibres, so assessment of the right ventricular free wall motion is useful. Assessment of right ventricular function is of prognostic significance even in animals with 'left heart' diseases. Methods of assessing the right ventricular systolic function are shown in Figure 2.23.

Transmitral flow

Acquisition of the image

- From left apical view, make sure the heart is vertical and the cursor is aligned with the long axis of the heart
- Put a colour flow region of interest over the MV
- Position sample volume of the cursor between MV leaflets cusps
- Record the mitral inflow pattern as a PW Doppler spectrum

Measurements and calculations

- From the transmitral PW Doppler spectrum, identify the E waves (early diastole) and A waves (associated with atrial contraction, following the P wave of the ECG)
- Measure peak E and A wave velocities
- Can calculate mitral E:A ratio
- There should be no respiratory variation in mitral inflow velocities (the presence of variation indicates increased ventricular interdependence, such as with pericardial disease)
- Other measurements include:
  - Mitral E wave duration
  - Mitral E wave deceleration time
  - Mitral A wave duration

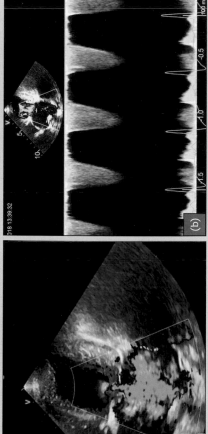
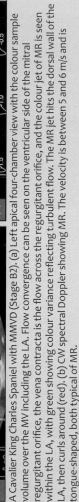

(a) From a left apical four-chamber view, a colour sample volume is placed over the MV. Red indicates blood moving towards the transducer. (b) A PW Doppler sample volume is placed between the tips of the MV to record transmitral flow. Note that for sinus rhythm there are two phases of diastolic filling, giving the two waves of mitral inflow. Early passive filling results in the E wave, and flow subsequent to atrial contraction gives the A wave (following the P wave of the ECG).

Mitral regurgitation

Acquisition of the image

- Use colour flow Doppler to identify the direction and size of the MR jet
- Normally, alignment with the jet is best from the left apical four-chamber view
- Occasionally, with asymmetric jets, other views are acquired. In cats with MR due to SAM of their anterior mitral valve leaflet, the MR jet projects to the posteriolateral wall of the LA, and alignment may actually be optimal from the RPS four-chamber view
- Use CW Doppler to record the MR spectral signal. Make sure the velocity scale is set at over 4 m/s
- The denseness of the spectral Doppler can give an indication of the severity of MR. With mild MR, spectra may be faint or incomplete
- MR is usually a tongue-shaped spectral signal; t can be more pointed in the presence of left-sided CHF

Measurements and calculations

- From the colour flow Doppler signal, the severity of MR can be semi-quantitatively assessed from jet area compared with LA area as: Trivial; + (<25% of LA); 2+ (25–50% of LA); 3+ (50–75% of LA); or 4+ (>75% of LA);
  Note: Jet area is not reliable at indicating severity of MR, since it is also affected by transducer frequency, gain settings, image quality etc.
- Measure peak MR velocity: normal is 5–6 m/s
- Use the modified Bernoulli equation to determine the PG between the LV and LA
- From the acceleration slope of the MR signal, $+dP/dt$ can be calculated (see 'Assessment of left ventricular diastolic function', below)
- From the deceleration slope of the MR signal, $-dP/dt$ can be calculated (see 'Assessment of left ventricular diastolic function', below)

A Cavalier King Charles Spaniel with MMVD (Stage B2). (a) Left apical four-chamber view with the colour sample volume over the MV including the LA. Flow convergence can be seen on the ventricular side of the regurgitant orifice, the vena contracta is the flow across the regurgitant orifice, and the colour jet of MR is seen within the LA, with green showing colour variance reflecting turbulent flow. The MR jet hits the dorsal wall of the LA, then curls around (red). (b) CW spectral Doppler showing MR. The velocity is between 5 and 6 m/s and is tongue-shaped, both typical of MR.

2.18 Spectral and colour flow Doppler echocardiography. Ao = aorta; AoO = aortic outflow; AoR = aortic regurgitation; CHF = congestive heart failure; CW = continuous wave; dP = pressure difference; dt = time difference; dv = velocity difference; ECG = electrocardiogram; ET = left ventricular ejection time; HCM = hypertrophic cardiomyopathy; HOCM = hypertrophic obstructive cardiomyopathy; HPRF = high pulse repetition frequency; IVS = interventricular septum; LA = left atrium; LAA = left atrial appendage; LPS = left parasternal; LV = left ventricle; LVOT = left ventricular outflow tract; MMVD = myxomatous mitral valve disease; MPA = main pulmonary artery (pulmonic trunk); MV = mitral valve; PDA = patent ductus arteriosus; PEP = pre-ejection period; PG = pressure gradient; PI = pulmonic insufficiency (regurgitation); PW = pulsed wave; RA = right atrium; R-CHF = right-sided congestive heart failure; RPS = right parasternal; RV = right ventricle; RVOT = right ventricular outflow tract; SAM = systolic anterior motion; TR = tricuspid regurgitation; TV = tricuspid valve; v = velocity; VSD = ventricular septal defect; VTI = velocity time integral. (continues)

Left ventricular outflow and aortic flow

Acquisition of the image

- **Subcostal view:** align CW Doppler cursor with the ascending Ao
- Record CW spectral Doppler. In most dogs, peak aortic velocities are obtained by this view
- In small dogs and a low frequency transducer, PW or HPRF Doppler signals may be possible
- Alignment for aortic flow by the subcostal view is not usually good in cats
- **Left apical view:** (three-chamber, or five-chamber view). Work at getting the cursor as parallel as possible to aortic flow (must be within 20 degrees)
- Use colour flow Doppler to assess the character of flow and any turbulence, and to identify the presence of any AoR
- Position the sample volume, just beyond the aortic valves, within the Ao
- Record spectral PW Doppler signals of aortic flow
- **Assessing step-up in velocity.** If aortic stenosis is suspected, the PW sample volume can be positioned in the LVOT before the possible obstruction, and LVOT peak velocity recorded by PW spectral Doppler. The sample volume is then moved back into the Ao, and peak aortic velocity recorded beyond the valve. A significant (>0.5 m/s) step-up of velocity suggests increased aortic velocities are due to aortic stenosis and not a high output state (increased stroke volume)

Measurements and calculations

- Measure peak velocity of aortic flow
- Calculate the PG across the aortic valve using the modified Bernoulli equation
- If aortic stenosis is present, it can be classified as: mild (PG <40 mmHg); moderate (PG = 40–80 mmHg); or severe (PG >80 mmHg)
- Trace around the aortic outflow spectrum to measure the VTI. From this, the forward stroke volume can be calculated. (See Figure 2.19)
- Systolic time intervals can be determined:
  - PEP is start of QRS complex of ECG to onset of flow
  - ET is the duration of the aortic outflow spectrum
- From the acceleration slope of the aortic spectrum, the following measurements can be made:
  - Peak acceleration from the initial, steepest part of the slope $(dv/dt \text{ max})$
  - Mean acceleration; the slope from baseline to peak velocity $(dv/dt \text{ mean})$
  - Acceleration time

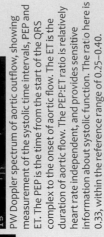

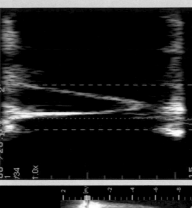

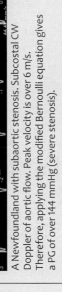

(a) Left apical three-chamber view optimizing alignment with aortic outflow. Ao = aorta; AO = aortic outflow; LAA = left atrial appendage; LV = left ventricle. (b) PW Doppler sample volume placed within the Ao, just beyond the aortic valves, to record aortic flow. Note that although the peak velocity is slightly above reference values at 1.72 m/s, there is no spectral dispersion and this spectral envelope indicates laminar flow.

A Newfoundland with subaortic stenosis. Subcostal CW Doppler of aortic flow. Peak velocity is over 6 m/s. Therefore, applying the modified Bernoulli equation gives a PG of over 144 mmHg (severe stenosis).

PW Doppler spectrum of aortic outflow, showing measurement of the systolic time intervals, PEP and ET. The PEP is the time from the start of the QRS complex to the onset of aortic flow. The ET is the duration of aortic flow. The PEP:ET ratio is relatively heart rate independent, and provides sensitive information about systolic function. The ratio here is 0.33, within the reference range of 0.25–0.40.

2.18 (continued) Spectral and colour flow Doppler echocardiography. Ao = aorta; AoO = aortic outflow; AoR = aortic regurgitation; CHF = congestive heart failure; CW = continuous wave; dP = pressure difference; dt = time difference; dv = velocity difference; ECG = electrocardiogram; ET = left ventricular ejection time; HCM = hypertrophic cardiomyopathy; HOCM = hypertrophic obstructive cardiomyopathy; HPRF = high pulse repetition frequency; IVS = interventricular septum; LA = left atrium; LAA = left atrial appendage; LPS = left parasternal; LV = left ventricle; LVOT = left ventricular outflow tract; MMVD = myxomatous mitral valve disease; MPA = main pulmonary artery (pulmonic trunk); MR = mitral regurgitation; MV = mitral valve; PDA = patent ductus arteriosus; PEP = pre-ejection period; PG = pressure gradient; PI = pulmonic insufficiency (regurgitation); PW = pulsed wave; RA = right atrium; R-CHF = right-sided congestive heart failure; RPS = right parasternal; RV = right ventricle; RVOT = right ventricular outflow tract; SAM = systolic anterior motion; TR = tricuspid regurgitation; TV = tricuspid valve; v = velocity; VSD = ventricular septal defect; VTI = velocity time integral. (continues)

Dynamic left ventricular outflow tract obstruction

Acquisition of the image

- Useful in, for example, cats with HOCM
- To confirm the scimitar shape typical of dynamic LVOT obstruction, the sample volume should be positioned at the site of colour variance, within the LVOT, not just beyond the aortic valves
- Both LVOT and aortic regions should be sampled by spectral Doppler

Measurements and calculations

- Record both LVOT and aortic velocities in cats with HOCM

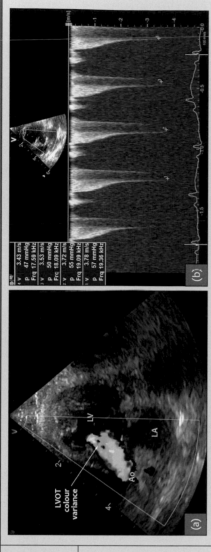

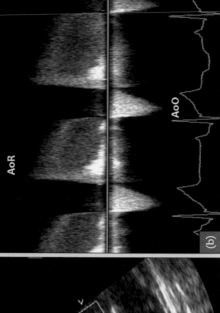

A Domestic Shorthaired cat with HOCM. (a) Left apical five-chamber view. Colour variance in the LVOT is associated with SAM and a basal septal bulge. (b) CW Doppler aligned with the turbulent flow in the LVOT. The biphasic acceleration to flow (scimitar appearance) is typical of dynamic LVOT obstruction, typically associated with SAM and HOCM.

Aortic regurgitation

Acquisition of the image

- Colour flow Doppler echocardiography is used to screen for the presence of AoR from the RPS five-chamber view, the right and left cranial long-axis views, examining the aortic valves, and the left apical three- and five-chamber views
- Spectral Doppler (CW) recording of the diastolic AoR signal is obtained from the apical three- or five-chamber views, wherever alignment is optimized

Measurements and calculations

- The presence of AoR is suspicious in breeds of dog susceptible to aortic stenosis. However, small amounts of AoR can be recognized in certain breeds such as Great Danes, without identified aortic valve pathology
- Measure peak AoR velocity
- Can determine the PG between the Ao and the LV in early diastole, provided alignment is good

2.18 (continued) Spectral and colour flow Doppler echocardiography. Ao = aorta; AoO = aortic outflow; AoR = aortic regurgitation; CHF = congestive heart failure; CW = continuous wave; dP = pressure difference; dt = time difference; dv = velocity difference; ECG = electrocardiogram; ET = left ventricular ejection time; HCM = hypertrophic cardiomyopathy; HOCM = hypertrophic obstructive cardiomyopathy; HPRF = high pulse repetition frequency; IVS = interventricular septum; LA = left atrium; LAA = left atrial appendage; LPS = left parasternal; LV = left ventricle; LVOT = left ventricular outflow tract; MMVD = myxomatous mitral valve disease; MPA = main pulmonary artery (pulmonic trunk); MR = mitral regurgitation; MV = mitral valve; PDA = patent ductus arteriosus; PEP = pre-ejection period; PG = pressure gradient; PI = pulmonic insufficiency (regurgitation); PW = pulsed wave; RA = right atrium; R-CHF = right-sided congestive heart failure; RPS = right parasternal; RV = right ventricle; RVOT = right ventricular outflow tract; SAM = systolic anterior motion; TR = tricuspid regurgitation; TV = tricuspid valve; v = velocity; VSD = ventricular septal defect; VTI = velocity time integral. (continues)

(a) A Maine Coon cat with severe aortic stenosis. RPS long-axis five-chamber view. The aortic valves were also incompetent and the diastolic AoR jet is shown by colour flow mapping. (b) A German Shepherd Dog puppy with moderately severe subaortic stenosis. CW Doppler spectrum obtained from a left apical three-chamber view, optimizing alignment with the LVOT and Ao. AoO is displayed below the baseline and AoR is displayed above the baseline.

Tricuspid flow

Acquisition of the image

- The left apical four-chamber view is normally used to assess the TV, with more cranial positioning to optimize the right heart
- In some cases, the right or left cranial short-axis views of the right ventricular inflow and outflow tract show good tricuspid flow
- Use colour flow Doppler to assess the valve
- Position the PW sample volume just within the leaflets of the TV
- Record PW spectral Doppler of tricuspid inflow
- Note that there is normally considerable respiratory and heart rate variation in the tricuspid inflow pattern
- The ECG may be required to interpret the pattern; often a forward systolic wave, corresponding to right ventricular outflow, is recorded if the sample volume is within the RV side of the valve

Measurements and calculations

- Measure TV E and A velocities
- The tricuspid E:A ratio can be calculated, but this will vary beat to beat due to the respiratory variation

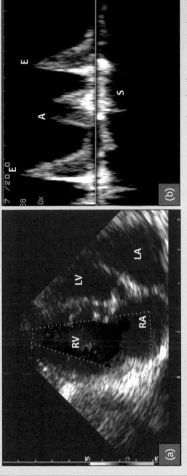
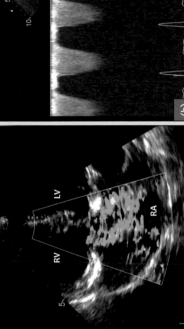

(a) Left apical four-chamber view, optimized for alignment with transtricuspid flow (red). A PW Doppler sample volume is positioned at the tips of the TV. (b) PW Doppler spectrum of transtricuspid flow. There is a peak corresponding to early passive RV filling (the E wave) and the A wave follows the P wave on the ECG, resulting in RV filling associated with atrial contraction. Note that in normal animals, the E and A wave velocities, and their ratio, show considerable respiratory variation. 'S' shows some forward systolic flow towards the RVOT.

Tricuspid regurgitation

Acquisition of the image

- Colour flow Doppler is used to assess the competence of the TV from the RPS long-axis four-chamber view, RPS short-axis view showing right ventricular inflow and outflow, the left apical four-chamber view and the left cranial short-axis view, optimizing the RA
- Use PW (or CW) spectral Doppler to align with the TR jet, and record the TR

Measurements and calculations

- Peak velocity of the TR jet is measured
- The PG between the RV and RA in systole can be calculated by the modified Bernoulli equation (Normal <30 mmHg)
- In the absence of pulmonic stenosis, the derived RV pressure is approximately equal to MPA systolic pressure (so the severity of pulmonary hypertension can be non-invasively assessed) (right atrial pressure is considered negligible if no signs of R-CHF)

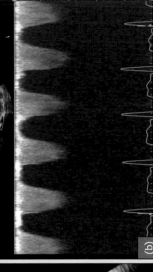

A Cavalier King Charles Spaniel with uncontrolled, biventricular CHF. Pulmonic stenosis was excluded. (a) Left apical four-chamber view optimizing the right heart. Colour flow shows severe TR. (b) CW Doppler of the TR. It is a: high velocity, about 4 m/s, so the RV–RA PG estimated by the modified Bernoulli equation is about 64 mmHg. As the dog had overt R-CHF, the RA pressure will be increased, so the estimated MPA systolic pressure is well over 64 mmHg. However, it is not usual to correct for right atrial pressure (actual or estimated).

2.18 (continued) Spectral and colour flow Doppler echocardiography. Ao = aorta; AoO = aortic outflow; AoR = aortic regurgitation; CHF = congestive heart failure; CW = continuous wave; dP = pressure difference; dt = time difference; dv = velocity difference; ECG = electrocardiogram; ET = left ventricular ejection time; HCM = hypertrophic cardiomyopathy; HOCM = hypertrophic obstructive cardiomyopathy; HPRF = high pulse repetition frequency; IVS = interventricular septum; LA = left atrium; LAA = left atrial appendage; LPS = left parasternal; LV = left ventricle; LVOT = left ventricular outflow tract; MMVD = myxomatous mitral valve disease; MPA = main pulmonary artery (pulmonic trunk); MV = mitral valve; PDA = patent ductus arteriosus; PEP = pre-ejection period; PG = pressure gradient; PI = pulmonic insufficiency (regurgitation); PW = pulsed wave; RA = right atrium; R-CHF = right-sided congestive heart failure; RPS = right parasternal; RV = right ventricle; RVOT = right ventricular outflow tract; SAM = systolic anterior motion; TR = tricuspid regurgitation; TV = tricuspid valve; v = velocity; VSD = ventricular septal defect; VTI = velocity time integral. (continues)

Pulmonic flow

Acquisition of the image

- The pulmonic valves are best imaged, and assessed by colour flow Doppler, from the right cranial short-axis view optimizing the pulmonic trunk
- Note that the pulmonic trunk is difficult to become aligned with from this view in most animals, as it wraps around the Ao
- Abnormalities of the RVOT are also best imaged from this view (e.g. double chambered RV)
- Some cats with HCM have dynamic RVOT obstruction, and the colour variance associated with this is best seen from the RPS cranial short-axis view. Spectral Doppler is guided from the colour flow signal to record the velocity of the RVOT
- Optimal alignment with pulmonary flow is normally achieved from a left cranial short-axis view, optimizing the pulmonic trunk
- The sample volume is positioned just beyond the pulmonic valves within the pulmonic trunk, and PW spectral Doppler is recorded

Measurements and calculations

- Measure peak velocity of the pulmonic flow
- The pulmonic outflow VTI is calculated by tracing around the pulmonic outflow spectrum
- The right ventricular stroke volume or cardiac output can be calculated, after determining the pulmonic cross-sectional area from the MPA diameter
- Shunt ratios, such as with a VSD, can be calculated
- Note that there should be no diastolic flow within the MPA. If diastolic flow is identified, it is important to search for a PDA

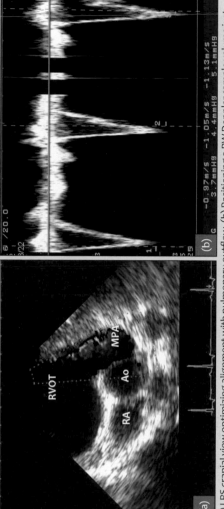

(a) LPS cranial view optimizing alignment with pulmonary outflow. (b) Positioning a PW Doppler sample volume just beyond the pulmonic valves allows recording of the pulmonic flow. Normal laminar flow is shown.

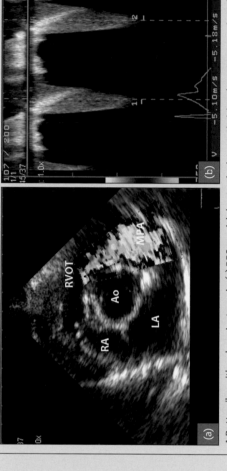

A Rottweiler with pulmonic stenosis. (a) RPS cranial short-axis view, optimizing flow in the MPA. Note the colour variance indicating high velocity and turbulent flow in the MPA. (b) CW spectral Doppler of the pulmonic flow shows a mean peak velocity of 5.0 m/s, corresponding to a PG between the RV and MPA of 100 mmHg (according to the modified Bernoulli equation), indicating severe pulmonic stenosis. Note that there is also a second, late accelerating peak of approximately half the peak velocity. This appearance on the spectrum is suggestive of concurrent dynamic infundibular obstruction.

2.18 (continued) Spectral and colour flow Doppler echocardiography. Ao = aorta; AoO = aortic outflow; AoR = aortic regurgitation; CHF = congestive heart failure; CW = continuous wave; dP = pressure difference; dt = time difference; dv = velocity difference; ECG = electrocardiogram; ET = left ventricular ejection time; HCM = hypertrophic cardiomyopathy; HOCM = hypertrophic obstructive cardiomyopathy; HPRF = high pulse repetition frequency; IVS = interventricular septum; LA = left atrium; LAA = left atrial appendage; LPS = left parasternal; LV = left ventricle; LVOT = left ventricular outflow tract; MMVD = myxomatous mitral valve disease; MPA = main pulmonary artery (pulmonic trunk); MR = mitral regurgitation; MV = mitral valve; PDA = patent ductus arteriosus; PEP = pre-ejection period; PG = pressure gradient; PI = pulmonic insufficiency (regurgitation); PW = pulsed wave; RA = right atrium; R-CHF = right-sided congestive heart failure; RPS = right parasternal; RV = right ventricle; RVOT = right ventricular outflow tract; SAM = systolic anterior motion; TR = tricuspid regurgitation; TV = tricuspid valve; v = velocity; VSD = ventricular septal defect; VTI = velocity time integral. (continues)

Pulmonic regurgitation/pulmonic insufficiency

Acquisition of the image
- Pulmonic regurgitation is normally best identified from the RPS views using colour flow Doppler, as on the left side, the valve and RVOT is within the near field of the ultrasound image
- Note that it is normal physiologically to identify a trivial amount of pulmonic regurgitation. More significant amounts may be seen in association with pulmonic stenosis or pulmonary hypertension
- Position the PW sample volume within the PI jet in the RV, and record spectral Doppler

Measurements and calculations
- Measure peak velocity of the PI jet
- The modified Bernoulli equation is used to estimate the PG between the MPA and the RV in early diastole
- Thus, diastolic MPA pressures can be estimated, which is useful to determine the severity of pulmonary hypertension non-invasively
- The peak velocity at the start of diastole is more likely to reflect mean MPA pressure, and the velocity at the end of the PI jet to reflect diastolic MPA pressure. Both could be measured, but usually just peak velocity is required
- The PI jet should gradually decelerate throughout diastole. Sudden deceleration, or termination prior to the end of diastole is consistent with pulmonary hypertension

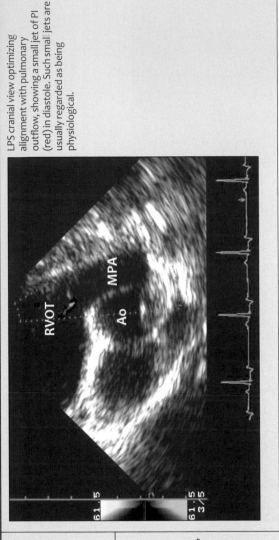

LPS cranial view optimizing alignment with pulmonary outflow, showing a small jet of PI (red) in diastole. Such small jets are usually regarded as being physiological.

2.18 (continued) Spectral and colour flow Doppler echocardiography. Ao = aorta; AoO = aortic outflow; AoR = aortic regurgitation; CHF = congestive heart failure; CW = continuous wave; dP = pressure difference; dt = time difference; dv = velocity difference; ECG = electrocardiogram; ET = left ventricular ejection time; HCM = hypertrophic cardiomyopathy; HOCM = hypertrophic obstructive cardiomyopathy; HPRF = high pulse repetition frequency; IVS = interventricular septum; LA = left atrium; LAA = left atrial appendage; LPS = left parasternal; LV = left ventricle; LVOT = left ventricular outflow tract; MMVD = myxomatous mitral valve disease; MPA = main pulmonary artery (pulmonary trunk); MR = mitral regurgitation; MV = mitral valve; PDA = patent ductus arteriosus; PEP = pre-ejection period; PG = pressure gradient; PI = pulmonic insufficiency (regurgitation); PW = pulsed wave; RA = right atrium; R-CHF = right-sided congestive heart failure; RPS = right parasternal; RV = right ventricle; RVOT = right ventricular outflow tract; SAM = systolic anterior motion; TR = tricuspid regurgitation; TV = tricuspid valve; v = velocity; VSD = ventricular septal defect; VTI = velocity time integral.

M-mode assessment of systolic function

Fractional shortening (%)

- FS = [(LVIDd − LVIDs)/LVIDd] x 100%
- This relies on normal wall motion
- It is a one-dimensional measurement
- It will give a falsely favourable impression of contractility in the presence of reduced afterload (e.g. severe MR)
- It is important to note whether the LVIDs measurement is within reference ranges; if LVIDs is increased above expected range for breed or weight, it indicates systolic dysfunction, regardless of the FS measurement

Ejection fraction (%)

- EF = [(EDV − ESV)/EDV] x 100%
- Teichholz formula for calculating EDV (ESV) from LV M-mode dimensions:
  EDV = [7/(2.4 + LVIDd)] x LVIDd³
  (for ESV, substitute LVIDd for LVIDs)
- There are various formulae to derive LV volumes from M-mode dimensions, and therefore EF
- The Teichholz formula is usually more accurate than the others
- However, there is no advantage to these compared with M-mode when a single dimensional method is being used, and volumes derived are very inaccurate in a dilated, rounded LV chamber

Percentage thickening of the IVS or LVFW (%th IVS, %th LVFW)

- %th IVS = ((IVSs − IVSd)/IVSd x 100%
- %th LVFW = (LVFWs − LVFWd)/LVFWd x 100%
- No longer commonly used

Velocity of circumferential fibre shortening

- Vcf = FS/ET
  (FS as a fraction, not a %)
- Units: circumferences/second
- This is another systolic time interval

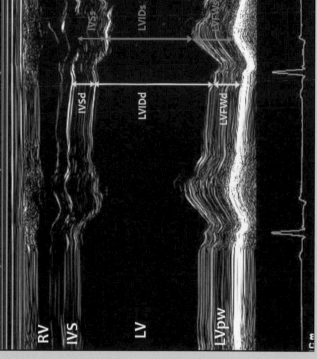

RV

IVS

LV

LVpw

IVSd

IVSs

LVIDd

LVIDs

LVFWd

LVFWs

cm

Measurement of the LV using M-mode. Diastolic measurements are taken at the end of diastole, at the start of the ECG QRS complex. Systolic measurements are taken at the nadir of septal motion (or the smallest LV cavity), which usually corresponds to the end of the T wave. Note the 'leading edge to leading edge' method of measurement: the proximal endocardium is included in each measurement, but not the distal endocardium. Thus, each measurement is not influenced by the effect of gain settings on endocardium thickness.

2.19 Assessment of left ventricular systolic function. Ao = aorta; BSA = body surface area; CO = cardiac output; csa = cross-sectional area; CW = continuous wave; DCM = dilated cardiomyopathy; dP = pressure difference; dt = time difference; dv = velocity difference; ECG = electrocardiogram; EDV = end-diastolic volume (of the left ventricle); EF = ejection fraction; EPSS = mitral valve E point to septal separation; ESV = end-systolic volume; ESVI = end-systolic volume index; ET = left ventricular ejection time; FS = fractional shortening; HCM = hypertrophic cardiomyopathy; HR = heart rate; IVS (with d or s) = interventricular septum (in diastole or systole); LA = left atrium; LV = left ventricle; LVFW (with d or s) = left ventricular free wall (in diastole or systole); LVID (with d or s) = left ventricular internal diameter (in diastole or systole); LVOT = left ventricular outflow tract; Lvpw = left ventricular posterior wall; MAPSE = mitral annulus plane systolic excursion; MR = mitral regurgitation; PEP = pre-ejection period; PG = pressure gradient; PW = pulsed wave; RA = right atrium; RPS = right parasternal; RV = right ventricle; SV = stroke volume; Vcf = velocity of circumferential fibre shortening; VSD = ventricular septal defect; VTI = velocity time integral. (continues)

M-mode assessment of systolic function *continued*

Mitral M-mode EPSS

- Measure mitral E point, up to endocardium of the IVS
- Reduced CO, and therefore opening of the mitral valve leaflets, is one of the causes of increased EPSS in animals with impaired systolic function

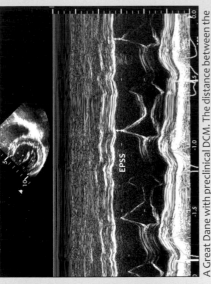

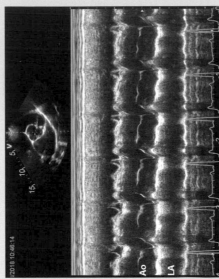

A Great Dane with preclinical DCM. The distance between the mitral E peak and the IVS is increased.

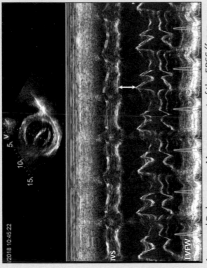

A normal Dobermann. Measurement of the EPSS (from anterior leaflet of mitral valve when open in early diastole – the E peak). This is simply the vertical distance between the two points. The EPSS should be <7 mm in any dog breed.

Assessment of aortic root excursion

- Subjective assessment of degree of anterior aortic root excursion during systole
- Animals with impaired contractility have flat aortic root motion

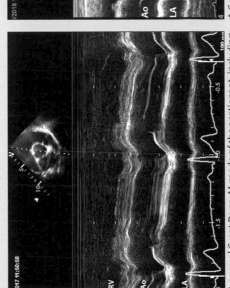

A normal Great Dane. M-mode of the aortic root, including aortic valves. The cursor was positioned on an RPS short-axis view at the level of the heart base. Note that the aortic root moves anteriorly (cranially) during each systole.

A Great Dane with preclinical DCM. The cursor was positioned on an RPS short-axis view at the level of the heart base. The aortic root with the aortic valve can be seen during the cardiac cycle. It does not move anteriorly during systole but remains fairly flat.

2.19 (continued) Assessment of left ventricular systolic function. Ao = aorta; BSA = body surface area; CO = cardiac output; csa = cross-sectional area; CW = continuous wave; DCM = dilated cardiomyopathy; dP = pressure difference; dt = time difference; dv = velocity difference; ECG = electrocardiogram; EDV = end-diastolic volume (of the left ventricle); EF = ejection fraction; EPSS = mitral valve E point to septal separation; ESV = end-systolic volume; ESVI = end-systolic volume index; ET = left ventricular ejection time; FS = fractional shortening; HCM = hypertrophic cardiomyopathy; HR = heart rate; IVS = (with d or s) = interventricular septum (in diastole or systole); LA = left atrium; LV = left ventricle; LVFW (with d or s) = left ventricular free wall (in diastole or systole); LVID (with d or s) = left ventricular internal diameter (in diastole or systole); LVOT = left ventricular outflow tract; LVpw = left ventricular posterior wall; MAPSE = mitral annulus plane systolic excursion; MR = mitral regurgitation; PEP = pre-ejection period; PG = pressure gradient; PW = pulsed wave; RA = right atrium; RPS = right parasternal; RV = right ventricle; SV = stroke volume; Vcf = velocity of circumferential fibre shortening; VSD = ventricular septal defect; VTI = velocity time integral. (continues)

M-mode assessment of systolic function continued

Systolic time intervals from aortic valve M-mode

- Measure the PEP
- Measure the ET
- Calculate the PEP:ET ratio
- Normal PEP:ET ratio is 0.25–0.4
- Systolic dysfunction is evident when the PEP:ET is >0.4
- Can identify premature closure of aortic valves in some patients with severe systolic dysfunction
- See Figure 2.17

MAPSE

- This is recorded from a vertical heart in a four-chamber view from the left apical windows (*can also use a two-chamber view, thus giving four different points of the mitral annulus*)
- Position the M-mode cursor at the mitral annulus, parallel to each wall, record M-mode and measure the maximum excursion from diastole to systole
- Calculate the average motion from the two or four points recorded
- Need to be perpendicular to the mitral annulus
- Sometimes, the lateral/posterior annulus is difficult to image due to lung interference
- Note if there is a wall motion abnormality at one of these points
- Normal mean MAPSE is >10 mm in medium and large breeds of dog
- This has prognostic value in cats with HCM
- This corresponds to apicobasilar contractility of the longitudinal fibres
- See Figure 2.17

2D assessment of LV systolic function

Ejection fraction (%)

- EF = [(EDV − ESV)/EDV] × 100%
- Simpson's rule (method of discs) is the preferred formula to calculate the LV volumes in systole (ESV) and diastole (EDV), using the software on the ultrasound machine
- The LV length is divided into 20 discs. From the volume of each disc, the sum of discs corresponds to the LV volume
- The modified Simpson's rule only requires one plane of the LV (four-chamber view)
- The full Simpson's rule, as used in humans, requires the apical four and two-chamber views (two orthogonal planes through the LV)
- There are several formulae for deriving LV volumes from the 2D images
- For all of these, it is very important to optimize the LV length and area; a foreshortened LV will lead to marked underestimation of volumes
- In dogs, the RPS long-axis four-chamber view normally gives the maximum volumes, rather than the left apical view (as used in humans)
- Simpson's rule is the most accurate method of determining LV volumes, as it is independent of geometrical assumptions or wall motion abnormalities
- Note: in conditions of reduced afterload, such as severe MR, the EF does not reflect contractility
- See also Chapter 9

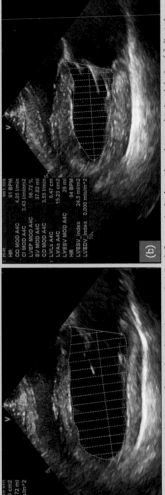

2.19 (continued) Assessment of left ventricular systolic function. (a) Assessment of left ventricular systolic function. (b) systole. The left ventricular area from the mitral hinge points is traced and closed along the mitral annulus line. The length of the LV is then indicated from midpoint of the annulus to the LV apex. The software divides this length into a number of discs and sums the calculated volume of each disc to give the total left ventricular volumes in diastole and systole. The EF can be calculated, and the LV volumes in diastole and systole indexed to BSA (or exponent of bodyweight, the latter being more mathematically appropriate).

A normal Dobermann. RPS long-axis four-chamber views optimizing left ventricular length and area obtained during (a) diastole and (b) systole.

Ao = aorta; BSA = body surface area; CO = cardiac output; csa = cross-sectional area; CW = continuous wave; DCM = dilated cardiomyopathy; dP = pressure difference; dt = time difference; dv = velocity difference; ECG = electrocardiogram; EDV = end-diastolic volume (of the left ventricle); EF = ejection fraction; EPSS = mitral valve E point to septal separation; ESV = end-systolic volume; ESVI = end-systolic volume index; ET = left ventricular ejection time; FS = fractional shortening; HCM = hypertrophic cardiomyopathy; HR = heart rate; IVS (with d or s) = interventricular septum (in diastole or systole); LA = left atrium; LV = left ventricle; LVFW (with d or s) = left ventricular free wall (in diastole or systole); LVID (with d or s) = left ventricular internal diameter (in diastole or systole); LVOT = left ventricular outflow tract; LVpw = left ventricular posterior wall; MAPSE = mitral annulus plane systolic excursion; MR = mitral regurgitation; PEP = pre-ejection period; PG = pressure gradient; PW = pulsed wave; RA = right atrium; RPS = right parasternal; RV = right ventricle; SV = stroke volume; Vcf = velocity of circumferential fibre shortening; VSD = ventricular septal defect; VTI = velocity time integral. *(continues)*

2D assessment of LV systolic function *continued*

End-systolic volume index

- The ESV is determined from 2D measurements that optimize the left ventricular length and area (e.g. Simpson's rule)
- The animal's bodyweight is converted to BSA in m² (consult tables or a formula)
- The ESVI is calculated (ml/m²)
- It is commonly cited that dogs with normal systolic function have an ESVI of <30 ml/m²
- However, indexing LV volume to BSA is not linear – very small dogs have low values, and large or giant breeds of dog have higher values. Breed-specific reference intervals should be consulted where available
- LV volumes including ESVI are more sensitive at identifying Dobermanns with DCM than M-mode criteria. In Dobermanns, ESVI >55 ml/m² is abnormal
- Values significantly above the ESVI reference interval indicate impaired systolic function
- ESVI is useful to assess systolic function in the setting of reduced afterload such as severe MR, where FS and EF cannot be used to indicate contractility
- See also Chapter 9

Doppler assessment of LV systolic function from aortic outflow

Peak aortic velocity

- Measure peak velocity of aortic flow
- In the absence of aortic stenosis, peak velocity of aortic outflow correlates with systolic function
- See Figure 2.18

Aortic flow acceleration

- Mean acceleration (dv/dt mean) is the slope from onset of aortic flow to peak velocity
- Maximum acceleration (cv/dt max) is the initial, steepest part of the slope
- Difficult to accurately measure, especially if very fast spectral Doppler sweep speeds are not available (>100 mm/s). This results in repeatability issues

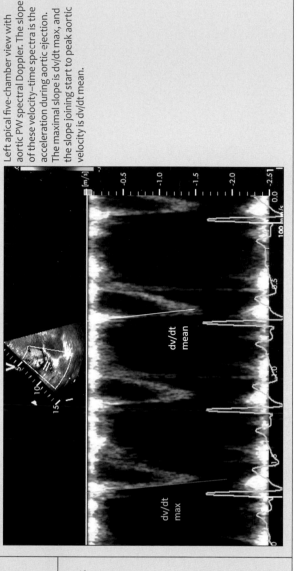

Left apical five-chamber view with aortic PW spectral Doppler. The slope of these velocity–time spectra is the acceleration during aortic ejection. The maximal slope is dv/dt max, and the slope joining start to peak aortic velocity is dv/dt mean.

2.19 (continued) Assessment of left ventricular systolic function. Ao = aorta; BSA = body surface area; CO = cardiac output; csa = cross-sectional area; CW = continuous wave; DCM = dilated cardiomyopathy; dP = pressure difference; dt = time difference; dv = velocity difference; ECG = electrocardiogram; EDV = end-diastolic volume (of the left ventricle); EF = ejection fraction; EPSS = mitral valve E point to septal separation; ESV = end-systolic volume; ESVI = end-systolic volume index; ET = left ventricular ejection time; FS = fractional shortening; HCM = hypertrophic cardiomyopathy; HR = heart rate; IVS (with d or s) = interventricular septum (in diastole or systole); LA = left atrium; LV = left ventricle; LVFW (with d or s) = left ventricular free wall (in diastole or systole); LVID (with d or s) = left ventricular internal diameter (in diastole or systole); LVOT = left ventricular outflow tract; LVpw = left ventricular posterior wall; MAPSE = mitral annulus plane systolic excursion; MR = mitral regurgitation; PEP = pre-ejection period; PG = pressure gradient; PW = pulsed wave; RA = right atrium; RPS = right parasternal; RV = right ventricle; SV = stroke volume; Vcf = velocity of circumferential fibre shortening; VSD = ventricular septal defect; VTI = velocity time integral. (continues)

Doppler assessment of LV systolic function from aortic outflow continued

Velocity time integral

- The aortic outflow spectrum is traced, and the area under its curve determined
- Calculation of forward SV and CO:
  - Forward SV = Ao csa x Ao VTI
  - Ao csa is determined by measuring the aortic diameter (d) in systole (at valve level; see Figure 2.15)
  - Ao csa = $\pi(^d/_2)^2$
  - Forward SV = Ao csa x Ao VTI
  - CO = SV x HR
- HR is calculated from the ECG:
  - HR = 60/R–R interval (in seconds)
- The VTI is also known as the stroke distance (units = cm)
- In cases of severe MR, forward SV can be subtracted from total left ventricular SV (e.g. from Simpson's rule: SV = EDV – ESV) to calculate MR volume and, therefore, regurgitant fraction
- In cases of a shunt such as a VSD, the pulmonic to systemic flow quotient can be calculated (Qp/Qs), where pulmonic flow is calculated in a similar way, using pulmonic VTI and csa of the pulmonic annulus

Left apical five-chamber view with aortic PW spectral Doppler. The VTI is measured by tracing around the modal velocity of the spectral Doppler envelope (shaded green). The area under the curve is stroke distance (measured in cm).

Systolic time intervals

- The PEP is the start of the ECG QRS complex, to the onset of aortic flow
- The ET is the duration of aortic flow
- Calculate the PEP:ET ratio
- The PEP:ET ratio is an index of contractility that is relatively independent of HR and load
- Normal ratio is 0.25–0.4
- Values above 0.4 suggest systolic dysfunction
- See Figure 2.18

Doppler assessment of LV systolic function from mitral regurgitant jet

MR jet peak velocity

- Measure peak velocity of MR jet
- MR jet velocity reflects the systolic PG between the LV and LA
- Where LA pressures are high (left heart failure) and/or in the presence of systolic impairment, this velocity will be reduced
- In dogs with DCM, MR velocity of <4 m/s is a negative prognostic indicator for survival

2.19 (continued) Assessment of left ventricular systolic function. Ao = aorta; BSA = body surface area; CO = cardiac output; csa = cross-sectional area; CW = continuous wave; DCM = dilated cardiomyopathy; dP = pressure difference; dt = time difference; dv = velocity difference; ECG = electrocardiogram; EDV = end-diastolic volume (of the left ventricle); EF = ejection fraction; EPSS = mitral valve E point to septal separation; ESV = end-systolic volume; ESVI = end-systolic volume index; ET = left ventricular ejection time; FS = fractional shortening; HCM = hypertrophic cardiomyopathy; HR = heart rate; IVS (with d or s) = interventricular septum (in diastole or systole); LA = left atrium; LV = left ventricle; LVFW (with d or s) = left ventricular free wall (in diastole or systole); LVID (with d or s) = left ventricular internal diameter (in diastole or systole); LVOT = left ventricular outflow tract; LVpw = left ventricular posterior wall; MAPSE = mitral annulus plane systolic excursion; MR = mitral regurgitation; PEP = pre-ejection period; PG = pressure gradient; PW = pulsed wave; RA = right atrium; RPS = right parasternal; RV = right ventricle; SV = stroke volume; Vcf = velocity of circumferential fibre shortening; VSD = ventricular septal defect; VTI = velocity time integral. (continues) ▲

Doppler assessment of LV systolic function from mitral regurgitant jet *continued*

LV +$^{dP}/_{dt}$ from CW Doppler trace of MR jet

- Good quality mitral regurgitant spectral Doppler signals are acquired
- They must have a clean acceleration slope
- From the acceleration slope of an MR spectral Doppler signal, two points are selected on this slope, e.g. at 1 m/s and at 3 m/s
- The modified Bernoulli equation is used to calculate the instantaneous pressure gradients at these two points (i.e. 1 m/s is 4 mmHg, and 3 m/s is 36 mmHg)
- The pressure difference between them is calculated (in this example, dP = 32 mmHg)
- The time between the two points is measured (= dt)
- $^{dP}/_{dt}$ can therefore be calculated
- This is reported to correlate well with the gold-standard of contractility, the catheterization derived +$^{dP}/_{dt}$
- It is difficult to measure short time durations accurately, unless the ultrasound machine is able to display spectral images at very high sweep speed (>100 mm/s)

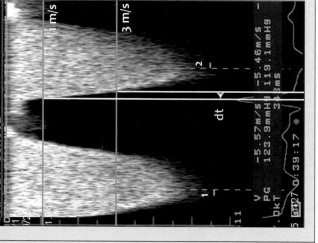

From the CW spectral Doppler of a clean MR jet at high speed, $^{dP}/_{dt}$ can be calculated as shown. From two points across the acceleration slope, the instantaneous pressures can be determined to give the pressure difference (dP). The time is measured between the two points (dt). Note that the peak velocity is about 5.5 m/s in this dog with MMVD and adequate systolic function.

2.19 (continued) Assessment of left ventricular systolic function. Ao = aorta; BSA = body surface area; CO = cardiac output; csa = cross-sectional area; CW = continuous wave; DCM = dilated cardiomyopathy; dP = pressure difference; dt = time difference; dv = velocity difference; ECG = electrocardiogram; EDV = end-diastolic volume (of the left ventricle); EF = ejection fraction; EPSS = mitral valve E point to septal separation; ESV = end-systolic volume; ESVI = end-systolic volume index; ET = left ventricular ejection time; FS = fractional shortening; HCM = hypertrophic cardiomyopathy; HR = heart rate; IVS (with d or s) = interventricular septum (in diastole or systole); LA = left atrium; LV = left ventricle; LVFW (with d or s) = left ventricular free wall (in diastole or systole); LVID (with d or s) = left ventricular internal diameter (in diastole or systole); LVOT = left ventricular outflow tract; LVpw = left ventricular posterior wall; MAPSE = mitral annulus plane systolic excursion; MR = mitral regurgitation; PEP = pre-ejection period; PG = pressure gradient; PW = pulsed wave; RA = right atrium; RPS = right parasternal; RV = right ventricle; SV = stroke volume; Vcf = velocity of circumferential fibre shortening; VSD = ventricular septal defect; VTI = velocity time integral.

PW Doppler measurement of isovolumic relaxation time

- From an apical five-chamber view, use colour Doppler to show red of transmitral flow and blue of left ventricular outflow
- Position a large sample volume so both mitral inflow (above the baseline) and left ventricular outflow (below the baseline) are recorded at the maximum sweep speed possible; obtain PW Doppler signals
- It is useful if valve clicks are acquired on the PW signal to assist timing, but not essential. A CW spectral Doppler signal may assist acquisition of valve clicks
- Measure the time from end of left ventricular outflow to onset of mitral flow; this is the IVRT
- The measurement is affected by heart rate; the corresponding R–R interval should be recorded so measurements can be corrected for heart rate if appropriate
- It is difficult to measure small time durations accurately and repeatably
- IVRT should not be significantly influenced by respiration (if it increases in inspiration and decreases with expiration, constrictive pericardial disease may be suspected)
- Make sure the low velocity reject is minimized, so that the intersection of the spectral Doppler traces and the baseline can be accurately identified (ideally with valve clicks)
- If poor quality spectral Doppler makes it difficult to define the IVRT, try also with CW (especially in larger dogs)

PW Doppler assessment of transmitral flow

- Mitral inflow E and A waves are recorded
- Measure peak velocity of mitral E and A waves
- The E wave deceleration time can also be measured (time from peak E until baseline)
- Mitral E wave and A wave durations can be measured
- The pressure half-time can be calculated using ultrasound machine software; this may be prolonged in the presence of mitral stenosis (uncommon)
- The ratio of E:A wave velocities should be >1 but <2
- Ageing influences this ratio and decreases the E:A ratio
- A pattern of *impaired relaxation* is identified by:
  - E:A ratio <1 (i.e. increased dependence on atrial contraction for ventricular filling)
  - Prolonged E wave deceleration time
  - Prolonged IVRT

Left apical five-chamber view with PW spectral Doppler from the LVOT showing transmitral inflow (E and A waves above the baseline) to the LV as well as left ventricular outflow (below the baseline). The time from end of left ventricular outflow to onset of mitral E wave (between green lines) is the IVRT.

Transmitral flow pattern from a Rottweiler with marked left ventricular concentric hypertrophy due to severe aortic stenosis. Note the A wave velocity exceeds the E wave (E:A reversal) and there is a long E wave deceleration time. These features are associated with impaired relaxation of the LV.

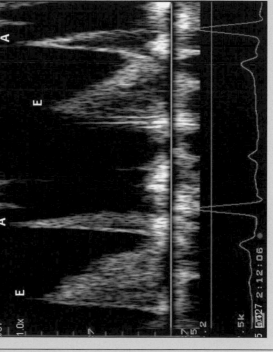

2.20 The Doppler assessment of left ventricular diastolic function. Ao = aorta; Ar = atrial reversal wave; CHF = congestive heart failure; CW = continuous wave; D = diastolic flow (PVF); dP = pressure difference; dt = time difference; ECG = electrocardiogram; ET = left ventricular ejection time; HCM = hypertrophic cardiomyopathy; HOCM = hypertrophic obst`uctive cardiomyopathy; HPRF = high pulse repetition frequency; IMP = index of myocardial performance (Tei index); IVCT = isovolumic contraction time; IVRT = isovolumic relaxation time; LA = left atrium; L-CHF = left-sided congestive heart failure; LPRF = low pulse repetition frequency; LV = left ventricle; LVOT = left ventricular outflow tract; MR = mitral regurgitation; MV = mitral valve; MVC = mitral valve closure; MVC = mitral valve opening; PVF = pulmonary venous flow; PW = pulsed wave; RA = right atrium; RPS = right parasternal; RV = right ventricle; S = systolic flow (PVF); Se = early flow; SI = main flow wave); Vp = left ventricular early flow propagation velocity. (continues) ▲

PW Doppler assessment of transmitral flow continued

- Cats with asymptomatic HCM often show an impaired relaxation pattern provided that separate transmitral E and A waves can be identified reliably

Transmitral flow from a cat with HCM with only mild dilatation of the LA. The A waves are slightly higher in velocity than the E waves, which is consistent with an impaired relaxation pattern. Note however that there is mild partial summation, which means the A wave starts prior to completion of the E wave deceleration (E at A; E@A; green line), which will make the A wave higher in velocity. If the mitral E wave deceleration is less than 0.2 m/s before the A wave starts, the transmitral flow pattern can be accepted as indicative of LV diastolic function.

- As a disease such as feline HCM progresses, the LA pressure increases, then the early diastolic pressure gradient between the LA and LV is increased. Therefore, E wave velocities increase again, giving a pseudonormal transmitral flow pattern (E:A >1)

Transmitral flow from a cat with HOCM and CHF that was receiving treatment. The mitral E:A wave velocity ratio is between 1 and 2 – a pseudonormal filling pattern.

2.20 (continued) The Doppler assessment of left ventricular diastolic function. Ao = aorta; Ar = atrial reversal wave; CHF = congestive heart failure; CW = continuous wave; D = diastolic flow (PVF); dP = pressure difference; dt = time difference; ECG = electrocardiogram; ET = left ventricular ejection time; HCM = hypertrophic cardiomyopathy; HOCM = hypertrophic obstructive cardiomyopathy; HPRF = high pulse repetition frequency; IMP = index of myocardial performance (Tei index); IVCT = isovolumic contraction time; IVRT = isovolumic relaxation time; LA = left atrium; L-CHF = left-sided congestive heart failure; LPRF = low pulse repetition frequency; LV = left ventricle; LVOT = left ventricular outflow tract; MR = mitral regurgitation; MV = mitral valve; MVC = mitral valve closure; MVO = mitral valve opening; PVF = pulmonary venous flow; PW = pulsed wave; RA = right atrium; RPS = right parasternal; RV = right ventricle; S = systolic flow (PVF); Se = early flow; SI = main flow wave); Vp = left ventricular early flow propagation velocity. (continues) ▲

PW Doppler assessment of transmitral flow continued

- Restrictive filling is due to increased LA pressure, reduced LA function and a stiff, poorly compliant LV. It is identified by:
  - E:A ratio >2
  - Brief duration E wave, with short deceleration time
  - Short IVRT
- Note: the restrictive filling pattern can be seen in any condition resulting in severe diastolic dysfunction; it is not specific for restrictive cardiomyopathy
- In tachycardic animals, such as many cats, summation of the E and A waves means that diastolic function cannot be assessed
- A vagal manoeuvre (e.g. gentle pressure on the nose in a cat) may separate E and A waves enough to acquire a couple of cardiac cycles to enable assessment
- Animals with atrial fibrillation also cannot have diastolic function assessed by transmitral flow pattern as they only have E waves

PW Doppler assessment of pulmonary venous flow

- From an apical four-chamber view, a sample volume is positioned in one of the pulmonary veins (this is easier in animals with left-sided failure, as the veins are dilated)
- Other views can also be used, provided a pulmonary vein is visible and parallel to the cursor (e.g. RPS short-axis view optimizing the LA; cranial left parasternal view of the left atrial appendage)
- Ensuring LPRF is used (not HPRF), PVF is recorded. There are three major components to PVF:
  - The Ar. During atrial systole, retrograde flow in the pulmonary veins is detected following the P wave of the ECG
  - Following atrial relaxation, some early forward flow is recorded (Se). During ventricular systole, the mitral annulus moves apically, and the main systolic (Sl) PVF wave results. Although partial separation of Se and Sl may be identified, in most animals, the peak S velocity is measured and a single peak is usually recorded
  - During diastole, the LA is merely a conduit between the pulmonary veins and the LV as it relaxes; this gives the diastolic (D) forward wave of the PVF pattern
- Measure peak velocity of S, D and Ar
- Measure the duration of Ar
- The durations of S and D can be measured

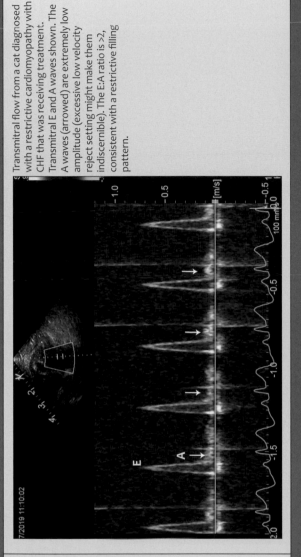

Transmitral flow from a cat diagnosed with a restrictive cardiomyopathy with CHF that was receiving treatment. Transmitral E and A waves shown. The A waves (arrowed) are extremely low amplitude (excessive low velocity reject setting might make them indiscernible). The E:A ratio is >2, consistent with a restrictive filling pattern.

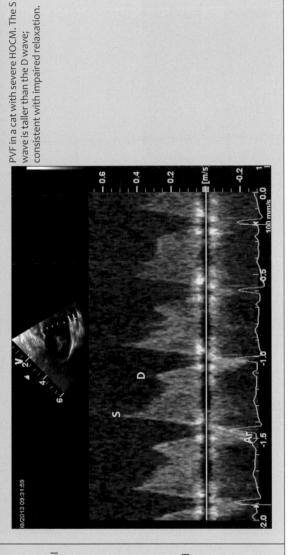

PVF in a cat with severe HOCM. The S wave is taller than the D wave; consistent with impaired relaxation.

2.20 (continued) The Doppler assessment of left ventricular diastolic function. Ao = aorta; Ar = atrial reversal wave; CHF = congestive heart failure; CW = continuous wave; D = diastolic flow (PVF); dP = pressure difference; dt = time difference; ECG = electrocardiogram; ET = left ventricular ejection time; HCM = hypertrophic cardiomyopathy; HOCM = hypertrophic obstructive cardiomyopathy; HPRF = high pulse repetition frequency; IMP = index of myocardial performance (Tei index); IVCT = isovolumic contraction time; IVRT = isovolumic relaxation time; LA = left atrium; L-CHF = left-sided congestive heart failure; LPRF = low pulse repetition frequency; LV = left ventricle; LVOT = left ventricular outflow tract; MR = mitral regurgitation; MV = mitral valve; MVC = mitral valve closure; MVO = mitral valve opening; PVF = pulmonary venous flow; PW = pulsed wave; RA = right atrium; RPS = right parasternal; RV = right ventricle; S = systolic flow (PVF); Se = early flow; Sl = main flow wave; Vp = left ventricular early flow propagation velocity. (continues)

PW Doppler assessment of pulmonary venous flow continued

- D deceleration time can be measured
- The relevant R–R intervals should be measured as measurements will be influenced by heart rate
- The velocity time integrals of S and D can be calculated by tracing the waveforms
- In normal dogs, S has lower velocity than D; S and D are usually of similar velocity in cats
- With ageing, D may decrease, and reversal may be identified
- In impaired relaxation, the S:D ratio is >1, and there is often a large Ar
- In a restrictive filling pattern, S velocity may be low, and D high but rapidly decelerating. Ar may be normal or reduced (depending on atrial function)
- The mitral A wave duration may be compared with the PVF Ar
- In normal animals, mitral A duration > Ar duration
- In situations of elevated filling pressures, duration of Ar > A
- In dogs with severe MR, reverse systolic flow (MR coursing up the pulmonary veins) may compromise assessment of diastolic function by PVF

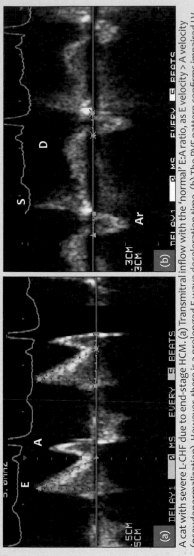

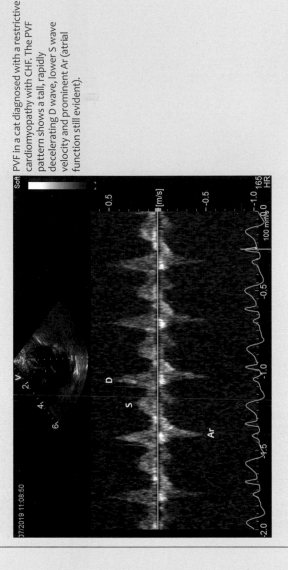

A cat with severe L-CHF due to end-stage HCM. (a) Transmitral inflow with the 'normal' E:A ratio, as E velocity > A velocity (pseudonormalization). However, there is a prolonged E wave deceleration time. (b) The PVF pattern confirms impaired LV relaxation, with high Ar velocity and S wave > D wave. Note the confirmation of elevated filling pressures as PVF Ar duration is > mitral A wave duration (see below).

PVF in a cat diagnosed with a restrictive cardiomyopathy with CHF. The PVF pattern shows a tall, rapidly decelerating D wave, lower S wave velocity and prominent Ar (atrial function still evident).

2.20 (continued) The Doppler assessment of left ventricular diastolic function. Ao = aorta; Ar = atrial reversal wave; CHF = congestive heart failure; CW = continuous wave; D = diastolic flow (PVF); dP = pressure difference; dt = time difference; ECG = electrocardiogram; ET = left ventricular ejection time; HCM = hypertrophic cardiomyopathy; HOCM = hypertrophic obstructive cardiomyopathy; HPRF = high pulse repetition frequency; IMP = index of myocardial performance (Tei index); IVCT = isovolumic contraction time; IVRT = isovolumic relaxation time; LA = left atrium; L-CHF = left-sided congestive heart failure; LPRF = low pulse repetition frequency; LV = left ventricle; LVOT = left ventricular outflow tract; MR = mitral regurgitation; MV = mitral valve; MVC = mitral valve closure; MVO = mitral valve opening; PVF = pulmonary venous flow; PW = pulsed wave; RA = right atrium; RPS = right parasternal; RV = right ventricle; S = systolic flow (PVF); Se = early flow; SI = main flow wave); Vp = left ventricular early flow propagation velocity. (continues)

Diastolic function from mitral regurgitant jet

- LV $-^{dP}/_{dt}$ from CW Doppler trace of MR jet
- Good quality MR spectral Doppler CW signals are obtained
- From the deceleration slope of the signal, two points are identified (e.g. at 3 m/s and 1 m/s) corresponding to instantaneous LV:LA pressure gradients at these two points of 36 mmHg and 4 mmHg. The pressure difference is therefore 32 mmHg (=dP)
- The time between the two points is measured (= dt)
- $-^{dP}/_{dt}$ is then calculated
- No data of reference values available so far in the veterinary literature
- It is difficult to measure short time durations accurately, unless the ultrasound machine is able to display spectral images at very high sweep speed (>100 mm/s)

MR jet from a cat with HCM. If there is a clean deceleration slope, $-^{dP}/_{dt}$ can be calculated, as shown.

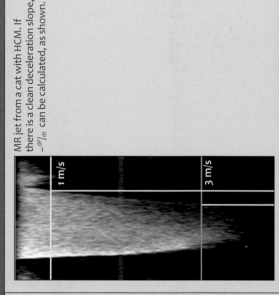

Velocity of propagation of mitral flow from mitral annulus towards the LV apex

- From the apical four-chamber view, colour flow Doppler is used to assess the column of blood corresponding to mitral inflow to the LV apex
- The colour Nyquist limit and/or baseline are altered so that there is a central aliased blue core in this colour signal
- The M-mode cursor is positioned within this column, aligning the M-mode cursor with the flow
- M-mode at maximum sweep speed is recorded. The distance this column of blood moves is plotted against time. This corresponds to the mitral flow E wave as it courses towards the LV apex
- The slope of the wave front or the aliased core of this column is the velocity it moves from mitral annulus to the apex (Vp); this can be measured from M-mode software
- Normal (in cats) is about 64 cm/s
- The steeper the slope, the better the diastolic function. Lower velocities indicate impaired diastolic function (without separating abnormal relaxation from restrictive physiologies)
- The ratio of mitral E wave velocity to Vp correlates with LV end-diastolic pressure (especially in cats)

Left apical four-chamber view with a colour sample volume from the MV towards the LV apex. The M-mode cursor is positioned within this column of blood of mitral flow into the LV. M-mode shows the column of blood corresponding to early filling moving from the mitral annulus to the LV apex. The slope of this line (Vp) reflects the diastolic properties of the LV.

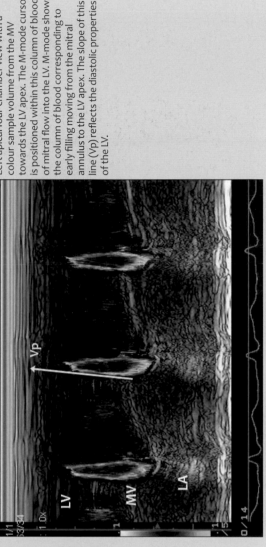

2.20 (continued) The Doppler assessment of left ventricular diastolic function. Ao = aorta; Ar = atrial reversal wave; CHF = congestive heart failure; CW = continuous wave; D = diastolic flow (PVF); dP = pressure difference; dt = time difference; ECG = electocardiogram; ET = left ventricular ejection time; HCM = hypertrophic cardiomyopathy; HOCM = hypertrophic obstructive cardiomyopathy; HPRF = high pulse repetition frequency; IMP = index of myocardial performance (Tei index); IVCT = isovolumic contraction time; IVRT = isovolumic relaxation time; LA = left atrium; L-CHF = left-sided congestive heart failure; LPRF = low pulse repetition frequency; LV = left ventricle; LVO⁺ = left ventricular outflow tract; MR = mitral regurgitation; MV = mitral valve; MVC = mitral valve closure; MVO = mitral valve opening; PVF = pulmonary venous flow; PW = pulsed wave; RA = right atrium; RPS = right parasternal; RV = right ventricle; S = systolic flow (PVF; Se = early flow; Sl = main flow wave); Vp = left ventricular early flow propagation velocity. (continues)

Index of myocardial performance (the Tei index)

- Transmitral inflow is recorded, so that the time from MV closure to opening is recorded
- Aortic flow is recorded, to measure the ejection time
- IMP = (IVCT + IVRT)/ET
- The time from MVC to MVO = IVCT + ET + IVRT
- To determine IVCT + IVRT, subtract ET from MVC–MVO
- IMP can then be calculated
- This is a combined index of systolic and diastolic function
- It could also be applied to the RV, from recordings of tricuspid flow and pulmonic flow

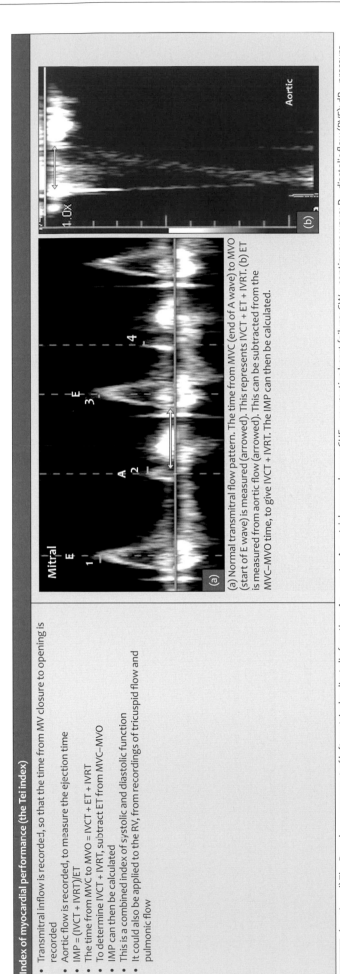

(a) Normal transmitral flow pattern. The time from MVC (end of A wave) to MVO (start of E wave) is measured (arrowed). This represents IVCT + ET + IVRT. (b) ET is measured from aortic flow (arrowed). This can be subtracted from the MVC–MVO time, to give IVCT + IVRT. The IMP can then be calculated.

2.20 (continued) The Doppler assessment of left ventricular diastolic function. Ao = aorta; Ar = atrial reversal wave; CHF = congestive heart failure; CW = continuous wave; D = diastolic flow (PVF); dP = pressure difference; dt = time difference; ECG = electrocardiogram; ET = left ventricular ejection time; HCM = hypertrophic cardiomyopathy; HOCM = hypertrophic obstructive cardiomyopathy; HPRF = high pulse repetition frequency; IMP = index of myocardial performance (Tei index); IVCT = isovolumic contraction time; IVRT = isovolumic relaxation time; LA = left atrium; L-CHF = left-sided congestive heart failure; LPRF = low pulse repetition frequency; LV = left ventricle; LVOT = left ventricular outflow tract; MR = mitral regurgitation; MV = mitral valve; MVC = mitral valve closure; MVO = mitral valve opening; PVF = pulmonary venous flow; PW = pulsed wave; RA = right atrium; RPS = right parasternal; RV = right ventricle; S = systolic flow (PVF); Se = early flow; SI = main flow wave; Vp = left ventricular early flow propagation velocity.

Acquisition of the image	Interpretation of the image	Measurements and calculations
• The left apical four-chamber view is acquired, ensuring the heart is as parallel with the ultrasound beam as possible. Longitudinal fibres at both the septal and lateral mitral annulus can be interrogated • When the right heart is optimized with more cranial positioning, PW-TDI can be used to assess velocity of right ventricular wall motion • Ensure the cursor is parallel to the longitudinal motion of the wall under interrogation (colour flow Doppler usually superimposed on the 2D image first) • Position the sample volume at the annulus • Change to PW-TDI Doppler, recording at maximum sweep speed	• There are three major phases to the longitudinal fibre motion: • In systole, the longitudinal fibres contract from the mitral annulus towards the apex, giving an S' wave (the velocity of which is an indicator of systolic function) • During early diastole, the active relaxation process of the longitudinal fibres gives the E' wave • Following atrial contraction, the resulting changes in the longitudinal fibres give the A' wave • There are also PW-TDI signals corresponding to IVC and IVR. These are biphasic, brief duration shifts in opposing directions from the preceding and following major waves; IVC is therefore positive/negative preceding the S' wave and IVR is negative/positive following S' and preceding E'. The IVCT and IVRT can be measured	• The S' wave velocity can be measured, which correlates with systolic function • The E' and A' wave velocities can be measured • The left-sided E':A' ratio may be <1 when there is impaired relaxation (including ageing change); more likely to be identified in the septum than the LVFW. (This parameter is less influenced by loading conditions than the mitral E:A ratio) • Left-sided PW-TDI can therefore unmask a pseudonormal transmitral flow pattern 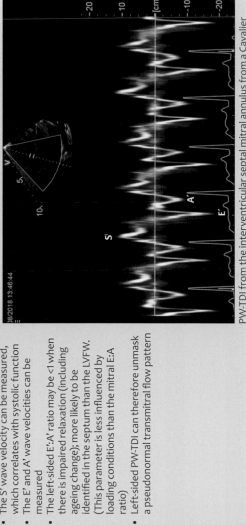 PW-TDI from the interventricular septal mitral annulus from a Cavalier King Charles Spaniel with Stage B2 MMVD but no systolic or diastolic dysfunction identified. The S' is seen above the baseline, E' and A' below the baseline. At a faster sweep speed, the rapid bidirectional shifts associated with IVC and IVR may be more evident. • The ratio of mitral E wave velocity to E' velocity is relatively load-independent and corresponds to filling pressures in humans. However, it is less reliable in dogs and cats. The normal ratio is about 8 in cats and humans and a ratio above 15 may predict elevated left-sided filling pressure • Right heart PW-TDI velocities tend to be much higher than the IVS or LVFW velocities 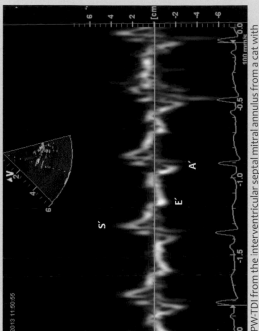 PW-TDI from the interventricular septal mitral annulus from a cat with HCM. All velocities are relatively low (<5 cm/s). The A' velocity is higher than the E' velocity, consistent with impaired relaxation.

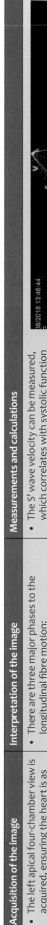

2.21 Pulsed wave tissue Doppler imaging (PW-TDI) assessment of myocardial function (longitudinal fibres). HCM = hypertrophic cardiomyopathy; IVC = isovolumic contraction; IVCT = isovolumic contraction time; IVR = isovolumic relaxation; IVRT = isovolumic relaxation time; IVS = interventricular septum; LV = left ventricle; LVFW = left ventricular free wall; MMVD = myxomatous mitral valve disease.

Acquisition of the image	Interpretation of the image	Observations, measurements and calculations
2D assessment		
• RPS long-axis four-chamber view, optimizing the left atrial diameter and including the PVe and RPA to compare these	• If interatrial septum is bulging (not just flaring) to the right, increased left atrial pressure can be inferred • When the PVe is much more dilated than the corresponding RPA, pulmonary venous hypertension is inferred	• Predominantly subjective assessment, although PVe diameter and RPA diameter can be measured RPS long-axis four-chamber view from a Cavalier King Charles Spaniel with advanced Stage B2 MMVD. The LA is very dilated and left atrial pressure is likely to be increased, as inferred from the bulging to the right (arrowed). The PVe (double-headed arrow) is much more dilated than the RPA. Even though there was no overt clinical or radiological evidence of cardiogenic pulmonary oedema, these findings suggest it is imminent and the dog should be closely monitored.
Mitral E wave velocity		
• Obtain from left apical four-chamber view, cursor aligned with transmitral flow • Measure peak velocity of early diastolic E wave	• The higher the mitral E velocity (provided no mitral stenosis), the higher the left-sided volume overload and/or left atrial pressure	• Mitral E velocity >1.2 m/s in MMVD is consistent with severe mitral regurgitation and/or increased left-sided filling pressure
Mitral E:IVRT ratio		
• Measure mitral E wave velocity • Left apical five-chamber view with large sample volume in LVOT over red of mitral and blue of LVOT flows • PW (or CW): record transmitral flow and left ventricular outflow • Make sure envelopes are clearly defined and intersect with the baseline (no excessive low-velocity reject setting) • Measure IVRT between valve clicks if present	• The ratio is less heart rate dependent than each variable on its own • The mitral E:IVRT ratio is the most accurate echocardiographic assessment of canine left-sided congestive heart failure	• Calculate mitral E:IVRT ratio • >2.5 is consistent with left-sided congestive heart failure in dogs with MMVD • >1.8 is consistent with left-sided congestive heart failure in dogs with DCM

2.22 Estimation of left-sided filling pressures. Ar = atrial reversal wave; CW = continuous wave; DCM = dilated cardiomyopathy; IVRT = isovolumic relaxation time; IVS = interventricular septum; LA = left atrium; LPRF = low pulse repetition frequency; LV = left ventricle; LVFW = left ventricular free wall; LVOT = left ventricular outflow tract; MMVD = myxomatous mitral valve disease; MV = mitral valve; PVe = pulmonary vein; PVF = pulmonary venous flow; PW = pulsed wave; PW-TDI = pulsed wave tissue Doppler imaging; RPA = right pulmonary artery; RPS = right parasternal; Vp = left ventricular early flow propagation velocity. (continues)

Acquisition of the image	Interpretation of the image	Observations, measurements and calculations
Mitral E:Vp ratio		
• Measure mitral E wave velocity • Vp: Flow propagation of early mitral flow towards left ventricular apex. Colour M-mode aligned with transmitral flow in the LV, between MV level and the LV apex. Reduce Nyquist limit to show an aliased core. Measure the slope of the red–blue interface of the aliased core ('Vp)	• Aim for separate, non-summated E and A waves for both E and Vp velocities • Mitral E:Vp ratio is considered the most accurate echocardiographic assessment of increased left-sided filling pressures in the cat • Vp may not be preload independent	• Calculate mitral E:Vp ratio • Baseline normal ratio in healthy anaesthetized cats is 1.2; values >1.6 likely to be abnormal (no data from naturally occurring diseased cats)
Mitral E:PW-TDI E' ratio		
• Measure mitral E wave velocity • Align in turn with IVS and LVFW, as parallel to each wall as possible. PW-TDI sample volume at base of each wall, mitral annulus level • Measure the velocity of the E' wave	• Aim for separate mitral E and A waves and PW-TDI E' and A' waves if possible (not summated waves) • Although E:E' ratio is a useful estimate of left-sided filling pressure in humans, it does not seem to be as useful in dogs or cats	• Calculate the E:E' ratio for either or both the IVS and LVFW • Values >15 likely to be abnormal
Pulmonary venous flow Ar duration compared with mitral A wave duration		
• Obtain transmitral flow as above from the left apical four-chamber view. PW Doppler • Provided there are separate E and A waves, measure the duration of the mitral A wave (avoid excessive low-velocity reject so the A wave intersects with the baseline) • Obtain PVF spectral Doppler (usually left apical four-chamber view). Must be LPRF pulsed wave Doppler (single sample volume). Avoid excessive low-velocity reject, so spectral Doppler envelopes intersect with the baseline. Identify the Ar • Measure the PVF Ar duration	• Make sure that the heart rates are similar during acquisition of transmitral and PVF spectral Doppler • Need good quality PVF spectral Doppler. This might be difficult to achieve in very large dogs or in dogs with mitral regurgitation entering the pulmonary veins • Not applicable in patients with atrial fibrillation, as there will not be an A wave or Ar	• The mitral A duration should be longer than the PVF Ar duration • If PVF Ar > mitral A duration, this is abnormal and is consistent with increased left-sided filling pressures • See Figure 2.20

2.22 (continued) Estimation of left-sided filling pressures. Ar = atrial reversal wave; CW = continuous wave; DCM = dilated cardiomyopathy; IVRT = isovolumic relaxation time; IVS = interventricular septum; LA = left atrium; LPRF = low pulse repetition frequency; LV = left ventricle; LVFW = left ventricular free wall; LVOT = left ventricular outflow tract; MMVD = myxomatous mitral valve disease; MV = mitral valve; PVe = pulmonary vein; PVF = pulmonary venous flow; PW = pulsed wave; PW-TDI = pulsed wave tissue Doppler imaging; RPA = right pulmonary artery; RPS = right parasternal; Vp = left ventricular early flow propagation velocity.

Acquisition of the image	Interpretation of the image	Observations, measurements or calculations
Tricuspid annular plane systolic excursion		
• Left apical four-chamber view, which optimizes the right heart • Make sure M-mode cursor is parallel to the RVFW longitudinal motion and therefore perpendicular to the lateral tricuspid annulus as it moves towards the apex during systole • M-mode: make sure the line of the tricuspid annulus can be seen throughout the cardiac cycle	• Reduced RV longitudinal contraction will result in lower value of TAPSE • Lower values of TAPSE than reference limits are of prognostic value • In cats with CHF, cats with pleural effusion are more likely to have low TAPSE value	 • Measure TAPSE from the end of diastole to the peak of systole • Values are influenced by the size of dog; weight-based reference intervals or allometric scaling for bodyweight can be used • In cats, normal values cited are 7.4–10.2 mm. Lower values are of little prognostic significance • See also Figure 2.17 TAPSE from a Sphinx cat with ascites (protein-rich transudate). The cat had preclinical HCM, but a cardiac cause for the ascites was unlikely. TAPSE was 8.4 mm (reference 7.4–10.2 mm), so RV function did not seem to be impaired.
Right ventricle fractional area change		
• Left apical four-chamber view, optimizing the right heart • Make sure the right ventricular length is optimized and it is a true long-axis view (not directed cranially towards the RVOT) • Freeze image at end of diastole (start of QRS complex). Trace area of the RV, closing at level of tricuspid annulus; this is the diastolic RV area (RVAd) • Freeze image at end of systole (smallest RV cavity). Trace area; this is the systolic RV area (RVAs)		• RV FAC = (RVAd – RVAs)/RVAd • Expressed as a percentage • Normal values have been cited as 45–48% A normal Dobermann. Left apical four-chamber views optimizing the right heart. (a) Diastolic and (b) systolic areas have been traced to allow calculation of FAC (one method of assessing right ventricular function). In this example, the RV diastolic area was 10.95 cm² and the RV systolic area was 5.05 cm². The FAC is therefore calculated: FAC = [(10.95 – 5.05)/10.95] × 100% = 53.9%.

2.23 Assessment of right ventricular systolic function. CHF = congestive heart failure; FAC = fractional area change; HCM = hypertrophic cardiomyopathy; PW-TDI = pulsed wave tissue Doppler imaging; RV = right ventricle; RVA (with s or d) = right ventricle area (in systole or diastole); RVFW = right ventricular free wall; RVOT = right ventricular outflow tract; TAPSE = tricuspid annulus plane systolic excursion. (continues)

Acquisition of the image	Interpretation of the image	Observations, measurements or calculations
PW-TDI S' velocity from the RVFW		
• Left apical four-chamber view, optimizing the right heart • Make sure the ultrasound beam is parallel to the RVFW • PW-TDI sample volume placed at the base of the RVFW, tricuspid lateral annulus • Obtain PW-TDI spectra • Measure the velocity of the S' wave		• There is an influence of body size, so may need to be corrected for bodyweight • In most dogs, S' is over 10 cm/s

A Cavalier King Charles Spaniel with confirmed pulmonary thromboembolism. PW-TDI with cursor aligned with the RVFW at the tricuspid annulus. The S' velocity is over 10 cm/s, consistent with adequate RV systolic function. The RV diastolic function shows a possible impaired relaxation pattern, with the A' waves higher in velocity than the E' waves. However, there are no reference values or accepted methods of assessing right ventricular diastolic function.

2.23 (continued) Assessment of right ventricular systolic function. CHF = congestive heart failure; FAC = fractional area change; HCM = hypertrophic cardiomyopathy; PW-TDI = pulsed wave tissue Doppler imaging; RV = right ventricle; RVA (with s or d) = right ventricle area (in systole or diastole); RVFW = right ventricular free wall; RVOT = right ventricular outflow tract; TAPSE = tricuspid annulus plane systolic excursion.

Other echocardiography techniques

These are only briefly mentioned here, as they are beyond the scope of a standard Doppler echocardiographic examination in clinical patients. See also 'Endoscopic thoracic ultrasonography', below.

Colour tissue Doppler imaging: Most echocardiography machines with PW-TDI have superimposed colour tissue Doppler to allow cursor placement before switching to PW-TDI. Offline analysis of the colour tissue Doppler on the myocardial walls can give some additional information. As with any Doppler technique, the structure (myocardial wall) under interrogation must be parallel to the ultrasound beam. Colour tissue Doppler can provide information about:

- Longitudinal motion of the ventricular walls. There is a velocity gradient between the base and apex (higher velocities at the base)
- Radial motion of the interventricular septum and the left ventricular free wall. There is also a gradient between the endocardium and epicardium (higher velocities at the endocardium). Only the segment parallel to the ultrasound probe can be assessed.

Despite a number of veterinary publications in the late 1990s and first decade of the 2000s, interest has recently waned and most investigators prefer speckle tracking echocardiography (STE).

Speckle tracking echocardiography: This is an offline analysis technique applied to greyscale images of the myocardium. The unique specular pattern of each segment of myocardium can be followed through the cardiac cycle. There is no angle dependence since this is not a Doppler method. Myocardial deformation (e.g. shortening in systole, lengthening in diastole) (strain) is directly assessed and expressed as a percentage. Strain rate can be calculated. This can be applied to the different myocardial fibre orientations:

- Longitudinal fibres
- Radial fibres (around the whole of the LV short axis)
- Circumferential fibres (around the whole of the LV short axis)
- Rotation and torsion can be determined (the left ventricular base and apex move in opposing directions, giving twist or 'wringing out' of the LV during systole)
- Different myocardial layers can be assessed (e.g. endocardial to epicardial).

Although the LV was originally studied, a number of more recent publications describe the utility of STE in detailed assessment of the RV and left atrium. STE remains a research tool rather than a routinely used clinical tool at present. It should be noted that STE software on machines by different manufacturers does not generate the same results and is not interchangeable.

Four-dimensional echocardiography: Three-dimensional ultrasonography requires a dedicated transducer, which images in two orthogonal planes. With the image displayed in real time through the cardiac cycle, this is four-dimensional echocardiography (4DE). It requires specific software and considerable time offline. The transducers are bulky to hold, have lower frequency and slow frame rates, so they are better suited to larger canine patients. Transoesophageal transducers with 4D are also available. 4DE can facilitate planning prior to cardiac interventions. In the future, the role of 4DE may become even more important (e.g. to facilitate minimally invasive mitral valve repair). For cardiac chambers, quantification of chamber volume may be more accurate from 3D images.

Summary of overall approach

A systematic and logical approach to obtaining standard echocardiographic images and measurements is essential in the evaluation of a cardiac patient. A good understanding of the pathophysiology of cardiac disease is required to interpret echocardiographic abnormalities (see Chapter 9).

Comparison with reference ranges is essential, although breed-specific reference ranges are not available for all breeds. Weight-based reference indices are available for dog and cat breeds without their own reference values, based on allometric scaling.

Assessment of overall left ventricular systolic performance requires integration of 2D, M-mode and Doppler methods. Assessment of diastolic function and left-sided filling pressures may be challenging especially with tachycardia or arrhythmias. An integrated approach and comprehension of the influence of heart rate and loading condition are essential.

Endoscopic thoracic ultrasonography

Indications

Endoscopic ultrasonography (EUS) has many potential indications and the ability to overcome some of the limitations of standard transthoracic ultrasonography. EUS is a versatile procedure that has evolved in human medicine from a purely diagnostic tool to an interventional and even therapeutic one. EUS is used in humans to perform endobronchial fine-needle aspiration of lung lesions and mediastinal lymph nodes as an alternative to mediastinoscopy and thoracoscopy techniques; however, this has not been described in clinical veterinary practice yet.

Although standard transthoracic ultrasonography has become a valuable diagnostic procedure for the assessment of thoracic disease in small animals (see above), it is unrewarding for examining some intrathoracic anatomy. This includes the tracheobronchial lymph nodes, the oesophagus and lesions in the caudal mediastinum. Lesions not in contact with the thoracic wall are also difficult to detect as they are hidden from view by the aerated lungs or bony thorax. Obesity poses an additional barrier. These obstacles to visualizing intrathoracic structures can be overcome by the use of EUS.

EUS is a form of endoluminal scanning which allows high-frequency ultrasound transducers to be brought directly to the region of interest via conventional endoscopes placed in the oesophagus or bronchus. This imaging modality provides detailed images of pathological processes both within and outside the luminal wall. It has found most success in humans for staging of lung, gastric and oesophageal cancer. Although it was originally designed to improve diagnostics in clinical human gastroenterology, applications for endoscopic ultrasound technology have evolved to become multifaceted and include thoracic imaging.

Potential veterinary indications for EUS of the thorax include:

- Dysphagia of unknown origin
- Tumour staging
- Evaluation of tracheobronchial lymph nodes
- Investigation and localization of radiographic soft tissue opacities that do not have contact with the thoracic wall
- Evaluation of intrathoracic paravertebral masses
- Cardiac imaging (transoesophageal echocardiography)
- Assessment of infiltration of the oesophageal wall
- Differentiation of mediastinal *versus* pulmonary masses
- Detection of small amounts of pleural fluid
- EUS-guided fine-needle aspiration of intrathoracic and oesophageal lesions.

EUS examination of the thorax is advantageous for determining the origin of intrathoracic soft tissue lesions and masses. Soft tissue opacities in the caudal thorax may be of pulmonary, mediastinal, oesophageal, paravertebral or vertebral origin. Observation of the movement of solid lesions during respiration under anaesthesia often provides a clue as to their origin. Pulmonary lesions move with the lung's direction during inspiration and expiration, whereas mediastinal lesions and vertebral lesions do not. It can also be determined whether solid lesions in the region of the caudal lung lobes have attachments to the lungs or the diaphragm by observing their excursions during respiration. In addition, radiographic lesions of soft tissue opacity can be differentiated as being solid or fluid-filled using EUS.

Pyrexia of unknown origin may be a potential indication for EUS of the thorax (Figure 2.24). Oesophageal and perioesophageal lesions can also be further examined with EUS (Figure 2.25). Determination of oesophageal wall involvement in solid and cavitary masses is very helpful for presurgical planning and prognosis. Endoscopic ultrasound-guided transoesophageal tissue sampling of pulmonary, perioesophageal, mediastinal and oesophageal wall lesions in both cats and dogs can also be performed.

In humans, transoesophageal EUS is considered to be superior to CT in the detection of enlarged mediastinal lymph nodes. Malignant lymph nodes as small as 3 mm, which were not detected with CT, have been detected using EUS. The implementation of EUS and endoscopic ultrasound-guided fine-needle aspiration have allowed a less invasive and more cost-effective means of diagnosing metastasis in mediastinal disease compared with CT. EUS may have potential in veterinary oncology for accurate staging of thoracic metastases.

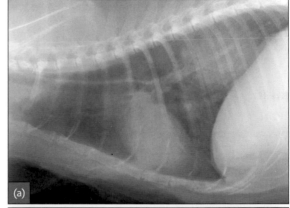
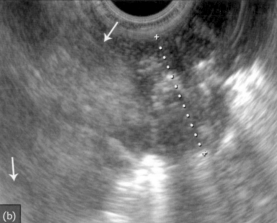

2.25 (a) Lateral thoracic radiograph of a 3 kg, 17-year-old neutered female cat with regurgitation and weight loss. A fairly well circumscribed soft tissue opaque lesion in the caudal thorax is shown with air-filled dilation of the oesophagus cranial to it. The lesion was shown to be midline on a ventrodorsal radiograph and suspected to originate in the mediastinum, most likely the oesophagus. (b) Endoscopic ultrasound image of a 5 cm homogeneous space-occupying lesion (between arrows), which involved the adjacent lung (indicated by calipers) as well as the oesophageal wall. Cytology of an endoscopic ultrasound-guided fine-needle aspirate of the lesion resulted in the diagnosis of oesophageal adenocarcinoma.

Restraint and patient preparation

EUS, like conventional endoscopy or CT, requires general anaesthesia. Patients should be prepared as for any routine endoscopic procedure. Positioning in left lateral recumbency is generally acceptable and once a position is

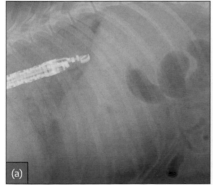
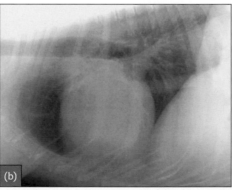
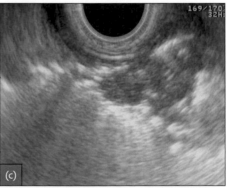

2.24 (a) Lateral thoracic radiograph of a canine cadaver, showing placement of the ultrasound endoscope for examination of the caudal lung lobes and mediastinum. (b) Lateral thoracic radiograph of a 76 kg, 5-year-old neutered male mixed-breed dog with recurrent pyrexia of unknown origin. The lungs were radiographically unremarkable and both transabdominal and transthoracic ultrasonography were unrewarding due to the large size of the dog. (c) Endoscopic ultrasound image of the dog in (b), showing a heterogeneous space-occupying lesion within the right caudal lung lobe. The margins are irregular and there is an expansile nature to the lesion seen by the pattern of air surrounding it. Lobectomy was performed and a chronic suppurative process with foreign material at its centre was diagnosed histologically.

adopted, it should be used repeatedly. This aids the beginner endosonographer in developing their endoscopic examination technique and recognition of important landmarks. Positioning in right lateral or ventral recumbency may be required, however, depending on the location of the lesion.

Technique

Equipment

Ultrasound endoscopes are similar to conventional endoscopes but with an ultrasound transducer attached at the tip (Figure 2.26). They also include the standard endoscopic features: optic, light source, working channel and video capabilities.

Ultrasound endoscopes can either be purchased for attachment to a compatible ultrasound machine or as all-in-one dedicated units. Two types of multifrequency transducers are available, radial and linear. High-quality colour and power Doppler ultrasonography is available on most scopes. Both large- and small-breed dogs, as well as cats, can be examined with the endoscope.

Transoesophageal examination method

In the EUS examination, intrathoracic structures are examined transoesophageally. Important landmarks include the thoracic inlet, cranial mediastinum and its great vessels, the base of the heart, bifurcation of the trachea, caudal vena cava, the thoracic vertebrae and intrathoracic aorta. Direct contact between the transducer and the oesophageal mucosa allows sufficient acoustic coupling in most cases. A condom-like stand-off balloon covering the transducer can be filled with water using the conventional buttons for suctioning and filling located on the scope handle.

Unlike conventional endoscopes, the echoendoscope has a much larger range of movement. The tip may be turned up to 90 degrees perpendicular to the long axis and in a 360-degree circle around it. This allows scanning in a large number of different planes.

Interpretation of the ultrasound views and anatomy is not as intuitive as in conventional transthoracic or transabdominal ultrasonography and a certain learning curve is required even for experienced ultrasonographers.

Fine-needle aspiration

Several aspiration needles of 22 G for solid organ sampling are available with a working handle. EUS can be used for fine-needle aspiration of various structures, including mediastinal and perioesophageal lymph nodes, aspiration of pleural fluid and pulmonary lesions. The aspiration technique is performed by endoscopic ultrasound-guided

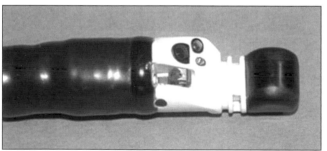

2.26 Olympus video endoscope. The scope is 1.25 m long with a multifrequency (5–10 MHz) linear transducer, 11.8 mm outer scope diameter at the insertional end and a 2.8 mm biopsy channel. Note that the endoscope is side-viewing (optics mounted at the side rather than the tip).

transoesophageal puncture and is generally performed with linear scanners. With radial scanners it is more difficult to visualize the tip of the needle because it appears only as a single point in the 360-degree image.

Many studies have been performed in humans and endoscopic ultrasound-guided fine-needle aspiration has been proven as feasible and safe. Bleeding, when it does occur, is usually self-limiting and appears as an echo-poor area adjacent to the sampled region. When this is detected, patients are typically treated with antibiotics and observed. Complications related to bacteraemia or infections have not been reported following transluminal fine-needle aspiration.

References and further reading

Affi A, Vazquez-Sequeiros E, Norton ID, Clain JE and Wiersema MJ (2001) Acute extraluminal hemorrhage associated with EUS-guided fine-needle aspiration: frequency and clinical significance. *Gastrointestinal Endoscopy* **53**, 221–225

Baron Toaldo M, Romito G, Guglielmini C *et al.* (2017) Assessment of left atrial deformation and function by 2-dimensional speckle tracking echocardiography in healthy dogs and dogs with myxomatous mitral valve disease. *Journal of Veterinary Internal Medicine* **31**, 641–649

Boon JA (2011) Veterinary Echocardiography, 2nd edn. Wylie-Blackwell, Ames

Bouvard J, Thierry F, Culshaw GJ *et al.* (2019) Assessment of left atrial volume in dogs: comparisons of two-dimensional and real-time three-dimensional echocardiography with ECG-gated multidetector computed tomography angiography. *Journal of Veterinary Cardiology* **24**, 64–77

Caivano D, Rishniw M, Birettoni F *et al.* (2018) Left atrial deformation and phasic function determined by two-dimensional speckle-tracking echocardiography in dogs with myxomatous mitral valve disease. *Journal of Veterinary Cardiology* **20**, 102–114

Caivano D, Rishniw M, Patata V *et al.* (2016) Left atrial deformation and phasic function determined by 2-dimensional speckle tracking echocardiography in healthy dogs. *Journal of Veterinary Cardiology* **18**, 146–155

Chetboul V, Gouni V, Sampedrano C *et al.* (2007) Radial strain and strain rate by two-dimensional speckle tracking echocardiography and the tissue velocity based technique in the dog. *Journal of Veterinary Cardiology* **9**, 69–81

Choi M, Lee N, Kim A *et al.* (2014) Evaluation of diaphragmatic motion in normal and diaphragmatic paralyzed dogs using M-mode ultrasonography. *Veterinary Radiology & Ultrasound* **55**, 102–108

Cornell CC, Kittleson MD, Della Torre P *et al.* (2004) Allometric scaling of M-mode cardiac measurements in normal adult dogs. *Journal of Veterinary Internal Medicine* **18**, 311–321

Dancygier H, Lightdale CJ and Stevens PD (1999) Endoscopic ultrasonography of the upper gastrointestinal tract and colon. In: *Endosonography in Gastroenterology. Principles, Techniques, Findings*, ed. H Dancygier and CJ Lightdale, pp. 13–168. CJ Thieme, New York

Domenech O and Oliveira P (2013) Transoesophageal echocardiography in the dog. *Veterinary Journal* **198**, 329–338

Doocy KR, Saunders AB, Gordon SG and Jeffery N (2018) Comparative, multidimensional imaging of patent ductus arteriosus and a proposed update to the morphology classification system for dogs. *Journal of Veterinary Internal Medicine* **32**, 648–657

Esser LC, Borkovec M, Bauer A *et al.* (2020) Left ventricular M-mode prediction intervals in 7651 dogs: Population-wide and selected breed-specific values. *Journal of Veterinary Internal Medicine* **34**, 2242–2252

Fries RC, Gordon SG, Saunders AB *et al.* (2019) Quantitative assessment of two- and three-dimensional transthoracic and two-dimensional transesophageal echocardiography, computed tomography, and magnetic resonance imaging in normal canine hearts. *Journal of Veterinary Cardiology* **21**, 79–92

Gaschen L, Kircher P and Lang J (2003) Endoscopic ultrasound instrumentation, applications in humans and potential veterinary applications. *Veterinary Radiology & Ultrasound* **44**, 665–680

Gaschen L, Kircher P, Hoffmann G *et al.* (2003) Endosonographic diagnosis of intrathoracic lesions. *Veterinary Radiology & Ultrasound* **44**, 292–299

Gress FG, Hawes RH, Savides TJ, Ikenberry SO and Lehman GA (1997) Endoscopic ultrasound-guided fine-needle aspiration biopsy using linear array and radial scanning endosonography. *Gastrointestinal Endoscopy* **45**, 243–250

Häggström J, Andersson AO, Falk T *et al.* (2016) Effect of body weight on echocardiographic measurements in 19,866 pure-bred cats with or without heart disease. *Journal of Veterinary Internal Medicine* **30**, 1601–1611

Hansson K, Häggström J, Kvart C and Lord P (2002) Left atrial to aortic root indices using two-dimensional and M-mode echocardiography in Cavalier King Charles Spaniels with and without left atrial enlargement. *Veterinary Radiology & Ultrasound* **43**, 568–575

Hwang TS, Yoon YM, Jung DI *et al.* (2018) Usefulness of transthoracic lung ultrasound for the diagnosis of mild pneumothorax. *Journal of Veterinary Science* **19**, 660–666

Konde LJ and Spaulding K (1991) Sonographic evaluation of the cranial mediastinum in small animals. *Veterinary Radiology & Ultrasound* **32**, 178–184

Lang RM, Badano LP, Mor-Avi V *et al.* (2015) Recommendations for cardiac chamber quantification by echocardiography in adults: an update from the American Society of Echocardiography and the European Association of Cardiovascular Imaging. *European Heart Journal Cardiovascular Imaging* **16**, 233–270

LeBlanc N, Scollan K and Sisson D (2016) Quantitative evaluation of left atrial volume and function by one-dimensional, two-dimensional, and three-dimensional echocardiography in a population of normal dogs. *Journal of Veterinary Cardiology* **18**, 336–349

Lisciandro GR, Lagutchik MS, Mann KA *et al.* (2008) Evaluation of a thoracic focused assessment with sonography for trauma (TFAST) protocol to detect pneumothorax and concurrent thoracic injury in 145 traumatized dogs. *Journal of Veterinary Emergency and Critical Care* **18**, 258–269

Menciotti G, Borgarelli M, Aherne M *et al.* (2016) Assessment of mitral valve morphology using three-dimensional echocardiography. Feasibility and reference values. *Journal of Veterinary Cardiology* **18**, 156–167

Nagueh SF, Smiseth OA, Appleton CP *et al.* (2016) Recommendations for the evaluation of left ventricular diastolic function by echocardiography: An update from the American Society of Echocardiography and the European Association of Cardiovascular Imaging. *Journal of the American Society of Echocardiography* **29**, 277–314

Pedro B, Stephenson H, Linney C *et al.* (2017) Assessment of left ventricular function in healthy Great Danes and in Great Danes with dilated cardiomyopathy using speckle tracking echocardiography. *Journal of Veterinary Cardiology* **19**, 363–375

Reichle JK and Wisner ER (2000) Non-cardiac thoracic ultrasound in 75 feline and canine patients. *Veterinary Radiology & Ultrasound* **41**, 154–162

Rishniw M and Erb HN (2000) Evaluation of four 2-dimensional echocardiographic methods of assessing left atrial size in dogs. *Journal of Veterinary Internal Medicine* **14**, 429–435

Rishniw M, Caivano D, Dickson D *et al.* (2019) Two-dimensional echocardiographic left- atrial-to-aortic ratio in healthy adult dogs: a re-examination of reference intervals. *Journal of Veterinary Cardiology* **26**, 29–38

Sahn DJ, DeMaria A, Kisslo J and Weyman A (1978) Recommendations regarding quantitation in M-mode echocardiography: results of a survey of echocardiographic measurements. *Circulation* **58**, 1072–1083

Santarelli G, Baron Toaldo M, Bouvard J *et al.* (2019) Variability among strain variables derived from two-dimensional speckle tracking echocardiography in dogs by use of various software. *American Journal of Veterinary Research* **80**, 347–357

Sargent J, Muzzi R, Mukherjee R *et al.* (2015) Echocardiographic predictors of survival in dogs with myxomatous mitral valve disease. *Journal of Veterinary Cardiology* **17**, 1–12

Schober KE and Chetboul V (2015) Echocardiographic evaluation of left ventricular diastolic function in cats: Hemodynamic determinants and pattern recognition. *Journal of Veterinary Cardiology* **17** Suppl 1, S102–S133

Schober KE, Bonagura JD, Scansen BA *et al.* (2008) Estimation of left ventricular filling pressure by use of Doppler echocardiography in healthy anesthetized dogs subjected to acute volume loading. *American Journal of Veterinary Research* **69**, 1034–1049

Schober KE, Hart TM, Stern JA *et al.* (2010) Detection of congestive heart failure in dogs by Doppler echocardiography. *Journal of Veterinary Internal Medicine* **24**, 1358–1368

Schober KE, Luis Fuentes V and Bonagura JD *et al.* (2003) Comparison between invasive hemodynamic measurements and noninvasive assessment of left ventricular diastolic function by use of Doppler echocardiography in healthy anesthetized cats. *American Journal of Veterinary Research* **64**, 93–103

Schober KE, Stern JA, DaCunha DN *et al.* (2008) Estimation of left ventricular filling pressure by Doppler echocardiography in dogs with pacing-induced heart failure. *Journal of Veterinary Internal Medicine* **22**, 578–585

Sieslack AK, Dziallas P, Nolte I *et al.* (2014) Quantification of right ventricular volume in dogs: a comparative study between three-dimensional echocardiography and computed tomography with the reference method magnetic resonance imaging. *BMC Veterinary Research* **10**, 242

Spalla I, Boswood A, Connolly DJ and Luis Fuentes V (2019) Speckle tracking echocardiography in cats with preclinical hypertrophic cardiomyopathy. *Journal of Veterinary Internal Medicine* **33**, 1232–1241

Spalla I, Payne JR, Borgeat K *et al.* (2017) Mitral annular plane systolic excursion and tricuspid annular plane systolic excursion in cats with hypertrophic cardiomyopathy. *Journal of Veterinary Internal Medicine* **31**, 691–699

Spalla I, Payne JR, Borgeat K *et al.* (2018) Prognostic value of mitral annular systolic plane excursion and tricuspid annular plane systolic excursion in cats with hypertrophic cardiomyopathy. *Journal of Veterinary Cardiology* **20**, 154–164

Strohm LE, Visser LC, Chapel EH *et al.* (2018) Two-dimensional, long-axis echocardiographic ratios for assessment of left atrial and ventricular size in dogs. *Journal of Veterinary Cardiology* **20**, 330–342

Suzuki R, Mochizuki Y, Yoshimatsu H *et al.* (2016) Myocardial torsional deformations in cats with hypertrophic cardiomyopathy using two-dimensional speckle-tracking echocardiography. *Journal of Veterinary Cardiology* **18**, 350–357

Suzuki R, Mochizuki Y, Yoshimatsu H *et al.* (2019) Layer-specific myocardial function in asymptomatic cats with obstructive hypertrophic cardiomyopathy assessed using 2-dimensional speckle-tracking echocardiography. *Journal of Veterinary Internal Medicine* **33**, 37–45

Thomas WP, Gaber CE, Jacobs GJ *et al.* (1993) Recommendations for standards in transthoracic two-dimensional echocardiography in the dog and cat. Echocardiography Committee of the Specialty of Cardiology, American College of Veterinary Internal Medicine. *Journal of Veterinary Internal Medicine* **7**, 247–252

Tidwell AS (1998) Ultrasonography of the thorax (excluding the heart). *Veterinary Clinics of North America: Small Animal Practice* **28**, 993–1015

Visser LC, Ciccozzi MM, Sintov DJ and Sharpe AN (2019) Echocardiographic quantitation of left heart size and function in 122 healthy dogs: A prospective study proposing reference intervals and assessing repeatability. *Journal of Veterinary Internal Medicine* **33**,1909–1920

Visser LC, Scansen BA, Schober KE and Bonagura JD *et al.* (2015) Echocardiographic assessment of right ventricular systolic function in conscious healthy dogs: repeatability and reference intervals. *Journal of Veterinary Cardiology* **17**, 83–96

Visser LC, Sloan CQ and Stern JA (2017) Echocardiographic assessment of right ventricular size and function in cats with hypertrophic cardiomyopathy. *Journal of Veterinary Internal Medicine* **31**, 668–677

Ward JL, Lisciandro GR, Ware WA *et al* . (2018) Evaluation of point-of-care thoracic ultrasound and NT-proBNP for the diagnosis of congestive heart failure in cats with respiratory distress. *Journal of Veterinary Internal Medicine* **32**, 1530–1540

Ward JL, Schober KE, Luis Fuentes V and Bonagura JD (2012) Effects of sedation on echocardiographic variables of left atrial and left ventricular function in healthy cats. *Journal of Feline Medicine and Surgery* **14**, 678–685

Wess G, Domenech O, Dukes-McEwan J *et al.* (2017) European Society of Veterinary Cardiology screening guidelines for dilated cardiomyopathy in Doberman Pinschers. *Journal of Veterinary Cardiology* **19**, 405–415

Wess G, Keller LJ, Klausnitzer M *et al.* (2011) Comparison of longitudinal myocardial tissue velocity, strain, and strain rate measured by two-dimensional speckle tracking and by color tissue Doppler imaging in healthy dogs. *Journal of Veterinary Cardiology* **13**, 31–43

Wess G, Maurer J, Simak J and Hartmann K (2010) Use of Simpson's method of disc to detect early echocardiographic changes in Doberman Pinschers with dilated cardiomyopathy. *Journal of Veterinary Internal Medicine* **24**, 1069–1076

Westrup U and McEvoy FJ (2013) Speckle tracking echocardiography in mature Irish Wolfhound dogs: technical feasibility, measurement error and reference intervals. *Acta Veterinaria Scandinavica* **55**, 41

Wood EF, O'Brien RT and Young KM (1998) Ultrasound-guided fine-needle aspiration of focal parenchymal lesions of the lung in dogs and cats. *Journal of Veterinary Internal Medicine* **12**, 338–342

Zoghbi WA, Adams D, Bonow RO *et al.* (2017) Recommendations for noninvasive evaluation of native valvular regurgitation: A report from the American Society of Echocardiography developed in collaboration with the Society for Cardiovascular Magnetic Resonance. *Journal of the American Society of Echocardiography* **30**, 303–371

Zois NE, Olsen NT, Moesgaard SG *et al.* (2013) Left ventricular twist and circumferential strain in dogs with myxomatous mitral valve disease. *Journal of Veterinary Internal Medicine* **27**, 875–883

Zois NE, Tidholm A, Nagga KM *et al.* (2012) Radial and longitudinal strain and strain rate assessed by speckle-tracking echocardiography in dogs with myxomatous mitral valve disease. *Journal of Veterinary Internal Medicine* **26**, 1309–1319

Chapter 3

Basics of thoracic computed tomography

Tobias Schwarz

Indications

Computed tomography (CT) can be used in dogs and cats with suspected thoracic disease as a first-line diagnostic tool or in combination with other imaging modalities. CT is more sensitive than radiography for the identification of many specific disease processes, their extent and organ involvement as well as progression. Combining thoracic CT with radiography and ultrasonography is often useful for time-efficient monitoring of disease and sampling procedures. CT is especially helpful for traumatic, infectious/inflammatory, neoplastic and developmental disorders, as these conditions frequently produce morphological changes that are readily observed on CT images.

Thoracic boundaries

Determination of the extent of palpable thoracic wall masses is essential for surgical planning. This determination often cannot be made accurately using radiography alone. Examples include vaccine-related feline fibrosarcomas or rib tumours with unknown expansion into the thoracic cavity (Figure 3.1). CT is also helpful for diagnosing and characterizing herniations of abdominal viscera into the pleural and pericardial cavities associated with defects in the diaphragm.

Pleural space

CT is very useful for the investigation of pleural abnormalities such as pleural effusion and masses. It can distinguish soft tissue masses from fluid, and identify and differentiate collapsed and consolidated lung lobes. CT is often not very helpful for identifying the cause of pneumothorax and offers little additional information over radiography.

Mediastinum including heart and major vessels

CT is an excellent imaging modality for many mediastinal disorders. Cardiovascular CT has gained a foothold in veterinary medicine, but the gold standard for most cardiac conditions is echocardiography. CT has been shown to be particularly useful to demonstrate:

- Sternal, cranial mediastinal and tracheobronchial lymphadenopathy, for oncological staging and presurgical planning

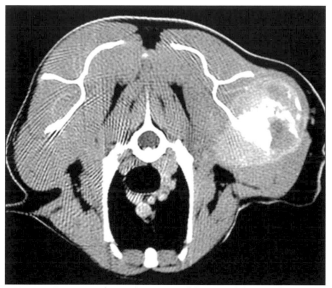

3.1 Contrast-enhanced CT image of the cranial thorax of an 8-year-old Domestic Longhaired cat with a mineralized sarcoma arising from the caudal aspect of the left scapula. This image is set with a narrow window (level 65 HU, width 187 HU) to emphasize the peripheral contrast enhancement of the mass at the expense of creating increased visibility of image noise and streak artefacts. The lungs cannot be appropriately assessed with this window.

- Cranial and caudal mediastinal masses and cysts (Figure 3.2)
- Oesophageal masses (spirocercosis, neoplasia)
- Aortic mineralization, aneurysm and parasitic infection (spirocercosis)
- Pericardial rupture and cardiac herniation
- Caval thrombosis and obstruction (Budd–Chiari-like syndrome)
- Heart base tumours
- Pneumomediastinum.

Airways and lungs

CT is an excellent modality to investigate suspected airway and lung pathology. Particularly useful indications are:

- Tracheal obstruction and rupture
- Bronchial obstruction, rupture and thickening, peribronchial infiltrate
- Oncological staging and presurgical planning (Figure 3.3)

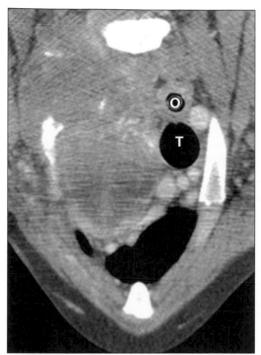

3.2 Contrast-enhanced CT image of the cranial mediastinum in a 6-year-old Labrador Retriever with an extraskeletal osteosarcoma. The image is set with a narrow window (level 70 HU, width 220 HU). The mass extended from the mid-cervical region to the cranial mediastinum where it deviated and compressed contrast-enhanced blood vessels, the trachea (T) and the oesophagus (O). There is also compression of the cranial lung lobes.

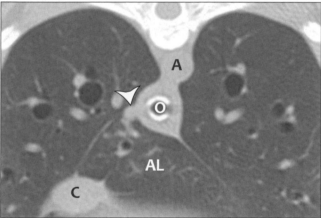

3.3 High-resolution CT image (1 mm slice width, 1 second rotation time, high spatial algorithm) of the caudodorsal thorax of a 10-year-old Miniature Poodle with a salivary adenocarcinoma. The image is set with a centre in the negative HU range and a wide window (level -744 HU, width 2456 HU). There is a single small lung nodule (arrowhead) in the dorsal aspect of the accessory lung lobe (AL) assessed as a potential metastasis. This nodule was not seen on thoracic radiographs. A post-chemotherapy treatment follow-up CT examination 4 weeks later revealed no growth of the nodule. A = aorta; C = caudal vena cava; O = catheterized oesophagus.

- All interstitial lung diseases
- Exact location, nature and extent of pulmonary masses and bullae
- Pulmonary thromboembolism
- Lung lobe torsion
- Differentiation between collapsed and consolidated lung lobes.

Restraint and patient preparation

Modern multislice helical CT scanners with 16 or more detector rows enable scanning of the canine and feline thorax in 10–30 seconds. This has changed the patient preparation requirements over the last 10 years.

- Sedation with additional physical restraint is adequate for most thoracic CT examinations in dogs (Figure 3.4).
- Cats can be placed in a custom designed restraining device (Figure 3.5). The VetCat Trap device allows safe and diagnostic quality CT imaging of cats and other similar sized animals, including intravenous contrast-enhanced CT. In dyspnoeic cats, conscious CT allows acquisition of diagnostic quality images within 10 to 30 seconds with minimal additional stress to the patient. Sedation is beneficial in cats who are bright, alert and responsive, or in pain. Diagnostic quality images can be reliably achieved in cats for all body parts except the head and neck, in which motion or non-symmetrical posture can hamper interpretation.
- General anaesthesia is required for patients undergoing CT-assisted interventional procedures such as fine-needle aspiration (FNA) and in critically ill patients, in which general anaesthesia is deemed safer than sedation. In patients with severe hyperpnoea, the constant movement of the lungs can lead to marked motion artefacts, rendering the CT study non-diagnostic. This is particularly relevant for pulmonary angiography CT studies. In these patients, general anaesthesia might be necessary to reduce the respiration rate or create temporary apnoea.
- Anaesthetic and monitoring equipment should be placed in such a way that the tubes and lines connecting it to the patient do not cross the gantry of the CT scanner, since they create major artefacts. This means equipment should be placed behind the CT scanner in a 'head first' set-up and in front of the scanning unit in a 'tail first' set-up (Figure 3.6).

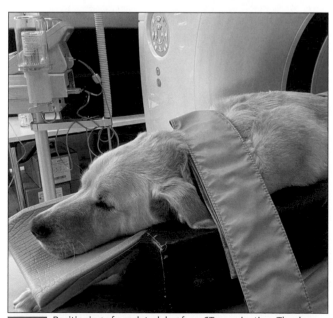

3.4 Positioning of a sedated dog for a CT examination. The dog has been safely anchored to the table in ventral recumbency with the help of a foam trough, a foam wedge for the head and Velcro bands.

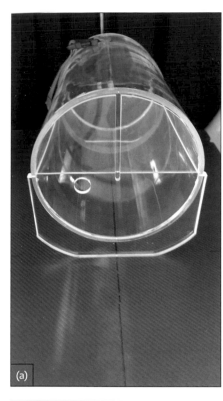

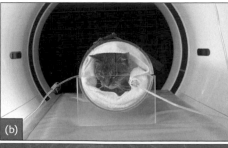

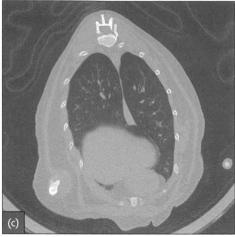

3.5 (a) The VetCat Trap CT device positioned on the CT table and aligned with the positioning laser lights. (b) A sedated Domestic Shorthaired cat undergoing a CT examination in a VetCat Trap device for cancer restaging. The cat is cushioned with towels and the device is closed with a strap. Intravenous contrast medium is delivered from a power injector via the left tube and oxygen is supplied via the connected tube on the right. (c) High-resolution CT image of the same cat showing the lungs along with parts of the device and cushioning material.
(b, courtesy of Misha Jarrett)

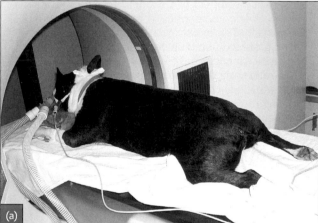

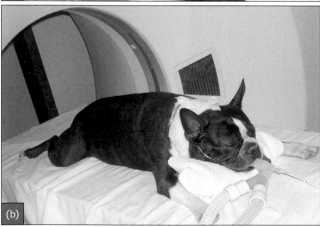

3.6 (a) An anaesthetized Boston Terrier in ventral recumbency and 'head first' position on the CT table. Notice the anaesthetic tubing and pulse oximetry cable crossing the gantry, which can create significant artefacts. (b) The same dog in ventral recumbency and 'tail first' position. When the thorax is scanned, the anaesthetic equipment will not cross the gantry and artefacts will be avoided. Notice the extended thoracic limbs are positioned outside the scanning area. Electrocardiography clips (not seen here) should be placed well cranial or caudal to the scanning area.

Regardless of patient position, there should always be sufficient length of the connections to allow adequate bed movement during the scan.

- CT is a modified X-ray technique that emits relatively high levels of ionizing radiation. Therefore, patient restraint must be sufficient for all personnel to be able to leave the CT room for the duration of the scan. It is possible to use mobile shielding devices that are designated for CT use for interventional procedures, provided all radiation safety measures are observed.
- It is imperative to securely anchor the patient to the CT table with large Velcro straps or other positioning devices designed for CT. Sandbags and other radiopaque positioning devices used in conventional radiography are usually unsuitable because they create major artefacts when located in the scan field and tend to fall off the CT table, which is much narrower than a conventional X-ray table.
- Care must be taken to avoid overt restriction of thoracic expansion, particularly in patients that already have compromised respiration. The use of an appropriately sized radiographic trough can be very helpful in this respect (see Figures 3.4 and 3.7).
- The patient should be positioned according to the nature of the study:
  - In general, ventral recumbency works best for thoracic wall, pleural, mediastinal, cardiovascular and airway studies
  - For abnormalities close to the thoracic vertebral column, dorsal recumbency is preferred because the recumbent side is not affected by respiratory movement
  - For studies focusing on lung parenchyma, physiological hypostatic lung collapse during anaesthesia should be considered. For example, if ventral lung disease is suspected, then dorsal recumbency is preferable (if tolerated by the patient). This will avoid the development of atelectasis in the area of interest. If lung changes consistent with atelectasis are seen on initial CT images, the scan

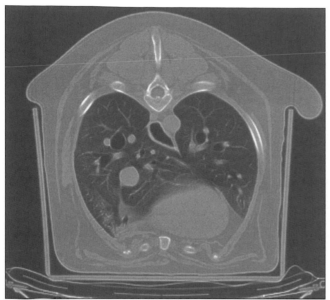

3.7 The 'canine muffin' sign. Occasionally, CT offers completely unexpected new vistas. This 4-year-old Saint Bernard was positioned for a thoracic CT scan in the largest trough available. The CT image of the caudal thorax reveals a muffin-shaped cross-sectional anatomy of the dog, indicating that the trough was not big enough and was potentially restricting respiration.

should be repeated with the patient positioned so that non-aerated lung lobes are non-dependent. In cases of hypostatic atelectasis, the affected lung tissue will regain aeration; if pathologically altered, it will remain atelectatic (see Chapter 12)

- If CT-guided biopsy or aspiration is planned, then the patient should be positioned with the biopsy side up or on the side
- Whether the dog is positioned 'head first' or 'tail first' is of little consequence for a thoracic CT examination other than for the anaesthetic set-up (see above).
- The thoracic limbs should be extended and placed parallel to the cervical vertebral column. Limb extension can be secured with the help of tape. Metallic monitoring devices such as electrocardiography clips should be positioned outside the scan area (see Figure 3.6).
- Respiratory control used to be critical for a diagnostic CT examination; however, with modern CT scanners, the examination time is very short, reducing the chance of significant motion artefacts. If the patient is under general anaesthesia, there are several strategies to achieve respiratory control:
  - Natural respiratory pause imaging. Each exposure is manually acquired at the onset of the respiratory pause at end-expiration. Tape markers on the patient can be helpful to identify the pause in the respiratory cycle. This is technically the simplest method and sometimes the only practical means to achieve a diagnostic scan. However, it is difficult to achieve consistently high image quality. It cannot be used for a helical CT scan
  - Induced respiratory pause imaging. The patient is hyperventilated rigorously for several minutes immediately prior to starting the scan. Most patients will then not breathe for 30–60 seconds, which is sufficient for most CT scans to be completed. This is the most commonly used technique for helical thoracic CT scans in

anaesthetized animals. The scan can also be interrupted should breathing commence and the manoeuvre repeated. Prolonged hyperventilation can be difficult to achieve with certain anaesthetic systems. Hyperventilation should not be performed unless it is safe to do so

- End-inspiratory breath-hold imaging is the standard for most human lung CT studies but is difficult to achieve with animals who are rarely trained to hold their breath on command. Maintaining a breath hold at inspiration can be achieved with a specific anaesthetic set-up that allows complete X-ray shielding for the monitoring anaesthetist
- Pharmacological control of respiration has been mainly used in research studies so far. In expert hands it can be a valuable tool.

Technique

Techniques for thoracic CT depend on the organ of interest. A study on a single animal may include several image sequences to evaluate the pulmonary parenchyma, mediastinal structures, ribs and thoracic wall.

- For mediastinal and other soft tissue structures, a 2–5 mm slice width, narrow window (level 50–100 HU, width 180–300 HU) should be used. The same is true for any contrast medium enhanced study to maximize contrast resolution (see Figures 3.1 and 3.2).
- For high-resolution pulmonary parenchymal imaging, a narrow slice width (0.5–1 mm), high kVp and mA, high-resolution reconstruction algorithms and small field of view should be chosen. A wide window (level -800 to -400 HU, width 1500–3000 HU) should be used for viewing (see Figures 3.3 and 3.5c).
- For CT screening of pulmonary metastatic disease, a high-resolution technique can be used to achieve maximal detail of potential lung nodules (0.5–1 mm slice width, helical respiratory pause imaging). Sufficient detail can also be achieved with thicker slices (5 mm), but the exact threshold of detectable nodule size with the different techniques has not been established.
- The tube rotation time should be kept at minimum (usually less than 1 second) for any thoracic study, to reduce the effect of motion.
- If induced respiratory pause imaging is used (see above), then it is always advantageous to scan the thorax in a caudocranial direction. This ensures the area of the highest respiratory motion amplitude is scanned first while the patient is still apnoeic.
- Sagittal and dorsal reconstructions are very useful to assess lesions identified on transverse images if a high image quality can be achieved. The image quality of orthogonal reconstructions depends on the slice width and interval (pitch in helical CT) (Figure 3.8).

CT-assisted fine-needle thoracic aspiration

CT-assisted FNA (Figure 3.9) is a valuable diagnostic tool where samples cannot be obtained via direct or ultrasound-guided techniques, such as from abnormalities that are surrounded by aerated lung. Compared with ultrasound-guided FNA, the sampling is not performed under real-time imaging control and the set-up is more time consuming. The manual technique involves several steps:

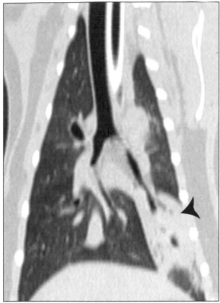

3.8 Dorsal plane CT image of an 11-year-old Domestic Shorthaired cat with a cavitated mass in its left caudal lung lobe (arrowhead). The image was reconstructed from a helical CT series with 1 mm slice thickness and a pitch of 1, resulting in an image resolution close to the transverse plane images. The main advantages of this plane are better alignment of the lesion with the bronchial and vascular tree and increased viewing area.

1. Identify lesion with CT scan and surgically prepare adjacent thoracic wall.
2. Place and secure needle along the transverse plane of the patient with tip subcutaneously inserted. The needles should be aligned with the positional laser lights along the transverse plane of the patient (Figure 3.9a).
3. CT scan the area of interest of anaesthetized patient with preliminary needle placement.
4. Assess from CT image the anticipated angle and depth of needle placement to hit the target and avoid vital structures (Figure 3.9b).
5. It is beneficial to hyperventilate the patient prior to the procedure to create a prolonged respiratory pause to minimize the chance of lung laceration. However, no further hyperventilation should be performed after the first aspiration.
6. Connect syringe, advance needle, harvest sample and retrieve needle as planned without direct CT monitoring.
7. Repeat entire procedure for the next sample, except for the hyperventilation.
8. Recheck CT scan for complications such as bleeding or pneumothorax (Figure 3.9c).

The author does not recommend performing full-core thoracic biopsies with the technique described above.

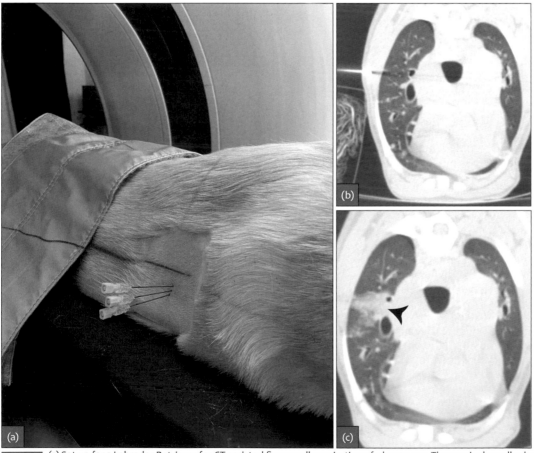

3.9 (a) Set-up for a Labrador Retriever for CT-assisted fine-needle aspiration of a lung mass. Three spinal needles have been placed with the needle tips in the thoracic wall muscles aligned with the laser light, along the transverse image plane of the patient. (b) Mid-thoracic CT image of a 3-year-old crossbreed dog with tracheobronchial lymphadenopathy, demonstrating the set-up for CT-assisted transpulmonary fine-needle lymph node aspiration. The needle is supported by a box, aligned with the image plane, and advanced subcutaneously (left side of image). A black streak artefact emanates from the needle tip. From this image, the depth and angle of needle advancement can be planned, and aspiration then pursued accordingly. (c) CT image from a recheck scan of the same dog as in (b). There is a small area of pulmonary haemorrhage along the needle track (arrowhead) and a small pneumothorax (not seen here). The dog recovered uneventfully from anaesthesia and a granulomatous lymphadenopathy was diagnosed.

References and further reading

Johnson VS, Corcoran BM, Wotton PR, Schwarz T and Sullivan M (2005) Thoracic high-resolution computed tomographic findings in dogs with canine idiopathic pulmonary fibrosis. *Journal of Small Animal Practice* **46**, 381–388

Johnson VS, Ramsey IK, Thompson H *et al.* (2004) Thoracic high-resolution computed tomography in the diagnosis of metastatic carcinoma. *Journal of Small Animal Practice* **44**, 134–143

Nemanic S, London CA and Wisner ER (2006) Comparison of thoracic radiographs and single breath-hold helical CT for detection of pulmonary nodules in dogs with metastatic neoplasia. *Journal of Veterinary Internal Medicine* **20**, 508–515

Oliveira CR, Mitchell MA and O'Brien RT (2011) Thoracic computed tomography in feline patients without use of chemical restraint. *Veterinary Radiology & Ultrasound* **52**, 41–52

Oliveira CR, Ranallo FN, Pijanowski GJ *et al.* (2011) The VetMouseTrapTM: A device for computed tomographic imaging of the thorax of awake cats. *Veterinary Radiology & Ultrasound* **52**, 368–376

Saunders J and Schwarz T (2011) Principles of CT image interpretation. In: *Veterinary Computed Tomography*, ed. T Schwarz and J Saunders, pp. 29–34. Wiley-Blackwell, Oxford

Schwarz T and O'Brien R (2011) CT acquisition principles. In: *Veterinary Computed Tomography*, ed. T Schwarz and J Saunders, pp. 9–28. Wiley-Blackwell, Oxford

Vignoli M, Ohlerth S, Rossi F *et al.* (2004) Computed tomography-guided fine-needle aspiration and tissue-core biopsy of bone lesions in small animals. *Veterinary Radiology & Ultrasound* **45**, 125–130

Chapter 4

Basics of thoracic magnetic resonance imaging

Maurizio Longo and Anthony Fischetti

Indications

In small animals, thoracic magnetic resonance imaging (MRI) is indicated for further investigation of thoracic wall lesions and intrathoracic masses detected with other imaging techniques, especially if computed tomography (CT) is not available. Cardiac MRI is a more recent clinical application, more often applied in human medicine, that is non-invasive and provides morphological and functional information about the heart.

Thoracic wall

MRI is indicated in the evaluation of thoracic wall lesions, such as lipomatous masses, migrating foreign bodies, soft tissue malignancies (e.g. feline injection site sarcoma) or rib tumours, particularly for surgical planning.

* Lipomatous masses can be readily recognized by hyperintensity on T1-weighted and T2-weighted sequences, along with signal suppression in fat-saturated images and short tau inversion recovery (STIR).
* Foreign bodies typically appear hypointense relative to muscle and fat on both T1-weighted and T2-weighted sequences, often with a geometrical shape, and hypointense to signal void on T2* gradient echo images. The chronic presence of a foreign body is associated with a surrounding inflammatory response, characterized by hypointensity on T1-weighted images and hyperintensity on T2-weighted images with a marked contrast enhancement, which might help with localization of the foreign body. Other possible features are the presence of fluid pockets, fistulae with a ring-enhancing wall and purulent or necrotic luminal content, chronic haemorrhage and gas pocketing.
* Abscesses appear hypointense on T1-weighted images, as do fluid collections and necrosis, with a typical ring enhancement on post-contrast T1-weighted sequences and mass effect on surrounding structures.
* Feline injection site sarcomas are usually heterogeneously hyperintense relative to local muscles on T1-weighted and T2-weighted images with a predilection for mineralization in larger masses, appearing as signal voids. Overall, a moderate to marked heterogeneous contrast enhancement

characterizes this type of neoplasia. The use of fat-saturated contrast-enhanced T1-weighted images could be helpful in delineating the macroscopic extension of the tumour with more accurate delineation of the number of muscles infiltrated by the neoplasm (Figure 4.1).
* Rib lesions are characterized by loss of the normal shape and margin of the thoracic cage by a well defined mass surrounding the rib and displacing adjacent bony structures (Figure 4.2). Often pleural effusion is also present.

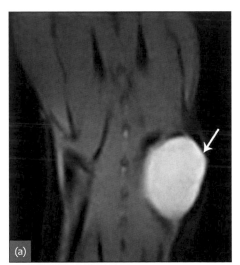

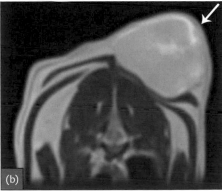

4.1 (a) Dorsal STIR and (b) transverse T2-weighted images of an adult Domestic Shorthaired cat in ventral recumbency with an injection-site sarcoma in the left interscapular region (arrowed). These images were acquired with a low-field MRI magnet (0.2 Tesla).

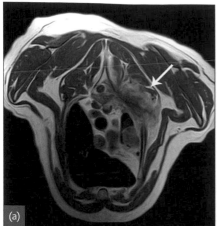

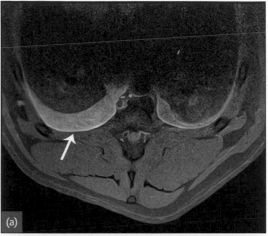

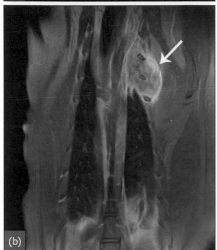

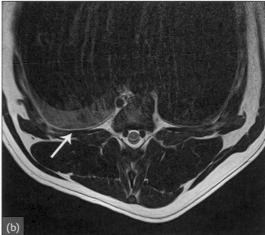

4.2 (a) Transverse T2-weighted and (b) dorsal STIR images of an 8-year-old Maine Coon cat in ventral recumbency with a left thoracic wall mass (arrowed). On the transverse image, severe rib osteolysis is visible.

4.3 (a) Transverse T1 fat-saturated and (b) T2-weighted images of a 2-year-old adult Borzoi in dorsal recumbency. Pleural effusion is present, with different intensity compared with the chest wall and lungs on both sequences (arrowed).

Diaphragm

MRI is discouraged for the investigation of traumatic diaphragmatic hernias due to respiratory motion and longer examination time compared with other imaging techniques. However, herniated content through congenital or traumatic diaphragmatic defects may be observed as an incidental finding during MRI examination of other regions, such as the back.

Pleural space

MRI may be used to evaluate the pleural interface, characterize pleural effusion and identify exudate and haemorrhages.

- In human medicine, the reported MRI findings suggestive of pleural malignancies are circumferential pleural thickening, nodularity and infiltration of the chest wall or diaphragm.
- Unlike CT, MRI may improve the identification of parenchymal and pleural lesions in the presence of pleural effusion, which allows a better depiction of the different signal intensities within the thoracic cavity (Figure 4.3).
- Pyothorax is associated with particulate pleural effusion, most commonly with a unilateral distribution due to the inspissated nature of the content, characterized by higher T1-weighted and lower T2-weighted signal intensity compared with other types of fluids which usually display a high T2 signal intensity.

Non-vascular mediastinum

MRI can be used to evaluate mediastinal structures, such as the oesophagus, thoracic duct, thymus and lymph nodes.

- Lymph nodes show peripheral low to intermediate signal intensity on T1-weighted and T2-weighted images, with a hyperintense central fatty hilus that is generally compressed in the case of metastatic or neoplastic disease (Figure 4.4). Specific lymphotrophic contrast media, such as ultra-small paramagnetic iron oxide particles, have been developed in animal experimental models for the detection of nodal metastasis for tumour staging.
- The canine thoracic duct and the cisterna chyli can be identified as hyperintense linear structures on fluid-sensitive sequences, such as T2-weighted transverse images and three-dimensional single-shot fast spin echo (3D SS-FSE) images with respiratory gating. The use of T2-weighted fat-saturated images may also improve their identification, suppressing the signal intensity from the surrounding mediastinal fat.
- The oesophagus can be seen as a tubular structure with low signal intensity surrounded by a thin fat-tissue hyperintensity. MRI can be used to assess oesophageal masses (neoplasia, granuloma) as well as the presence of incidental oesophageal reflux, which is

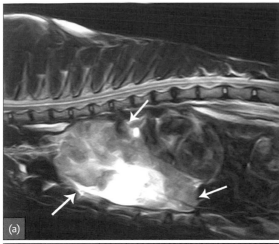

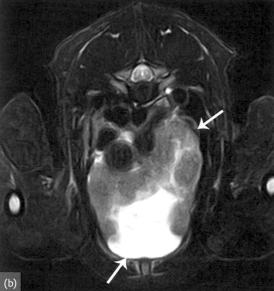

4.4 (a) Sagittal and (b) transverse T2-weighted images of a 15-year-old Domestic Shorthaired cat with a mediastinal expansile mass compatible with a diagnosis of thymoma (arrowed).

a common finding due to the dorsal recumbency commonly used to investigate the vertebral column.

- In human imaging, the MRI appearance of the thymus changes with age as it is replaced by fatty tissue, characterized by a progressive T1 shortening while T2 hyperintensity remains constant. The thymic signal can appear similar to lymph nodes, making identification of the latter challenging especially in the absence of pathology.

Heart and major vessels

In 20 years, cardiac MRI of dogs and cats has grown from experimental studies modelling human conditions to be clinically applicable to naturally occurring diseases common in veterinary medicine.

Cardiac image acquisition

- Standardized imaging protocols for cardiac MRI have only recently been addressed in publications; protocol and scan plane depend on whether cardiac structure or function is to be assessed. Performed properly, cardiac MRI examinations provide exquisite contrast of soft tissues and fluid, unparalleled by other modalities.

- *Black blood studies* (spin echo sequences) assess heart structure by providing unparalleled contrast between the lumen and surrounding soft tissues. By suppressing the signal of flowing blood, regional tissues like the heart walls and pericardium appear as varied shades of high signal contrasting against the lumen (Figure 4.5). These spin echo sequences have inherent drawbacks in temporal resolution; cine images are not feasible.
- *Bright blood studies* (gradient echo sequences) assess heart function such as blood flow volume, velocity and disruption (e.g. regurgitation); laminar flow has a higher signal (more bright) than turbulent flow. Cine images can be acquired rapidly for excellent temporal resolution (Figure 4.6). Because of the higher signal in the lumen, contrast between the blood and walls is lower than it is in black blood studies.

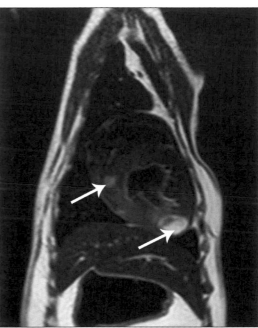

4.5 Dorsal cardiac image (black blood study) identifying two hyperintense lesions in the heart wall of a dog (arrowed) – a larger nodule at the apex and a small nodule associated with the interventricular septum. Only the larger lesion was identified on echocardiography. The lesions were presumed to be metastases from a confirmed splenic haemangiosarcoma.

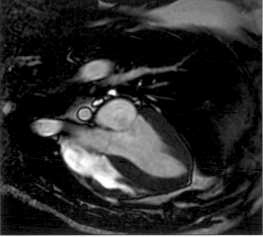

4.6 Bright blood study of a normal canine heart, single image of a cine loop. Image plane optimized for assessing mitral and aortic valves.
(Courtesy of Chris Warren-Smith)

- As with other protocols in ill patients, the greater number of signals acquired improves resolution, but at the expense of time. A balance must be reached between image quality to answer a specific question and length of anaesthesia for acquiring images.
- Specific hardware and software requirements for cardiac MRI include electrocardiogram (ECG)-gating (signal triggered usually on the R wave) and respiratory triggers/breath holds to reduce motion artefact, as well as MRI-safe anaesthesia equipment and coils that surround the thorax (e.g. wraparound chest coil or surface coil).

Indications

- Thoracic radiography and echocardiography remain the dominant imaging modalities for evaluation of the heart but cardiac MRI can provide additional information regarding extent of disease (e.g. pericardial involvement, great vessel invasion) for surgical or radiation planning (Figure 4.7). Structural details of congenital cardiac anomalies have also been described with cardiac MRI, supplementing echocardiographical findings.
- Cardiac MRI can be used to assess the extent of cardiac tumour involvement but, in clinical practice, CT angiocardiography is more often preferred due to cost, availability and shorter image acquisition time. In humans, cardiac MRI is the modality of choice for evaluation of cardiac tumours.
- Cardiac MRI can be used to assess abnormalities seen on radiographs that are not seen or are less defined on echocardiograms (e.g. aneurysmal right auricle, Figure 4.8).

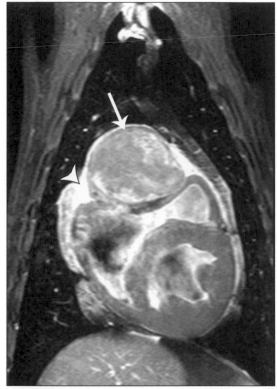

4.7 Dorsal, fat-saturated T2-weighted cardiac image (black blood study) of a large right atrial and auricular mass in a dog. In this plane, the mass compresses the free wall of the right ventricle (arrowed). Concurrent pericardial effusion surrounds the mass and heart (arrowhead). Complete suppression of blood flow could only be achieved for the most centrally located laminar blood in the ventricles.

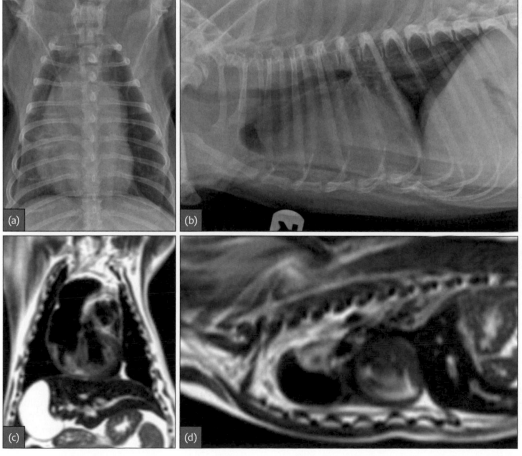

4.8 (a) Ventrodorsal and (b) right lateral thoracic radiographs of a dog. Notice the increased soft tissue opacity of the cranial mediastinum continuous with the cardiac silhouette. The soft tissue has a rounded cranial border and may be contributing to some degree of rightward displacement of the trachea at the level of the heart base. (c) Dorsal and (d) sagittal cardiac MR images (black blood study) show the source of the increased radiographic soft tissue opacity as a focal right auricular dilatation. The pericardium is intact cranially, outlined by hyperintense intrapericardial and mediastinal fat. Suppression of blood flow is nearly complete in all the visible heart chambers.

- More technically challenging indications for cardiac MRI involve assessment of cardiac function, including measurement of chamber volume, quantification of blood flow and determination of mitral regurgitant fraction. These quantitative measures benefit most from standardized plane acquisitions and sequencing. In humans, cardiac MRI is the non-invasive gold standard for cardiac function and the preferred imaging modality when precise quantification is needed.
- Contrast-enhanced cardiac MRI, including myocardial T1 mapping, may help to assess myocardial tissue non-invasively in cats and dogs, though clinical research remains in its infancy.

Airways and lungs

MRI is considered suboptimal for investigation of the lungs because of motion artefacts and inherent paramagnetic properties of air. Lung lesions, such as nodular lesions, masses, pulmonary infiltrate, lobar torsion, pulmonary emphysema, bronchiectasis and migrating foreign bodies, can be incidentally observed during MRI examination. In human oncology, MRI might help with characterizing pulmonary nodules using diffusion-weighted imaging to differentiate malignant from benign lung lesions.

Limitations and comparison with CT

In veterinary medicine, the main limitations associated with MRI are:

- The need for general anaesthesia
- A longer acquisition time compared with CT or radiology
- The presence of susceptibility artefacts produced by microchips and metallic foreign bodies which could impact on the diagnostic quality of the images
- The presence of motion artefact due to cardiopulmonary activity
- Patients with non-MRI-compatible pacemakers, protheses or implants which may move or warm up during the examination.

Motion artefacts associated with the respiratory and cardiac cycle could represent a limiting factor for thoracic MRI; however, they may be reduced with fast imaging sequences, gating MRI and altered phase-encoding directions.

Some advantages offered by MRI compared with CT are:

- Excellent soft tissue detail
- The possibility of characterizing tissue composition even without the use of contrast media
- The possibility of obtaining functional and cine-based sequences (cardiac MRI)
- Unlimited possible acquisition planes.

MRI represents the gold-standard examination for staging soft tissue masses and investigation of the cardiovascular system, while CT provides a more precise anatomical detail of bone, airways and lungs. Currently, CT is still considered the main cross-sectional advanced imaging modality for the thorax.

The longer acquisition time of MRI compared with CT also impacts clinical management, with a longer anaesthetic period and increased personnel usage and risks for the patient, and has economic consequences for the overall balance of the imaging unit compared with more efficient techniques such as CT.

Restraint and patient preparation

MRI examination is performed under general anaesthesia to limit motion artefacts. Drug delivery and anaesthetic equipment should be arranged in advance before positioning the patient to avoid moving the patient during the examination. Preparation includes:

- Removal of any external metallic material (e.g. collars, leads, etc.) from the animal prior to entering the MRI examination room
- Placement of a peripheral venous line for administration of contrast medium
- Preparation of MRI-compatible equipment for anaesthetic delivery and monitoring
- Setting of respiratory bellows, pulse oximeter or ECG before positioning the patient in the coil for gated MRI. For cardiac-gated MRI, animals should be clipped before positioning of electrodes.

Patient positioning for thoracic MRI depends on gantry type and dimensions, available coils and the investigated structures. The area of interest should be centred within the coil. A general thoracic scan may be centred just caudal to the scapula.

- To investigate cranial mediastinal masses and lungs, ventral recumbency should be used to minimize respiratory movements as well as reduce dependency-related pulmonary atelectasis.
- Giant breeds and deep-chested dogs may need to be in lateral recumbency to fit in the scanner. MRI-compatible (non-ferrous) positioners might allow accurate positioning of the patient.
- Small dogs and cats may be placed in ventral recumbency within a head or extremity coil, while medium and large-breed dogs may be positioned in a body or torso coil. Flexible coils might be used in combination to increase the signal intensity from the region of interest.
- For thoracic wall lesions, the patient should be positioned with the area of interest dependent to reduce motion artefact. A surface coil should be placed on the identified lesion.
- An oil capsule or syringe filled with a paramagnetic contrast medium could be used as a marker to aid the localization of swelling, scars or draining tracts.

Technique

After patient positioning and receiver imaging coil placement, a set of three-plane (dorsal, sagittal and transverse), low-resolution localizer images are obtained. These images will be used as a map to allow planning of the following scans. If the patient appears to be incorrectly positioned, it should be adjusted and the localizers must be repeated. Protocol parameters such as field of view, slice thickness and orientation, directions of phase and frequency encoding might be modified according to the investigated region to limit the presence of artefacts in the images.

- The field of view should be sufficiently large to include all the body, avoiding phase-wrap artefact.
- Slice thickness depends on the size of the patient, ranging from 4–7 mm, with 10% gap.

- Three-plane images can be obtained by orienting the slices perpendicular or parallel to the long axis of the animal. For rib lesions, oblique sagittal images aligned with the rib cage on the dorsal localizer may prove to be helpful, depending on the body conformation.

The selected sequences depend on the object of the study and can be divided into anatomical, functional and cine-based images. Anatomical sequences include standard T1-weighted and T2-weighted images, which aim to represent the anatomy and tissue signal properties. Functional sequences are used for the characterization of specific parameters, such as diffusion-weighted imaging (DWI), while cine-based images are dynamic sequences, used for example in ECG-gated cardiac MRI.

- T1-weighted images provide adequate anatomical detail and can be used with administration of intravenous paramagnetic contrast material to improve the conspicuity of lesions and the characterization of vessels.
- T2-weighted images are useful in the evaluation of the presence of fluid components such as oedema or fluid collections.
- The adipose tissue signal can be suppressed using fat-saturated spin echo sequences or, in T2-weighted images only, using STIR sequences. Furthermore, fat-saturated sequences are critical for evaluating uptake of contrast with a null-adipose signal, which is not possible with STIR. Both sequences may help in characterization of lipomatous, muscular and bony lesions, as well as highlighting lymph nodes and fluid-filled structures.
- DWI uses functional sequences that measure the movement of water molecules within tissues and can be used for characterization of lung nodules/masses, although information is lacking in veterinary medicine. In human radiology, the latter technique is beneficial for cancer staging. In general, lung malignancies present increased cellularity and increased extracellular space tortuosity, producing general restriction of interstitial water diffusion compared with benign nodules.

As mentioned above, motion artefacts generated by respiratory movement and the cardiac cycle may represent a limitation for thoracic MRI, resulting in ghosting and image degradation. Motion artefacts extend in the phase-encoding direction, regardless of movement orientation. To reduce their impact on image quality, the phase and frequency encoding can be oriented based on the region of interest.

- For lateral wall lesions, phase encoding for dorsal plane images should be set in a craniocaudal direction, while a dorsoventral direction should be set for transverse plane images.
- For cranial mediastinal masses, phase encoding should be oriented dorsoventrally for sagittal plane images and right–left for dorsal plane images.

Besides phase encoding, the use of presaturation bands, short echo time and fast imaging sequences can minimize the effects of motion artefacts. Special equipment can be also employed to actively reduce these artefacts, performing respiratory or cardiac gating and phase reordering and associating the image acquisition with the respiratory or cardiac cycle.

References and further reading

Bouvard J, Longo M, Schwarz MA et al. (2020) Accessory left ventricular chamber in a cat: multimodality imaging description by cardiac magnetic imaging and echocardiography. *Journal of Veterinary Cardiology* **28**, 55–61

Boxt LM (1999) Cardiac MR Imaging: A guide for the beginner. *Radiographics* **19**, 1009–1025

Schwarz T, Willis R, Summerfield NJ et al. (2005) Aneurysmal dilation of the right auricle in two dogs. *Journal of the American Veterinary Medical Association* **226**, 1512–1515

Dennis R (2018) MRI of non-cardiac thoracic conditions. In: *Diagnostic MRI in Dogs and Cats*, ed. W Mai, pp. 710–722. CRC Press, Boca Raton

Gilbert SH, McConnell FJ, Holden AV et al. (2010) The potential role of MRI in veterinary clinical cardiology. *Veterinary Journal* **183**, 124–134

Johnson VS and Seiler G (2006) Magnetic resonance imaging appearance of the cisterna chyli. *Veterinary Radiology & Ultrasound* **47**, 461–464

Kutara K, Kanda T, Maeta N et al. (2020) Combining non-contrast enhanced magnetic resonance thoracic ductography with vascular contrast-enhanced computed tomography to identify the canine thoracic duct. *Open Veterinary Journal* **10**, 68–73

Pessôa FMC, de Melo ASA, Souza AS et al. (2016) Applications of magnetic resonance imaging of the thorax in pleural diseases: A state-of-the-art review. *Lung* **194**, 501–509

Raptis CA, Ludwig DR, Hammer MM et al. (2019) Building blocks for thoracic MRI: Challenges, sequences, and protocol design. *Journal of Magnetic Resonance Imaging* **50**, 682–701

Rousset N, Holmes MA, Caine A et al. (2013) Clinical and low-field MRI characteristics of injection site sarcoma in 19 cats. *Veterinary Radiology & Ultrasound* **54**, 623–629

Sargent J, Connolly DJ, Watts V et al. (2015) Assessment of mitral regurgitation in dogs: comparison of results of echocardiography with magnetic resonance imaging. *Journal of Small Animal Practice* **56**, 641–650

Venkatesh V, Verdini D and Ghoshhajra B (2011) Normal magnetic resonance imaging of the thorax. *Magnetic Resonance Imaging Clinics of North America* **19**, 489–506

Wu LM, Xu JR, Hua J et al. (2013) Can diffusion-weighted imaging be used as a reliable sequence in the detection of malignant pulmonary nodules and masses? *Magnetic Resonance Imaging* **31**, 235–246

Chapter 5

Basics of thoracic nuclear medicine

Federica Morandi

Nuclear medicine, or nuclear scintigraphy, is a branch of medical imaging that uses radiopharmaceuticals (pharmaceuticals labelled with radioactive atoms) to evaluate physiological processes and diagnose a variety of diseases. Nuclear medicine differs from other imaging modalities in that it shows primarily the function of the system being investigated, as opposed to its anatomy. During planar scintigraphic studies, images are created using a radiation detector (the gamma camera) after the application of a radiopharmaceutical of choice, for example rectally or intravenously. Because scintigraphy employs radioactive compounds, radiation safety is of the utmost importance when handling the radiopharmaceutical dose, the animal being injected and waste products, such as urine and faeces. In small animal thoracic diagnostic nuclear medicine, the typical radiopharmaceutical dose is small (ranging between a minimum of 30 and a maximum of 740 MBq), resulting in minimal exposure from the animals and their excreta. Nevertheless, adherence to national radiation safety regulations is mandatory.

Indications

Indications for first pass radionuclide angiocardiography using sodium 99mTc-pertechnetate (Na99mTcO$_4$), 99mTc-diethylene-triamine-pentaacetate (DTPA) or 99mTc-mebrofenin include:

* Diagnosis of congenital cardiac shunt and determination of the direction of shunting (left-to-right versus right-to-left); especially useful in cases where radiographic and echocardiographic findings are equivocal
* Quantification of left-to-right cardiac shunts
* Follow-up evaluation after surgical correction of a shunt (patent ductus arteriosus (PDA)).

Indications for pulmonary scintigraphy using 99mTc-macroaggregated albumin (MAA) include:

* Evaluation of pulmonary perfusion in cases of suspected pulmonary thromboembolism (PTE)
* Evaluation and quantification of right-to-left shunts (reverse PDA, tetralogy of Fallot)
* Follow-up evaluation after surgical correction of a shunt (reversed PDA).

Indications for ciliary scintigraphy using 99mTc-MAA include:

* Evaluation of mucociliary function (ciliary dyskinesia).

Indications for static images using sodium 99mTc-pertechnetate scintigraphy include:

* Evaluation of cranial mediastinal masses (determining whether a mass is thyroidal in origin).

Restraint and patient preparation

First pass radionuclide angiocardiography

This study is easy and quick to perform and does not require sedation or general anaesthesia; however, sedation may be used in particularly fractious animals. Prior to the study, radiographs of the thorax should be obtained to check for left heart failure, which would render the study invalid. An animal with evidence of pulmonary oedema and/or pulmonary venous congestion should be treated until resolution of the decompensation before the study is conducted.

The radionuclide must be injected intravenously in a bolus fashion; therefore, prior to the study, a large-gauge, short-length intravenous catheter must be placed in the cephalic vein.

The animal is positioned in left lateral recumbency over the gamma camera and restrained by one or two assistants. It is vital that the animal remains still during the few seconds of the dynamic acquisition of the first pass, or the study will be non-diagnostic.

Pulmonary scintigraphy

No sedation or anaesthesia is necessary; however, sedation may be used in particularly fractious animals.

It is important to assess whether the animal may have pulmonary hypertension. Pulmonary hypertension is a contraindication for the use of 99mTc-MAA, since the particles will occlude a portion of the pulmonary capillary bed and, therefore, could potentially exacerbate this condition. If pulmonary hypertension is suspected, the particle dose must be reduced as much as possible. In cases of severe pulmonary hypertension, the study risks must be weighed against the benefit of achieving a diagnosis.

When evaluating for PTE, radiographs of the thorax should be obtained immediately prior to the study and interpreted in conjunction with the scintigraphic images. This is especially important because ventilation scintigraphy using inert radioactive gases or ^{99m}Tc-DTPA radio-aerosol is virtually never performed in practice due to its technical difficulty and radiation safety concerns.

Since the MAA particles can adhere to plastic tubing, it is best to inject directly into the vein – no intravenous catheter is needed.

The animal can be restrained in opposite lateral, dorsal and ventral recumbent positions over the gamma camera by an assistant.

^{99m}Tc-MAA scintigraphy for evaluation of mucociliary function

General anaesthesia is necessary, and a short endotracheal (ET) tube must be used to ensure that the tube terminates no further than the thoracic inlet. Radiographs can be obtained immediately prior to the study to confirm the position of the ET tube.

^{99m}Tc-pertechnetate scintigraphy for evaluation of cranial mediastinal masses

Anaesthesia is unnecessary, but sedation is generally required. If the study includes images of the thyroid using a pinhole collimator, then anaesthesia is needed. An intravenous catheter should be placed in the cephalic or saphenous vein to facilitate administration of the radionuclide. The animal can be restrained in opposite lateral, dorsal and ventral recumbent positions over the gamma camera by an assistant.

It is important to remember that if the animal has recently undergone a contrast study with intravenous injection of iodinated contrast material, the scintigraphy will be negative because iodine reduces thyroid uptake of ^{99m}Tc-pertechnetate: a delay of 3–4 weeks is recommended from the time of intravenous iodinated contrast material injection to the time of scintigraphy to avoid a false-negative result.

Technique
First pass radionuclide angiocardiography

The set-up for first pass radionuclide angiocardiography is easy and the acquisition time is short. Most commercially available nuclear medicine software has a programme that permits the calculation of pulmonary:systemic flow ratio (QP:QS), which allows for quantification of the magnitude of the shunt. Although the precise steps for image analysis will vary slightly depending on the software used, the principle behind the analysis is the same.

The only requirement for the radiopharmaceutical used in this study is that it must flow passively through the central circulation of the heart and lung. ^{99m}Tc-pertechnetate is the most used radionuclide; ^{99m}Tc-DTPA or ^{99m}Tc-mebrofenin are also frequently used, especially if rapid clearance from the soft tissues is needed, for instance if the study needs to be repeated on the same day. A dose of 185–740 MBq is adequate for a dog; 74–185 MBq is sufficient for a cat.

It is necessary to set up a dynamic acquisition, with at least four (ideally eight) frames per second to have temporal resolution of the various phases of the cardiac cycle. A total acquisition time of 60 seconds is more than adequate. A low-energy, all-purpose collimator is used; matrix size is set at 64x64×16 or 128×128×16.

After positioning the patient on the gamma camera in left lateral recumbency and centring over the heart, the dynamic acquisition is started simultaneously with the bolus injection. To perform the injection, it is best to use a short extension tube connected to the intravenous catheter, and a three-way stopcock connecting the extension tube to the syringe containing the radiopharmaceutical dose and to a syringe of saline solution. The radiopharmaceutical can be loaded in the extension tube (it is important that the volume of radiopharmaceutical is no larger than the volume of the extension tube) and injected as a bolus using the saline to flush.

Before analyzing the study, it is necessary to perform a control step to ensure that the injection was performed in a bolus fashion and that the study is of acceptable quality. To do this, a region of interest (ROI) is drawn over the cranial vena cava (CrVC) from which the computer creates a time activity curve (TAC) that plots the counts in the CrVC ROI over time. An acceptable bolus shows a curve with a tall peak and a narrow base, with the width of the peak at half the maximum counts (full width half maximum (FWHM)) measuring <2 seconds (Figure 5.1).

The evaluation of the study starts with a visual inspection: a normal first pass study is characterized by sequential passage of the radionuclide through the CrVC, right atrium, right ventricle (dextrophase), pulmonic trunk, lung, pulmonary veins (lung phase), left atrium, left ventricle and aorta (levophase). During the levophase, it should be possible to see the aorta clearly, because the lungs should be almost completely clear of the radiopharmaceutical (Figure 5.2).

In a left-to-right shunt, the lungs do not clear because of recirculation of the radiopharmaceutical through the shunt into the pulmonary circulation. It should be noted that incomplete clearance of the lungs is also observed with left heart failure, therefore evaluation of thoracic radiographs prior to the study is mandatory to rule out this differential. If the injection of radiopharmaceutical is performed too slowly, this will simulate slow lung clearance; moreover, if too much pressure is used during the injection, the bolus can split between the cephalic or omobrachial vein and the axillobrachial vein, creating a double peak in the TAC, which may mimic a recirculation peak (Figure 5.3). In a right-to-left shunt, the aorta becomes visible at the same time as the pulmonic trunk.

Quantitative analysis is performed by calculating the QP:QS. This is done by drawing an ROI over the caudodorsal lung field, avoiding the aorta, main pulmonary blood vessels and liver, and asking the computer to create a TAC that displays the lung counts over time. In a normal animal, there will be a peak as the bolus travels through the lungs, followed by a rapid fall (Figure 5.4). In an animal with a left-to-right shunt, a second peak is visible immediately after the first one, representing the recirculation of radionuclide into the lungs through the shunt (Figure 5.5). The computer software can then calculate a ratio of the area under the first, pulmonary curve (QP) and the second, recirculation (systemic) curve (QS). In a normal animal, the QP:QS ratio is <1.2. It has been shown that the QP:QS ratio correlates well with shunt fraction. A QP:QS ratio of about 3, for instance, corresponds to a shunt fraction of about 50%.

If the nuclear medicine computer does not have software for QP:QS analysis, an alternative procedure is to calculate the C2:C1 ratio. To calculate the C2:C1 ratio, an

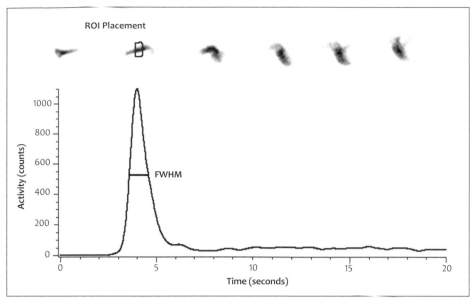

5.1 TAC from the CrVC in a normal dog illustrating a good bolus injection. The curve was obtained by drawing an ROI over the CrVC and plotting the counts in the ROI (y axis) over time in seconds (x axis). Notice the tall and narrow-based peak of the curve. The width of the peak at 50% of the peak maximum height (FWHM) is 1 second, indicating an excellent bolus.

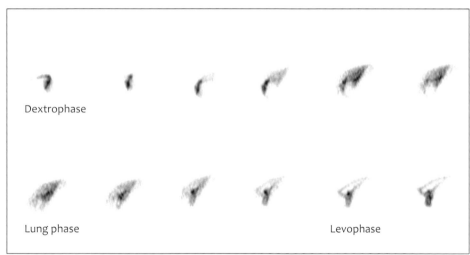

5.2 Serial left lateral scintigraphic images illustrating normal first pass radionuclide angiography in a dog. The images are taken at a rate of four frames per second, representing the 3 seconds immediately after the intravenous injection of ^{99m}Tc-DTPA. The radionuclide outlines the CrVC (top left), right heart, lungs, left heart and aorta. Notice that the margins of the aorta are distinct and the lung field clears completely during the levophase (last two images, bottom right).

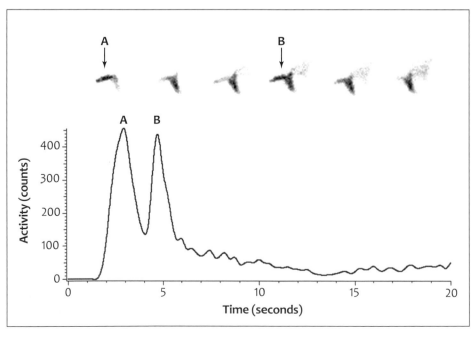

5.3 TAC from the CrVC in a normal dog illustrating a split bolus. This is an example of a biphasic bolus: the first peak in the TAC (A) is followed by a second peak (B), which may be erroneously interpreted as a recirculation peak compatible with a left-to-right shunt. This mistake is easily avoided by evaluating the TAC in conjunction with the dynamic acquisition.

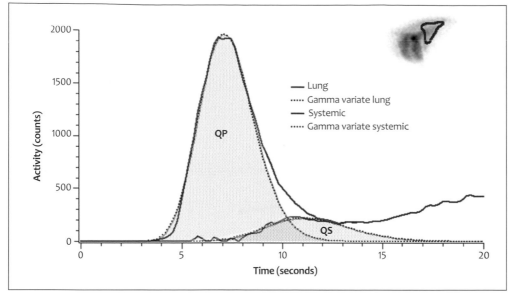

5.4 Pulmonary TAC (blue) in a normal dog showing an initial increase and successive sharp fall of the pulmonary counts as the radioactive bolus passes through the pulmonary circulation (QP). The curve in red represents systemic activity in the lungs (QS), which is due to blood flow in the bronchial branches of the broncho-oesophageal artery. The dotted lines represent fitted curves, which were generated by the computer during the analysis and calculation of QP:QS ratio. The image in the top right corner illustrates positioning of the pulmonary ROI in the caudodorsal aspect of the lungs.

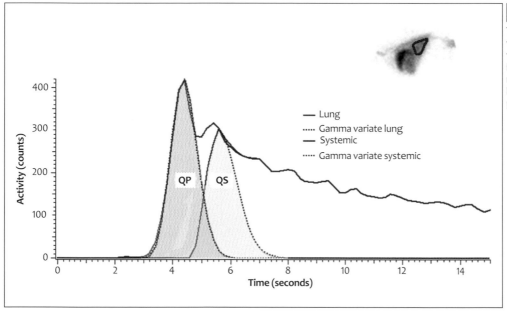

5.5 Pulmonary TAC in a dog with a left-to-right shunt. The curve was generated in the same way as the one in Figure 5.4. Notice the large systemic peak (QS), indicating recirculation of the radiopharmaceutical through the left-to-right shunt. QP = pulmonary peak.

ROI is placed in the caudodorsal lung field in the same way as for QP:QS analysis and a lung TAC is created. From the TAC, it is necessary to identify three points: C1, the maximum pulmonary counts, obtained at the peak of the pulmonary curve; Tmax, the time from the initial appearance of the bolus until the peak of the pulmonary curve (C1); and C2, the pulmonary counts at 2xTmax (Figure 5.6). A normal C2:C1 ratio is <0.5 (the counts at C2 must be less than half the counts at C1). While this method is easy to use, it is less accurate than the QP:QS ratio in distinguishing normal animals from animals that have a left-to-right shunt.

Pulmonary scintigraphy

Pulmonary scintigraphy for the evaluation of PTE and right-to-left shunts is easily performed and requires only the acquisition of static images; no particular software is necessary for image analysis.

Pulmonary perfusion imaging using the radiopharmaceutical ^{99m}Tc-MAA is based on physical blockade of the MAA particles in the first capillary bed encountered after intravenous injection. Because the MAA particles have a mean diameter of 10–40 μm, in a normal animal the particles lodge in the pulmonary capillaries and the distribution is proportional to blood flow. The particles have a biological half-life of 4–6 hours, reflecting their removal by pulmonary macrophages. The capillary embolization is therefore reversible.

A dose of 17.5 MBq is adequate for a cat or small dog, with up to 74 MBq for a large dog. For ^{99m}Tc-MAA, it is important to estimate how many particles will be injected into the patient. Most commercially available kits contain 4–12 million particles: the typical dose in a 70 kg human patient is 10% of the kit, which is estimated to result in embolization of <0.1% of the pulmonary capillaries. In small animals, no more than 5–10% of the kit should be used. It is especially important to use the smallest possible particle dose when evaluating for a possible right-to-left shunt, and when pulmonary hypertension is suspected. In cases of documented severe pulmonary hypertension, the study is contraindicated. It is also better not to perform the study if adequate particle dilution cannot be reached, for instance in a very small dog or cat.

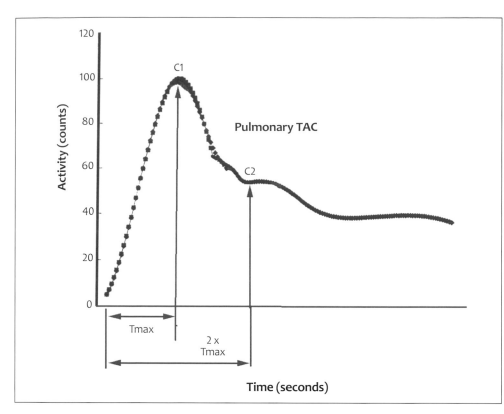

5.6 TAC in a dog with a left-to-right shunt, showing the reference points necessary for calculation of the C2:C1 ratio. C1 is the point of maximum pulmonary counts; Tmax is the time after the beginning of the pulmonary upslope at which C1 occurs; C2 is the point on the curve at 2xTmax. The C2:C1 ratio in normal dogs should be <0.5.

As the particles remain in position for several hours, the intravenous injection can be performed away from the gamma camera. It is better to acquire images 1–5 minutes after the injection because some particles begin to be removed by macrophages and the label begins to dissociate as time elapses.

The radiopharmaceutical should be injected directly into the cephalic or saphenous vein; ^{99m}Tc-MAA tends to form clots when mixed with blood in the syringe prior to injection, which can happen if the operator has difficulty in finding a vein and blood is withdrawn and allowed to remain in the syringe for a short period. The ^{99m}Tc-MAA clot does not represent a danger for the animal, but it will localize to the lungs creating an artefactual 'hot spot' that can be confusing during image interpretation (Figure 5.7). It is best to perform the injection with the animal in ventral recumbency to avoid collapse of the dependent lung and ensure even distribution to both lungs; it is important to remember that the distribution is proportional to blood flow.

When investigating possible right-to-left shunts, static right and left lateral, ventral and dorsal images of the whole body should be acquired. When the study is performed to evaluate for PTE, images are limited to the thorax and include additional oblique views. Matrix size is set at 256x256x16. Images should be acquired for 250,000–500,000 counts. A low-energy, all-purpose collimator is adequate.

In normal animals, radioactivity is distributed exclusively to the lungs, which have uniform intensity (Figure 5.8). In animals with right-to-left shunts, radioactivity is seen in the systemic circulation and is especially noticeable in the capillaries of the renal cortices and cerebral hemispheres. In patients with PTE, wedge-shaped pleural-based perfusion defects are present; the corresponding radiographs are normal or occasionally show focal oligaemia and smaller than normal pulmonary blood vessels. Shunt fraction can be easily calculated by dividing the total extrapulmonary counts by the total body counts.

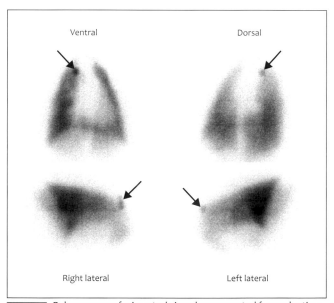

5.7 Pulmonary perfusion study in a dog presented for evaluation of possible pulmonary thromboembolism. Note the small but intense focus of activity in the apex of the right cranial lung lobe (arrowed). This was a ^{99m}Tc-MAA clot.

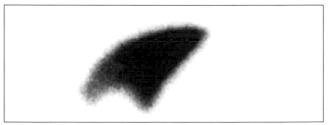

5.8 Left lateral scintigram of the lungs of a normal dog after intravenous injection of approximately 37 MBq of ^{99m}Tc-MAA. Notice the uniform radiopharmaceutical distribution within the lungs, with no evidence of distribution outside the pulmonary capillaries. The smooth photopenic area seen cranioventrally represents the cardiac notch.

99mTc-MAA scintigraphy for evaluation of mucociliary function

Scintigraphy with 99mTc-MAA can also be used for the evaluation of mucociliary function in cases of suspected ciliary dyskinesia. The study is easy to perform and does not require specific software for image analysis, but does require general anaesthesia.

The animal is positioned in ventral recumbency on a table and the gamma camera is positioned immediately dorsal to it and centred over the thorax. A low-energy, all-purpose collimator is adequate. A short ET tube must be used so that the tube does not interfere with 99mTc-MAA movement; a 90-degree connector with port is ideal to connect the ET tube to the anaesthetic machine.

Two external radioactive markers (57Co or 99mTc) are placed along the side of the animal, one at the level of the caudal margin of the scapula or fifth intercostal space, which corresponds to the location of the carina, and the other 20 cm cranially. These markers will assist in the accurate deposition of the 99mTc-MAA droplet.

A sleeved catheter must be used to deposit a droplet of 99mTc-MAA within the tracheal lumen at the tracheal bifurcation: a 10 Fr male urinary catheter with the tip removed works well as the outer sleeve, and a 5 Fr catheter can be used as the inner catheter. A small droplet of 99mTc-MAA (<30 MBq in 30 µl volume) is aspirated into the inner catheter; the inner catheter is then withdrawn into the outer catheter to avoid contamination of the trachea during positioning. The catheter is then advanced into the ET tube through the port at the right-angle connection, or the anaesthetic machine is momentarily disconnected to allow placement of the catheter. The catheter is advanced until the radioactive 99mTc-MAA droplet is just cranial to the level of the caudal external radioactive marker (level of the carina); the persistence scope is used to assess the location of the catheter with respect to the external radioactive markers. The internal catheter is then advanced about 1 cm beyond the outer sleeve and a small volume of air is injected, resulting in deposition of the radioactive droplet in the trachea. At this point the inner catheter is retracted into the outer catheter, both catheters are removed together from the trachea and, if necessary, the anaesthetic machine is reconnected.

A series of 60-second dorsal static images is then acquired, starting just after radiopharmaceutical deposition, and then every 5 minutes for a total of 40 minutes afterwards. Matrix size is set at 256x256x16.

In a normal animal, the radiopharmaceutical droplet is cleared by the mucociliary apparatus and moves cranially as a discrete 'hot spot' (Figure 5.9). Movement usually starts 1–2 minutes after deposition. Sometimes a residual lower-intensity focus remains at the original site of deposition. In an animal with non-functional cilia, there will be no movement throughout the entire study. This is an 'all or nothing' evaluation: either the droplet moves, or it does not. The velocity at which the droplet moves varies greatly from animal to animal, even in healthy dogs and cats in the same age groups.

99mTc-pertechnetate scintigraphy for evaluation of cranial mediastinal masses

99mTc-pertechnetate scintigraphy can be used in the evaluation of cranial mediastinal masses, to determine whether a mass detected radiographically and/or ultrasonographically is thyroidal in origin. The technique is the same as for thyroid scintigraphy.

The administered dose is 74–185 MBq of 99mTc-pertechnetate in the dog and 37–148 MBq in the cat. A low-energy, all-purpose collimator is used; matrix size is set at 256×256×16. Image acquisition is best performed 20–30 minutes after injection. The animal is placed over the gamma camera and opposite lateral, ventral and possibly dorsal static images of the thorax are acquired for a minimum of 250,000 counts. A mass of thyroidal origin will show radionuclide uptake much like the thyroid gland does.

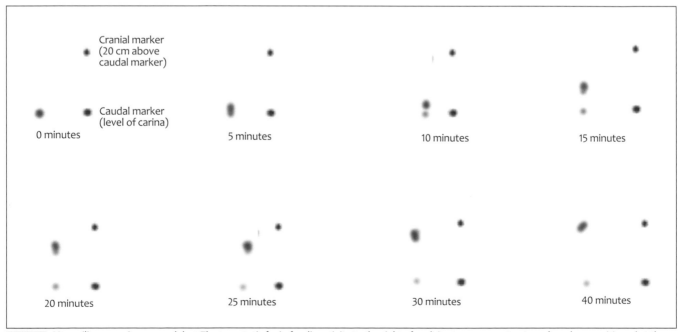

5.9 Mucociliary scan in a normal dog. The two static foci of radioactivity to the right of each image represent external markers positioned at the caudal border of the scapula and 20 cm cranial to it. The images are dorsal views obtained at 0, 5, 10, 15, 20, 25, 30 and 40 minutes after deposition of a small droplet of 99mTc-MAA just cranial to the carina. The radioactive droplet is at the level of the caudal external marker at 0 minutes (top left image); subsequently, the droplet moves cranially and is almost at the level of the cranial marker at 40 minutes (bottom right image).

References and further reading

Alderson PO and Martin EC (1987) Pulmonary embolism: diagnosis with multiple imaging modalities. *Radiology* **164**, 297–312

Bahr A, Miller M and Gordon S (2002) First pass nuclear angiocardiography in the evaluation of patent ductus arteriosus in dogs. *Journal of Veterinary Internal Medicine* **16**, 74–79

Brawner WR and Daniel GB (1993) Nuclear imaging. *Veterinary Clinics of North America: Small Animal Practice* **23**, 379–398

Daniel GB and Berry CR (2006) Pulmonary and mucociliary scintigraphy. In: *Textbook of Veterinary Nuclear Medicine, 2nd edn*, ed. GB Daniel and CR Berry, pp. 303–327. ACVR Publications, Tennessee

Daniel GB and Brawner WB (2006) Thyroid scintigraphy. In: *Textbook of Veterinary Nuclear Medicine, 2nd edn*, ed. GB Daniel and CR Berry, pp. 181–198. ACVR Publications, Tennessee

Daniel GB and Bright JM (1999) Nuclear imaging, computed tomography and magnetic resonance imaging of the heart. In: *Textbook of Canine and Feline Cardiology*, ed. PR Fox, D Sisson and NS Moise, pp. 193–203. WB Saunders, Philadelphia

Daniel GB and Morandi F (2006) First pass radionuclide angiocardiography. In: *Textbook of Veterinary Nuclear Medicine, 2nd edn*, ed. GB Daniel and CR Berry, pp. 257–273. ACVR Publications, Tennessee

Morandi F, Daniel GB, Gompf RE and Bahr A (2004) Diagnosis of congenital right-to-left shunts with ^{99m}Tc-MAA. *Veterinary Radiology and Ultrasound* **45**, 97–102

Thrall DE, Badertscher RR, Lewis RE and McCall JW (1979) Scintigraphic evaluation of pulmonary perfusion in dogs experimentally infected with Dirofilaria immitis. *American Journal of Veterinary Research* **40**, 1426–1432

Wolff RK (1987) Comparison of two methods of measuring tracheal mucous velocity in anesthetized Beagle dogs. *American Review of Respiratory Disease* **20**, 137–142

Chapter 6

Practical applications of artificial intelligence in thoracic radiology

Neil Shaw, Ben van Klinken and Tobias Schwarz

The value of artificial intelligence in clinical care

With the number of proposed healthcare applications for artificial intelligence (AI) exploding in recent years, it is critical to consider which challenges could be addressed by AI and how it can add significant value to veterinary practices. Despite AI having intersected with veterinary medicine many years ago, its use for diagnostic applications in veterinary medicine is relatively new.

How AI applications for radiology help veterinary practice

The value of AI for radiology has been more comprehensively demonstrated in human medicine, but interest in the analogous potential for AI in veterinary medicine has gained traction. Some of the benefits of AI include:

- Reducing errors: errors in interpretations of plain radiographs are common in veterinary medicine and have been observed to occur due to human experiences such as fatigue, distraction and cognitive biases. This was addressed by the development of several techniques, such as structured reports, checklists, standardization of the process for interpretation and approaches to de-bias interpretation, as well as the development of certain AI techniques
- Reducing costs: using AI to evaluate plain radiographs can help to establish diagnoses without dependency on the limited availability of advanced technologies such as computed tomography and ultrasonography. At the same time, because many veterinary practices do not have board-certified radiologists in house, AI applications can prevent the costs associated with daily consultations with external specialists. Radiology consultations can then be prioritized for more complex cases
- Faster assessments: demand for veterinary radiologist consultations exceeds the ability of specialists to supply these services. Relying solely on specialists for imaging analysis can delay diagnosis, precluding immediate treatment and potentially enhancing anxiety in both pets and their caregivers

- Convenience: developers have recognized the market importance of delivering AI applications that not only provide reliable predictive readouts but also fit seamlessly into clinical workflows. Software applications are therefore increasingly convenient to use in veterinary practice, addressing not only clinical challenges but also those related to office efficiencies
- Tighter feedback loops: it has always been the responsibility of veterinary surgeons (veterinarians) to provide the best possible care but clients now expect better customer service than previously. This trend, driven by the emphasis in customer satisfaction in other industries, means clients want accurate answers faster and at lower cost. Diagnostic AI applications can help meet this growing demand.

AI opportunities and challenges in thoracic radiology

Thoracic radiology is uniquely positioned for the application of AI. Thoracic radiographs are more technically demanding and challenging to interpret than other radiographs. This opens opportunities for AI applications, but also creates challenges:

- Variation in radiographic image quality
- Anatomical variations in thoracic conformation
- Dynamic changes in thoracic organ size and shape (due to inspiration, expiration, systole, diastole, swallowing).

Building effective AI solutions

Creating AI that can reliably read thoracic plain radiographs and provide fast, accurate assessments of the clinical implications of these images is a long, laborious and expensive process. It requires deconstructing radiographs, teaching the AI system how to understand normal anatomy across species, breeds and body-type variation in similar animals, and teaching the AI system how to identify abnormalities in these same contexts. Successfully achieving this level of understanding in an AI system requires significant trial and error and an ongoing iterative process that enables the system to continue to learn through the input of new data.

Learning of lower-dimensional ground truth data manifolds

To produce a dataset that AI can accurately model, the high-dimensional data of a radiograph must first be simplified (its dimensionality must be reduced). There are several staple techniques for dimensionality reduction and visualization outside of biomedical applications, but they all have shortcomings when it comes to radiography.

- *Principal component analysis (PCA)* is a projection algorithm, trying to preserve the overall structure of the data. It does not try to determine the existence of a lower-dimensional manifold to which the data can be mapped, representing a more fundamental ground truth pattern behind the data.
- *t-distributed stochastic neighbour embedding (t-SNE)* is a manifold learning technique trying to predict the shape of a lower-dimensional manifold. In addition to taking a long time to compute even with multi-core computing, the outputs are highly unstable and dependent on the initial parameters of the t-SNE run.
- *Uniform manifold approximation and projection (UMAP)* improves upon t-SNE's stability and compute time by a wide margin, but it can still be hampered by noisy data to the point where it suffers from the same subjectivity problem as t-SNE.

Using a combination of existing manifold learning techniques combined with custom-tuned, diffusion-aware manifold learning approaches, it is possible to build models with single-channel images of points representing 3D objects. This assumption turns out to work in practical implementation due to the translucency of most objects in X-ray images. In addition to their usefulness in visualization and preserving data structure, the denoising steps make for plots that can cluster data even when they have come from different instruments with highly varied image quality. This combined approach provides high visualization quality and preserves global structure to an extent that is arguably superior to other machine learning techniques. Figure 6.1 demonstrates the data generated by this technique for pleural effusion.

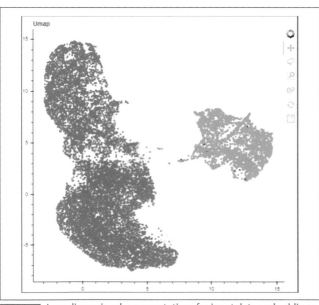

6.1 Low-dimensional representations for input data embeddings and output labels for detecting pleural effusion. The green masses represent the separation of data points that reflect normal *versus* abnormal anatomy.

Entropy-aware model interpretability

Machine learning techniques commonly lack transparency (they are sometimes referred to as 'black boxes' because it is hard to see how they work). Two criteria are critical to improve clinician comfort with relying on these models for predictive information:

- *Explainability* refers to how well one can establish the function of each part of a network, for example what purpose each node in a neural network or each branch in a decision tree serves in the overall function
- *Interpretability* refers to how well one can establish cause and effect in how a machine learning model operates (e.g. which part of an input contributed to a given decision). Methods such as heat mapping (Figure 6.2) can improve interpretability. If explainability cannot be provided, then machine learning model decisions must at least be interpretable.

Consider the task of interpreting a classification decision about an input image. While an entire image is fed into a model all at once, not all parts of an image are equal in each decision. Deep neural network training involves teaching a model how to ignore certain parts of the input while focusing on others. There are plenty of tools that focus on using activation- and gradient-centric approaches to decision interpretability. However, more than just the model needs to be considered in this decision. Consider the equation for the entropy of a greyscale image, where n is the number of grey levels (256 for 8-bit images), p_i is the probability of a pixel having grey level i and b is the base of the logarithm function:

$$-\sum_{i=0}^{n-1} p_i \log_b p_i$$

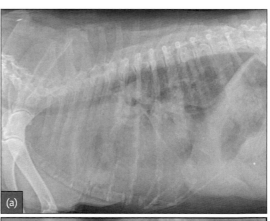

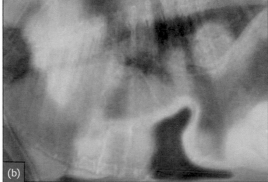

6.2 Translation of (a) a plain radiograph to (b) a heat map image. The pathological pleural fluid is red.

In this naive function, the probability assumes a uniform distribution of probabilities (i.e. each being just as likely as the others). For real-world applications this is not the case and is better represented by conditional probability rather than unconditional (i.e. the probability of a given pixel value is partly conditionally dependent on the surrounding pixels). Using this knowledge, an interpretability tool can be created that weights the changes in a model's activations with the changes to the input decision image.

The result of this in turn is a pixel-specific map of the image, acting as a proxy for which parts of the input image are most important for a given binary classification decision. Figure 6.2 illustrates a heat map (colour) generated from a plain radiograph (black and white). The colours indicate the clinical information captured through the process described above. Warmer colours represent regions classified as abnormal anatomy, while cooler colours represent normal regions.

Current practical applications of AI software for thoracic radiography

The first comprehensive AI software for small animal radiography was developed by SignalPET®. It provides instantaneous processing that produces actionable information at the point of care, limited only by the need for a digital machine, and can thus be used anytime and anywhere in the world. The system displays a range of defined pathologies as tabs with a probability bar for presence (red) or absence (green) of the specified abnormality (Figure 6.3). The radiographs still need to be interpreted by a veterinary surgeon for a meaningful diagnosis. This is similar to laboratory analysis software, where the results are complemented by a laboratory reference range of normality. Any test result needs to be interpreted in the context of the clinical patient.

AI-driven assisted radiography allows an optimization of workflow in the veterinary practice. Veterinary nurses or technicians frequently obtain and check the technical quality of radiographs, whereas the veterinary surgeon oversees interpretation. In other institutions, radiographs are obtained by nurses, technicians or non-specialized veterinary surgeons, but are interpreted by veterinary radiologists. This can be optimized by using initial AI results as a triaging tool to ensure that a clinical diagnosis is reached quicker, or that animals with diagnosed critical conditions are prioritized for final interpretation.

Future developments for AI in thoracic radiology and related fields

Although computers are superior to humans in recognizing patterns on images, currently teaching of AI applications is based on what humans perceive. Given the vast amount of data available for training these systems, these applications will continue to improve in their accuracy and precision over time. Software technologies will therefore continue to be refined.

While the performance of clinical applications will improve, the applications themselves will also expand. While the outputs of existing AI systems will complement work in veterinary medicine, eventually they may also be able to drive new types of clinical decision making that are impossible without machine learning. The next era of AI applications in thoracic radiology is likely to be driven by pattern recognition beyond the capabilities of even the most highly trained human eye and offer new ways of predicting health-related conditions. With these data in hand, we will have a deeper understanding of health status in asymptomatic animals (i.e. risk assessment) and have greater power to offer protective guidance and enhance longevity.

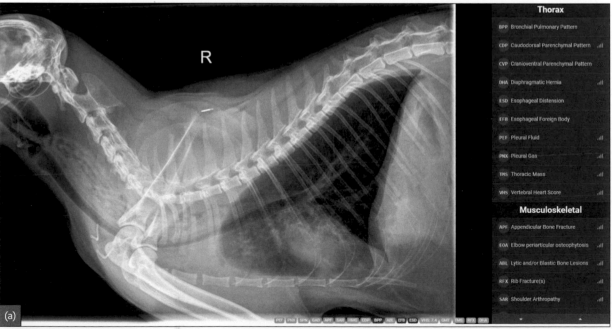

6.3 Thoracic radiographs analysed with the SignalPET® AI software. (a) Lateral radiograph of the neck and thorax of a cat with an obstructive oesophageal foreign body and secondary aspiration pneumonia. The AI system flags 'Bronchial Pulmonary Pattern', 'Cranioventral Parenchymal Pattern', 'Esophageal Distension' and 'Esophageal Foreign Body' as abnormal (red tabs) with a 4-out-of-4 probability index. All other listed pathological entities are listed as 4-out-of-4 normal. Interpretation by a veterinary radiologist concurs with these results. (continues) ▶

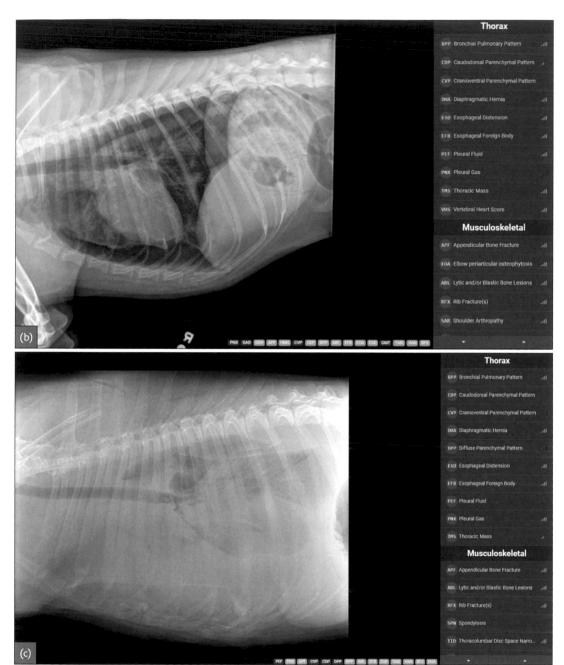

6.3 (continued) Thoracic radiographs analysed with the SignalPET® AI software. (b) Lateral thoracic radiograph of a dog with pneumothorax. The AI system flags 'Cranioventral Parenchymal Pattern' and 'Pleural Gas' as abnormal (red tabs) with a 4-out-of-4 probability index. 'Caudodorsal Parenchymal Pattern' is listed as normal (green) with a 2-out-of-4 probability index. All other listed pathological entities are listed as 4-out-of-4 normal. Interpretation by a veterinary radiologist concurs with the diagnosis of pneumothorax. The cranioventral and caudodorsal lung AI interpretation requires application of context by the veterinary surgeon. In pneumothorax, secondary lung collapse is a consequence of increased pleural pressure and unlikely to be an independent disease such as pneumonia. (c) Lateral thoracic radiograph of a dog with pleural effusion. The AI system flags 'Caudodorsal Parenchymal Pattern', 'Cranioventral Parenchymal Pattern', 'Diffuse Parenchymal Pattern' and 'Pleural Fluid' as abnormal (red tabs) with a 4-out-of-4 probability index and 'Spondylosis' as 2-out-of-4 abnormal. 'Thoracic Mass' is listed as normal (green) but only with a 2-out-of-4 probability index. All other listed pathological entities are listed as 4-out-of-4 normal. Interpretation by a veterinary radiologist concurs with the diagnosis of pleural effusion. Applying context, the lung changes are most likely due to effusion-related collapse and not an independent pathology. There is no obvious visible cause of the effusion, including a distinct mass. However, there is a slight dorsal deviation of the cranial thoracic trachea that would be consistent with a cranial mediastinal mass. Reflecting on the AI results is crucial to achieve a correct diagnosis or undertake further diagnostic tests if necessary.

References and further reading

Alexander K (2010) Reducing error in radiographic interpretation. *Canadian Veterinary Journal* **51**, 533

Alvarez-Melis D and Jaakkola TS (2018) On the robustness of interpretability methods. arXiv:1806.08049

Burti S, Longhin Osti V, Zotti A and Banzato T (2020) Use of deep learning to detect cardiomegaly on thoracic radiographs in dogs. *The Veterinary Journal* **262**, 105505

Croskerry P (2009) Clinical cognition and diagnostic error: applications of a dual process model of reasoning. *Advances in Health Sciences Education* **14**, 27–35

Li S, Wang Z, Visser LC, Wisner ER and Cheng H (2020) Pilot study: Application of artificial intelligence for detecting left atrial enlargement on canine thoracic radiographs. *Veterinary Radiology & Ultrasound* **61**, 611–618

Lustgarten JL, Zehnder A, Shipman W, Gancher E and Webb TL (2020) Veterinary informatics: forging the future between veterinary medicine, human medicine, and One Health initiatives—a joint paper by the Association for Veterinary Informatics (AVI) and the CTSA One Health Alliance (COHA). *JAMIA Open* **3**, 301–317

Markopoulos PP, Kundu S, Chamadia S and Pados DA (2017) Efficient L1-norm principal component analysis via bit flipping. *IEEE Transactions on Signal Processing* **65**, 4252–4264

McInnes L, Healy J and Melville J (2020) UMAP: Uniform manifold approximation and projection for dimension reduction. arXiv:1802.03426

Moon KR, van Dijk D, Wang Z *et al.* (2019) Visualizing structure and transitions in high-dimensional biological data. *Nature Biotechnology* **37**, 1482–1492

Pfau D, Higgins I, Botev A and Racanière S (2020) Disentangling by subspace diffusion. arXiv:2006.12982

Roberts N, Prabhu VU and McAteer M (2019) Model weight theft with just noise inputs: The curious case of the petulant attacker. arXiv:1912.08987

Sidarta-Oliveira D and Velloso L (2020) Comprehensive visualization of high-dimensional single-cell data with diffusion-based manifold approximation and projection (dbMAP). Available from: ssrn.com/abstract=3582067 [preprint]

van der Maaten L and Hinton G (2008) Visualizing data using t-SNE. *Journal of Machine Learning Research* **9**, 2579–2605

Waite S, Scott J, Gale B *et al.* (2017) Interpretive error in radiology. *American Journal of Roentgenology* **208**, 739–749

Chapter 7

Basics of thoracic image interpretation

Peter Scrivani and Tobias Schwarz

Overview of thoracic image interpretation

Following image acquisition, veterinary surgeons (veterinarians) must evaluate the images and provide an interpretation of the study. Image interpretation goes beyond lesion detection: it is the process of identifying signs and patterns and explaining their meaning in each patient. When possible, the interpretation should explicitly address any clinical question that prompted the study. Veterinary surgeons achieve best practice by basing the interpretation on extensive clinical experience, a good working knowledge of how patients are managed, and a strong knowledge of the patient's history, normal anatomy and physiology, pathology, imaging technology and epidemiological principles.

The reading environment

- Images should be evaluated in a quiet ergonomically appropriate environment that maximizes workflow, supports a healthy posture, avoids repetitive stress injuries, circumvents burnout and distraction, and improves efficiency and accuracy (Figure 7.1). It is particularly important to avoid visual fatigue due to glare and a mismatch between the ambient room light and monitor brightness. For a screen brightness of at least 350 cd/m², ambient light should be about 20–40 lux. Users should allow their eyes to adjust for about 15 minutes prior to image evaluation and take breaks from staring at the monitor.
- Medical display devices: digital display monitors are the modern standard for viewing imaging studies (Rubin *et al.*, 2019).
  - Primary diagnostic displays are used mostly by radiologists or other health professionals to generate medical reports.
    - Minimal recommended resolution = 3 megapixels.
    - Minimal recommended luminance range = 1–350 cd/m².
    - Regularly calibrated to within 10% of the DICOM Grayscale Standard Display Function.
  - Clinical review displays are used by a range of health professionals to view and interpret images to direct patient care and are often used in conjunction with the report.
    - Minimal recommended resolution = 2 megapixels.
    - Minimal recommended luminance range = 0.8–250 cd/m².
    - Annually calibrated to within 20% of the DICOM Grayscale Standard Display Function.
- Mobile device displays are typically handheld, compact and lightweight devices that perform many of the functions of other display options. Due to the range of devices available and difficulty in controlling the reading environment, these displays should be used mainly in the absence of a primary diagnostic display.

Patient information

- The signalment, history and available clinical information are required to establish prior probability of disease. If these are unknown, then it is the interpreter's responsibility to obtain this information.

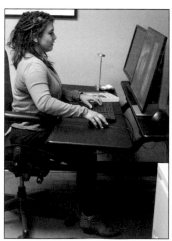
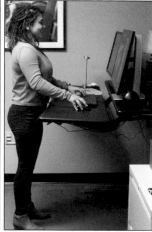

7.1 Improved work efficiency and avoiding repetitive injury is possible with an ergonomic workstation. The optimal desk height varies with the size of the user and different tasks. Adjustable desks allow users to make small height modifications for different tasks and larger variations to shift between sitting and standing positions. When sitting, it is important to have a comfortable chair that supports the spine. For both sitting and standing, the display monitor should be tilted 10–20 degrees, positioned about an arm's length away and a couple of inches below eye level. The keyboard should be flat or have a slight negative incline to avoid wrist extension and be wide enough for hands to be about shoulder-width apart. The mouse should be easy to move and comfortable to grip. Good ambient lighting is essential and can be achieved with a combination of natural light, overhead light and task lighting. When possible, extraneous stressors (e.g. background noise) should be eliminated and items that promote a calm pleasant workplace introduced.

- The reason for performing the examination must be identified (i.e. treatment planning or diagnosis). For treatment planning studies, the interpreter must ensure that the report provides the necessary information (e.g. anatomical location and extent of the abnormality). For diagnostic studies, the conclusion should be one of the following:
  - A definitive diagnosis
  - A short, prioritized differential diagnosis
  - If neither is possible, that the study did not answer the clinical question (further study may be necessary).

Image quality and appropriateness of the examination

- The interpreter should conduct an initial assessment of the imaging examination:
  1. Confirm that the images belong to the correct patient.
  2. Determine how the patient was oriented during image acquisition (e.g. standing, recumbent). In small animals, assume that the X-ray beam is oriented vertically (perpendicular to the floor) unless otherwise indicated.
  3. If possible, use the anatomy and history to confirm that marker placement is correct. For lateral radiographic views where the left and right sides summate with each other, the 'L' or 'R' marker indicates the point of exit of the X-ray beam was on the patient's left or right side, respectively. For other thoracic images where it is possible to discern left and right, the 'L' or 'R' marker indicates the patient's left or right side.
  4. Review any previous imaging studies and reports.
- The interpreter should then review the history and determine whether the imaging examination is likely to answer the clinical question.
  1. Was the appropriate study performed to answer the clinical question?
  2. Is the examination of sufficient quality? The study does not have to be perfect to answer the clinical question and imperfect studies are acceptable when there are extenuating circumstances related to cost, efficiency, patient safety, technician safety and availability of equipment. Careful consideration should be given to anything that might adversely influence the final interpretation, such as insufficient views, poor patient positioning, underexposure and respiratory motion.
  3. If the study is unlikely to answer the clinical question, additional images should be acquired when possible or the study limitations should be taken into consideration when making the final interpretation.

Systematic evaluation of the imaging study

- Displaying images consistently and according to convention facilitates the development of a single mental picture of normal anatomy and recognition of abnormal conditions and patient orientation.
  - The conventional hanging protocol for lateral thoracic radiographs is to place the patient's dorsum at the top of the image and the patient's cranial aspect towards the viewer's left.
  - The conventional hanging protocol for dorsoventral and ventrodorsal thoracic radiographs is to place the patient's cranial aspect at the top of the image and the patient's left side towards the viewer's right.
- Once the images are organized and prepared for viewing, observers should systematically inspect them for imaging signs.
  - Most experienced radiologists are immediately drawn to, and spend most of their time looking at, the most important finding(s). They are also very adept at looking at the rest of the image(s) to detect any additional findings that may have minor or major consequence. Early in the training period, novices may benefit from using a systematic approach to consciously evaluate every aspect of the study. For example, one may look at all the organs or areas in the same order each time.
  - If multiple images are provided together, they should not be viewed in isolation. If something catches the eye on one image, then that finding should be fully evaluated on multiple images before evaluation of the rest of the image. Displaying multiple images simultaneously (e.g. orthogonal views, different windows) or clicking back and forth between different images helps streamline this type of evaluation.
  - The search for abnormalities must not end after one is found as additional abnormalities might be present.
- Although inefficient, looking at images at different times (now and later) can yield important new information on the second viewing. Similarly, opinions from other people can help.

Subconscious biases during interpretation

Despite the best efforts to interpret imaging studies in a completely systematic and unbiased way, the default mode of human thought processing relies on biases to facilitate a quick response such as a fight or flight reaction. This can be overcome by analytical thinking, but this does not occur naturally in the first instance as it is slow and laborious (Kahneman and Patrick, 2011). In the image interpretation process, this way of thinking manifest commonly in different scenarios:

- Being locked in to a tunnel vision of a limited differential diagnosis once a pattern is recognized. If on retrospective assessment this turns out to be the wrong diagnosis, it is often difficult to comprehend why the correct pathology, that was a well known entity to the observer, was not included in the original differential diagnosis (Figure 7.2)
- Being unable to complete a systematic review of an imaging study in the presence of a very prominent anatomical or pathological structure. This could be described as 'the power of the obvious'. By being constantly drawn to this feature, the observer is unable to concentrate on the systematic review (Figure 7.3)
- Subconscious pattern recognition relies on the visible and obvious. A radiographic sign of the absence of a certain feature, such as the normally non-visible pleural space and mediastinal vessels, usually requires analytical thinking and is therefore often missed in the initial intuitive interpretation process. Similarly, when the cardiac silhouette is effaced by neighbouring structures, the intuitive approach usually homes in on the opacity and not the visible absence of the cardiac silhouette which is often the key to diagnosis (Figure 7.4)

- Intuitive thinking is a natural cognition process that cannot simply be replaced by analytical thinking as the first modal response. All people with some image interpretation experience will use an intuitive pattern recognition approach at the beginning of the image interpretation process consciously or subconsciously, whether they think they interpret the image systematically or not. It is therefore best to accept and manage this. It is also important to understand that there is a certain reward basis for the thinking process. Human thinking drives on the feeling of satisfaction, when identifying a potential diagnosis for a detected pattern. The authors find the following approaches useful to deal with this during the interpretation process:

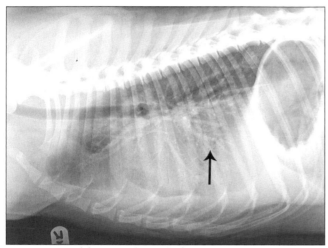

7.2 Lateral thoracic radiograph of a 3-year-old Labrador Retriever cross with dyspnoea. There is partial effacement of the cardiac silhouette by pleural fluid and opacification of the accessory lung lobe, containing some gas bubbles (arrowed). Based on these signs, a very reasonable diagnosis is pyothorax and pneumonia secondary to a migrating foreign body. However, a diagnosis of accessory lung lobe torsion was made at surgery. Although the accessory lung lobe infrequently undergoes torsion, the combination of pleural effusion and lung consolidation with vesicular pattern is a classic radiographic pattern of lung lobe torsion. Failure to include relevant differentials can occur when subconscious pattern recognition bias influences the 'best match'.

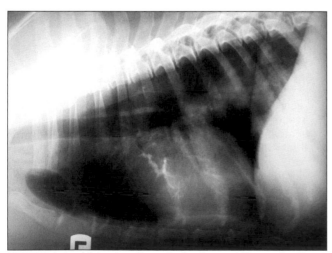

7.3 Lateral thoracic radiograph of an 8-year-old Rottweiler. The linear mineralization summating with the cardiac silhouette craves the attention of the viewer ('power of the obvious'). It is difficult to concentrate on other areas, such as the gas-distended oesophagus, until this obvious lesion has been dealt with. It is therefore best to describe the mineralization first. This is incidental aortic mineralization, commonly seen in older dogs.

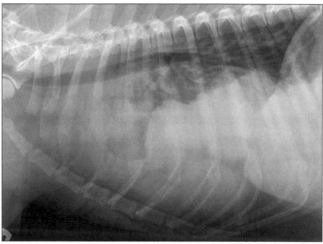

7.4 Lateral thoracic radiograph of an 8-year-old Golden Retriever with dyspnoea and lethargy. Most observers are initially drawn to the multiple soft tissue opacities in the ventral thorax. However, the key to resolving this case is recognizing that the cardiac silhouette is not visible. It can be assumed that the heart is present in a living dog. Therefore, border effacement is the likely cause for this, which can only be caused by a soft tissue structure in direct contact with the heart, such as the pericardial sac, pleural fluid or masses, lungs that have the opacity of soft tissue, herniated abdominal content or mediastinal masses. Eliminating the least likely candidates first and using context from other views and other radiographic signs such as the dorsal deviation of the trachea, a cranial mediastinal mass is the most likely and is consistent with the confirmed diagnosis of thymoma.

- A first round of interpretation in which a spontaneous diagnosis is made ('shooting from the hip'). This gives a feeling of satisfaction ('I am so clever') and makes the observer more open to analytical thinking. This round is then followed by a round of reflection ('Let's check my amazing blitz diagnosis') which is the analytical process of systematic review
- Interpreting the cardiac silhouette first or early in the interpretation process. It is big, in the middle of the image and impossible not to look at during interpretation. It craves attention, distracting from the assessment of other structures. Once it is assessed, a feeling of satisfaction occurs, making the observer ready to move on in the interpretation
- Interpreting large or obvious pathological lesions first or early in the interpretation process for the same reasons as for the cardiac silhouette
- When performing the systematic review, making a conscious effort to reflect on non-visible structures as signs of normality or pathology
- Breaking down the task into very small, seemingly trivial steps makes it less challenging to engage analytical thinking. For example:
  - The cardiac silhouette is not visible → the heart can be assumed to be present → it must be effaced by neighbouring structures → neighbouring structures are the pericardium, pleural space, mediastinum and some lung lobes, or abdominal herniated content → eliminate the least likely of these five options
  - The lung opacity is either normal, decreased or increased → if increased, describe any mass lesions → if lesion is too diffuse to describe as a mass, apply other characteristics such as lung patterns

- Writing down the main findings and differential diagnoses at every round of interpretation. The act of writing stimulates reflection, as does reading notes. For this, handwriting is more powerful than typing or dictating. Where possible, for the same reasons, vocalizing initial thoughts is helpful

- Cherishing reviewing thought processes (for which it is useful to have them written down). In addition to the satisfaction found in the initial intuitive process, there is satisfaction to be found in reviewing it ('I have learned something today'). Doing this will also further fine-tune pattern recognition in intuitive thinking ('I will never forget this one'), and thereby improve future performance.

Making use of the entire available spectrum of image resolution

Image resolution refers to the amount of information captured in an image (The Royal College of Radiologists, 2012). The maximum image resolution is determined at the time of image acquisition and may or may not be displayed during evaluation.

The displayed image is affected by many factors including screen size and luminance, viewing angle, distance and post-processing of the image. Some post-processing decisions are made at the time of image reconstruction, such as applying a computer algorithm to increase edge sharpness, which improves the acutance (perceived *versus* actual sharpness). Other post-processing decisions are made locally at workstations during the image evaluation using software tools such as zooming and windowing.

Optimizing spatial resolution

If a digital radiograph cannot be displayed fully on the monitor at the original resolution, then the image should be evaluated twice to optimize use of the available spatial resolution (Figure 7.5). First, the entire image should be displayed within the maximum available screen area – this optimizes pattern recognition of non-spatially limited abnormalities. Second, the entire radiograph should be systematically evaluated (part by part) at the original resolution using zoom and magnification tools. Additional magnification can be helpful but does not add to the information that was initially captured.

In contrast to radiographs, most other types of medical images are small enough to be viewed on a monitor without interpolation below the acquisition resolution, even when multiple scans are displayed side by side.

Optimizing contrast resolution

The amount of grayscale information that can be displayed at one time is limited. To optimize evaluation of all structures relative to differences in signal intensity, digital images should be evaluated multiple times using different windows and levels (Figure 7.6). The window level (or centre) is the midpoint of the grayscale. It should be selected to optimize viewing of the desired tissue. The window width is the number of grey shades that are displayed. It should be selected to optimize whether the image contrast is high or low.

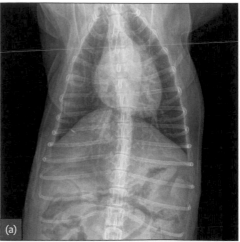

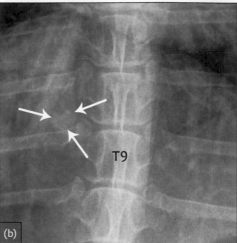

7.5 Making use of the available spatial resolution by using the pan and magnification tools: the same dorsoventral thoracic radiograph of a 13-year-old Miniature Poodle displayed at (a) 25% resolution and (b) 100% resolution. If the entire digital radiograph cannot be displayed on the monitor at the original resolution, then the image should be evaluated at least twice. Firstly, the entire image should be displayed within the maximum available screen area. Secondly, each part of the image should be evaluated at the original resolution. The pulmonary nodule (arrowed) is more noticeable in (b). T9 = ninth thoracic vertebra.

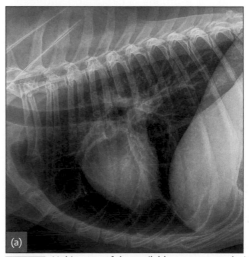

7.6 Making use of the available contrast resolution by adjusting the window centre and width: the same lateral thoracic radiograph of a 4-year-old Labrador Retriever cross is shown using different display windows. In (a), the window and level are optimized for evaluating the skeleton; in (b), the lungs. The cardiac silhouette is dorsally located due to dehydration. In (a), this finding could be erroneously attributed to pneumothorax. (continues)

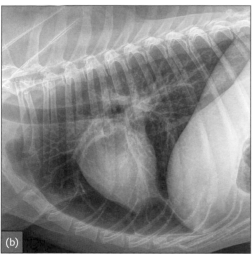

7.6 (continued) Making use of the available contrast resolution by adjusting the window centre and width: the same lateral thoracic radiograph of a 4-year-old Labrador Retriever cross is shown using different display windows. In (a), the window and level are optimized for evaluating the skeleton; in (b), the lungs. The cardiac silhouette is dorsally located due to dehydration. In (b), the pulmonary blood vessels are clearly seen extending to the periphery of the thoracic cavity. Images should be evaluated using different windows and levels to make use of all the available grayscale information.

Anatomy

The animal body comprises five parts: head, neck, trunk, tail and limbs. The trunk encompasses the back (dorsum), thorax, abdomen and pelvis. The thorax, abdomen and pelvis are conceptually similar as they each have a musculoskeletal (somatic) wall that encloses a major body cavity. The major body cavities are the thoracic, abdominal and pelvic cavities. They are ventral to the back, contain internal organs (i.e. viscera) and are generally subdivided into smaller cavities and spaces by serous membranes.

Thoracic cavity

The thorax is located between the neck and abdomen and chiefly contains the major organs of circulation and respiration. The thoracic boundaries define the thoracic cavity.

- The thoracic inlet is the cranial aperture or opening.
- The thoracic outlet is the caudal aperture or opening and mostly comprises the diaphragm.
- The dorsal boundary is formed by the back.
- The ventral boundary is formed by the:
  - Chest (pectoral region)
  - Breast (sternal region)
  - Left thoracic body wall (costal region)
  - Right thoracic body wall (costal region).

Thoracic viscera

The thoracic cavity houses the thoracic viscera. The basic unit of a living organism is the cell. Cells combine to form tissues. There are two embryonic tissue types based on morphology: epithelium and mesenchyme. There are four fetal and postnatal tissue types: epithelial, connective, muscular and nervous. Tissues with a similar function combine to form organs. An internal organ is a viscus. Organs are either solid (e.g. thymus, lymph nodes) or hollow (e.g. heart). Most thoracic organs are hollow and their lumens may contain fluid (blood vessel), air (trachea),

ingesta or nothing (oesophagus). The lungs are unique because of the bidirectional airflow and presence of multiple tiny lumens that may be regionally different or may act collectively as one unit.

- Molecular imaging focuses on imaging cellular and subcellular pathways.
- Morphological imaging focuses on tissues, organs, spaces and cavities.
- Functional imaging provides physiological information regardless of morphology.

During radiography, both solid and hollow organs can form a silhouette in the image. In hollow organs, a silhouette generally appears when the lumen is fluid-filled (same opacity as the wall) or collapsed and empty. In this situation, appropriate descriptors generally relay information about the overall silhouette (overall size, shape and opacity) and not internal components (Figure 7.7). Occasionally, comments can be made specifically about wall or lumen content (e.g. the wall is mineralized, the lumen contains centrally located gas, the lumen contains a foreign body). Cross-sectional imaging and contrast radiographic studies might allow for additional descriptors of wall thickness, wall architecture (e.g. layering, cortex/medulla) and lumen diameter, and of internal components such as parenchymal nodules or cysts.

Hollow organs may change in size because of normal muscle contractions and relaxations that constrict or dilate the lumen. Hollow organs may also be surgically enlarged by dilation. Solid organs and the walls of hollow organs may enlarge due to the influx of fluid, fibre or cells, or the enlargement of cells. Hollow organs can also enlarge due to increased intraluminal pressure (e.g. venous distention, gas distention) and may appear taut when this is severe.

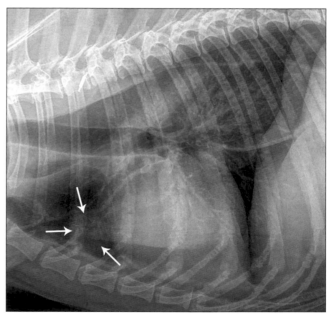

7.7 Lateral thoracic radiograph of a 9-year-old Beagle with myasthenia gravis associated with thymoma. The myasthenia gravis has caused megaoesophagus. Notice the oesophageal diameter is severely diffusely increased and the lumen contains a large volume of gas. The thymoma (arrowed) forms a small mass-like tumour, which is circumscribed, round, and has a homogeneous soft tissue opacity. Viscera are either solid or hollow. During radiography, it is impossible to determine whether the thymic mass is solid or hollow (cystic and fluid-filled) as both would produce a silhouette. For similar reasons, the heart, which is a hollow organ, is often described in terms of the cardiac silhouette. The trachea and oesophagus are hollow and gas-filled, and cross-sectional imaging is required to determine their internal architecture.

Solid organs and the walls of hollow organs may shrink due to loss of fluid or cells, reduced size of cells or fibrosis. Hollow organs can also shrink due to external compression or when internal pressure is lost and then may appear collapsed or flaccid.

Hollow organs that contain intraluminal gas and fluid may have a gravity-dependent air–fluid interface visible on cross-sectional imaging or during radiography using a horizontally oriented X-ray beam (Figure 7.8). Suspended or trapped gas suggests caseous, organizing or foreign material.

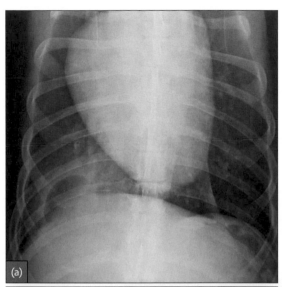
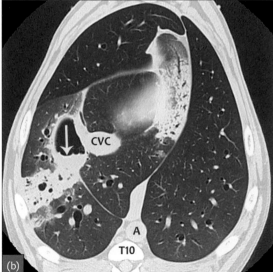

7.8 (a) Ventrodorsal thoracic radiograph and (b) transverse thoracic CT image of a 6-month-old mixed-breed dog with a right caudal lung lobe abscess and pneumonia due to a migrating plant awn. On the radiograph, no air–fluid interface is observed because a vertically oriented X-ray beam was used. CT was performed in dorsal recumbency and an air–fluid interface (arrowed) is detected due to gravity-dependent distribution of gas and fluid. Gravity-dependent distribution of gas and fluid in the lungs is also evident on the CT image: the lungs are more lucent and the pulmonary blood vessels are smaller ventrally. To the right of and dorsal to the abscess and in the ventral tip of the accessory lung lobe, there are patches of lung consolidation without volume loss attributed to the infiltration of fluid and inflammatory cells into the lung parenchyma (i.e. pneumonia). The right caudal lung lobe also has a diffuse ground-glass opacity and larger pulmonary blood vessels due to increased blood flow typical of inflammation. Increased blood flow to poorly ventilated lung can produce a ventilation:perfusion mismatch (physiological right-to-left shunting). The plant awn is not seen. A = aorta; CVC = caudal vena cava; T10 = tenth thoracic vertebra.

Connective tissues

Connective tissue supports all tissues (Figure 7.9). The topography of thoracic viscera is partly determined by specialized connective tissues (i.e. serosa, adventitia and fascia) that hold organs in place or allow motion. These connective tissues also determine the imaging appearance of many types of thoracic disease.

Serosa (serous membrane): This is a smooth thin sheet-like membrane that consists of a secretory squamous epithelial layer (mesothelium) and a supporting connective tissue layer.

* The outer layer of thoracic organs is the tunica serosa (visceral layer of a serous membrane) or tunica adventitia (tunica externa).
* A serous cavity (e.g. pleural cavity) is formed when a serous membrane reflects upon itself producing a mesothelial-lined space. Normally, the cavity is only a potential space as it only contains a small volume of fluid derived from serum. This fluid provides lubrication and allows movement of organs. Abnormal expansion of a body space/cavity is most commonly due to an influx of fluid, gas or cells and may be influenced by the internal pressure (e.g. tension pneumothorax). Reduced size of a body space/cavity is usually due to a loss of volume or compression.
* A double fold of serosa that does not produce a mesothelial-lined cavity and connects viscera together or to the body wall is either a mesentery, omentum or ligament (e.g. pulmonary ligament).
* Serous membranes are typically characterized as parietal when covering a body wall or visceral when covering an organ.

Adventitia: This is loose connective tissue that lacks mesothelium and binds structures together and may store fat. Most of the structures within the mediastinum are connected and covered by adventitia. The heart is an exception.

Fascia: The fascia also may contain fat and is a casing of connective tissue that surrounds and stabilizes the position of organs including muscles, blood vessels, bones and nerves. Fascia tends to form bands or sheets and can create pathways for nerves and blood vessels as well as for the spread of disease. In the thoracic cavity, the outermost membrane is the endothoracic fascia. It contains a variable amount of fat and attaches the parietal pleurae to the internal surface of the thoracic body wall. In the neck, back and thoracic body wall, superficial and deep fasciae lie between skin, muscle and viscera (i.e. oesophagus and trachea). Products of disease such as gas, inflammation/infection, neoplasms and haemorrhage can travel through these pathways, and some routes lead into the thoracic cavity.

Body regions

The external surface descriptions for the thorax are detailed below and shown in Figure 7.10:

* Thoracic vertebral region: overlying the thoracic vertebrae
  * Interscapular region: between the dorsal borders of the scapulae
* Pectoral region: regions on the surface of the chest
  * Presternal region: overlying the superficial pectoral muscle (especially the descending part), between the median and lateral pectoral grooves

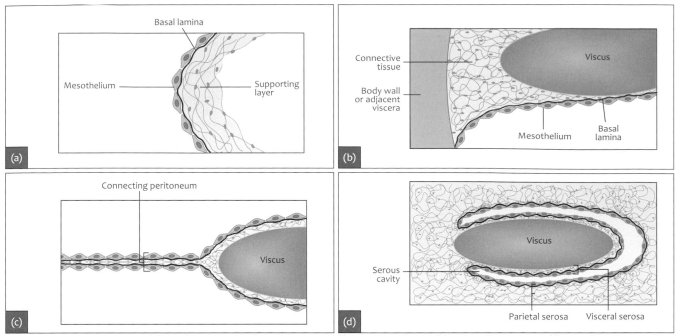

7.9 Connective tissues and their relationships to adjacent structures. (a) Serous membrane. (b) Body wall and organs. (c) Formation of connecting peritoneum (ligaments, mesenteries and omenta). (d) Serous cavity (e.g. pleural cavity). In the thorax, the parietal pleura attaches to the body wall via the endothoracic fascia, a third type of connective tissue.

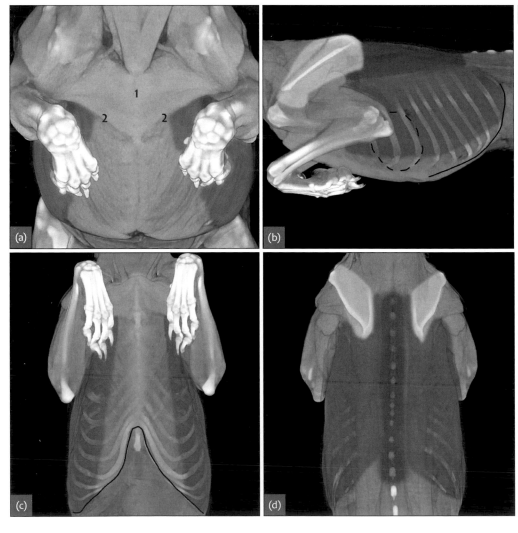

7.10 Volume-rendered CT images of a 9-year-old mixed-breed dog showing the (a) cranioventral, (b) left, (c) ventral and (d) dorsal aspects of the thorax, back and thoracic limbs. The surface regions of the thorax and back are identified. The ventral surface of the thorax is called the pectoral region or chest. It is divided into: the presternal region (orange) that overlies the descending pectoral muscles between the median (1) and lateral (2) pectoral grooves, the sternal region (green) that overlies the sternum, the region of the thoracic mammary glands (not shaded), the scapular region (yellow) that overlies the scapulae, the costal region (blue) that overlies the osseous portion of the ribs, and the cardiac region (dotted line in (b)) that overlies the heart caudal to the moveable tricipital line. The solid line in (b) and (c) indicates the costal arch, which is formed by the cartilaginous portions of the asternal ribs connecting the most caudal rib to the sternum. Dorsally, the surface regions of the back (regions of the dorsum) are the lumbar region (unmarked) and the thoracic vertebral region (red); the portion between the dorsal borders of the scapulae is further characterized as the interscapular region (withers).

- Sternal region: overlying the sternum
- Thoracic mammary gland region
- Scapular region: overlying the scapulae
- Costal region: overlying the ribs, excluding the costal cartilages
  - Intercostal space: space between ribs
  - Costal arch: formed by costal cartilages of the asternal ribs and connecting the ventral end of the last rib to the sternum
  - Cardiac region: overlying the heart, caudal to the tricipital margin.

Orientation and direction terminology

- Object planes (e.g. organ, tissue) (Figure 7.11).
  - Long axis (longitudinal): a line drawn through the structure along its largest dimension.
  - Short axis (transverse or transversal): perpendicular to the long axis.
  - Note that multiple short or long axes through an object are possible depending on the overall shape.
- Body planes (Figure 7.12). It should be noted that imaging modalities designed for humans use terms appropriate for bipeds.
  - Median: a plane that divides the thorax into equal left and right halves.
  - Sagittal (paramedian): all planes parallel to the median plane dividing the thorax into asymmetrical left and right sections.
  - Transverse (transversal): all planes perpendicular to the longitudinal axis dividing the thorax into cranial and caudal sections. In bipeds, the axial plane divides the thorax into superior and inferior (cranial and caudal) sections.
  - Dorsal: all planes perpendicular to both the median and transverse planes, parallel to the dorsum, and dividing the thorax into dorsal and ventral sections. In bipeds, the coronal or frontal plane divides the thorax into anterior and posterior (ventral and dorsal) sections.
  - Oblique: any plane at an angle to the above planes.
- Directions.
  - Cranial/caudal: towards/away from the head.
  - Dorsal/ventral: towards/away from the back.
  - Medial/lateral: towards/away from the median plane.
  - Intermediate/middle: between two similar structures or midway between positions (intermediate, especially between medial and lateral).
  - External/internal and superficial/deep: closer to/farther from the external surface of the body.
  - Median: in the median plane.
  - Dorsal midline/ventral midline: longitudinal line in the median plane on the dorsal/ventral surface of the thorax.

Recommendations are available for how to combine directional terms in a standardized fashion when naming radiographic views (Smallwood *et al.*, 1985). These same recommendations may be used to provide consistent anatomical descriptions of the thorax. When using left or right, these terms should come first (e.g. left cranial, right caudal). Cranial and caudal otherwise should take priority (e.g. cranioventral, caudodorsal) and medial and lateral should be last (e.g. craniodorsomedial, caudoventrolateral).

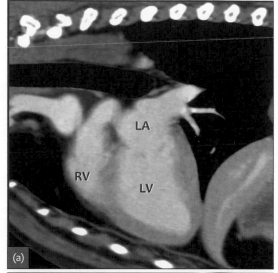

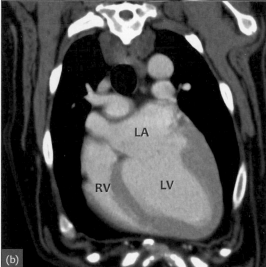

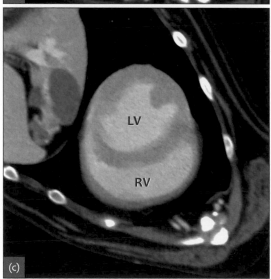

7.11 Object planes. Contrast-enhanced thoracic CT images (soft tissue window) of a 9-year-old mixed-breed dog. All three images are oriented at 90 degrees to each other. (a, b) Long-axis and (c) short-axis images of the heart. The terms long-axis (longitudinal axis) and short-axis (transverse axis) describe planes through a specific organ or tissue. The long and short axes of a structure might not correspond to the three conventional planes that divide the thorax. For example, (a) may also be called a sagittal oblique image of the thorax, (b) a transverse oblique image and (c) a dorsal oblique image. Both terms for each image are correct, but the former indicates that the emphasis is on the heart *versus* the thorax. LA = left atrium; LV = left ventricle; RV = right ventricle.

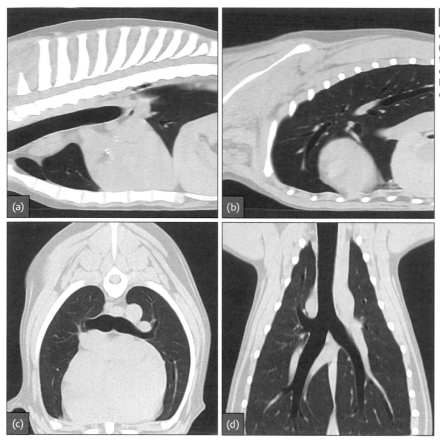

7.12 Body planes. Thoracic CT images (lung window) of a 9-year-old mixed-breed dog depicting (a) the median plane, (b) a sagittal plane, (c) a transverse plane and (d) a dorsal plane. These terms of orientation are used primarily when describing planes through the entire thorax *versus* individual thoracic structures. Images representing oblique planes are also possible.

Body systems

The body systems (groups of organs sharing a common function) that comprise the thorax include:

- Integumentary system
  - Skin (epidermis, dermis and subcutaneous tissue), hair, skin glands and thoracic mammary glands
- Digestive system
  - Oesophagus: part of the alimentary canal connecting the pharynx and stomach
- Respiratory system (lower respiratory tract only)
  - Lower airway: the passageway from the rima glottidis to respiratory bronchioles
    - Large airways (caudal part of laryngeal lumen, trachea and bronchi)
    - Small airways (bronchioles)
  - Lungs: the site of gas exchange between the body and the external environment (the parenchyma or airspace)
  - Alternatively, the respiratory tracts may be divided functionally into the 'conducting zone' and 'exchange zone.' The conducting zone also includes the upper respiratory tract
- Circulatory system
  - Cardiovascular system: the network is pressurized and closed as blood never leaves the confines of heart, arteries, veins and capillaries. The pulmonary circulation involves the right heart and lungs: it is where blood is oxygenated. The systemic circulation involves the left heart and entire body: it is where oxygenated blood is delivered
  - Lymphatic system: this network does not have a central pump like the heart and is open because interstitial fluid collects into thin valveless vessels

before being returned to the veins near the heart. Large lymphatic vessels are called ducts. Lymph is filtered by lymph nodes. A collection of lymph nodes occurring at a predictable location and draining a similar region is a lymph centre
  - Extracellular fluid is called interstitial fluid when in the interstitium, lymph when in lymphatic vessels and serum when in blood vessels (Figure 7.13)
  - The thoracic duct is the chief channel for returning lymph from the body to the systemic circulation: collecting lymph from the head, neck, abdominal viscera, pelvis and limbs
  - There are three major thoracic lymph centres. The major lymph nodes in these centres are the cranial sternal, cranial mediastinal and tracheobronchial lymph nodes
  - T-lymphocyte production and maturation occurs in the thymus, which is in the cranial mediastinum and regresses with age
- Skeletal system
  - The portion of the axial skeleton consisting of the rib cage, sternum and thoracic vertebral column. Includes red and yellow bone marrow
- Muscular system (skeletal muscle)
  - Epaxial muscles primarily comprise the intrinsic back muscles, are innervated by the dorsal branch of the spinal nerves and are predominantly located dorsal to the transverse processes of the vertebrae, attaching to the vertebral column, ribs and skull
  - Hypaxial muscles are innervated by the ventral branch of the spinal nerves, are predominantly located ventral to the vertebral column, and include the thoracic and abdominal wall muscles, diaphragm, and all limb and girdle muscles

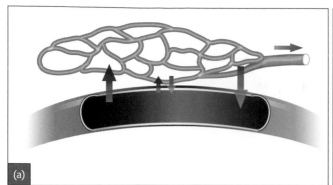

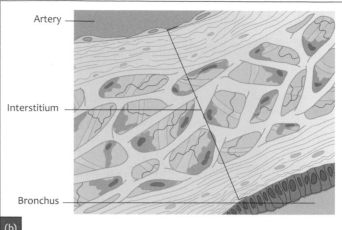

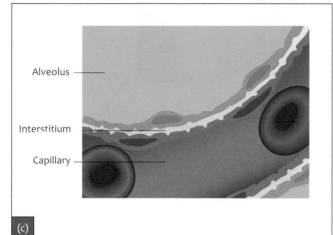

7.13 (a) Movement of extracellular fluid between the interstitium, capillary and lymphatic vessels. The systemic circulation (*versus* the pulmonary circulation) is depicted. The interstices collectively form the interstitium and are filled with extracellular fluid. There is a constant movement of fluid between the interstitium, capillary lumen and lymphatic vessel lumen. The movement of extracellular fluid between the blood vessel and interstitium is governed by a balance of hydrostatic (red arrows) and oncotic (colloid osmotic; blue arrows) pressure gradients, described as Starling forces. The brown arrow denotes drainage of the interstitial fluid as lymph by the lymphatic system. (b) The interstitium between a bronchus and a pulmonary artery is thick where connective tissue joins two adventitia and creates fluid-filled spaces called interstices. (c) The alveolar interstitium is a much thinner shared membrane between the alveolus and capillary that allows for gaseous exchange.
(Redrawn after Lauren D. Sawchyn, DVM, CMI)

- Nervous system
  - The central nervous system (CNS) encompasses the brain and spinal cord, assimilates sensory information about the external environment and internal body and sends coordinated motor responses to other parts of the CNS or the rest of the body
  - The peripheral nervous system (PNS) connects the body to the CNS, providing both sensory information and motor responses, and comprises cranial and spinal nerves (e.g. vagus, recurrent laryngeal, phrenic), ganglia (e.g. cervicothoracic, sympathetic trunk, middle cervical) and organs like the aortic bodies
  - The PNS includes the somatic nervous system for innervation relating to voluntary muscle control (e.g. body wall movement) and the autonomic nervous system (ANS) that innervates internal organs (e.g. to control heart rate). The efferent portion of the ANS allows the body to be in two different functional states: sympathetic and parasympathetic.

Embryology

Formation of the thoracic boundaries and serous cavities

The intraembryonic coelom begins as one continuous space that forms between the outer somatic (parietal) and inner splanchnic (visceral) layers of the lateral plate mesoderm. The somatic layer and ectoderm combine to form the somatopleure, which will expand, fuse with the same on the opposite side, and give rise to the body wall, parietal pericardium, parietal pleurae and parietal peritoneum. The splanchnic layer and endoderm combine to form the splanchnopleure, which will give rise to the gut (e.g. oesophagus), outgrowths from the gut (e.g. lungs), visceral pericardium, visceral pleurae and visceral peritoneum.

Subsequently, the intraembryonic coelom is partitioned into the thoracic and abdominopelvic cavities, and then further divided into the major serous cavities by folding of the embryo, growth of the heart and lungs, and development of the paired pleuropericardial membranes and diaphragm. The major serous cavities are the pericardial, pleural and peritoneal cavities. In carnivores, a fenestrated mediastinum separates two pleural cavities (left and right). A minor serous cavity, the mediastinal serous cavity (also called the Sussdorf's space), forms in the caudal mediastinum adjacent to the right side of the oesophagus due to expansion of the right pneumoenteric recess cranial to the diaphragm (see Chapter 10). The diaphragm forms from the septum transversum (central tendon), dorsal oesophageal mesentery (crura), paired pleuroperitoneal folds (periphery) and ingrowth of body wall muscle (periphery).

Osseous development

The ribs and sternebrae develop by endochondral ossification where bone replaces a hyaline cartilage model. Ribs are derived from the sclerotome portion of the paraxial mesoderm and form the costal process of the vertebrae. The sternum develops from the somatic mesoderm in the ventral body wall. The vertebrae form via multiple mechanisms. The vertebral arch forms as part of neurulation. The vertebral body forms as part of somitogenesis, somite segmentation and endochondral ossification.

Aerodigestive tract formation

The endoderm-lined foregut gives rise to the oesophagus and lower respiratory tract. The latter arises from a median outpouching of the foregut (ventral surface) called the laryngotracheal (respiratory) diverticulum. The respiratory diverticulum separates the upper and lower airways and gives rise to the caudal larynx, trachea and lungs. The developing trachea produces buds and then divides forming branching and progressively smaller bronchi and bronchioles. Associated with the terminal bronchioles, the developing lung undergoes a series of four maturation periods to form functional alveoli.

Cardiovascular development

Ab initio, the heart arises cranial to the brain and then is repositioned caudoventrally into the thoracic cavity due to growth and folding of the embryo. The heart arises from two endocardial tubes that come together and fuse into a single cylindrical tube with unidirectional flow and five regions: sinus venosus, primordial atrium, ventricle, bulbus cordis and aortic sac. This tube folds to form the bulbo-ventricular loop and eventually transforms into four chambers and two circuits (systemic and pulmonary) maintaining unidirectional flow.

The sinus venosus transfers to the right side so blood flow across the atrium is right-to-left. Growth of the septum primum partially divides the primordial atrium into two atria and the persistent opening is the ostium primum. With growth of the endocardial cushions, the ostium primum closes and an ostium secundum develops in the same septum. In addition, a septum secundum develops. The gap remaining in the wall is the foramen ovale. After birth, the foramen is no longer patent. The endocardial cushions forming the primordial atrioventricular (AV) septum separate the common AV canal into left and right AV canals. The developing interventricular septum divides the primordial ventricle into two chambers and eventually fuses with the endocardial cushions creating a four-chamber heart.

The pericardium is a fibroserous sac that envelops the heart and reflects around the roots of the great vessels. The outer part is the fibrous pericardium and the inner part is the serous pericardium. The serous pericardium comprises a parietal layer that is firmly fused to fibrous pericardium, a serous cavity called the pericardial cavity and a visceral layer that is also called the epicardium (Figure 7.14). The fibrous pericardium is derived from the septum transversum, its apex attaches to the ventral part of the diaphragm via the phrenicopericardial ligament and its cranial surface variably contacts the thymus. The phrenic nerves arise from the mid-to-caudal cervical spinal cord segments and innervate the diaphragm. In the thorax, these nerves primarily run along the mediastinal pleurae, but caudally the right nerve runs through the plica venae cavae. In the middle mediastinum, the nerves run between the mediastinal pleural and fibrous pericardium.

The aortic arch and major arteries to the head, neck and thoracic limbs arise from six paired aortic arches that form sequentially between the dorsal and ventral aortae. The embryonic aortic arches are initially symmetrical and subsequently undergo changes that result in the final asymmetrical form of the adult. The paths of the recurrent laryngeal nerves vary due to this developmental process. In adults, the left recurrent laryngeal nerve loops around the aortic arch and the right recurrent laryngeal nerve loops around the right subclavian artery.

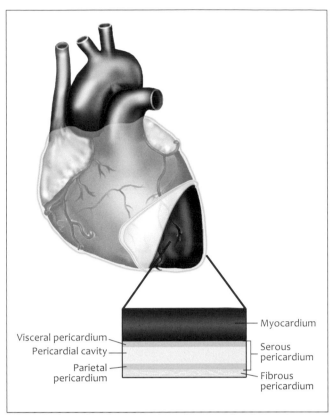

7.14 The pericardium comprises a fibrous pericardium and serous pericardium. The serous pericardium can be further divided into the visceral pericardium, pericardial cavity and parietal pericardium.

The descending aorta is in the midline, divided into thoracic and abdominal parts, and forms when the two embryonic dorsal aortae fuse. The thoracic aorta has parietal and visceral branches. Parietal branches supply the thoracic back and dorsal part of the body wall. Ventrally, the internal thoracic arteries also supply the body wall. Visceral branches supply the intrathoracic oesophagus, bronchi, mediastinum and pericardium. They transport only a small portion of blood from the left ventricle and represent the structural blood flow to the lungs that provides nutrients. The chief blood flow to the oesophagus and bronchi is via the broncho-oesophageal artery.

The pulmonic trunk and left and right pulmonary arteries arise from the truncus arteriosus and sixth pharyngeal arches. The pulmonary blood flow comprises all blood from the right ventricle and represents the functional blood flow to the lungs where gas exchange occurs. In the fetus, the ductus arteriosus connects the pulmonic trunk to the aortic arch. After birth, this vessel closes and forms the ligamentum arteriosum.

The systemic and portal venous systems that bring deoxygenated blood to the heart arise from three pairs of embryonic venous systems (umbilical, vitelline and cardinal). A fourth venous system drains the lungs and conveys oxygenated venous blood to the left side of the heart.

Interpretation principles

The thorax comprises mostly hollow organs or potential spaces, which produce different interpretation paradigms from solid structures. Frequently, the most important factor that informs differential diagnosis is the anatomical localization of the abnormality (e.g. pneumonia occurs in the lung and not the pleural cavity nor the mediastinum).

The precision of a differential diagnosis list often relates to the exactitude of anatomical localization, but there are limits to what is possible. There is a big difference between localizing an abnormality to the caudodorsal thorax, caudodorsal lung field and left caudal lung lobe. The first description is deliberately vague and indicates that the abnormality may be in the lung, pleural cavity, body wall, diaphragm or mediastinum. The latter two descriptions are more exact, imply that the abnormality is in the lung, but differ by how precisely the abnormality can be localized within the lung. The latter information can be important when a disease preferentially affects a specific part of the lung.

When determining the anatomical position of a thoracic abnormality, it is helpful to begin by localizing the abnormality to one of five broad anatomical compartments (listed below). This early step is helpful because it quickly allows one to eliminate unlikely diagnostic considerations that affect other compartments (Figure 7.15).

- Thoracic boundaries:
  - Some signs of disease in this anatomical compartment are discontinuous rib margin, vertebral malalignment, extrapleural sign and herniation of abdominal viscera into the thoracic cavity.
- Pleural cavities:
  - Some signs of disease in this anatomical compartment are retraction of lung margin away from the body wall, pulmonary blood vessels not extending to the periphery of the thoracic cavity, scalloped lung margins and wide pleural fissures.
- Lungs:
  - Some signs of disease in this anatomical compartment are altered lung size, pulmonary opacification, linear patterns, nodular patterns, air bronchogram, border effacement of pulmonary blood vessels and lobar sign.
- Mediastinum:
  - Some signs of disease in this anatomical compartment are localization to the median plane, increased width, tracheal stripe sign, oesophageal enlargement and lymph node enlargement.
- Cardiac silhouette:
  - Some signs of disease in this anatomical compartment are increased size, altered shape (globoid or focal bulging) and altered opacity.

Some animals have disease in multiple anatomical compartments due to the same disease affecting multiple compartments or multiple diseases affecting different compartments. Anatomical localization to specific structures within the broad anatomical compartment can further assist narrowing and prioritizing the differential diagnosis. For example, different lung diseases affect the parenchyma (airspace), bronchi (airways) and stroma (connective tissue, blood vessels). Chapters 8–12 are organized by these five broad anatomical compartments and address this process of further localizing disease to more precise anatomical compartments.

Cardiopulmonary physiology

Maintaining a constant internal environment (homeostasis) is a fundamental principle that underlies much of physiology. The body has several control systems that maintain its internal environment and comprise positive and negative feedback control loops. These loops feature a sensor, control centre, effector and feedback mechanism: information is mainly transmitted through nervous impulses or chemical messengers (hormones).

- Circulatory system function:
  - Circulate fluid throughout the body for the removal of waste and the delivery of nutrients, chemicals and cells.
- Respiratory system function:
  - Conducting zone: conveys, moistens and warms the air from outside the body as it makes its way to the lungs. In the thorax, the trachea, bronchi and bronchioles conduct air between the lungs and the external environment
  - Respiratory zone: gas exchange occurs in the pulmonary parenchyma or airspace (i.e. pulmonary acinus or the lung distal to a terminal bronchiole).

Cardiac conduction and cardiac cycle

In the right atrium, the sinoatrial node acts as a normal biological pacemaker controlling heart rate and rhythm. Electrical excitation originates at this location and then depolarization propagates through both atria, the atrioventricular node, the bundle of His and the Purkinje fibres

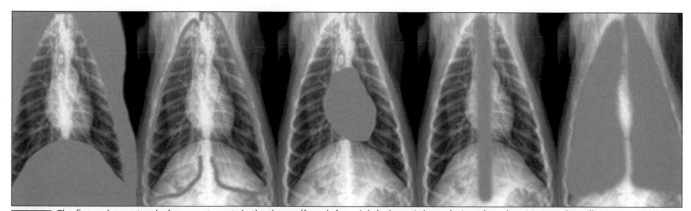

7.15 The five major anatomical compartments in the thorax (from left to right): thoracic boundaries, pleural cavities, cardiac silhouette, mediastinum and lungs. During image interpretation, once an abnormality is identified, it is helpful to first localize the abnormality to one or more of these major anatomical compartments. Subsequent evaluation may further define the anatomical location within the anatomical compartment or reveal additional findings that help prioritize the differential diagnosis.

of the left and right bundle branches, resulting in activation of all ventricular muscle. Pathological conditions that disrupt or alter this pathway can lead to arrhythmias and cardiac dysfunction.

The cardiac cycle refers to the phases that describe the path blood takes through the heart (Klabunde, 2021):

- Atrial contraction with closed semilunar valves (aortic and pulmonic) and open atrioventricular valves (mitral and tricuspid)
  - P wave of electrocardiogram (ECG) (atrial depolarization)
  - Fourth heart sound (S4)
  - 10–40% of ventricular filling by atria (rest *versus* exercise)
  - Ventricular volume is maximal after atrial contraction (end-diastolic volume)
- Isovolumetric phase: ventricular pressure increases without a change in volume because all valves are closed
  - QRS complex of ECG (ventricular depolarization)
- Ventricular emptying
  - Initial rapid ejection of blood into the aorta and pulmonic trunk by ventricular contraction with open semilunar valves and closed atrioventricular valves
    - Left atrial pressure initially decreases and then atrial pressure increases due to atrial filling
    - First heart sound (S1), systolic murmur may indicate valve disease or intracardiac shunt
  - Reduced ejection of blood as ventricular repolarization occurs
    - T wave of ECG
    - Atrial pressures continue to increase
  - Isovolumetric relaxation: ventricular pressure decreases without volume change because all valves are closed
    - Second heart sound (S2)
    - Blood remaining in the ventricle is end-systolic volume
    - Left atrial pressure continues to rise as blood returns from the lungs
- Ventricular filling
  - Initial rapid filling of the ventricles when the atrioventricular valves open (semilunar valves remain closed)
    - Ventricular pressure briefly falls as the ventricle is still undergoing relaxation but begins to rise due to atrial flow once relaxation is complete
    - No normal heart sound, a third heart sound (S3) might indicate ventricular dilatation
  - As ventricles continue to fill, intraventricular pressure increases and filling reduces because of a reduced pressure gradient across the atrioventricular valves
    - During rest, about 90% of ventricular filling is passive and occurs before atrial contraction Aortic and pulmonary arterial pressures continue to drop.

Perfusion

The chief function of the heart is to impart energy to blood and thereby create and sustain an arterial blood pressure that allows adequate perfusion, which is the delivery of blood to the capillary beds of tissues and organs for the exchange of gases, nutrients and waste products (Klabunde, 2021; Chaudhry *et al.*, 2022).

Perfusion throughout the body is via two circulatory loops:

- The pulmonary circulation provides deoxygenated blood from the right side of the heart to the lungs and returns oxygenated blood to the left side of the heart
- The systemic circulation provides oxygenated blood from the left side of the heart to most of the body and returns deoxygenated blood to the right side of the heart. This circuit is a larger and higher pressure system.

Blood is pumped through both circuits by muscular contractions of the heart. The velocity and amount of blood delivered to tissues and organs is controlled by several factors and blood vessels play a major role in controlling flow. Flow rate is the volume of fluid passing through an area during a specified amount of time. Flow depends on fluid characteristics (velocity, viscosity, density, compressibility) and blood vessel characteristics (radius (r), length, stiffness, elasticity). Flow is measured by the Poiseuille equation, which is pressure change divided by resistance.

$$\text{Resistance} = \frac{8 \times \text{viscosity} \times \text{length}}{\pi r^4}$$

Arteries have thick, elastic walls to accommodate high pressures. Arterioles have the biggest effect on blood pressure regulation by determining the resistance to blood flow, which ensures that blood flow to capillary beds is constant and not pulsatile (Chaudhry *et al.*, 2022). Abnormal arterial stiffening, narrowing, or inflammation can interfere with normal arteriolar function.

- Arteriolar smooth muscle constriction and dilation are under autonomic (involuntary) control. Baroreceptors and chemoreceptors associated with the aorta and carotid arteries provide afferent (sensory) information. Arteriolar constriction increases resistance so there is decreased blood flow and blood pressure at the level of the capillaries. Arteriolar dilation decreases resistance so there is increased blood flow at the level of the capillaries and a smaller decrease in blood pressure at this level.
- Diastolic blood pressure is directly proportional to total peripheral resistance and defined as the lowest arterial pressure when the ventricles are relaxing and filling. Recoil of the aortic wall also contributes to diastolic pressure.
- Systolic blood pressure is directly proportional to stroke volume and defined as the peak arterial pressure when the ventricles are contracting. Aortic compliance affects systolic pressure.
- Pulse pressure is the difference between systolic and diastolic pressures, proportional to stroke volume and inversely proportional to arterial compliance.
- Mean arterial pressure is the average pressure in the arteries throughout the cardiac cycle.

Most of the blood volume resides in the venous system, but the proportions of arterial and venous blood vary with total blood volume, intravascular pressures, cardiac output, vascular resistance and vascular compliance (Klabunde, 2021). The venous system is generally a lower pressure system due to low resistance and high compliance.

Some concepts necessary for understanding heart physiology

- Cardiac output is the volume of blood ejected from the left ventricle each minute (stroke volume x heart rate) and is normally equal to venous return (Chaudhry *et al.*, 2022).
- Stroke volume is the amount of blood pumped out of the heart after one contraction. It is the difference between end-diastolic and end-systolic volumes. It increases with increased contractility, increased preload and decreased afterload.
- Preload is the pressure on the ventricular muscle by the ventricular end-diastolic volume.
- The Frank–Starling law states that the heart attempts to equalize cardiac output with stroke volume, and therefore describes the relationship between the end-diastolic volume and the stroke volume. In other words, as more blood returns to the heart during diastole, the heart will contract harder and pump more blood during systole.
- Afterload is the pressure that is needed to eject blood during ventricular contraction (systole) and is proportional to the mean arterial pressure. It is estimated by the minimum pressure needed to open the aortic valve, which is equivalent to the diastolic pressure.
- Ejection fraction is an index for contractility and is equal to the stroke volume divided by the end-diastolic volume. A low ejection fraction indicates heart failure.

Starling forces describe the movement of extracellular fluids between the blood vessels and the interstices. Blood plasma volume and interstitial fluid volume are controlled by the balance of hydrostatic and oncotic (colloid osmotic) pressure gradients, which together define the net pressure that governs the direction of fluid movement (Taylor, 1981). Net pressure is the product of the difference in hydrostatic pressure between the capillaries and interstitium and the difference in osmotic pressure between the capillaries and interstitium.

- Blood oncotic pressure induced by proteins like albumin can draw fluid into blood vessels when it is greater than the interstitial oncotic pressure. A reduction in proteins can shift blood out of blood vessels.
- Blood hydrostatic pressure that is greater than interstitial fluid hydrostatic pressure can shift water and small molecules into the interstices.
- Interstitial fluid hydrostatic pressure is generally lower than capillary hydrostatic pressure due to continuous lymphatic drainage.

Ventilation

Ventilation is the movement of air between the lungs and environment that occurs during inhalation and exhalation. Lung inflation and deflation are a result of pressure changes that occur during breathing. Contraction and relaxation of the diaphragm and intercostal muscles alter the size of the thoracic cavity. Assuming that the larynx and lower airway are patent:

- During inhalation, expansion of the thoracic cavity creates a negative pressure (relative to atmospheric pressure) within the thoracic cavity that allows the lungs to fill with air
- During exhalation, reduction in the size of the thoracic cavity creates a positive pressure within the thoracic cavity that propels air out of the lungs.

Lung properties

- Elasticity refers to the ability of something to return to its normal shape after being stretched or compressed. Lung elasticity is a result of the collagen and elastin fibres in the connective tissue meshwork. Separation of the lung from the thoracic body wall during disease, as with pleural fluid and pneumothorax, will cause lung collapse due to its inherent elasticity.
- Surface tension is the tendency of liquid surfaces to form the minimum surface area possible because liquid molecules are more attracted to each other than to adjacent molecules in the air. Surface tension in the pleural cavities holds the lungs against the body wall and helps prevent the lungs from collapsing. In the lungs, the water lining the inner surface of the alveoli would lead to collapse of the alveoli because of this tendency except that type II pneumocytes produce surfactant. A surfactant is a surface-active agent that reduces surface tension, preventing collapse of the alveoli.
- Compliance is a characteristic of many body parts and is the relationship between changes in volume and changes in pressure (Desai *et al.*, 2022). In other words, it is a description of how well an elastic structure stretches. Lung compliance is a measure of lung expandability (how well it can stretch). An abnormally stiff lung (e.g. atelectatic, fibrotic, absent surfactant) has low compliance; this makes breathing more difficult as it requires more work. A lung with poor elastic recoil (e.g. emphysema) has too high compliance such that the alveoli have a high residual volume of gas making it difficult to expel air out of the lungs.

The relationship between ventilation and perfusion

The heart and lungs are inextricably linked (Powers and Dhamoon, 2021). Gas exchange occurs in the lungs between the alveolar air (from the environment) and pulmonary capillaries (circulatory system).

- Ventilation (V) refers to airflow into and out of the alveoli.
- Perfusion (Q) refers to blood flow in the alveolar capillaries.

Different portions of the lung experience variable degrees of ventilation and perfusion due to physiological, physical (e.g. gravity) and pathological conditions. Collective changes in ventilation and perfusion in the lungs are measured using the ratio of ventilation to perfusion (V:Q). V:Q mismatches can affect gas exchange and lead to hypoxaemia.

- Decreased V:Q ratio: right-to-left shunts (i.e. pulmonary arterial blood bypasses the alveoli).
  - Pulmonary arteriovenous malformations.
  - Congenital developmental cardiovascular anomalies (e.g. tetralogy of Fallot, Eisenmenger syndrome).
- Decreased V:Q ratio: physiological right-to-left shunts (i.e. non-ventilated lung is perfused).
  - Airway obstruction (e.g. asthma).
  - Decreased diffusion (e.g. pulmonary fibrosis, emphysema, pulmonary oedema, pneumonia).
- Increased V:Q ratio: physiological right-to-left shunts (i.e. ventilated lung is not perfused).
  - Pulmonary embolism may restrict blood flow to ventilated alveoli.
  - Overventilation of normally perfused lung, which may occur, does not usually lead to hypoxaemia.

Note that hypoxaemia may occur when there is normal ventilation and perfusion (e.g. high-altitude hypoxia, carbon monoxide toxicity). Also, poor perfusion elsewhere in the body can produce ischaemia and infarction in those locations. Hypoxic vasoconstriction, a normal physiological process, can minimize the effect of physiological right-to-left shunts by redirecting blood flow to better ventilated areas of the lungs for more efficient exchange.

Selected interpretation principles

Thoracic imaging is unique because cardiac and respiratory motion often have a considerable influence on image quality. To overcome some of this limitation, it may be necessary to sedate patients, position them in ventral recumbency, select a high sampling rate, or perform cardiac and respiratory gating so heart and lung motion are coordinated with image acquisition. For some dynamic studies, a trade-off between temporal and spatial resolution may be necessary.

Hypoxic vasoconstriction accounts for why there may not be detectable pulmonary opacification with atelectasis (there is a comparable reduction in blood flow to the lungs) (Figure 7.16). Hypoxic vasoconstriction is not as effective during general anaesthesia, which is why atelectasis may be more problematic (more right-to-left shunting due to more perfusion of poorly ventilated lung).

The interpretation of some pulmonary findings will depend on whether the patient is hypoxaemic or not. The body can compensate for some lung abnormalities (even extensive ones) and not develop hypoxaemia. Other causes are more likely to produce hypoxaemia. For example, the V:Q mismatch that occurs during pneumonia may be due not only to decreased ventilation because of decreased diffusion but also because of increased perfusion due to inflammation. Therefore, even minor lung abnormalities could produce greater than anticipated hypoxaemia (see Figure 7.8).

In patients with cardiac, pulmonary, vascular or pleural cavity disease, it is extremely helpful to consider the impact of volume, pressure and flow.

Congenital developmental anomalies

Congenital developmental cardiac anomalies tend to produce either volume overload or pressure overload to specific heart chambers or the great vessels (Figure 7.17). Volume overload is typically due to cardiovascular shunts

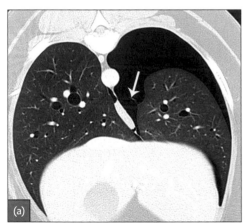
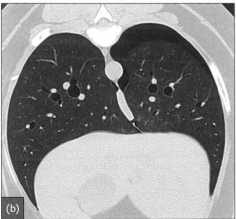

7.16 Transverse thoracic CT images of a 7-year-old Golden Retriever with pneumothorax. (a) The left pleural cavity contains a large volume of gas and the left caudal lung lobe is partially collapsed. The opacity of this lung lobe is only minimally increased because there is a comparable reduction in blood flow to that lung lobe due to hypoxic vasoconstriction (note the reduction in size and number of the pulmonary blood vessels). The left pulmonary ligament (arrowed) can be seen attaching the left lung to the mediastinum. (b) Following thoracocentesis, the volume of pleural gas is reduced and the left caudal lung lobe is expanded and aerated with an opacity that is similar to that of the right caudal lung lobe. In normal animals, the opacity of the lung parenchyma (airspace) reflects a balance between the amount of air and blood in the lung. During disease, pulmonary opacification is due to the infiltration of fluid, fibre or cells into the lung and/or reduced aeration. Pulmonary hyperlucency is generally due to increased spacing of the soft tissue structures of the lung (e.g. emphysema) or reduced blood flow (e.g. hypovolaemia).

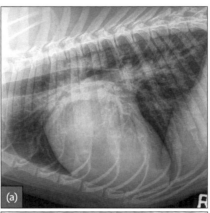
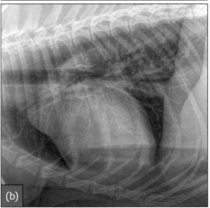

7.17 Right lateral thoracic radiographs of (a) a 10-month-old German Shepherd Dog with a patent ductus arteriosus and (b) an 8-year-old Golden Retriever with subaortic stenosis. Both dogs had echocardiographically confirmed left heart enlargement. (a) Left heart enlargement is easily seen as the cardiac silhouette is tall and wide with prominent bulges of the left atrium and left ventricle. This is due to volume overload causing eccentric hypertrophy of the left heart. Although the dog has a left-to-right shunt (aorta to pulmonic trunk), it is the left side of the heart that experiences the volume overload because of the pulmonary drainage: the affected cardiac chambers enlarge. (b) The left heart enlargement is not detected. This is due to pressure overload causing concentric hypertrophy of the left ventricle: the affected cardiac chamber decreases in size due to increased muscular thickness. In (a), there is loss of the cranial cardiac waist due to focal enlargement of the aortic arch and pulmonic trunk, and the pulmonary blood vessels are enlarged and numerous due to pulmonary overcirculation. In (b), there is loss of the cranial cardiac waist due to post-stenotic dilatation of the aortic arch, and a mediastinal fat pad mildly displaces the cardiac silhouette dorsally.

and induces eccentric hypertrophy in the affected structure. Typically, this produces a large heart chamber, which is easily detected during radiography unless the shunt is small. One can determine the type of shunt by knowing which chamber(s) or vessels blood is being shunted to. Pressure overload is typically due to an obstruction to flow (e.g. a stenosis) and induces concentric hypertrophy in the upstream chamber. Typically, this produces a thick myocardium at the expense of the lumen and, therefore, heart chamber enlargement may not be detected radiographically unless the obstruction is severe or long-standing. However, a post-stenotic dilatation is common and more easily seen during radiography. The type of stenosis can be determined by assessing whether there is bulging of the aortic arch or pulmonic trunk.

Pulmonary oedema

Pulmonary oedema has numerous causes and is often a result of altered Starling forces. Some causes include increased capillary hydrostatic pressure due to left heart failure or fluid overload (pulmonary venous distention may also be observed), increased capillary permeability due to acute respiratory distress syndrome or sepsis, decreased capillary osmotic pressure due to nephrotic syndrome or liver failure, and obstructed lymphatic drainage (Figure 7.18).

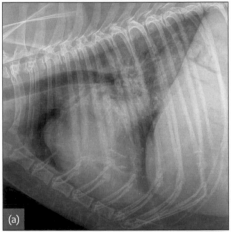

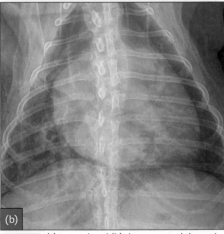

7.18 (a) Lateral and (b) dorsoventral thoracic radiographs of a 15-year-old mixed-breed dog with cardiogenic pulmonary oedema and postcapillary pulmonary hypertension due to a ruptured chorda tendina (confirmed via echocardiography). The cardiac silhouette is tall, long and wide with bulges of the left atrium, left ventricle and right atrium. The caudodorsal lung field has a severe ground-glass opacity due to elevated left atrial pressure and reduced pulmonary venous drainage causing left-sided congestive heart failure. Elevated left atrial pressure also increases systolic right ventricular pressure by increasing the load on the right ventricle.

Pulmonary thrombosis

Pulmonary thrombosis may produce reduced lung volume (atelectasis) due to surfactant disruption making it more difficult to expand the lungs (see Chapter 12).

Bronchial foreign bodies

Bronchial foreign bodies can cause increased lung size when acute if the foreign body acts like a one-way valve (obstructive air trapping). Bronchial foreign bodies can also cause decreased lung size when chronic because air in the lung gets absorbed and the lung cannot reinflate due to the obstruction (obstructive atelectasis) (Figure 7.19).

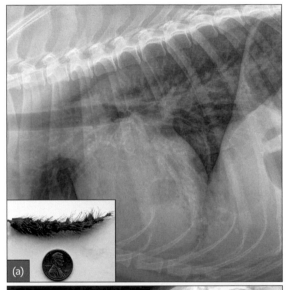

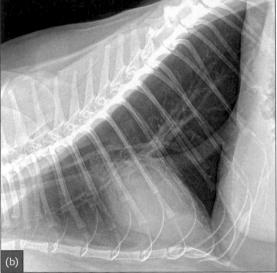

7.19 Lateral thoracic radiographs of (a) a 5-year-old Labrador Retriever with a chronic intermittent cough due to a bronchial foreign body and (b) an adult cat that was found dead. Assessing lung volume is one of the most important steps in the imaging interpretation of lung disease. (a) The dog has chronic obstructive atelectasis of the right middle lung lobe. The affected lung lobe is small and has patchy areas of consolidation. The foreign body is undetectable. The insert shows a plant awn that was endoscopically removed from the bronchus and an American penny as a size reference. (b) The cat has acute obstructive air trapping, diffusely affecting both lungs. Post-mortem lungs are frequently collapsed. In this cat, the lungs are severely expanded and the diaphragm is flat due to a valve-like tracheal foreign body seen cranial and dorsal to the cardiac silhouette, consistent with kibble.

((b) Courtesy of Lance Rozear)

Pulmonary hypertension

Pulmonary hypertension is abnormally increased pulmonary artery pressure (Reinero *et al.*, 2020). Echocardiography, especially Doppler echocardiography (e.g. to estimate pressure change across the tricuspid valve), can be used to support a diagnosis of pulmonary hypertension, but it is not a definitive test. During radiography, enlargement of the left and right pulmonary arteries, pulmonic trunk and right heart may also suggest pulmonary hypertension, especially when severe or long-standing.

Imaging plays an important role in assisting classification of the cause of pulmonary hypertension (Figure 7.20):

* Left heart disease
* Airway or parenchymal lung disease
* Pulmonary embolism
* Dirofilarial infection or angiostrongylosis.

There are several underlying mechanisms that may lead to the development of pulmonary hypertension:

* Increased pulmonary arterial blood flow (e.g. left-to-right shunt)
* Increased pulmonary vascular resistance (e.g. vasoconstriction, perivascular inflammation, lumen obstruction, increased blood viscosity, vascular hardening, pulmonary disease)
* Increased pulmonary venous pressure (e.g. left heart disease, compression of a large pulmonary vein)
* A combination of factors.

During radiography and computed tomography (CT), intravascularly administered contrast agents tend to be iodinated. Contrast enhancement is a combination of intravascular and extravascular mechanisms (Figure 7.21). Intravascular enhancement (angiography) occurs because

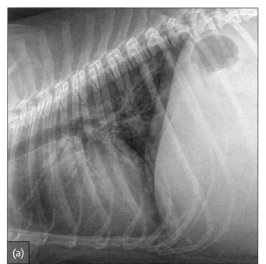

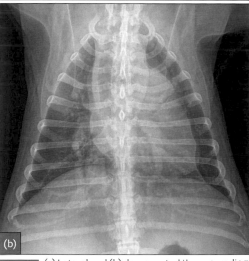

7.20 (a) Lateral and (b) dorsoventral thoracic radiographs of a 2-year-old dog with heartworm infection. This dog had pulmonary hypertension due to increased pulmonary arterial resistance. The pulmonary arteries are moderately enlarged and tortuous (best seen on the dorsoventral view), and the pulmonic trunk and the right heart are moderately enlarged. The dog also has caval syndrome as the presence of worms is interfering with tricuspid valve closure, obstructing blood flow through the right heart and increasing systemic venous pressure: there is enlargement of the caudal vena cava and abdominal distention with absent serosal contrast due to ascites (peritoneal fluid). Starling forces can lead to fluid moving out of the capillaries when blood hydrostatic pressure is high.

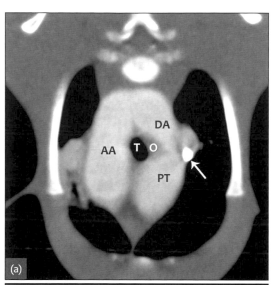

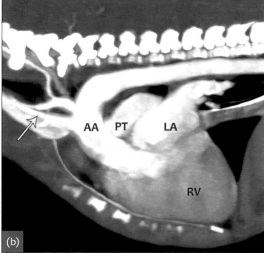

7.21 (a) Transverse and (b) sagittal thoracic CT angiograms of a 2-month-old Staffordshire Bull Terrier with a vascular ring anomaly. There is good opacification of the left heart, aorta and pulmonic trunk following a systemic venous injection of contrast material. (a) The vascular ring can be seen surrounding the trachea and oesophagus. The vascular ring anomaly comprises a persistent right fourth aortic arch and a patent ductus arteriosus. In normal dogs, the aortic arch is to the left of the trachea (not to the right as in this dog) and the ductus arteriosus does not contrast enhance because it forms a ligamentum arteriosum. Note that the ductus arteriosus is derived from the left sixth aortic arch and connects the aorta to the pulmonic trunk. (b) This image was acquired to the right of the midline (the ductus arteriosus is not included) and image acquisition was timed so that contrast material was in the levophase. Contrast material is present in the left atrium but not in the right ventricle. The cranial vena cava has an intravascular catheter (arrowed). AA = aortic arch; DA = ductus arteriosus; LA = left atrium; O = oesophagus; PT = pulmonic trunk; RV = right ventricle; T = trachea.

contrast material is present in the lumen of blood vessels. From a non-selective venous injection, image acquisition can be timed to preferentially show contrast material in the arteries (arterial phase) or arteries and veins (delayed phase). Most tissues generally show some degree of background contrast enhancement due to the normal blood supply.

- Increased intravascular enhancement is due to any process that increases blood flow or blood volume (e.g. neovascularization, vasodilation, hyperaemia, shunting).
- Decreased intravascular enhancement is due to insufficient dose, inappropriate timing of image acquisition or anything that decreases blood flow (e.g. vascular obstruction, hypotension).

Extravascular enhancement is also called interstitial enhancement because contrast material leaks out of the permeable capillary walls into the interstitial fluid. Other contrast agents are used for magnetic resonance imaging (MRI) and ultrasonography.

Pathology

Broad categories of disease

Disease may develop because of abnormal regulated or unregulated growth or because of internal or external forces that produce cell injury and loss. These factors are used to determine the four major categories of disease (i.e. developmental anomalies, neoplasia, inflammatory disease and degenerative disease). Some diseases may fall under multiple headings (e.g. feline hyperthyroidism is both a benign neoplasm and a metabolic disorder).

Developmental anomalies

These malformations are structural or functional abnormalities that are the result of some error in normal regulated growth and may be present at conception or arise during prenatal (congenital) or postnatal (acquired) development. These malformations may be due to genetic or environmental teratogens (e.g. ionizing radiation, infections, hyperthermia, toxins). The type of malformation usually depends more on the timing of the insult in relation to ontogenesis than on the underlying cause. Imaging is especially useful for characterizing developmental anomalies because many involve morphological change (Figure 7.22). Imaging may be performed specifically to characterize developmental anomalies when the malformation is associated with patient morbidity or is a potential risk factor for future disease. Many developmental malformations, however, are incidental findings of minor consequence and should not be mistaken as clinically significant.

Neoplasia

Neoplasia is *unregulated* growth in the body that is new: the new tissue is called a neoplasm. Neoplasms may be benign or malignant. Hyperplasia is reversible, whereas neoplasia is not.

- Benign neoplasms tend to progress slowly and rarely invade adjacent tissues or spread to distant sites.

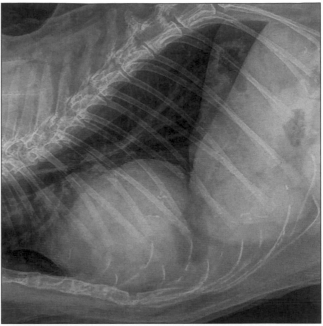

7.22 Lateral thoracic radiograph of a 12-year-old Maine Coon cat with nasal lymphoma. During staging, the cat was also diagnosed with a peritoneopericardial diaphragmatic hernia, which is a congenital developmental anomaly of variable clinical importance. The cardiac silhouette is enlarged with distorted shape and heterogeneous opacity. The ventral aspect of the diaphragm is effaced and the caudal sternebrae are fused. CT revealed herniation of liver lobes, choleliths, the gallbladder and the fatty falciform ligament through a defect in the ventral midline of the diaphragm into the pericardial cavity.

A benign neoplasm, however, may cause substantial morbidity when it physically interferes with an organ's function (e.g. bronchial obstruction) or releases substances such as hormones (e.g. thyroid adenoma causing feline hyperthyroidism).
- Malignant neoplasms tend to progress rapidly and frequently invade adjacent tissues or metastasize. A malignant neoplasm that physically or functionally disrupts normal processes is cancer. Some patients with cancer develop a paraneoplastic syndrome, which is a set of signs that occurs distant to the tumour. The signs may be due to:
  - The neoplasm releasing substances (e.g. proteins, hormones) that travel through the blood and affect distant organs
  - Immune responses meant to kill the tumour that also damage healthy cells
  - Unknown mechanisms (e.g. hypertrophic osteopathy secondary to intrathoracic vagus nerve injury).

During imaging, neoplasms are frequently seen because they form a space-occupying lesion, which is an abnormal swelling (Figure 7.23). Regardless of whether the neoplasm is benign or malignant, the swelling may be localized and organized forming a small (nodule) or large (mass) abnormality. Nodular and mass-like lesions may be solid, cystic or cavitary. Hollow lesions may contain fluids, gas or both. Alternatively, the swelling may be less organized (i.e. infiltrative) or unseen in the circulation (e.g. leukaemia). Organ infiltration may appear as regional swelling or diffuse enlargement depending on how widespread the distribution is. Linear patterns are possible when the neoplasm follows nerves, airways or vascular tracts.

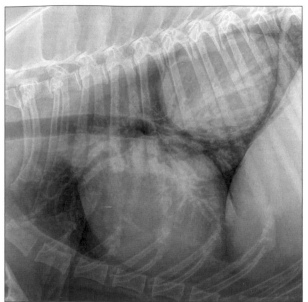

7.23 Lateral thoracic radiograph of a 7-year-old Labrador Retriever with a histologically confirmed pulmonary chondrosarcoma. The neoplasm forms a large solitary tumour in the left caudal lung lobe. The tumour is rounded, circumscribed and has a homogeneous soft tissue opacity. In addition, the tumour forms a positive summation shadow with the ribs, vertebral bodies and pulmonary blood vessels.

Inflammatory diseases

Exposure to harmful stimuli (e.g. infectious agents, allergens, trauma, ischaemia, chemical irritants, ionizing radiation) can cause cell damage and activate the inflammatory response. Inflammation is a collection of the body's reactive processes that initiates the healing process and may remove the offending stimuli, protect the body from further damage and ultimately return the body to normal.

Some of the molecular, vascular and cellular responses are:

- Coagulation
- Complement activation
- Fibrinolysis
- Increased vascular permeability
- Leucocyte extravasation
- Phagocytosis
- Vasodilation.

An insufficient inflammatory response can be fatal and lead to progressive tissue damage by the inciting stimulus.

- Acute inflammation is transitory (hours to weeks) and begins quickly after exposure to harmful stimuli and comprises a series of immune and vascular events that produces localized pain, loss of function, redness and heat. Chemically mediated systemic effects (e.g. fever, malaise, leucocytosis) are possible. Hyperaemia and swelling are common. Hyperaemia is due to increased blood flow and vasodilatation. Swelling is due to cellular infiltration and extracellular fluid accumulation. Extracellular fluid accumulation may be within body cavities, on epithelial surfaces (serous or fibrinous effusion) or within tissues (oedema). The outcome is usually elimination of the inciting factor and resolution of inflammation (i.e. return to normal) but fibrous scarring is possible. Fibrous scarring may be of minor consequence due to wound healing or may be a cause of ongoing dysfunction.

- Chronic inflammation occasionally follows acute inflammation and may be associated with progressive tissue damage, which might lead to organ failure. It may organize into a mass (e.g. abscess, granuloma).
- Inflammatory disease refers to an exaggerated inflammatory response that produces more tissue damage than would have been caused by the inciting stimulus. Extensive tissue remodelling and fibrosis can replace normal tissue to such an extent that there is organ failure and death (e.g. pulmonary fibrosis). It is broadly subdivided into:
  - Infectious inflammatory disease, which may have viral, bacterial, mycotic, algal or parasitic causes
  - Non-infectious inflammatory diseases, which are typically due to a defect in the immune system (e.g. allergy, autoimmune disease).

During imaging, signs of acute inflammation (e.g. hyperaemia, swelling), chronic inflammation (e.g. scarring, abscess, granuloma) and inflammatory disease (e.g. atrophy, fibrosis) may be seen (Figure 7.24).

- The shape of infiltrative disease tends to conform to the shape of the organ (e.g. bronchitis produces 'tram lines' and rings).
- Signs of inflammation and neoplasia may overlap (i.e. infiltration, masses). Abscesses tend to be hollow masses and granulomas tend to be solid. Abscesses may contain fluid, gas or both.

Degenerative diseases

Degenerative disease is a catch-all term for a broad group of diseases that disrupt the normal biochemical processes of differentiated cells, resulting in cell death, loss of cellular components or accumulation of intracellular products. Because of the large number of diseases included in this group, it is helpful to create subdivisions.

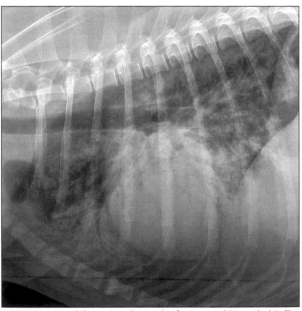

7.24 Lateral thoracic radiograph of a 5-year-old Bearded Collie with pneumonia. The results of the tracheal wash showed septic suppurative inflammation due to polymicrobial infection (Gram-positive cocci, Gram-positive rods and Gram-negative rods). In this case, the infiltration of fluid and inflammatory cells into the airspace displaced the air and caused a large portion of the cranioventral lung field to be consolidated. Border effacement of the pulmonary blood vessels and air bronchograms can be seen.

Although imperfect, one approach is based on the underlying pathological mechanism:

- Genetic: familial or hereditary
- Nutritional: dietary deficiencies
- Toxic: intoxication by exogenous (environmental) poisons
- Metabolic: endogenous (internal) insufficiencies or intoxications. More specifically, organ dysfunction or failure that affects the normal elimination of nitrogenous wastes, maintenance of normal electrolyte and glucose levels, or converting food to energy, proteins, lipids, nucleic acids and carbohydrates
- Trauma: blunt, penetrating, compressive or tensile tissue damage
- Ischaemic: poor tissue oxygenation (hypoxia) due to inadequate blood supply (abnormal perfusion) or low blood oxygen (hypoxaemia)
- Idiopathic: having no known cause (similar to cryptogenic, having an uncertain cause).

During imaging, the signs and patterns observed are incredibly diverse due to the scope of diseases included in this category (Figure 7.25). Signs may indicate the cause (e.g. a source of sepsis leading to hypoglycaemia) or result (e.g. uraemic pneumonitis secondary to renal injury) of disease.

With some exceptions (e.g. trauma), many degenerative diseases alter molecular pathways that take place at the cellular and subcellular levels and therefore do not produce detectable morphological changes at all or until late in the disease process. Imaging signs may be definitive, but frequently are not specific for the underlying cause. Soft tissue mineralization (e.g. lower airways, aortic valves, intervertebral discs, ossifying pulmonary metaplasia) is a common sign of degeneration that is often (but not always) an incidental finding of minor consequence. Signs of trauma are typically a result of compression, laceration, fracture or haemorrhage.

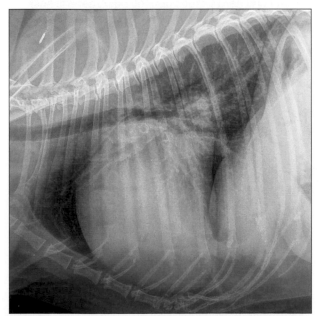

7.25 Lateral thoracic radiograph of a 12-year-old Tibetan Terrier with bilateral degenerative atrioventricular valve disease. The cardiac silhouette is tall with a large bulge of the left atrium. The results of this evaluation are negative for cardiogenic pulmonary oedema.

The relationship between imaging, gross pathology and histopathology

Based on the limits of what is achievable regarding image resolution, the results of morphological imaging are often equivalent to, and produce a similar differential diagnosis to, gross pathology. More specific diagnoses are typically attainable during advanced pathological examinations because more precise patterns of disease are obtainable, including histological, molecular (immunohistochemistry) and genetic patterns. As the same imaging pattern may be produced by several different diseases, knowing the pathological patterns associated with an imaging pattern helps determine the differential diagnosis. It can be challenging to determine even the broad category of disease based solely on imaging signs, and harder to determine the type of neoplasm (e.g. carcinoma, sarcoma) or inflammation (e.g. suppurative, granulomatous) (Figure 7.26). Advanced imaging techniques (e.g. molecular imaging, computer learning) might also provide more specific diagnoses.

Imaging alone, or the combination of imaging and pathology, may provide the most accurate diagnosis under certain conditions. Some abnormalities are detectable only because of physical or physiological properties like having internal pressure or blood flow, which may be absent in death or when an organ is removed from the body. In these circumstances, *in vivo* imaging is especially helpful. Imaging may depict abnormalities that go unnoticed during surgery or autopsy and *vice versa*. Imaging also may be performed after death, but post-mortem artefacts (e.g. inability to inflate lungs, tissue gas accumulation) can be problematic.

Imaging frequently complements biopsy because the collected pathological sample is often limited by not being able to convey information about gross morphology (e.g. whether the abnormality forms a mass) or regional and distant spread in the body (i.e. distribution). In some instances, the final diagnosis may only be reached by combining imaging, pathological and clinical findings. For example, some diseases may produce the same histological pattern but have a different distribution in an organ, body, sex or species.

Distribution

Distribution (spread) is important for prognosis, treatment planning and prioritizing the differential diagnosis. There are many different distributions that can be described, many of which are contextual. For example, in certain contexts, the word focal means solitary, circumscribed or small. Many terms also are synonyms, which can add confusion due to individual preferences. As distribution can refer to local and/or distant types of spread, descriptors of distribution are commonly used to convey the number of abnormalities, margination and possibly shape (see Chapter 12).

- Solitary abnormality:
  - Mass (space-occupying lesion or infiltrative/locally extensive)
  - Cyst (definition is contextual: in imaging, a round, fluid-filled abnormality circumscribed by a thin membrane; in pathology, the membrane is epithelium-lined)
  - Cavity
  - Disruption (e.g. laceration, dislocation, fracture).
- Multiple abnormalities:
  - Bilateral symmetrical
  - Asymmetrical (random).

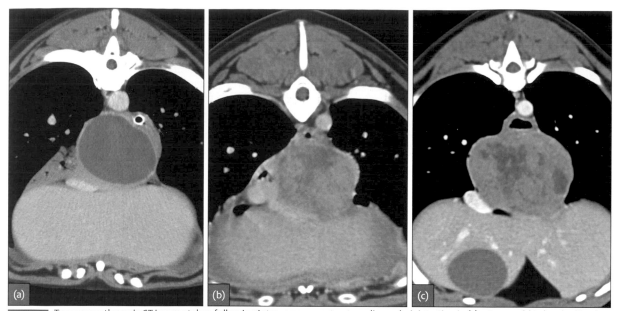

7.26 Transverse thoracic CT images taken following intravenous contrast medium administration in (a) a 7-year-old Labrador Retriever, (b) an 8-year-old Scottish Terrier and (c) a 9-year-old Rat Terrier. Each dog has a single round circumscribed mass that was localized to the dorsal part of the caudal mediastinum. In (a), inflammatory disease (specifically, mediastinal serous cavity empyema) was prioritized because the mass comprised homogeneous non-contrast-enhancing fluid. In (b) and (c), a neoplasm was prioritized because the mass contained contrast-enhancing tissue in addition to irregular non-contrast-enhancing cavities. Epithelial (mesothelioma, carcinoma) and mesenchymal (sarcoma) neoplasms were possible, and the tumours underwent histology and immunohistology in both dogs. In (b), the tumour is a mesothelioma of the mediastinal serous cavity. In (c), the tumour is a pulmonary adenocarcinoma. It can be difficult to differentiate whether a lesion is in the mediastinum or lung. Imaging patterns may help prioritize the broad category of disease (i.e. developmental, inflammatory, neoplastic or degenerative) or may provide a specific diagnosis. However, the same imaging patterns can commonly be produced by many different diseases. During radiography, simply observing a soft tissue mass in the caudal mediastinum would not have been sufficient to prioritize inflammatory *versus* neoplastic disease without additional clinical information.

- Widespread abnormality:
  - Diffuse: all parts of a tissue or organ are affected, not necessarily to the same degree
  - Generalized: the entirety or majority of a tissue or organ is affected, but there is normal tissue between abnormalities.

Diagnostic nomenclature

If the diagnosis is established, precise descriptions should be used. For example, if thoracic radiography is performed for staging of a biopsy-confirmed rib osteosarcoma, then the rib abnormality should be called an osteosarcoma and not a solitary aggressive bone lesion. Many diseases can be named simply by adding a meaningful suffix to the type of cell, tissue or organ that is abnormal (e.g. lymphocytosis, lymphadenitis, lymphoma). There are many common exceptions (e.g. pneumonia, pneumothorax, vascular ring anomaly, vertebral dislocation). There also are several eponymous diseases (e.g. Eisenmenger complex, tetralogy of Fallot). Prefixes and other descriptive modifiers also may be used to identify the disease (e.g. mononeuropathy, polyneuropathy, microcardia, embolic pneumonia).

The most common suffixes are -osis, -opathy, -itis and -oma:

- The suffixes '-osis' and '-opathy' indicate a condition, state, abnormal process or disease (e.g. kyphosis, pneumopathy) and alone do not specify a pathogenesis. They are often used with idiopathic (e.g. osteopathy) or degenerative diseases (e.g. systemic toxicosis). Further modifying these terms may increase the exactness of the diagnosis (e.g. thoracic kyphosis, systemic pyrethrin toxicosis)
- The suffix '-itis' refers to inflammatory disease (e.g. tracheobronchitis). Polymorphonuclear leucocytes (e.g. neutrophils) tend to predominate in acute inflammation, and macrophages and lymphocytes tend to predominate in chronic inflammation. These different histological patterns are typically indiscernible based only on imaging signs
- Determining the extent of suppurative inflammation is a common reason for performing imaging. Suppurative inflammation is typically associated with bacterial infections and characteristically produces pus, which may spread through various soft and hard tissues depending on several host and pathogen factors. This spread results in different types of superficial or deep tissue inflammation. The extent of disease spread is communicated by characterizing the types of tissue inflammation present (Figure 7.27)
  - Soft tissue (e.g. cellulitis, fasciitis, myositis, pleuritis, mediastinitis, myocarditis, oesophagitis, pneumonitis)
  - Bone (e.g. periostitis, osteitis, osteomyelitis)
- Suppurative inflammation also may accumulate within an existing body cavity (i.e. empyema, pyothorax) or in an abnormal cavity that is walled and deep in tissue (i.e. abscess). These distinct morphological forms of suppurative inflammation may be seen during imaging
- The suffix '-oma' typically refers to a neoplastic tumour (e.g. thymoma) but also is used to name some non-neoplastic masses (e.g. granuloma, haematoma). Additional naming conventions distinguish benign and malignant disease (e.g. thyroid adenoma *versus* thyroid adenocarcinoma, lipoma *versus* liposarcoma). Specifically, malignancy (i.e. cancer) is denoted by modifying the suffix to indicate the type of normal cell that the cancer cell resembles:
  - Epithelial cell: carcinoma

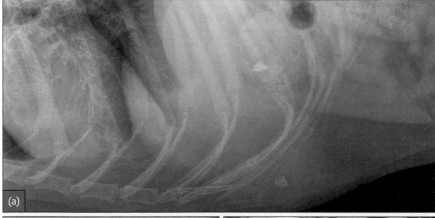

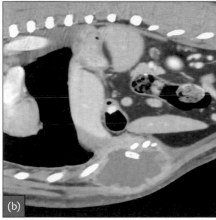 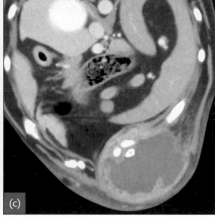

7.27 (a) Lateral thoracic radiograph, (b) transverse thoracic CT image and (c) sagittal CT image of an 8-year-old mixed-breed dog with cytologically confirmed suppurative inflammation. CT was performed with the dog in dorsal recumbency. In the sternal region, left caudoventral to the xiphoid process, the inflammation forms a large solitary mass with a thick irregular wall, large fluid-filled cavity and a small bone fragment. Adjacent to the mass, there is fat stranding in the body wall fasciae and body wall muscles. The superficial fascia is also mildly swollen with increased attenuation and indistinct margins. Both pleural cavities contain a small volume of gravity-dependent fluid. The adjacent cutaneous tissues also are thick and have a soft tissue attenuation. The imaging diagnosis is a presumed body wall abscess with locally extensive fasciitis, myositis and oedema; although direct extension into the serous cavities is not detected, pleuritis and pyothorax (pleural empyema) are possible given the presence of pleural fluid. The results of this evaluation are negative for osteomyelitis and peritonitis. The bone fragment is a segment of the costal cartilage and may be a sequestrum or nidus for infection.

- Mesenchymal cell (outside bone marrow): sarcoma
- Haematopoietic cell from bone marrow that matures in lymph nodes or blood: lymphoma or leukaemia, respectively.

During imaging, it is best to make a specific diagnosis whenever possible (e.g. diaphragmatic hernia, patent ductus arteriosus, rib fracture). When it is impossible to make a specific diagnosis, then a more general imaging diagnosis can be made by identifying the tissue or organ that is abnormal and using an appropriate prefix or suffix (e.g. neuropathy, pneumopathy) or by stating the imaging finding (e.g. wide cranial mediastinum, cranioventral lung consolidation, abnormal left third rib) (Figure 7.28).

Because many imaging patterns are not specific enough to make a definitive diagnosis, the suffixes '-osis' and '-opathy' are usually appropriate when making an imaging diagnosis (e.g. thoracic lymphadenopathy) but

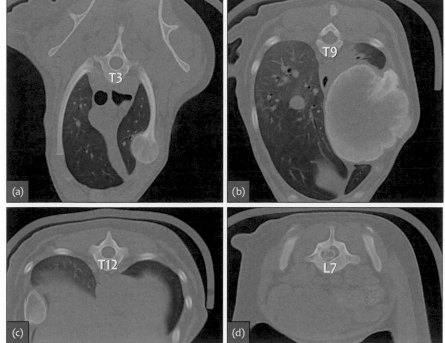

7.28 Transverse trunk CT images (bone window) at the level of the (a) third, (b) ninth and (c) twelfth thoracic vertebrae, and (d) the seventh lumbar vertebra of a 4-month-old mixed-breed dog with osteochondromatosis diagnosed on post-mortem examination. Based on the CT signs, the dog has a generalized random, non-aggressive polyosteopathy consistent with an imaging diagnosis of presumed osteochondromatosis (alternatively, presumed multiple cartilaginous exostosis). This idiopathic acquired developmental condition produces multiple benign masses containing cartilage and bone. These masses are typically clinically inconsequential except when causing intraluminal airway obstruction or compression of significant structures. (b) A large rib mass severely compresses the left lung. (d) A pedunculated vertebral mass extends into the vertebral canal compressing nerves of the cauda equina. Many more small masses were present throughout the skeleton.

other options exist (e.g. lymphadenomegaly). Imaging patterns are not as specific as histological patterns, but in some instances one can highly prioritize a pathogenic mechanism based on other information like test accuracy and clinical context. In this instance, it is helpful to use more specific terms when making an imaging diagnosis (e.g. neuritis, pneumonia, thymoma). It may be helpful to add the modifier 'presumed' to indicate the lack of definitive testing like cytology, histology or culture (e.g. presumed restrictive pleuritis, presumed infiltrative lipoma, presumed discospondylitis).

When the imaging diagnosis is not equivalent to a specific diagnosis, then either a prioritized differential diagnosis should be provided or it should be indicated that the results are too vague to be helpful. A differential diagnosis should only be provided when there are a few highly likely causes. Long lists are usually unhelpful. In general, when imaging is unable to answer the clinical question, then additional testing is necessary.

When the differential diagnosis list is long, it may be possible to prioritize the four basic pathogenic mechanisms like inflammation or unregulated growth instead of providing a list of diseases, which can be misrepresentative and unhelpful due to the sheer number of possibilities and lack of imaging specificity. It also may be possible to shorten the list by prioritizing whether the abnormality is more likely benign *versus* malignant or acute *versus* chronic.

Imaging information

Imaging signs

Images contain information in the form of fundamental units called signs. An imaging sign is simply any recognizable feature that may be detected in one or more images acquired during an imaging study. Imaging signs may be simple descriptors, tests, risk factors, prognostic indicators, or indicators of treatment response or disease progression.

As a diagnostic or screening test, the presence of a sign usually indicates the probable presence or occurrence of a disease (e.g. mitral valve dysplasia, myasthenia gravis, pulmonary adenocarcinoma) or pathological condition (e.g. left-sided congestive heart failure, megaoesophagus, pulmonary metastasis). The absence of a sign usually indicates the absence of these things. There are some exceptions in which the presence of a sign indicates the normal state, for example:

- A sail sign often refers to the normal thymus
- A glide sign indicates a normal pleural interface at that level and thus rules out pneumothorax.

Imaging signs may be qualitative or quantitative and are typically detected by visual inspection. Occasionally, imaging signs are detected by other methods like computer algorithms, palpation (3D prints) or hearing (Doppler sound conversion). The description of imaging signs should reflect the method by which they were detected. Examples of signs that can be seen include enlargement, irregular margins and altered opacity. Examples of signs that cannot be seen include hard and heavy. There are two broad categories of imaging signs: general and special.

- General imaging signs are alterations in normal opacity, size, shape, number, position, margination, alignment and function. These signs are 'general' because they apply to most organs and can be detected using most imaging modalities. For example, altered size – almost any organ can become enlarged or small, and this finding can be detected with most imaging modalities. General imaging signs tend to indicate that an organ is abnormal but may not be specific enough to determine the cause. Nonetheless, this information can be helpful and direct next steps in patient care (e.g. initially differentiating whether coughing is due to cardiac or respiratory disease). General imaging signs are also very helpful when the cause of an abnormality is not recognized. The anatomical location and distribution of the abnormality should be described first, followed by a description of the abnormality in terms of altered size, shape, opacity and margination (Figure 7.29).
- Special imaging signs are a vast collection of unique features that may be detected during evaluation of an imaging study. Examples include bronchial mineralization, osteolysis, mosaic pattern, enthesophyte formation, wide pleural fissure and air bronchograms. These signs are special because they are frequently associated with a specific organ, a specific imaging modality, or both. Like general imaging signs, many special imaging signs only indicate that an organ is abnormal. For example, an extrapleural sign typically indicates a body wall mass but not the exact diagnosis. However, some special imaging signs may indicate a precise cause. For example, simultaneous initial opacification of the aorta, ductus arteriosus and pulmonic trunk following contrast material injection into the left ventricle is a specific sign of patent ductus arteriosus. A pattern commonly refers to a recognizable feature or design, especially one that has repeated elements. This definition also applies to imaging; a pattern is a type of special imaging sign. An imaging pattern also may refer to a collection of signs that occur together. For example, an alveolar pattern comprises several signs including increased opacity, border effacement of pulmonary blood vessels and air bronchograms.

Imaging signs may be categorized as expected or unexpected.

- Expected signs are ones that the interpreter is specifically looking for based on the reason for performing the study. These signs are always pertinent and may be present or absent: both should be documented. For example:
  - Enlarged left atrium
  - No oesophageal foreign body.
- Unexpected signs are usually incidental findings because they are unrelated to the reason for performing the study. These findings vary in clinical importance, which also should be documented: minor consequence, major consequence or uncertain consequence. For example:
  - Incidental/minor consequence: spondylosis deformans
  - Incidental/major consequence: solitary pulmonary mass
  - Incidental/uncertain consequence: altered diaphragmatic contour.

Both types of finding should be documented, especially when the presence or absence of these signs will influence patient care or require monitoring (Figure 7.30). Changes from prior studies should also be documented.

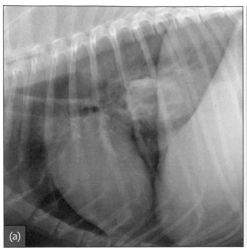
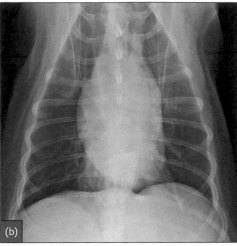

7.29 (a) Lateral and (b) ventrodorsal thoracic radiographs of an 11-year-old mixed-breed dog with an oesophageal foreign body. When the reason for the imaging study is to confirm an oesophageal foreign body and note the location and any other outcome, then it is appropriate to simply describe that the oesophageal foreign body is in the caudal oesophagus, immediately cranial to the diaphragm. Gas is not detected in the mediastinum and the rest of the thorax is normal, so the results of the evaluation are negative for oesophageal perforation and aspiration pneumonia. When the reason for performing the examination is to determine the cause of the clinical signs, then the abnormality should first be described in terms of imaging signs before a definitive or differential diagnosis is provided, or it is concluded that the clinical question is not answered by the study. When it is difficult to describe the findings of an imaging study because the results are not straightforward, then a failproof method is to first describe the abnormal anatomical structure, or the location of the abnormality, and then describe the general imaging signs (e.g. changes in size, shape, margination, opacity). For example: the thoracic oesophagus is diffusely enlarged and has a large, irregularly shaped, circumscribed mineral opacity that is just cranial to the diaphragm; cranially, the oesophageal lumen is gas-filled.

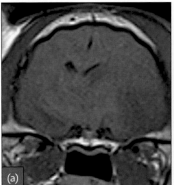
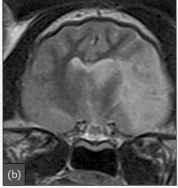
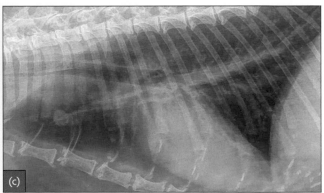

7.30 Transverse (a) T1-weighted and (b) T2-weighted brain MR images and (c) a lateral thoracic radiograph of a 15-year-old Domestic Longhaired cat with imaging diagnoses of a presumed territorial infarction of the left middle cerebral artery and an incidental pulmonary nodule of uncertain clinical importance. The pulmonary nodule was an incidental finding because it was unexpected and did not relate to the clinical signs nor the MRI diagnosis. The clinical importance of the pulmonary nodule was uncertain because the likely cause was not determined during imaging; the differential diagnosis included benign and malignant neoplasms and chronic inflammatory conditions (e.g. granuloma). Post-mortem examination confirmed cerebral infarction and diagnosed a pulmonary carcinoma that was unlikely to be related to the brain abnormality and clinical signs.

Technical elements that influence detection of imaging signs

Most medical images are a two-dimensional (2D) representation of a three-dimensional (3D) object, even when the image appears 3D due to perspective and shading. True 3D medical images are '3D prints'. Planar images are produced in radiography, fluoroscopy and scintigraphy and are 2D representations of the internal structure of non-uniformly composed 3D objects. Potential limitations include (Figure 7.31):

- Lack of depth perception, commonly accommodated for by obtaining at least two orthogonal views
- Summation of multiple structures creating unexpected shapes (summation shadows)
- Formation of unexpected shapes due to unfamiliar perspective (one reason why standardized patient positioning and X-ray beam orientation is important).

Cross-sectional images are produced in CT, MRI, ultrasonography, positron emission tomography (PET) and single-photon emission computed tomography (SPECT) and are 2D images that represent 3D slices through the patient. Depth perception is determined by the sequence of images.

Artefacts and technical complications

An image artefact is any anomaly in the image that does not represent the true nature of the original object that was examined. An image artefact may be due to some physical limitation or property of the technology (e.g. sampling rate) or some natural process or property of the examined object (e.g. respiratory motion). Artefacts may be detrimental by preventing evaluation of a structure (e.g. motion) or by being misinterpreted. Artefacts may be useful by providing a clue as to the composition of a structure (e.g. acoustic enhancement is seen with fluid). A technical complication is any anomaly in the image that is the result of

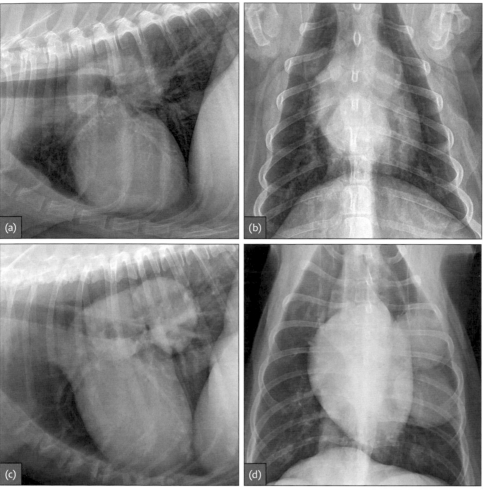

7.31 Orthogonal thoracic radiographs of (a, b) a 4-year-old Australian Shepherd Dog with lymphoma and (c, d) a 13-year-old Standard Poodle with multiple lung masses. One of the limitations of planar imaging is lack of depth perception within the displayed image. On the lateral views (a, c), both dogs have an abnormal soft tissue opacity that summates with the lung hilus: the opacity may be in the body wall, the mediastinum or either lung. One of the best ways to overcome the lack of depth perception is to obtain an orthogonal view. On the orthogonal views (b, d) the abnormality is localized to the mediastinum in the Australian Shepherd Dog and to the left lung in the Standard Poodle.

improper operation of the imager, equipment failure or an issue with patient compliance. It is important to be able to identify image artefacts and technical complications, understand how they occur, and know how to eliminate or correct for the problem. When the latter is impossible or impractical, then it is important to know how the artefact or technical complication will affect image interpretation.

Differential absorption of the X-ray beam

Differential absorption of the X-ray beam occurs when an X-ray beam passes through a non-uniform object such that the intensity of the X-ray beam that exits the object is different at different locations. The absorption or transmission of X-rays through the body depends on the energy of the X-rays and the composition, density and thickness of the tissues in the path of the X-rays. Nearly all aspects of the radiographic image are a result of differential absorption of the X-ray beam. Some other factors that contribute to the radiographic appearance of an object include magnification, distortion and geometric unsharpness. Because of magnification and distortion, it is usually recommended to obtain radiographic views such that the abnormality is as close to the detector as possible. However, when using a vertically oriented X-ray beam, lung abnormalities are frequently best seen when they are farther away from the detector because the non-gravity-dependent lung is better expanded providing greater contrast.

There are three phenomena that result from differential absorption of the X-ray beam that determine how the internal structure of an object is represented in a planar image, and that can create or obscure imaging signs (Figure 7.32):

- Contrast is the ability to differentiate different objects in the image due to differences in the intensity of the X-ray beam leaving the objects. Adjacent structures in the image that have similar absorption of the X-ray will be harder to differentiate than structures that have a larger difference. During radiography, five opacities may be differentiated and are a clue to the composition of the examined object. From least to most opaque these are: air, fat, fluid/soft tissue, mineral/bone and metal
- Summation shadows occur when multiple structures are encountered along the path of the X-ray beam. Therefore, the resulting image does not represent a single structure but rather a summation of all structures in that path
  - A positive summation shadow appears as an increased opacity
  - A negative summation shadow appears as a decreased opacity
- Border effacement (synonyms: border obliteration, silhouette sign) occurs when the borders between adjacent structures within the image cannot be differentiated because there is equal absorption of the X-ray beam resulting in a single shape (a silhouette) that represents multiple structures. Note, these objects may be adjacent in the image but not necessarily in the patient because planar images lack depth perception. In practice, the resulting silhouette almost always has a soft tissue or fluid opacity as this phenomenon rarely produces a silhouette of a different opacity.

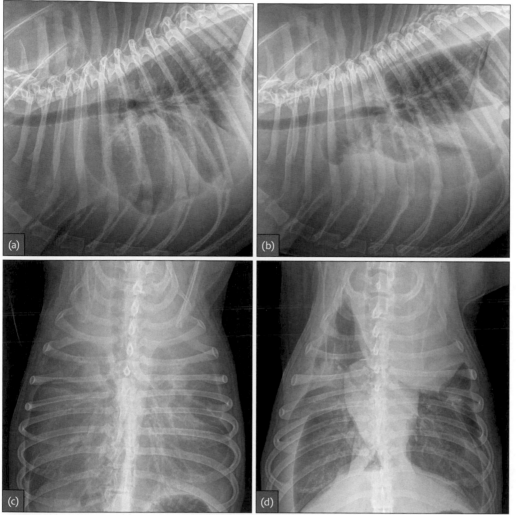

7.32 (a) Right lateral, (b) left lateral, (c) dorsoventral and (d) ventrodorsal thoracic radiographs of a 6-year-old Boxer with bilateral pleural fluid and a cranial thoracic mass. Each observable form in a radiograph is primarily the result of differential absorption of the X-ray beam. In (a), (b) and (c), the cardiac silhouette and mass are not seen. In (d), the cardiac silhouette and mass are visible because the pleural fluid shifted to the dorsal portion of the pleural cavities with the animal in dorsal recumbency. This allows for greater differential absorption of the X-ray beam across the image. To better understand this process, each image can be considered as a grid of tiny squares. Each square is the smallest picture element, or pixel. Each pixel has a shade of grey (opacity) that corresponds to the amount of absorption of the X-ray beam as it passed through the patient at that location. Whiter areas have greater absorption and blacker areas have less absorption. With radiography, there are five recognizable opacities, and adjacent pixels that have a similar opacity will result in identifiable forms (silhouettes) within the image. Ideally, these forms will signify a specific object within the patient. The ability to look at an image and differentiate structures due to differences in opacity is called contrast: the greater the contrast, the easier it is to differentiate structures. However, silhouettes do not always signify true objects within the patient. When objects that are adjacent in the image have a similar opacity, then there will be border effacement (silhouetting) between the objects creating a novel form (silhouette) that represents more than one object in the patient. Note, these objects may not be adjacent within the patient because planar images lack depth perception. All identifiable forms in the image are summation shadows that may be brighter (positive) or darker (negative). For example, the ribs form positive summation shadows and the lungs form negative summation shadows. Occasionally, summation shadows form that do not represent patient anatomy.

Image interpretation

The principal purpose of image interpretation is usually to answer clinical questions. Therefore, it is necessary to understand the reason for performing the imaging study. The same study may be performed for different reasons and show the same signs, but the interpretation may be different based on the information available prior to imaging and the information sought at the time of acquisition. For example, a study may be performed to determine the cause of clinical signs (e.g. suppurative inflammation) or to determine the extent or spread of suppurative inflammation of a known cause to plan treatment. This section focuses on studies performed to determine the cause of signs and considers the human element of image interpretation.

The evaluation of an imaging study comprises searching for the presence or absence of imaging signs and then determining the meaning of those results based on what is known about the patient. The entire process of selecting the imaging study, evaluating the images for signs and patterns, and interpreting their meaning to effect patient care is often referred to as clinical reasoning.

Clinical reasoning is a complex concept that has no generally accepted definition. It is roughly the process by which a health professional contextually integrates basic and clinical knowledge with initial patient information to form a case representation of the problem. Instead of general processes like 'reasoning skills' or 'critical thinking,' it is knowledge that is key to improving clinical reasoning (Gruppen, 2017). Clinical reasoning applies to both diagnostic and therapeutic reasoning; this manual focuses on diagnostic interpretation of thoracic images. Veterinary surgeons achieve best practice by basing interpretation on extensive clinical experience, a good working knowledge of how patients are managed, and a strong knowledge of the patient history, normal anatomy and physiology, pathology, imaging technology and epidemiological principles.

Thoracic imaging interpretation should provide information that explicitly addresses the inciting reason for the imaging performed. When the diagnosis is known, imaging is usually performed to plan or assist intervention (e.g. determine tumour boundaries, guide catheterization), establish the extent of disease (e.g. staging) or provide prognostic information that will help a client decide between management choices. When the diagnosis is unknown, imaging is primarily performed to reduce diagnostic uncertainty regarding an already established differential diagnosis based on signalment, history, physical examination and laboratory tests. The degree to which uncertainty must be reduced varies with many factors. Ideally, one would eliminate diagnostic uncertainty, but that frequently is unachievable due to associated costs, risks, lack of definitive tests and other variables.

Imaging may be performed in healthy individuals to screen for disease or to establish the risk of developing disease. It may be performed in patients with clinical signs of disease to rule out unlikely causes when the initial differential diagnosis list is long, rule in or confirm likely causes when the initial differential diagnosis list is short, or a combination of both. Imaging also may add new diseases to the initial differential diagnosis list.

Interpreting imaging test results

Searching for an imaging sign or pattern is equivalent to performing an imaging test. The best imaging tests are reliable (reproducible), valid (precise) and accurate (see below) Imaging signs are either detected or not detected.

- Detecting an imaging sign is a positive test result for the diseases that may produce that sign.
- Not detecting an imaging sign is a negative test result for the diseases that may produce that sign.

This informs differential diagnosis. Imaging test results are either positive or negative for a disease (Figure 7.33). Indicating that the result of an imaging study is positive or negative for a sign (versus a disease), although commonly done, can lead to confusion. Positive and negative test results are either true or false. The most important attributes for determining whether a positive or negative test result is likely to be true are the type and quality of the imaging study, disease severity, prior probability of disease, and the accuracy of the imaging test. The first two relate to the ability to detect signs (Figure 7.34).

Prior probability is the probability that a disease is present based on evidence available before the test was performed. In most instances, prior probability is determined by defining the patient population (using signalment, history and any other available clinical information) and knowing or estimating the prevalence of disease in that population (Figure 7.35). If the prevalence of disease is high, then a positive test result is more likely to be true

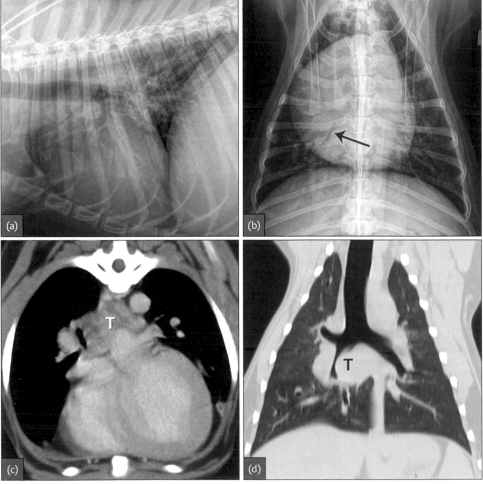

7.33 (a) Lateral and (b) dorsoventral thoracic radiographs, and (c) transverse and (d) dorsal thoracic CT images of a 9-year-old German Shorthaired Pointer with cytologically confirmed pulmonary carcinoma and neutrophilic inflammation. Imaging signs of disease are either detected or not detected. Evidence of the neoplasm is present on all four images. On the lateral thoracic radiograph, an indistinct perihilar opacity is detected. On the dorsoventral thoracic radiograph, narrowing of the bronchus to the right caudal lung lobe is detected (arrowed). On both CT images, a tumour (T) caudal to the carina and compression of the right caudal lobar bronchus are detected. In all images, pulmonary nodules are not detected, and the results of this evaluation are negative for pulmonary metastasis.

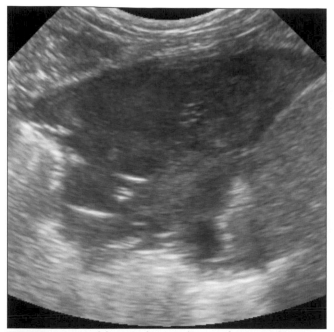

7.34 Intercostal thoracic ultrasound image of a 16-year-old Domestic Shorthaired cat. Imaging test results are either positive or negative for disease. Positive and negative test results are either true or false. In this cat, lung consolidation (an imaging sign) is detected in the ventral lung tip of one lobe. Lung consolidation occurs with many different conditions including pneumonia, haemorrhage, neoplasia and atelectasis. Therefore, the ultrasound test results are positive for each of these conditions: the results are not positive for lung consolidation, which is a sign and not a disease. Additional information (e.g. history, vital signs, blood analysis) is needed to prioritize whether the positive results are likely true or false because the test is not specific for one cause. Typically, only one result is true-positive, and the rest are false-positive.

and a negative test result is more likely to be false. If the prevalence of disease is low, then a positive test result is more likely to be false and a negative test result is more likely to be true.

Test accuracy refers to how well the test determines whether disease is present or absent. Two common measures of test accuracy are sensitivity and specificity (Figure 7.36). An ideal test is both sensitive and specific.

- Sensitivity is a measure of how well a test identifies an animal as having the disease when the disease is present. A sensitive test is associated with few false-negative results and is good at ruling out diseases.
- Specificity is a measure of how well a test identifies an animal as not having the disease when the disease is absent. A specific test is associated with few false-positive results and is good for ruling in a disease.

Errors in medical imaging interpretation

Experts typically formulate a diagnostic hypothesis through immediate recognition of the signs, using brain mechanisms that are fast, automatic and effortless (Melo *et al.*, 2011). While they are efficient and often sufficient, these heuristic approaches are subject to some types of medical errors (Brady, 2017; Busby *et al.*, 2018). The four most common types of error in medical imaging are listed below. The first two are especially prone to bias (a skewed liking in favour of or against one thing) and cause problems when the validity of an interpretation unavoidably comes down to 'expert opinion' because comparison to a gold standard is unattainable. The latter two relate to communication mistakes.

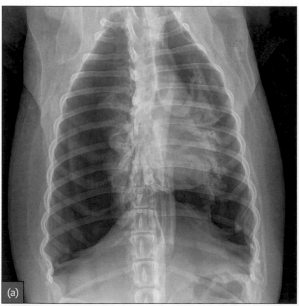

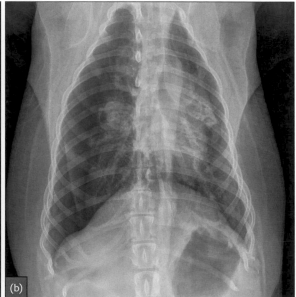

7.35 Dorsoventral thoracic radiographs of a 7-year-old Samoyed with a tension pneumothorax, obtained (a) before and (b) after thoracocentesis. In both radiographs, the pleural cavities contain gas and both lungs are collapsed. The pneumothorax is worst on the right side and there is a mediastinal shift to the left. Prior to thoracocentesis, the thoracic cavity was severely expanded causing a barrel-chested conformation: the ribs were spread farther apart and more perpendicular to the vertebral column. In addition, the diaphragm was displaced caudally and was flatter than normal. Pneumothorax is either open or closed. The results of this evaluation are negative for causes of open pneumothorax because no sign of body wall trauma (e.g. rib fracture, fascial gas) is detected and the prior probability is low as there was no history of trauma. The results of this evaluation also are negative for tracheal or oesophageal perforation as pneumomediastinum was not detected. The results of this evaluation are positive for causes of closed pneumothorax (e.g. lung neoplasia, pulmonary abscess rupture, grass awn migration, spontaneous). The results of this evaluation are indeterminate for a lung abnormality because any abnormality would be obscured by the lung collapse. However, spontaneous pneumothorax is most likely based on the imaging signs and high prior probability: spontaneous pneumothorax is common in northern dog breeds. This diagnosis was confirmed during CT, surgery and histology as there were ruptured lung bullae without underlying lung disease.

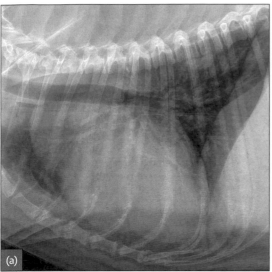
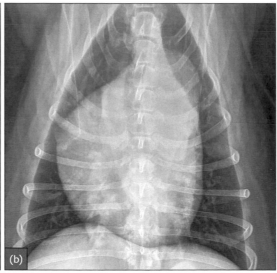

7.36 (a, b) Orthogonal thoracic radiographs of a 9-year-old Golden Retriever with a heart base tumour confirmed during echocardiography. There is a large soft tissue tumour at the cranial aspect of the heart base, left and ventral to the caudal fourth of the trachea. A sensitive test is one that produces few false-negative results. Radiographic signs are not sensitive for a chemodectoma arising from the aortic bodies because the tumour must be large before it is detectable. Echocardiographic and CT signs are more sensitive because smaller tumours are detectable. A specific test is one that produces few false-positive results. Imaging signs are moderately specific for a chemodectoma because there are very few other types of tumour that occur in this precise location. The accuracy of the imaging signs can be affected by how the imaging study was performed and evaluated (e.g. obtaining one view *versus* multiple views, using windowing and zoom).

- A perceptual error refers to not detecting an abnormality that is present or incorrectly identifying an abnormality as present when it is absent.
  - Misidentification.
- A cognitive or interpretative error refers to incorrectly understanding the importance of the presence or absence of an abnormality.
  - Misinterpretation.
- Communication errors are those in which the intended meaning of an imaging study is not faithfully conveyed.
  - May be a simple error such as transposing left for right, a misregistered dictation error or inappropriate punctuation.
  - May be a complicated or unorganized description that lacks clarity, brevity and pertinence.
- Lack of timeliness: not providing meaningful results in time to effectively influence clinical decisions.

Bias in image interpretation

- Anchoring bias: a predisposition to fixate on early impressions even when subsequent conflicting information becomes available; reluctance to change the initial impression or accept the new information.
- Framing bias: being improperly swayed to conclude something based on the way the information was presented.
- Availability bias: inclination to favour diagnoses that readily come to mind.
- Confirmation bias: tendency to seek evidence that supports an existing diagnostic hypothesis.
- Inattentional bias: predisposition to overlook discernible findings because they are in an unexpected location or circumstance.
- Satisfaction of search: tendency to stop searching for additional abnormalities once an abnormality that may explain the condition is identified.
- Premature closure: tendency to accept a preliminary diagnosis as final before sufficient evidence is acquired.
- Outcome bias: inclination to prefer a diagnosis with a favourable outcome based on empathy *versus* evidence.

- Zebra retreat: reluctance to diagnose an uncommon condition, even when there is supporting evidence, due to unfamiliarity.
- Attribution bias: inclination to ascribe findings based on stereotypical patient characteristics.
- Hindsight bias: reluctance to accept the difficulty in making the initial diagnosis once there is knowledge of the outcome.
- Satisfaction of report: propensity to perpetuate an impression from a prior report.

Ideally, the evaluation of an imaging study would always reveal a characteristic sign or pattern of a disease when the disease is present and only when the disease is present. In this way, there would be perfect agreement between the presence or absence of a sign and knowing whether a disease is present or absent. In reality, detecting signs and determining the meaning of their presence or absence is influenced heavily by other factors such as how the study was performed, history, prior diagnosis, fatigue and bias. Therefore, image interpretation is an educated opinion, subject to error and differences of opinion (Figure 7.37).

The determination of what is right or wrong is usually a legal decision (e.g. in cases of alleged negligence) and often based on expert opinion because a gold standard test is often unavailable. Because image interpretation is neither absolute nor indisputable, multiple legitimate interpretations may exist and contradict each other. In this situation, it is important to understand that the issue is not necessarily whether someone is right or wrong. The issue is whether they have provided a reasonable interpretation that is substantiated by the available evidence. As a simple example, an imaging study may consistently give the 'wrong' answer and thus correctly interpreting the study would yield the wrong answer. Image interpretation errors are inevitable and do not equate to malpractice. Therefore, realistic goals for image interpretation are to minimize causes of error, learn from mistakes and report errors as soon as possible to facilitate appropriate care.

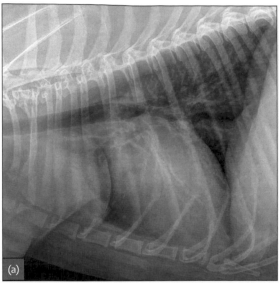
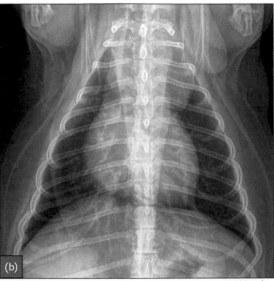

7.37 (a) Lateral and (b) dorsoventral thoracic radiographs of an 11-year old mixed-breed dog with a surgically and histologically confirmed pulmonary adenocarcinoma. Image interpretation is an educated opinion, subject to error and differences of opinion. It can be difficult to differentiate whether an abnormality localizes to the mediastinum or lung. Consequently, a perfectly reasonable and acceptable interpretation of this imaging study would have been to prioritize a cranial mediastinal mass over a lung mass, based on the midline location in the thoracic cavity (between the thoracic inlet, trachea and heart), undetected air bronchograms and a possible 'sail' sign. Understanding that errors may occur and factoring that in when making patient care decisions is part of best practice. When possible, causes of error should be minimized, mistakes should be learned from to reduce future errors and errors should be reported as soon as possible to facilitate appropriate patient care.

References and further reading

Brady AP (2017) Error and discrepancy in radiology: inevitable or avoidable? *Insights into Imaging* **8**, 171–182

Busby LP, Courtier JL and Glastonbury CM (2018) Bias in radiology: The how and why of misses and misinterpretations. *RadioGraphics* **38**, 236–247

Chaudhry R, Miao JH and Rehman A (2022) *Physiology, Cardiovascular.* Available from: www.ncbi.nlm.nih.gov/books/NBK493197. [Accessed on: 05/09/2023]

Desai JP and Moustarah F (2022) *Pulmonary Compliance.* Available from: www.ncbi.nlm.nih.gov/books/NBK538324. [Accessed on: 05/09/2023]

Gruppen LD (2017) Clinical reasoning: Defining it, teaching it, assessing it, studying it. *Western Journal of Emergency Medicine* **18**, 4–7

Kahneman D and Patrick E (2011) *Thinking, Fast and Slow.* Penguin Books, London

Klabunde RE (2021) *Cardiovascular Physiology Concepts, 3rd edn.* Wolters Kluwer, Philadelphia

Melo M, Scarpin DJ, Amaro E *et al.* (2011) How doctors generate diagnostic hypotheses: A study of radiological diagnosis with functional magnetic resonance imaging. *PLoS ONE* **6**, e28752

Powers KA and Dhamoon AS (2023) *Physiology, Pulmonary Ventilation and Perfusion.* Available from: www.ncbi.nlm.nih.gov/books/NBK539907. [Accessed on: 05/09/2023]

Reinero C, Visser LC, Kellihan HB *et al.* (2020) ACVIM consensus statement guidelines for the diagnosis, classification, treatment, and monitoring of pulmonary hypertension in dogs. *Journal of Veterinary Internal Medicine* **34**, 549–573

Rubin C, Fascia D and Harvey D (2019) *Picture Archiving and Communication Systems (PACS) and guidelines on diagnostic display devices.* Available from: www.rcr.ac.uk. [Accessed on 05/09/2023]

Smallwood JE, Shively MJ, Rendano VT and Habel RE (1985) A standardized nomenclature for radiographic projections used in veterinary-medicine. *Veterinary Radiology* **26**, 2–9

Taylor AE (1981) Capillary fluid filtration. Starling forces and lymph flow. *Circulation Research* **49**, 557–575

The Royal College of Radiologists (2012) *Picture archiving and communication systems (PACS) and guidelines on diagnostic display devices, 2nd edn.* Available from: www.rcr.ac.uk. [Accessed on 05/09/2023]

Chapter 8

Thoracic boundaries

Stacy Cooley and Peter Scrivani

Imaging anatomy

The four boundaries of the thoracic cavity are the thoracic inlet, back (dorsum), chest (pectoral region) and diaphragm. The cranial boundary is the thoracic inlet, which is delineated by the first rib pair, manubrium and first thoracic vertebra. The inlet provides passage for the trachea, oesophagus, longus colli muscles, and vessels and nerves coursing to the head, neck and thoracic limbs. The region between the shoulder joint and thorax, where the blood vessels and nerves pass to and from the thoracic limb, is the axilla (armpit) or axillary region. Adequately inflated lungs should extend to the thoracic inlet. The left pleural cupula commonly extends further cranially than the right and may normally extend cranial to the thoracic inlet during maximum lung inflation. The thoracic inlet can be used as an acoustic window to access the cranial mediastinum during ultrasonography. The dorsal boundary is the back and includes structures such as the thoracic vertebrae, spinal cord, associated muscles and skin. The ventral boundary is the chest, which encompasses the ribs, sternum, associated muscles and skin. The left and right sides are commonly called the 'thoracic body walls' and normally contain 13 rib pairs and the intercostal muscles. The caudal boundary is the thoracic outlet, which is principally defined by the musculotendinous diaphragm. The outlet provides passage for the oesophagus, caudal vena cava, aorta, thoracic duct, vagus nerves and psoas muscles.

Thoracic skeleton

The thoracic skeleton is the part of the axial skeleton that comprises the ribs, sternum and thoracic vertebrae. These osseous and cartilaginous structures enclose and protect the principal organs of respiration and circulation. The bones and associated fascia also serve as attachment sites for muscles of the shoulder girdles, thoracic limbs, neck, back, diaphragm, thoracic body wall and abdominal body wall.

Rib cage

In dogs and cats, the osseous and cartilaginous rib cage normally consists of 13 rib pairs that articulate with the thoracic vertebral column and sternum. The enclosure is generally narrower cranially than caudally and the dorso-ventral height may be longer than the left-to-right width (deep chested), shorter than the width (broad chested) or about the same (barrel chested). The ribs are identified by side (left, right, paired) and sequentially numbered cranio-caudally (1 to 13).

- The first 8–9 ribs connect directly to the sternum via synovial joints (sternocostal joints) and are the true or sternal ribs.
- The 9th–12th ribs connect indirectly to the sternum via the costal arch and are the false or asternal ribs. The costal arch is formed by the union of the costal cartilages of these ribs (Figure 8.1).
- The 13th ribs (and occasionally the 12th in cats) are not connected to the costal arch and are the floating ribs.
- Ribs consist of osseous and cartilaginous parts:
  - The wider osseous part has a cortex and medulla, comprises the dorsal two-thirds of the rib, and consists of the head, neck, body, tubercle and angle
  - The costal cartilage is the ventral third and is variably mineralized (mineralization generally increases with age and chondrodystrophy)
  - The costochondral junction is the intersection between osseous and cartilaginous parts and has a variable appearance.
- Each rib has two synovial articulations with the vertebral column (Figure 8.2):

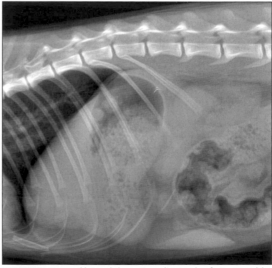

8.1 Normal lateral thoracic radiograph of a 1-year-old cat. The costal arch is formed by the union of the costal cartilages of the 9th–11th ribs. The costal cartilages of the 12th ribs do not connect with the costal arch and the 13th ribs lack costal cartilage; both sets are floating ribs.

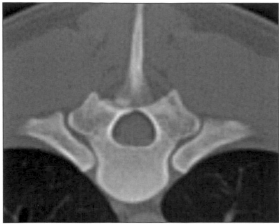

8.2 Normal transverse computed tomography image of a mid-thoracic vertebra in a dog. Each rib articulates with the vertebrae at two locations. On each side (bilaterally), the costovertebral joint lies between the rib head and costal fovea, and the costotransverse joint lies between the rib tubercle and transverse process.

- Costovertebral joints between the rib head, the cranial costal fovea (T1–T13) of the caudal vertebra and the caudal costal fovea (T1 to T10 or T11) of the cranial vertebra. Note that most rib heads articulate with two thoracic vertebrae
- Costotransverse joints between the rib tubercle and transverse fovea on the transverse process of the vertebra.
- Intercostal spaces are between ribs and are composed mostly of muscles. Blood vessels and nerves run along the caudal border of the ribs. There are 12 pairs of intercostal spaces, numbered sequentially craniocaudally.

Sternum

The sternum consists of eight bones arranged craniocaudally along the ventral aspect of the thorax in the midline. In dogs and cats, the sternebrae normally do not fuse as in some species. The sternum rotates ventrally during inspiration with the anchor point at the manubrium. The respiratory excursion is larger in cats than dogs. The sternebrae may be numbered craniocaudally, but sternebrae 1 and 8 have unique names.

- The cranial sternebra is the manubrium.
- The caudal sternebra is the xiphoid process, elongated caudally by the xiphoid cartilage.
- The individual sternebrae are joined by intersternal cartilages that form sternal synchondroses.
- The sternocostal joints are synovial joints that join the first 8–9 ribs with the sternum through the costal cartilages.
- Dogs generally have a mildly curved sternum and the individual sternebrae are square in cross-section (Figure 8.3a).
- Cats have straighter sternal alignment with cylindrical sternebrae and a flat xiphoid process (Figure 8.3b).

Vertebral column

The vertebral column forms the central axis of the skeleton and comprises all the vertebrae arranged in series from cranial to caudal. Dogs and cats normally have 13 thoracic vertebrae that are sequentially numbered craniocaudally (e.g. 12th thoracic vertebra or T12). Adjacent thoracic vertebrae are joined by a cartilaginous joint (i.e. intervertebral

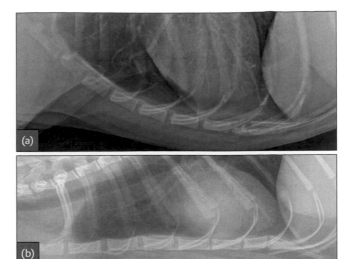

8.3 Normal lateral radiographs of the sternum in (a) a dog and (b) a cat. The sternum comprises eight bones. The cranial sternebra is the manubrium and the caudal is the xiphoid process. The canine sternum is more curved than the feline sternum.

disc) and paired synovial joints (i.e. joints of the left and right articular processes). Because these structures lie between vertebrae, their names designate both vertebrae (e.g. T11–T12). Each vertebra also has articulations with the ribs (as described above) and several ligaments and muscles attach to and stabilize the vertebral column. When counting ribs to identify the number of the vertebra, it is important to remember that most rib heads articulate with two consecutive vertebrae. However, the rib head more prominently attaches to the cranial aspect of the vertebra that has the same number as the rib. The typical vertebra is divided into dorsal (arch) and ventral (body) parts and is irregularly shaped due to the addition of several processes for muscle attachment.

- Dorsally, the vertebral arch comprises the paired pedicles and laminae, which define the boundaries of the vertebral foramen: collectively, the vertebral foramina form the vertebral canal through which passes the spinal cord. The intervertebral foramina, through which pass the spinal nerves and blood vessels, are between the pedicles of adjacent vertebrae.
- Ventrally, the vertebral body is relatively short and has flat cranial and caudal extremities (vertebral endplates) joined by intervertebral discs.
  - In cats, the 12th and 13th ribs articulate with the ventral aspect of the vertebral body (as opposed to the lateral aspect). This arrangement, along with the positioning of the psoas muscles and the fact that the pleural cavities do not extend as far caudally as in dogs, sometimes prevents the caudodorsal lung margin of cats from extending to the ventral aspect of the T12 and T13 vertebral bodies (Figure 8.4). This normal appearance should not be mistaken for a sign of pleural fluid.
- Each thoracic vertebra has an unpaired spinous process (spine) that arises from the dorsal aspect of the vertebral arch and is variable in shape and orientation:
  - Cranially, the spinous processes are largest (tallest) and oriented relatively perpendicular to the vertebral column (dorsoventrally)
  - In the mid-thoracic region, the spinous processes are smaller and angled caudally to the level of the

8.4 Normal lateral radiographs and transverse CT images of the vertebral column in (a) a dog and (b) a cat. The arrangement of the T12 and T13 rib pairs relative to the vertebral bodies and the size of the psoas muscles (*) in cats is such that the caudal lung tips may not extend all the way to the vertebral column on lateral radiographs (arrowed). This normal feline appearance should not be mistaken for a sign of pleural fluid.

10th or 11th thoracic vertebra, which has the first dorsoventrally oriented spinous process (anticlinal vertebra)
- Caudal to the anticlinal vertebra, the spinous processes are shorter, wider and angled mildly cranially.
- Thoracic vertebrae have paired transverse processes that are short.
  - In the caudal thoracic vertebral column, the transverse processes have additional mammillary (craniodorsally) and accessory (caudally) processes.
- Thoracic vertebrae have paired cranial and caudal articular processes, which are at the junctions of the pedicles and laminae. The caudal articular processes of one vertebra and the cranial articular processes of the adjacent vertebra articulate to form the paired

articular process joints, which change orientation at the anticlinal space (T10–T11).
- Cranially, the joint spaces are oriented in a dorsal plane with the cranial articular process ventral to the caudal articular process.
- Caudally, the joint spaces are oriented in a sagittal plane with the cranial articular process lateral to the caudal articular process.

Diaphragm

The diaphragm is a sheet-like musculotendinous structure that attaches to the rib cage and separates the thoracic and abdominal cavities. The muscular portion is peripheral and the tendinous portion is central. Cranially, the diaphragm is lined by endothoracic fasciae and pleurae except at the mediastinum. Caudally, the diaphragm is lined by the transverse fascia and peritoneum except at the bare area of the liver. The diaphragm is cranially convex, and the most cranial aspect of the convexity is the *cupula*, which lies between the middle and ventral thirds of the diaphragm. The diaphragm is also connected to the liver, heart and lungs by double sheets of peritoneum or pleura (e.g. falciform ligament, caudal mediastinal reflection).

The diaphragm develops from a framework formed by the growth of the septum transversum ventrally and the left and right pleuroperitoneal folds dorsally. These three structures fuse and separate the pleural and peritoneal cavities after the pericardial cavity has separated from the peritoneal cavity. Failure of the pleuroperitoneal folds to fuse with the septum transversum produces a congenital developmental defect that allows herniation of abdominal contents into the thoracic cavity. The central tendon is the most cranial aspect of the diaphragm and is formed from the septum transversum; the muscular portion is formed by the migration of muscle cells from somites that created the thoracic body wall.

- The central tendon has an opening for the caudal vena cava, the caval foramen. Unlike other structures that pass through openings in the diaphragm, the vessel is firmly adhered to the diaphragm by adventitia.
- The muscular portion of the diaphragm attaches to the ribs, sternum and lumbar vertebrae establishing costal, sternal and lumbar parts:
  - The costal and sternal parts connect the ventrolateral aspects of the central tendon to the medial aspects of the 8th–13th costochondral junctions, ribs and xiphoid process
  - The lumbar part joins the caudodorsal aspect of the central tendon to the ventral aspects of the 3rd and 4th lumbar vertebrae (L3 and L4) via long tendons, the left and right diaphragmatic crura
  - The right diaphragmatic crus is larger and has loosely connected muscle bundles medially that form the oesophageal hiatus for the passage of the oesophagus and vagus nerves; it also serves as a component of the caudal ('lower') oesophageal sphincter mechanism
  - In the dorsal aspect of the caudal mediastinum, the aortic hiatus lies between the two diaphragmatic crura and lumbar vertebrae and provides passage for the aorta, azygos vein and thoracic duct.
- From the lumbar attachment to the most caudal rib, the diaphragmatic margin is free ventral to the psoas muscles and gives passage to the sympathetic trunk. At this location, the lumbocostal arch, the pleura and peritoneum impinge upon one another dorsal to the diaphragm (Figure 8.5).
- The diaphragm is innervated by paired (right and left) phrenic nerves that arise from the 5th–7th cervical spinal nerves and course through the mediastinum along the oesophagus.

During radiography, the cranial margin of the diaphragm is well defined and contrasted by air-filled lungs, while most of the caudal margin forms a silhouette with the liver or gastric wall. The ventral margin, however, may be visible when contrasted by mediastinal (cranial) or falciform (caudal) fat. On lateral views, this ventral portion of the diaphragm is seen as a uniform thin band of soft tissue coursing dorsoventrally. Radiographically, the diaphragmatic silhouette is divided into the cupula (cranioventral), left crus (left caudodorsal) and right crus (right caudodorsal). The appearance of these three parts varies between radiographic views (Figure 8.6):

- On lateral views, the weight of the abdominal organs causes the gravity-dependent crus to be positioned cranially (e.g. the left crus is cranial to the right crus when the patient is in left lateral recumbency)
- On right lateral views, the caudal vena cava forms a silhouette with the more cranially positioned right crus and the crura are parallel
- On left lateral views, gas in the gastric fundus is commonly seen caudal to the left crus and the crura diverge dorsally
- On dorsoventral (DV) views, the cupula is cranially positioned and the crura are not typically observed
- On ventrodorsal (VD) views, the cupula is more caudally positioned and both crura are generally visible.

The diaphragm extends cranially into the thoracic cavity and forms recesses at insertion points on the thoracic body wall or back. The space between the ribs and the diaphragm is the costodiaphragmatic recess. The

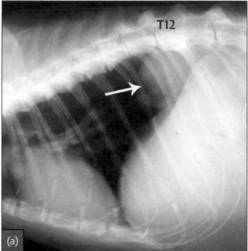

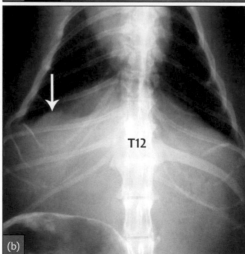

8.5 (a) Lateral and (b) ventrodorsal thoracic radiographs of an adult cat with multiple abdominal masses due to biopsy-confirmed abdominal carcinoma. Unrelated to that diagnosis, the costodiaphragmatic recesses are asymmetrical, the right 12th and 13th ribs articulate with the right side of the T12 vertebral body, the left 12th and 13th ribs are fused and articulate with the left side of the T12 vertebral body, and there is ultrasound-confirmed herniation of the right kidney cranial to the diaphragm (arrowed). This diaphragmatic hernia is presumed to be the result of abnormal development of the diaphragm and adjacent vertebrae, causing enlargement of the space dorsal to the lumbocostal arch. The diaphragmatic margin is normally free ventral to the psoas muscles; here, the pleura encroaches on the renal capsule through this space dorsal to the diaphragm.

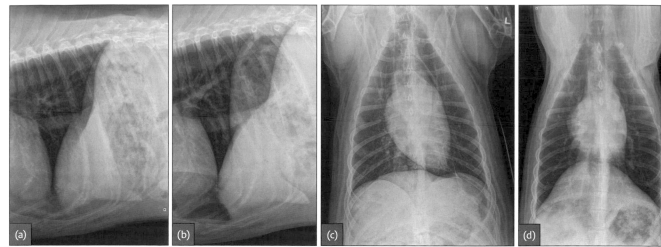

8.6 Normal thoracic radiographs of a dog. (a) On the right lateral view, the right diaphragmatic crus is cranial. (b) On the left lateral view, the left diaphragmatic crus is cranial. (c) On the VD view, both the crura and the cupula are visible. (d) On the DV view, the diaphragm is visible as a single dome. Note the gastric fundus is immediately caudal to the left diaphragmatic crus. On the VD and DV views, the locations of the costodiaphragmatic recesses are bilaterally symmetrical.

space between the psoas muscles (ventral to the lumbar vertebrae) and diaphragm is the lumbodiaphragmatic recess. Both recesses are bilateral. With adequate lung inflation, the left and right costodiaphragmatic recesses are positioned symmetrically at the same rib level (Figure 8.6cd).

Functional aspects

The thoracic cavities of cats and dogs are structurally and functionally different. For example, feline thoracic cavities have greater maximal respiratory excursion and compressibility. Consequently, reduced thoracic compressibility due to a thoracic mass is a more common physical examination finding in cats. During imaging, the degree of thoracic cavity expansion may be assessed by looking at the thoracic boundaries – particularly the diaphragm and ribs. Assessing thoracic cavity expansion is important because changes are chiefly due to normal respiration, pulmonary disease, pleural disease or abdominal distention.

Thoracic cavity volume may be assessed using many imaging modalities. During thoracic radiography, appropriate lung inflation is primarily assessed on DV and VD views by rib position: ribs that are more perpendicular to the vertebral column indicate well inflated lungs (see Figure 8.6). Animals with poorly inflated lungs will have smaller intercostal spaces and caudally rotated ribs (Figure 8.7). Other important indicators are the positioning of the mediastinal structures, symmetry of the diaphragm and enlargement of the costodiaphragmatic recesses (i.e. flat diaphragm). On lateral views, a flat diaphragm may be partly recognized as enlargement of the lumbodiaphragmatic recesses.

Whereas conventional radiography and computed tomography (CT) display the diaphragmatic and skeletal positions only at the precise moment of exposure, fluoroscopy allows assessment of these structures during inhalation and exhalation. Dynamic assessment may be important as the loss of normal motion might be a sign of disease.

- During inhalation, thoracic volume increases primarily due to contraction of the diaphragm but also by contraction of the intercostal muscles moving the ribs. Mild ventral displacement of the sternum also contributes to increased thoracic volume.
  - Diaphragmatic contraction causes the diaphragm to become flatter and caudally displaced. Interestingly,

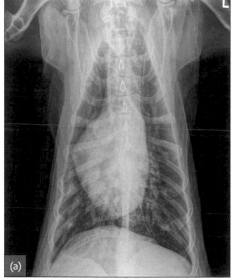

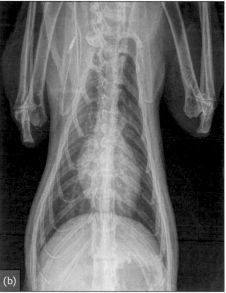

8.7 Normal VD thoracic radiographs of (a) a dog and (b) a cat with poor lung inflation. Note the ribs are angled caudally compared with Figure 8.6cd, which show well inflated lungs with ribs perpendicular to the vertebral column. In (a), the right lung is less inflated with increased opacity. In (b), the pulmonary blood vessel margins are poorly defined.

simultaneous stimulation of both phrenic nerves results in a greater change in thoracic pressure than the sum of pressure changes obtained by stimulating individual nerves, indicating a synergistic effect.
- Intercostal muscle contractions elevate and separate the ribs. During contraction, the position of the first rib pair is fixed by scalenus muscles that anchor the thoracic body wall, allowing for expansion.
- During exhalation, thoracic volume decreases primarily due to muscle relaxation. Exhalation is normally a passive process but can be enhanced by contraction of expiratory thoracic and abdominal musculature, usually in cases of obstructive pulmonary processes and coughing.
  - Diaphragmatic relaxation causes the diaphragm to move cranially and become cranially convex.
  - Intercostal muscle relaxation causes contraction of the rib cage, bringing the ribs closer together.

Interpretative principles

Distribution of osseous abnormalities

- One abnormal bone:
  - A single abnormality (solitary monostotic) is commonly due to a primary bone neoplasm, osteomyelitis, congenital developmental anomaly or trauma (e.g. fracture)
  - Multiple abnormalities (multiple monostotic) are uncommon but may be seen with cancer or osteomyelitis.
- Multiple abnormal bones:
  - Multiple abnormalities with an anatomically symmetrical distribution (symmetrical polyostotic) are uncommon and are most seen with congenital developmental anomalies and systemic conditions (e.g. bilateral hypoplastic ribs, hypertrophic osteopathy)
  - Multiple abnormalities with a generalized random distribution (asymmetrical polyostotic) are typically due to metastatic cancer or infection, multicentric neoplasia (e.g. multiple myeloma), multiple cartilaginous exostosis or insufficiency fractures
  - Multiple abnormalities affecting adjacent bones (locally extensive polyostotic) are typically due to local spread of a neoplasm, suppurative inflammation or trauma (e.g. severe bite wounds, migrating foreign body, discospondylitis)
  - Multiple fractured ribs with the fractures arranged in a row (linear polyostotic) are typically due to trauma.
- Widespread bone disease:
  - All parts of all bones are abnormal although not all parts may be affected to the same degree (diffuse distribution). This is commonly seen with metabolic bone disease (e.g. primary or secondary hyperparathyroidism, osteosclerosis). This distribution also may be termed 'generalized' or that may be reserved for when some parts of the bones are spared (there is some normal bone between abnormalities).

Radiographic patterns of aggressive bone lesions

- Bone abnormalities may be further characterized as aggressive or non-aggressive.

- Aggressive bone abnormalities are more strongly associated with bone neoplasms and infections (osteomyelitis).
- Differentiating between aggressive and non-aggressive bone lesions is based on evaluating several variables:
  - Presence and type of bone lysis
  - Presence and type of periosteal reaction
  - Zone of transition between normal and abnormal bone
  - Rate of progression (requires serial examinations).

Rib cage

Rib lesions can be overlooked easily for several reasons, including small size, peripheral location and low radiographic contrast. Therefore, deliberately performing a systematic evaluation to identify rib abnormalities, such as fractures or aggressive lesions, is crucial. Once a rib abnormality is identified, oblique radiographic views tangential to and collimated to the abnormality may improve lesion characterization.

Abnormal number of ribs

- Increased or decreased rib number is commonly caused by a congenital developmental anomaly that produces a transitional cervicothoracic or thoracolumbar vertebra. These findings are usually incidental and of minor consequence but documenting the anatomical variation may be important for surgical planning.
  - C7 may have small ribs ('cervical ribs') (Figure 8.8).
  - First and second ribs may be fused.
  - T13 may lack ribs, have small ribs, or have ribs that look like transverse processes (Figure 8.9).
  - L1 may have ribs or transverse processes that are long and rib-like.
  - Rib anomalies may be unilateral or bilateral.
- Certain diseases (e.g. a neoplasm) may obliterate a rib such that it is undetectable during imaging. Absence of rib that is not associated with a developmental anomaly is a finding of major consequence (Figure 8.10).

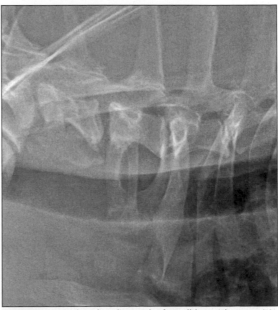

8.8 Lateral neck radiograph of a Bulldog with a transitional cervicothoracic vertebra that was an incidental finding of minor consequence. The C7 vertebra has a pair of small ribs that are incompletely fused with the first pair of thoracic ribs.

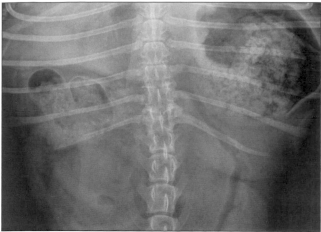

8.9 VD radiograph of the thoracolumbar junction in a dog with a transitional thoracolumbar vertebra. At T13, the right rib is normal in size and shape, and the left rib is thick, appearing like a long transverse process. The T13 vertebral body is also abnormal (butterfly vertebra).

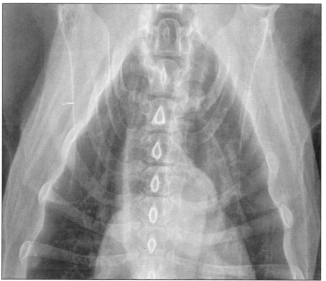

8.10 VD thoracic radiograph of a dog with a solitary aggressive bone lesion of the left third rib. The dorsal aspect of the rib is absent due to severe osteolysis and is surrounded by a soft tissue tumour with indistinct margins.

Altered rib opacity

- Decreased opacity:
  - Osteolysis: typically focal or multifocal decrease in opacity due to irreversible bone destruction. The bone destruction may involve the rib cortices, medulla or both. Punctate lucencies may be seen in the bone marrow (e.g. due to multiple myeloma, lymphoma). Lysis is typically due to an aggressive process such as cancer or osteomyelitis and may lead to pathological fracture
  - Osteopenia: decreased bone mineral density that may be generalized or regional. During imaging, the affected ribs have reduced opacity (reduced contrast with adjacent soft tissues), thin cortices and coarse trabecular markings (Figure 8.11). In animals, generalized osteopenia is often due to alterations in calcium homeostasis and is often reversible but may lead to insufficiency fractures (Figure 8.11). Osteopenia is usually associated with osteomalacia, as osteoporosis is less common in non-human animals.

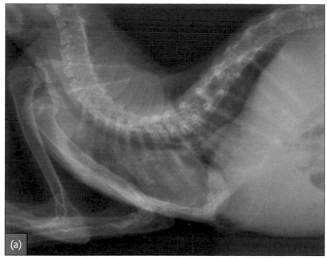

(a)

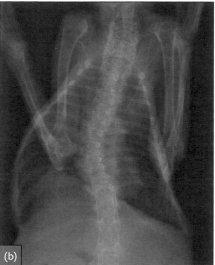

(b)

8.11 (a) Lateral and (b) DV thoracic radiographs of a cat with nutritional secondary hyperparathyroidism, scoliosis and lordosis. There is generalized osteopenia with reduced contrast between bone and soft tissue, reduced corticomedullary distinction and thin bone cortices. The thoracic vertebral column is misaligned, with right and ventral convexities.

- Increased opacity:
  - Periosteal reaction: a reparative or proliferative bone process that may be generalized (e.g. hypertrophic osteopathy) or regional (e.g. callus, neoplasm, osteomyelitis)
  - Osteosclerosis: abnormal hardening of bone, usually due to replacing normal tissue or adding connective tissue and mineral. Regional osteosclerosis is common in the appendicular skeleton (rare in the axial skeleton) and due to increased medullary bone secondary to applied stresses (Wolff's law). Generalized osteosclerosis is uncommon in animals but may be seen in association with feline leukaemia virus (Figure 8.12). Osteopetrosis, another cause of generalized osteosclerosis, is rare in animals and typically a generalized condition due to inherited or acquired genetic mutations leading to impaired osteoclastic activity and reduced bone resorption.
- Physiological anatomical variation:
  - Variable mineralization of the costal cartilages often increases with age
  - Well defined, rounded regions of mineral proliferation at the costochondral junctions without associated rib lysis (Figure 8.13).

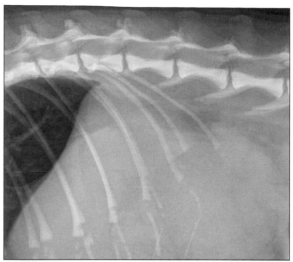

8.12 Lateral radiograph of a cat with severe diffuse osteosclerosis (presumed osteopetrosis). The ribs and vertebral bodies maintain a normal shape and are of homogeneous mineral opacity with absent corticomedullary distinction and trabecular markings.

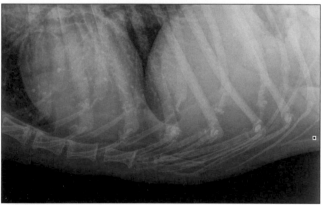

8.13 Lateral thoracic radiograph of a dog with degenerative remodelling. The costal cartilages are mineralized, and the costochondral junctions have irregular well defined margins. No rib lysis is detected. The dog also has ossifying pulmonary metaplasia, another degenerative change. All these findings are incidental and of minor consequence.

Altered rib size, margin and shape

- Small ribs are usually a congenital developmental anomaly associated with hypoplasia, aplasia or incomplete mineralization.
- Expanded enlarged ribs are usually due to aggressive disease but may be due to cartilaginous exostosis. Peripheral enlargement of ribs is usually due to periosteal proliferation which may be due to healing fracture callus or indicative of an aggressive bone lesion.
- Margin alteration is commonly due to a periosteal reaction; the underlying rib cortex may be continuous or discontinuous. Causes include:
  - A reparative or reactive process of bone
  - Active lesions characterized by ill-defined and/or irregular margins
    - Aggressiveness is more likely if lysis is also present
  - Chronic/non-aggressive lesions characterized by well defined and smooth margins.
- A discontinuous rib margin may be a subtle or obvious sign of disease (e.g. fracture, neoplasm, infection).

- Alterations in shape with loss of margin definition are usually due to trauma, infection or neoplasia.
- Alterations in shape with preservation of margin definition are usually due to trauma or developmental malformations.
- Ill-defined ribs with continuous cortical margins may be due to osteopenia.
- Symmetrical rib position indicates normal lung inflation and correct positioning to obtain diagnostic images.
- Narrow or wide intercostal spaces can be due to:
  - Oblique radiographic view (i.e. artefactual)
  - Rib or vertebral malformations (see Figure 8.11)
  - Trauma or previous surgery (Figure 8.14)
  - Pneumothorax
  - Lung expansion or collapse.
- 'Barrel chest' conformation is a normal anatomical variation in brachycephalic breeds (e.g. Bulldog, Boston Terrier); in these patients, the thoracic shape is rounded with equal and bilaterally symmetrical rib spacing. However, a 'barrel chest' conformation due to maximal thoracic expansion can be pathologically acquired (Figure 8.15) secondary to obstructive or space-occupying intrathoracic lesions, including:
  - Severe pleural fluid or pneumothorax
  - Large intrathoracic masses
  - Pulmonary hyperinflation
  - Feline lower airway disease
  - Restrictive pleuritis.

Altered soft tissues

The body wall soft tissues should be bilaterally symmetrical with well defined musculature when contrasted by fat in the superficial and deep fasciae; the thickness of the fat varies with body habitus (Figure 8.16). Skin folds are commonly seen during thoracic radiography (Figure 8.17) and should not be mistaken for pathology such as pleural fluid or pneumothorax. Skin folds can frequently be differentiated from such pathology because they extend beyond the thoracic margins. Summation of superficial objects leading to false diagnoses of lung pathology also arises from wet hair (including from ultrasound gel, Figure 8.18), debris in the hair, nipples and superficial nodules or masses. Orthogonal views, careful palpation of the body wall and placement of metal opaque markers or barium paste can help differentiate a summation shadow caused by superficial structures from lung pathology.

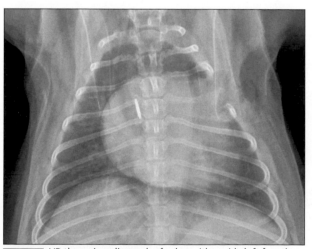

8.14 VD thoracic radiograph of a dog with a wide left fourth intercostal space secondary to a chronic displaced rib fracture and lung herniation into the body wall.

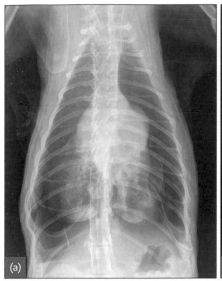

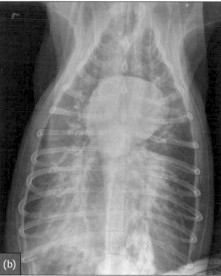

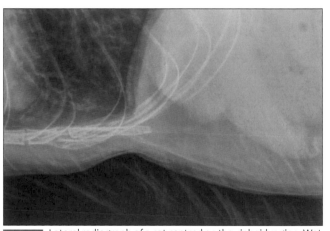

8.15 DV thoracic radiographs of (a) a cat with severe bilateral pneumothorax *ex vacuo* secondary to generalized restrictive pleuritis and (b) a Dobermann with left-sided congestive heart failure. Both animals have a pathological 'barrel chest' conformation due to maximal expansion of the thoracic cavity by different mechanisms.

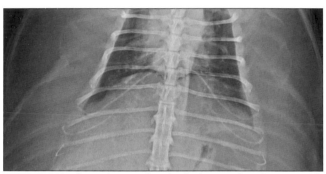

8.16 DV radiograph centred on the diaphragm of an obese cat with substantial bilaterally symmetrical fat within the body wall. The opaque body wall musculature is laterally displaced but remains well defined from the fat.

8.18 Lateral radiograph of a cat centred on the xiphoid region. Wet hair from ultrasound gel summates with the ventral thoracic and abdominal fat and could be mistaken for body wall swelling or peritoneal fluid but extends beyond the skin margin.

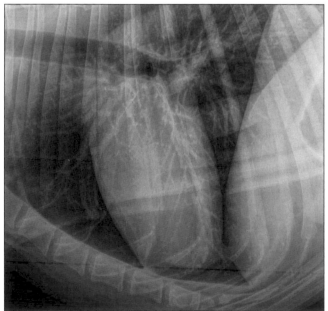

8.17 Normal lateral thoracic radiograph of a dog with obliquely oriented skin folds in the ventral part of the thorax. In this example, the skin folds produce multiple alternating opaque and lucent bands that are positive and negative summation shadows of the skin with the rest of the thorax. These lines may be distinguished from intrathoracic abnormalities because they extend beyond the margins of the thoracic cavity (they extend caudally over the abdomen and cranioventrally over the axilla).

Asymmetrical soft tissue swelling is typically a sign of pathology. The soft tissue swelling may be regional (focal, locally extensive) or widespread (multifocal, generalized, diffuse). The soft tissue swelling also may be infiltrative (e.g. haemorrhage, oedema, cellulitis, fasciitis) or form a mass-like lesion (e.g. neoplasm, abscess, haematoma). The swelling may project externally, internally (into the thoracic cavity) or both. A body wall or pleural abnormality may occasionally be mistaken for a pulmonary lesion. During thoracic radiography, these conditions may be differentiated when the abnormality produces an extrapleural sign, indicating a body wall abnormality (Figure 8.19). An extrapleural sign is produced when the abnormality is viewed tangentially to the X-ray beam and has oblique margins that gradually taper toward the body wall: a pulmonary lesion is expected to form an acute angle between the lesion and the lung periphery.

Trauma, particularly bite wounds, can introduce gas into the superficial and deep fasciae of the body wall (Figure 8.20). Gas also may dissect into the fascial planes following other injuries (e.g. tracheal laceration). Summation of body wall gas and thoracic viscera during radiography can be confusing and lead to the misidentification of abnormalities (either presence or absence).

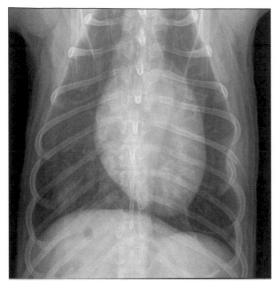

8.19 DV thoracic radiograph of a dog with an acute traumatic left rib fracture. Associated with the fracture, there is a focal soft tissue swelling that displaces the visceral pleura medially and has oblique margins that gradually taper towards the body wall (i.e. an extrapleural sign).

Orthogonal views can help localize the abnormal gas accumulation to the body wall or thoracic cavity (Figure 8.21); however, CT may be necessary for definitive localization of gas. Gas also may be observed with some infections. A rent in the body wall can lead to herniation of lung externally or fat internally (Figure 8.22).

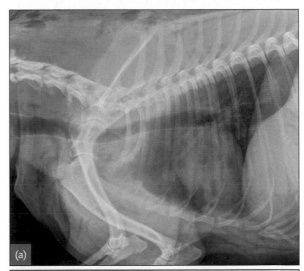

(a)

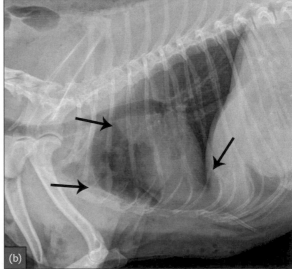

(b)

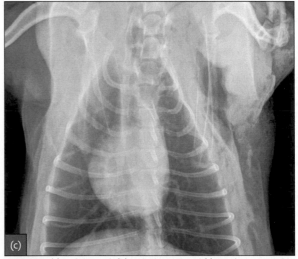

(c)

8.21 (a) Left lateral, (b) right lateral and (c) VD thoracic radiographs of a dog with bite wounds. (a, b) On the lateral views, body wall gas creates confusing apparent lung pathology (arrowed). (c) This can be accurately localized to the left body wall on the orthogonal view.

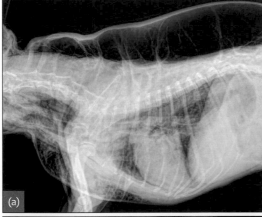

(a)

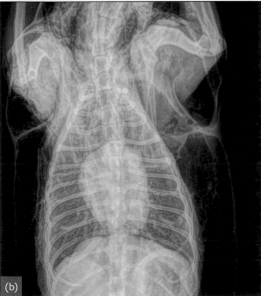

(b)

8.20 (a) Lateral and (b) VD thoracic radiographs of a dog with extensive body wall gas from a tracheal rupture secondary to severe bite wounds. The gas extends throughout the superficial fascia of the neck and thorax, visceral fascia of the ventral neck, and mediastinum.

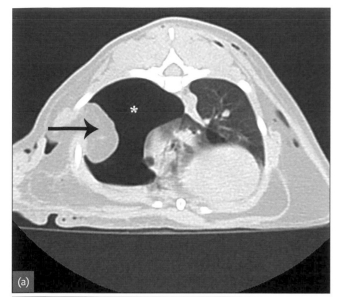

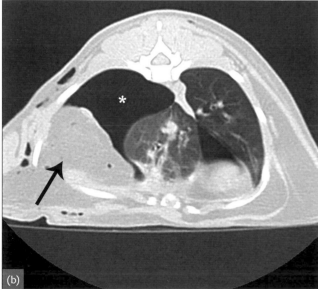

8.22 (a, b) Transverse thoracic CT images of a cat with major trauma causing herniation of body wall fat into the right pleural cavity through a large rent in the thoracic body wall (arrowed). The cat also has a tension pneumothorax (*), rib fractures (not shown), and gas dissection through the superficial and deep fasciae of the body wall.

Vertebral column

The dorsum, or back, is often included in thoracic imaging studies and needs to be evaluated. As spinal imaging is a specialized topic the description provided here, where it relates to thoracic imaging, is more general. Assessment of the vertebral column is optimized by careful patient positioning. On lateral thoracic radiographs, paired structures like transverse processes, rib heads and intervertebral foramina should summate with each other. On DV and VD views, the vertebral column should summate with the sternum and the 'tear-drop' shaped spinous processes (see Figure 8.10) should summate with the vertebral bodies.

Clinically important vertebral abnormalities that may be detected during thoracic radiography include fractures, dislocations, neoplasms, osteomyelitis and discospondylitis. Alignment of the vertebral column is also especially important to assess. Developmental abnormalities (e.g. malformed vertebral bodies, malformed vertebral arches, malalignment) are common, especially in some breeds, and may be clinically important or incidental findings of minor consequence. Degenerative changes (e.g. spondylosis deformans, vertebral osteoarthrosis) are common, typically of minor consequence and potentially misinterpreted as important abnormalities. Soft tissue swelling, as described for the body wall (see 'Altered soft tissues', above), is also possible.

Sternum

During thoracic radiography, the sternum and associated soft tissues are best examined on lateral views because there is no summation with the vertebral column. Oblique radiographic views, ultrasonography or CT also may be helpful when sternal abnormalities are incompletely evaluated with radiography.

Clinically important sternal lesions are rare and include costosternal and sternal dislocations, sternal fractures, neoplasms, osteomyelitis and developmental anomalies (e.g. pectus excavatum). Soft tissue swelling, as described for the body wall (see 'Altered soft tissues', above), is also possible. Conformational and degenerative lesions are common and potentially misinterpreted as clinically important abnormalities. Some common findings of no or minor consequence are:

- Well defined bridging bone between sternebrae
- Mild variations in overall curvature
- Increased or reduced number or fusion of adjacent sternebrae (Figure 8.23)
- Incomplete fusion (may be associated with other midline defects or congenital malformations)
- Minor malalignment of sternebrae, particularly the xiphoid process in cats
- Variation in the size and shape of sternebrae (particularly the manubrium and xiphoid process).

Diaphragm

Normal appearance

During radiography, the normal diaphragm is smooth, curved and has soft tissue opacity. The cranial margin is well defined and contrasted by gas in the lungs. The caudal margin is indistinguishable due to border effacement with the liver and gastric wall. The ventral portion of the diaphragm may be contrasted by mediastinal and

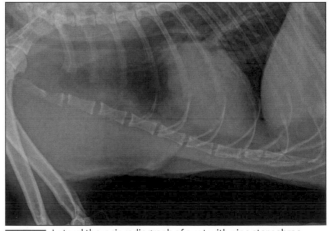

8.23 Lateral thoracic radiograph of a cat with nine sternebrae (rather than eight). This finding is an incidental congenital developmental anomaly of minor consequence.

falciform fat. Normal position of the diaphragm with good lung inflation (see Figure 8.6) can be assessed as follows:

- Lung tissue is frequently visible between the diaphragmatic cupula and cardiac silhouette
- The caudal vena cava should be approximately parallel to the vertebral column
- On VD views, the costodiaphragmatic angles should be approximately 45 degrees and located at the level of the 11th rib
- On lateral views, the lumbodiaphragmatic angle should be approximately 45 degrees and located at the level of the 11th thoracic vertebra
- On DV views, the cupula should be centrally positioned with respect to the median plane
- On VD views, the laterally positioned crura should be similar in size and location.

Several technical and patient factors may influence the appearance of the normal diaphragm:

- Shape varies with:
  - Patient recumbency and X-ray beam orientation (vertical *versus* horizontal)
  - Orientation of the central axis of the X-ray beam (e.g. centred over the thorax *versus* the abdomen)
  - Breed/conformation
  - Degree of lung expansion or collapse, including normal phases of respiration
  - Degree of pleural cavity expansion
  - Degree of abdominal distention (e.g. peritoneal fluid, organomegaly, obesity)
- Visibility varies with the presence of pleural fluid or lung disease.

Diaphragmatic asymmetry

DV or VD radiographs are best for assessment of dia-phragmatic symmetry. If diaphragmatic asymmetry is sus-pected on a DV view, a VD view should be obtained and vice versa. Diaphragmatic asymmetry is usually unrelated to primary diaphragmatic pathologies (e.g. paralysis, masses) because they are rare. More commonly, asym-metry is due to technical factors (i.e. positioning) or varia-bility in lung inflation, or is secondary to displacement of other associated organs (e.g. ribs).

- Radiographic findings of asymmetry include:
  - Asymmetric location (rib number) and size of the costodiaphragmatic recesses
  - Excessive cranial displacement of one crus that is repeatable on multiple views and between images obtained during inhalation and exhalation
  - Possible associated findings: rib fractures, body wall swelling, pleural fluid or gas, mediastinal shift.
- Non-pathological causes include:
  - Mild asymmetry, which is usually clinically unimportant
  - Oblique positioning.

Bilateral displacement

Bilateral displacement of the diaphragm is typically harder to identify than unilateral displacement, particularly when the normal shape of the diaphragm is maintained. Obtaining both DV and VD views may aid detection (Figure 8.24). As with diaphragmatic asymmetry, bilateral dia-phragmatic displacement is usually secondary to other

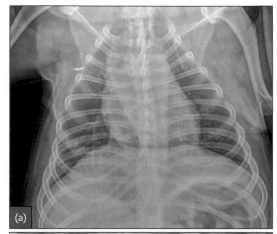
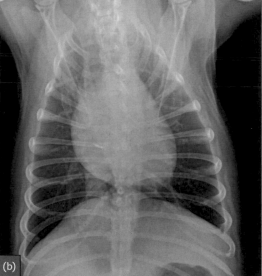

8.24 (a) DV and (b) VD thoracic radiographs of a dog. In (a), bilateral displacement of the diaphragm is suspected, but diaphragm location is normal in (b).

factors and uncommonly due to primary diaphragmatic disease. Cranial displacement of the diaphragm is most commonly due to increased size of the abdomen (e.g. peri-toneal fluid, pregnancy, abdominal mass, obesity) or reduced volume of both lungs (e.g. obstructive tracheal foreign body). Bilateral phrenic nerve paralysis is rare.

Diaphragmatic margin

The diaphragm is cranially convex with a smooth cranial margin that is normally well defined and contrasted by gas. Portions of the cranial margin may be effaced by normal structures (e.g. caudal vena cava) or by abnormal soft tissue structures in the thorax. The caudal margin should form a silhouette with the liver or be contrasted by fal-ciform fat. Loss of normal silhouetting is commonly observed in animals with pneumoperitoneum. Rarely, the diaphragmatic contour may be altered by lung hyperin-flation (e.g. tenting of the diaphragm), diaphragmatic masses or diaphragmatic eventration. During ultrasono-graphy, the cranial margin of the diaphragm is obscured by lung or pleural gas: the cranial margin may be observed when there is lung consolidation or pleural fluid.

Diaphragmatic motion (dynamic studies)

- Fluoroscopy and ultrasonography allow for dynamic evaluation.

- Normal motion: during inhalation, the diaphragm moves caudally, becomes flatter and increases the volume of the thoracic cavity. During exhalation, the diaphragm moves cranially, becomes rounder and decreases the volume of the thoracic cavity. This motion is often coordinated with motion of the rib cage (see 'Functional aspects', above).
  - Paradoxical motion: a portion or the entirety of the diaphragm moves cranially during inhalation and caudally during exhalation.
- The following parameters were observed in healthy Beagles under controlled respiratory conditions and general anaesthesia (Moon *et al.*, 2017):
  - Range of diaphragm excursion relative to T8: ½ to 1 vertebral body length (median ¾)
  - Symmetrical crural excursion in right lateral recumbency
  - Asymmetrical crural excursion in left lateral recumbency
  - Excursion is generally larger for the left crus.
- Using the liver as an acoustic window, transabdominal ultrasonography allows for unilateral sequential evaluation of the non-recumbent diaphragmatic crus. Ultrasonographic evaluation includes the assessment for normal *versus* paradoxical motion and the amount of excursion (the difference between left and right sides is less than 50% in normal dogs).

Diseases of the thoracic skeleton

Developmental anomalies

Chondrodysplasia

Chondrodysplasias are caused by a variety of genetic abnormalities leading to abnormal cartilage development and skeletal malformations. Chondrodysplasia may affect all skeletal structures (proportionate dwarfism) or primarily facial bones or the appendicular skeleton (disproportionate dwarfism).

- Proportionate dwarfism is usually caused by inadequate growth hormone production due to pituitary dysfunction. Pituitary dwarfism has an autosomal recessive mode of inheritance in the German Shepherd Dog and has recently been described in Saarloos and Czechoslovakian Wolfdogs. Clinical signs include retention of puppy coat and/or symmetrical alopecia, small stature and hunched posture. Imaging findings include signs of skeletal dysmaturity. Magnetic resonance imaging (MRI) of the brain may reveal a cyst in the location of the pituitary gland. Endocrine testing is necessary for confirmation as overlap of clinical and imaging findings can occur with other forms of chondrodysplasia and multiple endocrinological abnormalities may be concurrently present (e.g. growth and thyroid hormone abnormalities).
- Chondrodysplasia is commonly encountered as a breed standard (e.g. in Dachshunds, Figure 8.25) but has been sporadically described in other dog breeds (e.g. Alaskan Malamute, Norwegian Elkhound, Labrador Retriever, Boxer). A truncation mutation in a collagen-binding protein has been reported in Norwegian Elkhounds (Kyöstilä *et al.*, 2013).
- Congenital hypothyroidism, most described in Boxers, is a rare cause of disproportionate dwarfism due to

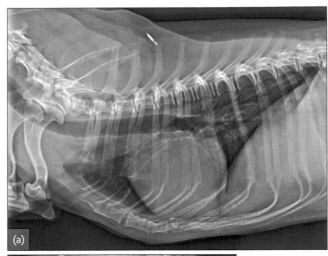

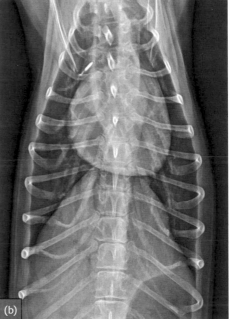

8.25 Normal (a) right lateral and (b) DV thoracic radiographs of a Dachshund. Note the short vertebral bodies, barrel chest conformation and internal curvature of the rib cage at costochondral junctions.

lack of thyroid hormone. Radiographic signs overlap with proportionate dwarfism and are primarily due to osseous dysmaturity that is most pronounced in the appendicular skeleton (e.g. non-uniform physes, abnormal curvature of long bones):
- Small, irregular epiphyses of vertebral bodies
- Short vertebral bodies
- Exaggerated rounding of thoracic shape ('barrel chest')
- Inward curvature of the ribs at the costochondral junctions.

Midline fusion defects

- Spinal dysraphism: a group of developmental anomalies of the vertebral arch due to incomplete closure of the neural tube (i.e. an error of neurulation). Clinically silent anomalies (spina bifida occulta) are occasional incidental findings during thoracic imaging. These vertebral arch malformations are typically covered by normal muscle and skin, and often only affect a single site (Figure 8.26). However, multiple sequential defects are possible, the cleft may be open

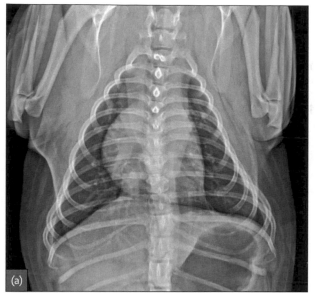

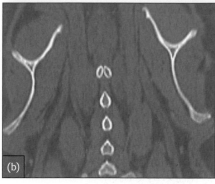

8.26 (a) DV thoracic radiograph and (b) dorsal CT image of a Bulldog with incomplete fusion of the T1 spinous process (spina bifida occulta).

Vertebral body anomalies

Vertebral body anomalies are due to abnormal somite formation or segmentation (somitogenesis) or abnormal endochondral ossification. Abnormal vertebral bodies (e.g. hemivertebrae) are typically small or abnormally shaped and commonly seen in the mid-thoracic vertebral column of 'screw-tail' breeds (e.g. Bulldogs) and sporadically in other breeds. Abnormalities may be focal or multifocal and unilateral or bilateral with shape and size variation based on the number and size of the osseous defects. Many of these anomalies are incidental findings of minor consequence, but the malformations can cause vertebral stenosis, abnormal alignment of the vertebral column, or both. Neurological deficits may be present when the severity of the anomaly leads to extradural spinal cord compression. Radiographic signs include:

- Non-uniformity of vertebral body length
- Fused vertebrae
- Short, angular, wedge and/or butterfly vertebrae (Figure 8.28)
- Variable vertebral column curvature, most commonly scoliosis or kyphosis
  - Unilateral and/or multiple defects typically cause more vertebral column curvature
- Reduced vertebral canal size (stenosis)
- Reduced intercostal space width that is worse dorsally
- MRI is the best modality for complete assessment of spinal cord compression secondary to vertebral malformations. Myelography can also be performed to assess for spinal cord compression (Figure 8.29).

to the environment, and neurological deficits may be present when there is concurrent herniation of meninges or neural tissue through the cleft (producing a meningocoele or meningomyelocoele). Cross-sectional imaging is usually required for characterization.
- Sternal dysraphism (Figure 8.27): may be clinically silent or associated with other malformations (e.g. peritoneopericardial diaphragmatic hernia (PPDH)).
  - Duplication (incomplete fusion) of the sternebrae is seen on the DV and VD views.

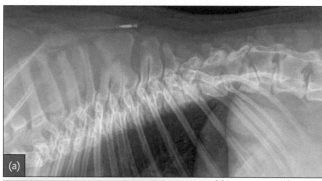

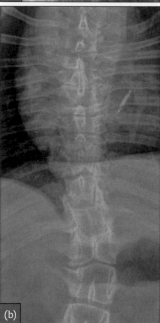

8.28 (a) Lateral and (b) VD radiographs of the thoracolumbar vertebral column in a neurologically normal French Bulldog with short, wedge and butterfly-shaped vertebrae, narrow intercostal spaces, fusion of spinous processes and mild scollosis.

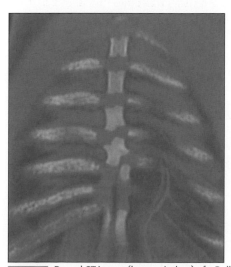

8.27 Dorsal CT image (bone window) of a Bulldog with sternal dysraphism, a midline defect. This patient also had pulmonic stenosis but no other midline fusion defect.

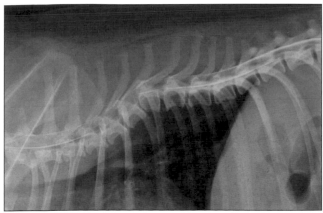

8.29 Lateral thoracic myelogram of a dog with congenital developmental kyphosis. The mid-thoracic vertebral column has malformed vertebral bodies and a focal dorsal convexity with attenuation of contrast material within the subarachnoid space at the level of the lesion, consistent with extradural spinal cord compression.

Articular process dysplasia

Articular process dysplasia is dysgenesis and/or abnormal ossification of articular processes causing them to be small or absent with incomplete formation of the synovial joints. Articular process dysplasia is commonly seen in the thoracic vertebrae. Dysplasia of the caudal articular processes is commonly reported in small-breed dogs such as Pugs, English Bulldogs and French Bulldogs, but occurs in many breeds. The malformation is commonly seen in neurologically normal dogs. However, it could lead to instability with secondary formation of fibrous bands, hypertrophy of surrounding soft tissues and/or intervertebral disc herniation that can cause chronic extradural spinal cord compression. Radiographic findings include (Figure 8.30):

- Small or absent articular processes
- Variably increased width of articular process joints
- Sclerosis of adjacent vertebral bodies
- Signs of intervertebral disc degeneration (see 'Intervertebral disc degeneration', below).

Myelography, Myelo-CT or MRI is required to demonstrate spinal cord compression.

Pectus excavatum

Pectus excavatum is dorsoventral narrowing of the thoracic cavity, possibly associated with a short diaphragm and closer apposition of the caudal portion of the sternum and vertebral column (Figure 8.31). Burmese cats and brachycephalic dogs, specifically Maltese and Bulldogs, are predisposed. Proposed reasons include genetic malformations, increased resistance to air flow due to conformation, or both. Mild cases are usually asymptomatic and do not require intervention. The malformation is most commonly a static congenital developmental anomaly, but pectus excavatum can be dynamic and acquired (Figure 8.32) secondary to upper airway obstruction (e.g. laryngeal paralysis, nasopharyngeal polyp) and paradoxical motion.

- On physical examination, the sternal region has a palpable concavity due to dorsal displacement of the caudal sternum, which is radiographically visible. The degree of malformation is variable.
  - When mild, the condition is clinically silent.
  - With severe displacement, respiratory and/or cardiovascular compromise is possible.
- Concurrent congenital malformations have been reported, including hypoplastic trachea, ventricular septal defect and PPDH.
- Radiographic signs include:
  - Dorsal displacement of the sternebrae and shorter distance to the vertebral column, most severe caudally
  - Dorsal curvature of the costal cartilages
  - Sternebrae positioned dorsal to the ventral curvature of the costal cartilages
  - Cardiac displacement: dorsal on lateral radiographs and lateral (usually leftward) on DV and VD radiographs.

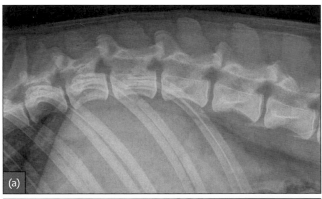

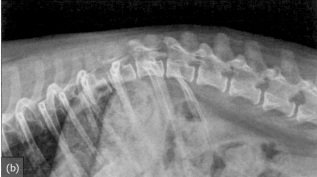

8.30 Lateral radiographs of the thoracolumbar vertebral column in (a) a normal dog and (b) a Pug with articular process dysplasia. In (b), from T10–T12, the caudal articular processes are small or absent and the intervertebral disc spaces are narrow ventrally.

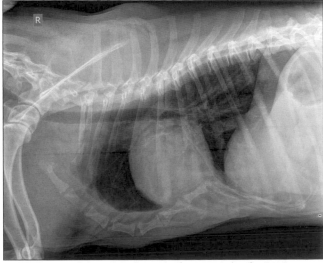

8.31 Lateral thoracic radiograph of a young Labrador Retriever with pectus excavatum. The congenital developmental sternal malformation caused mild displacement of the cardiac silhouette without cardiovascular dysfunction.

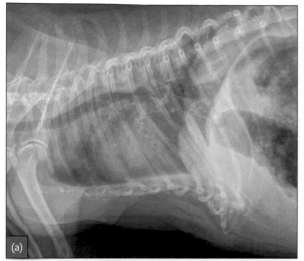

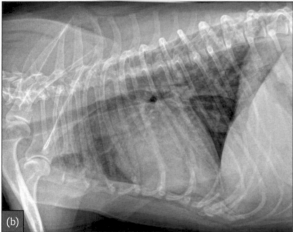

8.32 Lateral thoracic radiographs of a 13-year-old Yorkshire Terrier with progressive dyspnoea for 3 months that acutely decompensated due to laryngeal obstruction (epiglottic retroversion, swelling). (a) Thoracic radiographs on the day of decompensation demonstrated acquired pectus excavatum. (b) The sternum was normal 3 days prior.

- Surgical intervention may be required in cases with severe cardiovascular compromise. Sternal splinting reduces respiratory distress and right ventricular outflow tract obstruction in severe cases. Radiographic indices comparing the height of the thorax with the vertebral bodies (e.g. fronto-sagittal index, vertebral index) may help assess the severity of the malformation but decisions regarding surgical intervention should be based on clinical signs.
- Pectus excavatum should be differentiated from:
  - Flail sternum (rare): dynamic displacement of sternum (often paradoxical) due to bilateral rib cartilage fractures. Fluoroscopy or paired radiographs obtained at peak inhalation and exhalation can be used to demonstrate dynamic displacement
  - 'Flat pup syndrome' or 'swimmer puppy' (rare): malformation characterized by reduced thoracic height without dorsal displacement of the sternum. Affected puppies have abduction of the limbs and inability to walk. Prognosis is generally poor but successful medical management has been described
  - Pectus carinatum ('pigeon' or 'keeled' chest): outward displacement of the caudal sternum, leading to increased height of the thorax and usually incidental (Figure 8.33). Pugs and French Bulldogs are predisposed.

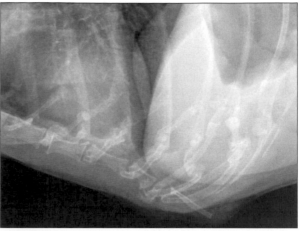

8.33 Lateral radiograph centred on the xiphoid region in a French Bulldog with pectus carinatum (ventral displacement of the caudal sternum).

Vascular malformations

Vascular malformations (rare) including angioma, hamartoma and arteriovenous malformation have been reported in dogs with neurological deficits. Vertebral angiomatosis, a specific type of hamartoma, has been described as a cause of expansile bone lesions, profound back pain and neurological deficits in young adult cats.

Vertebral stenosis

Vertebral stenosis is caused by any osseous or soft tissue malformation that causes reduced size of the vertebral canal (Figure 8.34). The stenosis may be focal, multifocal

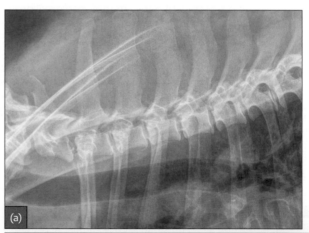

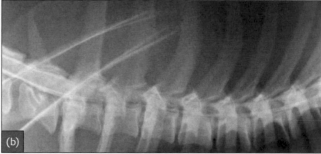

8.34 (a) Lateral cervicothoracic radiograph and (b) myelogram of a dog with neurological deficits due to 'Wobbler' syndrome (cervical spondylomyelopathy). At T1–T3, the vertebral canal is narrow with diffuse attenuation of contrast material in this region, consistent with vertebral stenosis. Vertebral stenosis may cause extradural spinal cord compression or predispose the spinal cord to injury following minor trauma.

or widespread. If stenosis is severe enough to cause spinal cord compression, neurological deficits will develop. Vertebral stenosis may predispose animals to spinal cord injury following minor trauma that would not normally result in neurological deficits. Vertebral stenosis in conjunction with cervical spondylomyelopathy may be recognized on the periphery of the thoracic radiograph and is common in the Dobermann and Great Dane, and also frequently diagnosed in other large and giant breeds (e.g. Mastiff). In the thorax, reduced height of the vertebral canal, most commonly of T2–T6, may be visible on survey radiographs. Specific imaging of the neck and back, ideally with cross-sectional imaging such as MRI, is necessary for complete characterization and is beyond the scope of this text.

Lysosomal storage diseases

Lysosomal storage diseases are inborn errors in metabolism due to genetic mutations in enzymes leading to accumulation of metabolic products within cellular lysosomes and, eventually, cell dysfunction and/or death. Mucopolysaccharidosis (MPS) comprises a group of lysosomal storage diseases described in dogs and cats, resulting from deficient degradation of glycosaminoglycans, leading to multifocal lesions including progressive skeletal deformities. Specific genetic mutations have been identified in a variety of dogs and cats (Haskins *et al.*, 1983; Spellacy *et al.*, 1983), including domestic cats and Plott hounds (MPS Type 1), Wire Haired Dachshunds and Schipperke (MPS Type 3) and Siamese cats, Miniature Pinschers and Miniature Schnauzers (MPS Type 6). Vertebrae are commonly affected. Prognosis is poor as dogs rarely live more than 1 year. However, promising recent research studies in both dogs and cats demonstrate that neonatal retroviral gene therapy can ameliorate the severity of musculoskeletal lesions, such as increasing long bone length and reducing cartilage erosions (Herati *et al.*, 2008; Ponder *et al.*, 2012). Radiographic signs include (Figure 8.35):

- Short, thick and abnormally shaped bones, particularly vertebrae
- Narrow intervertebral disc spaces
- Variable vertebral fusion (ankyloses)
- Degenerative joint disease (see 'Degenerative lesions', below), articular erosions
- Thick long bones and ribs.

Traumatic fractures

- Thoracic trauma is common in small animals and most fractures are traumatic, even in cases with unknown history.
- A traumatic fracture is a focal failure of bone due to rapidly applied high-grade force, typically to normal bone.
- Trauma may be blunt or penetrating and may cause soft tissue laceration or rupture, compression injury, haemorrhage and visible fractures. Tissue or organ displacements are also possible.
  - Bleeding may occur within a tissue (e.g. pulmonary contusions), body cavity (e.g. haemothorax) or externally.
  - Penetrating injuries produce an open wound in the body wall (e.g. open pneumothorax).
- Radiography is recommended prior to treatment because physical examination findings may be misleading.

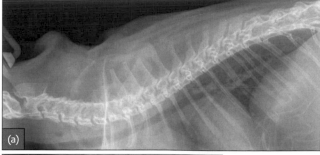

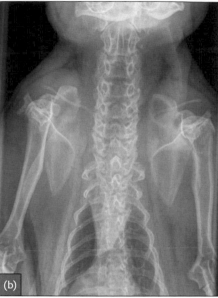

8.35 (a) Lateral and (b) VD cervical radiographs of a juvenile cat with mucopolysaccharidosis. The vertebral bodies and arches are thick, the vertebral endplates are irregular, the intervertebral disc spaces are narrow and the articular process joints are poorly defined due to bridging bone.

- Skin damage does not accurately reflect damage to underlying soft tissues, particularly with bite wounds.
- Patients with a thoracic lesion may have normal respiratory rate and effort.
- Small-breed dogs are at great risk of receiving substantial penetrating injuries from animal fights and bite wounds.
- Rib fractures are common radiographic lesions associated with trauma and are most often due to vehicular trauma or bite wounds (Figure 8.36).
  - Displaced fracture fragments can penetrate the thoracic wall, damaging the lungs or introducing gas or haemorrhage into the ipsilateral pleural cavity (or both pleural cavities).
  - Presence of rib fractures generally does not affect prognosis unless there is laceration of thoracic viscera.
  - Fractures from vehicular trauma are commonly located dorsally.
  - Fractures from bite wounds are variable in location but usually affect the middle portion of the thorax.
  - Segmental fractures are two complete fractures in the same rib that are separate from each other and can lead to body wall instability ('flail chest', see below).
- Vertebral fractures and dislocations are secondary to major trauma and frequently occur at junctions between vertebral segments (e.g. cervicothoracic, thoracolumbar).

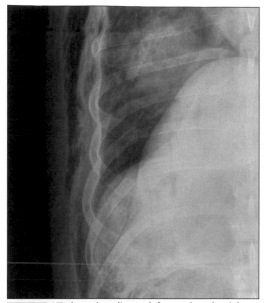

8.36 VD thoracic radiograph focused on the right costal region in a dog with recent vehicular trauma. The dog has multiple acute traumatic rib fractures, body wall gas and lung contusion. The rib fractures are subtle, arranged in a line, and characterized by discontinuous margins and abnormal angulation.

- Dogs with vertebral fractures secondary to vehicular trauma may have reduced survival.
- Vertebral fractures are relatively common in dogs with vehicular trauma and it is important to differentiate stable vertebral fractures (e.g. transverse process fracture) from fractures that cause vertebral column instability, which carry an increased risk of spinal cord injury.
- Substantial spinal cord trauma can occur without substantial vertebral trauma (e.g. concussion and contusion due to hyperflexion/hyperextension injury). Spinal cord trauma can also be exacerbated by positioning for radiography.
- Vertebral fractures can also occur in conjunction with annular rupture and intervertebral disc herniation.
- Subtle differences in technique and obliquity can affect lesion detection (Figure 8.37).
- Sternal fractures/dislocations are rare (Figure 8.38).
- 'Flail chest' (uncommon): two or more fractures in adjacent ribs can lead to instability of the thoracic wall and paradoxical movement of a segment (fragments are displaced inwards during inhalation and outwards during exhalation).
  - Abnormal body wall movement theoretically causes abnormal airflow leading to physiological 'dead space'; in combination with pain, associated lung contusion and incomplete lung expansion, this condition leads to hypoxaemia and respiratory distress.
  - It is most commonly secondary to bite wounds and is more common in male dogs.
  - 'Flail sternum' is a specific form of flail chest, causing paradoxical respiratory movement of the sternum (inwards during inhalation and outwards during exhalation) due to multiple fractures.
  - 'Pseudo-flail chest' can occur with a single rib fracture when there is substantial intercostal muscle damage.
- Radiographic signs of acute traumatic thoracic skeletal fractures may be obvious or subtle.

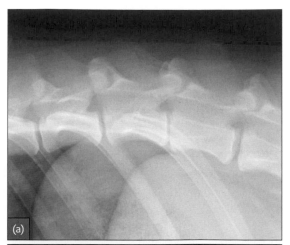

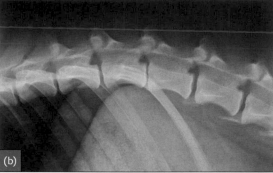

8.37 Lateral thoracolumbar radiographs of a dog with acute trauma. (a) Slight radiographic underexposure allows for detection of the fracture line in the T13 spinous process. (b) Slight obliquity and increased exposure better demonstrates the reduced size of the T13–L1 intervertebral foramen and collapse of the T13–L1 intervertebral disc space, suggestive of annular rupture and possible intervertebral disc herniation.

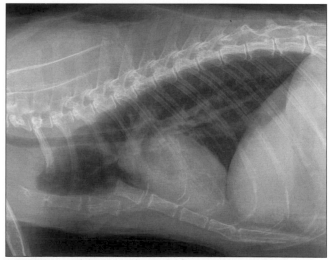

8.38 Lateral thoracic radiograph of a cat with a presumed (unwitnessed) traumatic sternal dislocation.

- Rib, vertebral or sternal displacement/malalignment.
- Increased width of synovial joints (joint dislocation).
- Increased or decreased width of intercostal spaces, intervertebral disc spaces or intersternal spaces.
- Discontinuity of cortical margins of the ribs, vertebrae or sternebrae:
  - Linear lucency traversing the rib
  - A focal increase in opacity if the fracture fragments are overriding.

- Vertebral physeal abnormalities in young animals: non-uniformity of physeal width (narrow or wide), cortical malalignment of epiphyses (Figure 8.39).
- Short vertebral body (compression fracture, Figure 8.39).
- Concurrent traumatic lesions:
  - Pulmonary contusions (most common)
  - Pleural fluid
  - Pneumothorax
  - Body wall swelling, loss of definition of body wall fascial planes (Figure 8.40)
  - Body wall gas (most commonly secondary to bite wounds)
  - Body wall debris/foreign material, metal ammunition
  - Visceral herniation (e.g. lung) through body wall; indicates complete rupture of the musculature (Figure 8.41).
- Multiple, oblique and/or collimated views in patients with known thoracic trauma may help to detect:
  - Non-displaced or minimally displaced fractures
  - Fractures at the costochondral junction or the dorsal aspects of the ribs
  - Costosternal dislocations.
- Wound extension into the pleural cavity is possible even when there is no specific radiographic abnormality (e.g. fluid, pneumothorax).
- Radiographs may underestimate the severity of body wall and visceral abnormalities.

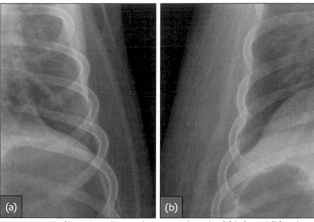

8.40 VD thoracic radiographs centred on the (a) left and (b) right costal regions in a dog with unilateral trauma. There is body wall asymmetry, with (a) the left body wall having normal thickness and well defined musculature. (b) The right body wall is swollen with wispy soft tissue within the fat and poorly defined musculature.

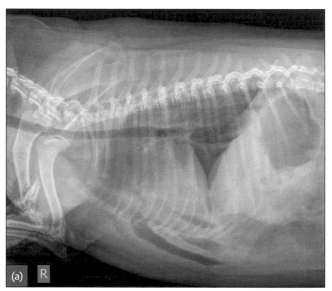

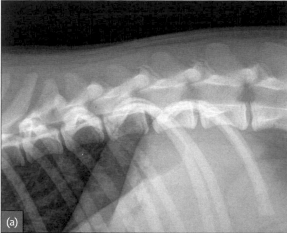

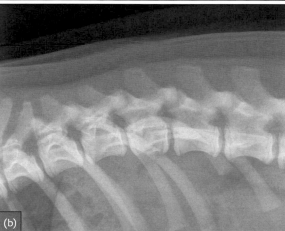

8.39 Lateral thoracolumbar radiographs of (a) a normal juvenile dog and (b) a juvenile dog with a T13 compression fracture following vehicular trauma. (b) The T13 vertebral body is short due to overriding fracture margins, and the ventral cortical margin is irregular and discontinuous.

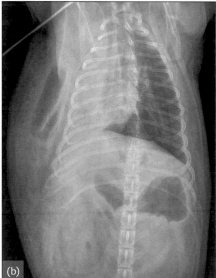

8.41 (a) Lateral and (b) VD trunk radiographs of a dog with traumatic herniation of intestine into the right thoracic body wall, which is severely swollen. Within the thoracic cavity, the right hemithorax has diffuse soft tissue opacity that was not present on referral radiographs from the same day and, thus, was attributed to progression of traumatic lesions, though not further localized to the pleural cavity or lung. Note the left humeral fracture on the lateral view.

- Treatment:
  - Single and non-displaced rib fractures are commonly treated conservatively (analgesia and rest)
  - In patients with bite wounds, thoracotomy is warranted when three or more of the following radiographic lesions are detected: lung contusion, rib fracture, pneumothorax, pleural fluid
  - Penetrating wounds, particularly bite wounds, generally have a good outcome when surgically explored
  - Multiple, internally displaced rib fractures may need surgical reduction and stabilization
    - Stabilization in cases of flail chest is controversial and patients can be successfully managed conservatively
  - Presence of respiratory distress does not correlate with mortality.
- Fracture healing depends on degree of displacement among other factors (e.g. patient age) and is impaired by normal respiratory motion.
  - With normal bone metabolism and mild displacement, fractures will heal with callus that is smooth and diminishes over time with remodelling.
  - With metabolic disturbances (e.g. endocrinopathy) or substantial displacement, non-union or malunion may occur with variable amount of callus.
- Differentiating trauma due to accidental blunt force (e.g. motor vehicle accidents (MVA)) and non-accidental injury (NAI) due to abuse can be challenging but several patterns have been recognized that can be helpful in the clinical setting:
  - Rib fractures are common due to both causes
  - Rib fractures due to MVA tend to be unilateral, multiple, sequential, most common cranially (ribs 1–4) and progressively less common caudally (least common in ribs 11–13)
  - Rib fractures due to NAI tend to be bilateral with no specific craniocaudal distribution
  - Rib fractures in various stages of healing suggest multiple traumatic events at different times (Figure 8.42)
  - NAI more commonly causes vertebral fractures than MVA. Outside the thorax, several additional lesions are indicative of NAI (e.g. damage to digits, scleral haemorrhage, teeth and skull fractures).
- Other imaging modalities:
  - CT and MRI are more accurate than radiography for subtle fractures and vertebral instability (Figure 8.43).

Atraumatic fractures

An atraumatic fracture, or rather, a minimally traumatic fracture, is a focal failure of bone caused by low-grade force. The affected bone may be normal or abnormal.

- Pathological fracture specifically refers to a fracture through a focal neoplasm (benign or malignant). Occasionally, the term is also applied to describe a fracture through osteomyelitis (see also insufficiency fracture).
  - Clinically, pathological fractures can present acutely but have radiographic signs of chronicity and/or aggressiveness. In the absence of major trauma, thorough evaluation of the radiographic abnormality for subtle osteolysis or periosteal reaction is important.

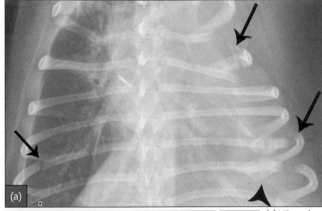
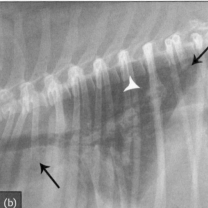

8.42 (a) VD and (b) lateral thoracic radiographs of a dog with multiple traumatic fractures at various stages of healing due to repeated episodes of abuse. The acute fractures have well defined angled margins (arrowed). The chronic (healing) fractures show bridging callus (arrowheads).

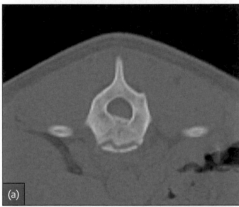
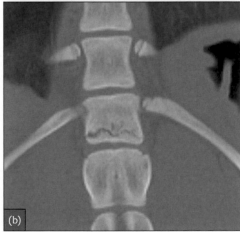

8.43 (a) Transverse and (b) dorsal back CT images (bone window) of a dog with a T13 vertebral body fracture. CT is more sensitive than radiography for subtle bone fractures that may determine whether the vertebral column is likely to be stable. CT can also provide information about neural injury, although MRI is more accurate.

- These fractures may be overlooked and obscured by more obvious changes associated with the underlying disease.
- Insufficiency fractures occur in abnormally weakened bone due to normal stresses. The bone may be weakened by several conditions including infection and metabolic bone diseases caused by conditions such as renal or nutritional secondary hyperparathyroidism. The abnormal bone may be softened or brittle depending on the underlying pathological mechanism.
- Fatigue (stress) fractures are due to repetitive low-grade stress but the underlying bone is normal. These fractures may appear different depending on whether they are in compact or spongy bone and are rare in the thoracic skeleton. Rib fractures may be observed when there is severe, often obstructive, respiratory disease causing excessive rib motion, particularly during exhalation. They are often serial, bilateral and have a caudodorsal preferential location at the edge of the serratus dorsalis caudalis muscle insertion, due to the shearing forces of this expiratory muscle. Underlying conditions include:
  - Feline lower airway disease, including feline asthma (Figure 8.44)
  - Chronic canine bronchial disease
  - Lobar emphysema.

Osteomyelitis (infection of the thoracic skeleton)

- Usually results from direct inoculation from penetrating trauma or migrating foreign bodies (e.g. grass awns).
  - Most commonly due to bite wounds; male, small-breed dogs are predisposed.
  - May be secondary to prior surgery (e.g. sternotomy, thoracotomy).
  - Haematogenous spread from a septic focus (e.g. urinary tract infection, pyometra) is possible and most common in discospondylitis.
- The vertebrae are the most common site of thoracic skeleton infection (i.e. vertebral osteomyelitis). The diagnosis can be made more specific when a precise component of the skeletal system is abnormal (e.g. vertebral physitis). In dogs, infection of the vertebrae is usually because of discospondylitis (Figure 8.45). Sternal osteomyelitis is least common (Figure 8.46).
- In dogs with systemic aspergillosis, thoracic lesions are mostly attributed to discospondylitis with fewer lesions observed in the ribs and sternum, or isolated to the vertebrae only.
- Radiographic signs of osteomyelitis:
  - Signs of aggressiveness, including:
    - Spongy (trabecular) bone lysis (geographical, moth-eaten or permeative)

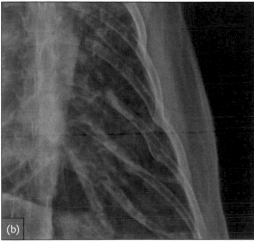

8.44 (a) Lateral and (b) VD thoracic radiographs centred on the left costal region in a cat with chronic cough secondary to severe lower airway disease. Note the chronic remodelling rib fractures.

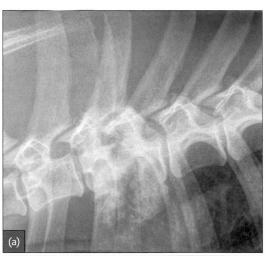

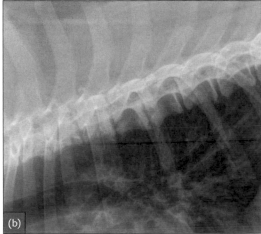

8.45 Lateral radiographs of the thoracic vertebral column in two dogs with discospondylitis. The imaging signs can range from (a) obvious to (b) subtle and are characterized by lysis of adjacent vertebral endplates, an active periosteal response and variable intervertebral disc space width.

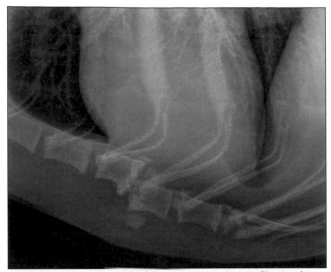

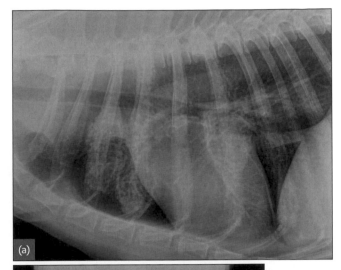

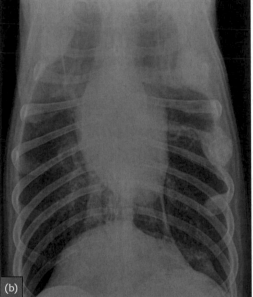

8.46 Lateral radiograph of the sternum in a German Shepherd Dog with locally extensive polyostotic sternal osteomyelitis and sternal dislocation, characterized by lysis and an active periosteal response. This patient also had discospondylitis secondary to aspergillosis (not shown).

- – Compact (cortical) bone destruction: thin and/or non-uniform cortical thickness
- – Poorly defined (i.e. active) periosteal proliferation, usually with a smooth or palisading pattern
- – Poor corticomedullary distinction
- Osteomyelitis of multiple, sequential ribs, sternebrae or vertebral bodies usually indicates spread of infection through bone and soft tissue
- Soft tissue swelling, gas and/or foreign material
- Discharge from a sinus tract (tunnelling wound under the skin) or fistula (a pipe-like connection between two hollow epithelialized spaces) may be present
- Randomly distributed aggressive bone lesions indicate haematogenous spread, most commonly due to fungal infection (Figure 8.47)
- Pleural fluid; less commonly mediastinal fluid (e.g. secondary to sternal infection)
- Focal soft tissue mass: abscess, granuloma
- Possible insufficiency/pathological fracture
- Radiographic signs overlap with neoplasia (see 'Neoplasia', below) and definitive differentiation may be radiographically impossible. However, patients with osteomyelitis tend to be younger and more commonly present with pain, fever and/or lethargy
- Possible underlying causes should be investigated (e.g. foreign body, sequestrum, surgical implant abnormality).
- Ultrasonography can be used to assess the bone surface and soft tissue components of a swelling including locating and removing foreign bodies, sampling tissues for cytology and culture, and aiding in therapeutic drainage of abscesses.
- Discospondylitis:
  - The most common and important infection of the thoracic skeleton is discospondylitis
    - More common than vertebral osteomyelitis (spondylitis) or vertebral physitis. The former involves only the vertebra (not the disc) and the latter is centred on the vertebral physis
  - Caused by haematogenous infection of the intervertebral discs and adjacent vertebral bodies

8.47 (a) Lateral and (b) VD thoracic radiographs of a dog with asymmetrical polyostotic aggressive bone abnormalities secondary to systemic coccidioidomycosis fungal infection. The bone abnormalities are consistent with osteomyelitis and are primarily proliferative. Thoracic lymphadenopathy is not detected. On the VD view, the two large cranial abnormalities are associated with an extrapleural sign.

- Most commonly secondary to bacterial infection of the urogenital tract with *Staphylococcus*, *Streptococcus* or *Escherichia coli*
- Brucellosis infection (zoonotic) in intact patients
- Fungal infection is also possible, most commonly aspergillosis
- Most common in middle-aged to older large-breed dogs, particularly German Shepherd Dogs, but also reported in juveniles (<6 months of age)
- Discospondylitis rarely occurs secondary to decompression surgery for intervertebral disc herniation
  - German Shepherd Dogs and dogs >20 kg have increased risk
- Radiographic signs of discospondylitis lack sensitivity, particularly with early infection, and cross-sectional imaging (especially MRI) may be required for diagnosis
- Fluoroscopy can aid in sampling of intervertebral discs

- In addition to the above radiographic signs, signs specifically associated with discospondylitis include:
  - Lysis of adjacent vertebral endplates
  - Sclerosis of vertebral bodies adjacent to the lysis
  - Increased width (secondary to lysis) or collapse of intervertebral disc spaces
  - Single or multiple disc spaces affected
  - The lumbosacral junction is most commonly affected
- Radiographic lesions may persist after clearance of active infection. Serial radiographs are valuable to assess response to treatment. Resolved discospondylitis will be seen as increased bone opacity with smooth and well defined vertebral margins; vertebral bodies may fuse
  - Progression of bone lysis may be observed initially after treatment, even when clinical signs improve.
- Treatment:
  - For traumatic wounds, depth of wound extension secondary to bite trauma is not associated with mortality rate when surgically explored; therefore, surgical wound exploration and debridement is warranted in all cases
  - For discospondylitis, long-term antibiotic or antifungal therapy is usually required. Therapy is continued until there are no longer radiographic signs of bone activity on radiographs, with an average duration of treatment around 1 year for bacterial infection. Aspergillosis has a poor prognosis; relapse is common and many dogs require lifelong antifungal treatment.

Neoplasia

- Primary bone, multicentric and metastatic neoplasms can affect any of the bones of the thoracic skeleton, most commonly the ribs. Tangential and oblique radiographs may help detect subtle lysis or periosteal proliferation (Dennis, 1993).
- Masses arising from the thoracic skeleton might produce an extrapleural sign or displace the adjacent visceral pleural margin away from the body wall (see Chapter 11).
- Primary malignant bone neoplasms are relatively rare in the axial skeleton despite being relatively common in the appendicular skeleton, particularly in dogs. Osteosarcoma and chondrosarcoma are most common; fibrosarcoma, haemangiosarcoma and other primary benign bone neoplasms (osteoma, chondroma) are rare (Pirkey-Ehrhart et al., 1995). Prognosis is very good after surgical resection of chondrosarcoma but is guarded for other types of malignancies, particularly osteosarcoma (Hammer et al., 1995).
  - Primary rib neoplasms are often located near the costochondral junction
  - Primary rib and sternal neoplasms are often clinically silent unless they impede the movement of the thoracic limbs or grow externally and become visible or palpable; rib tumours are often diagnosed late in the disease process due to minimal clinical signs.
  - Respiratory signs may be present if there is substantial intrathoracic extension.
- Primary vertebral neoplasms can cause neurological deficits secondary to extradural spinal cord compression.

- Radiographic signs:
  - A solitary mass-like tumour is typically present; cross-sectional imaging may be needed to see the actual tumour
  - Typically, there is monostotic lysis; can become locally extensive polyostotic with large masses (particularly rib neoplasms, Figure 8.48)
  - Aggressive vertebral lesions are often predominantly lytic and can be difficult to detect, particularly early (Figure 8.49)

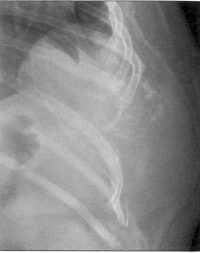

8.48 VD thoracic radiograph centred on the left costal region of a dog with a solitary primary bone neoplasm that arises from a rib and involves adjacent ribs (locally extensive polyostotic). The neoplasm forms a large mass-like tumour that is centred on the rib, extends medially into the thoracic cavity, extends laterally to form a bulge on the skin surface, and extends cranially and caudally displacing the adjacent ribs. The main rib affected has extensive osteolysis and an amorphous periosteal response. The adjacent displaced ribs are sclerotic or have a periosteal reaction.

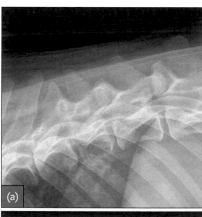
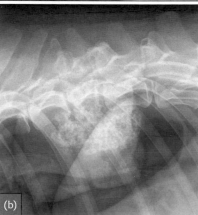

8.49 Lateral radiographs of the thoracic vertebral column in a dog with a solitary primary bone neoplasm that arises from a vertebra. (a) Initially, the abnormality is subtle, mostly affecting the vertebral body and characterized by lysis and poorly defined cortical margins. (b) After 1 year of radiation therapy, the mass is progressive with extensive periosteal proliferation and progressive lysis extending into the vertebral arch, and the vertebral body is short due to a pathological compression fracture. CT confirmed that the neoplasm has spread ventrally into the adjacent lung, causing pneumothorax. Note the contrast with the ventral soft tissue portion of the tumour.

- Periosteal proliferation is often more poorly defined compared with osteomyelitis (e.g. amorphous, 'sunburst')
- Expansile lesions with thinning of the cortices (Figure 8.50)
- Focal or locally extensive 'mass effect': displacement of adjacent ribs, wide adjacent rib spaces bulging of the body wall
- A large intrathoracic component of the mass may be visible, which can displace intrathoracic structures
- Pleural fluid
- Pulmonary metastasis may be present
- Oblique and/or collimated radiographs may be better at identifying lysis and/or periosteal proliferation (Figure 8.51).
- Primary sternal neoplasms are rare.
- Pathological fracture of the vertebral body can occur secondary to neoplasia and often leads to reduced size of the vertebral body and can be difficult to detect (Figure 8.52).
- Metastatic neoplasms:
  - Urogenital and mammary carcinoma are most common but other tumour metastasis is possible (e.g. osteosarcoma)
  - Often asymmetrical polyostotic
  - Ribs are the most common site for metastasis of the thoracic skeleton

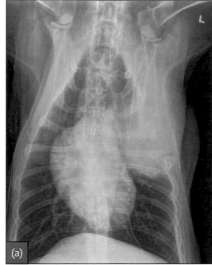

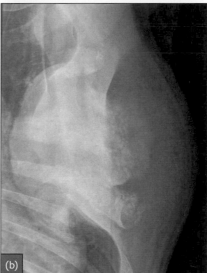

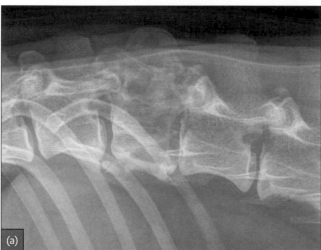

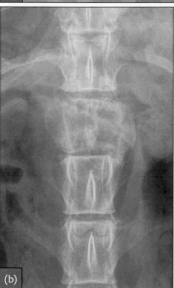

8.50 (a) Lateral and (b) VD radiographs of the thoracolumbar vertebral column in a dog with a solitary primary bone neoplasm that arises from a vertebra. The neoplasm forms an expansile bone lesion that affects both the vertebral body and arch. Notice the outward displacement and thinning of the cortices with moth-eaten lysis. The vertebral body is also short. (b) Loss of the pedicles can be observed on the VD view.

8.51 (a) VD and (b) oblique collimated VD thoracic radiographs in a dog with a palpable body wall mass. (a) The full extent of the rib involvement is not appreciated on the VD view. (b) The oblique view reveals that the neoplasm forms a mass-like tumour that extends medially producing an extrapleural sign, causes the skin to bulge laterally, and displaces the adjacent ribs cranially and caudally. In addition, the tumour is characterized as a locally extensive polyostotic aggressive bone lesion. Note the severe lysis and extensive palisading periosteal response that were not apparent on the initial radiograph.

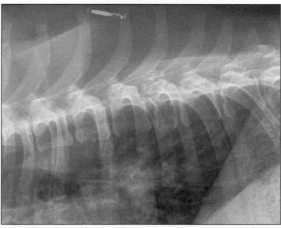

8.52 A lateral back radiograph in a dog with a pathological compression fracture secondary to a lytic, non-proliferative aggressive bone tumour. The vertebral body is short, which could be confused with a vertebral malformation if the subtle signs of an aggressive bone tumour and fracture were not observed.

- Usually small and located in the dorsal or middle portion of the rib
- Can be small, subtle (Figure 8.53) and/or mimic a healing rib fracture with a smooth, continuous periosteal reaction but without a fracture line.
- Multicentric or round cell neoplasms:
  - Multiple myeloma (Figure 8.54):
    - Typically polyostotic and asymmetrical due to multiple punctate to moth-eaten lytic lesions without periosteal proliferation in both ribs and vertebral bodies (often described as 'punched out' or 'cookie cutter' lesions)
    - Lysis may be easier to detect in the lumbar vertebrae due to reduced summation of structures
    - Pathological fracture may be present
    - Can also be seen in the sternum, scapulae and proximal humeri
    - Radiographs can be normal; MRI findings have been described but are beyond the scope of this text
    - Plasma cell tumours may be solitary monostotic
  - Lymphoma:
    - Lymphoma is one of the most common neoplasms in small animals but less commonly affects the musculoskeletal structures

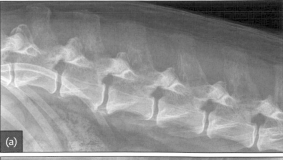

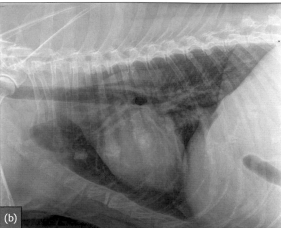

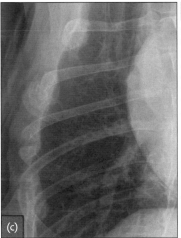

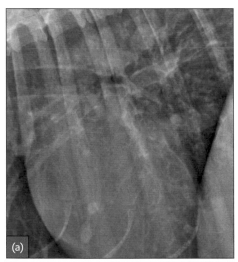

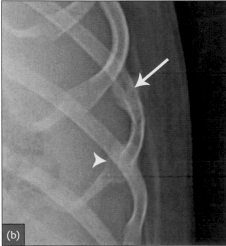

8.53 Orthogonal close-up thoracic radiographs of a dog with (a) pulmonary metastasis characterized by multiple generalized random soft tissue nodules and (b) rib metastasis characterized by a subtle solitary aggressive bone lesion (arrowed). It is important not to mistake the normal costochondral junction (arrowhead) for an expansile bone abnormality.

8.54 Lateral (a) back and (b) thoracic radiographs in a dog with multiple myeloma. (a) There are numerous moth-eaten lytic defects in the lumbar vertebrae. (b) The findings are more subtle but include moth-eaten lysis of T9, thin cortices in the ribs with heterogeneous trabecular bone and multiple pathological rib fractures with variable signs of healing. (c) The orthogonal view allows further characterization of the rib fractures.

- Recent MRI reports describe primarily osseous signal changes and soft tissue paravertebral lesions without vertebral cortical destruction; radiographs are likely poorly sensitive for vertebral lymphoma (Allett and Hecht, 2016)
- Most common vertebral tumour in cats
- May be monostotic or polyostotic
- Extensive bone marrow involvement possible, may require MRI to detect
- Variable radiographic appearance including normal; mixed lytic and proliferative lesions are possible. Minimal periosteal proliferation in vertebrae
- Metaphyseal distribution with pathological fractures may be seen in juveniles
- Histiocytic sarcoma:
  - Aggressive, mixed lytic and proliferative lesions of the joints, proximal humeri and vertebral column
  - Golden Retrievers and Rottweilers are predisposed to skeletal lesions associated with histiocytic sarcoma.

- Body wall neoplasms:
  - Lipoma is an extremely common neoplasm of the body wall and appendicular skeleton. Lipomas are most commonly mobile, slow growing and have little clinical consequence. However, they can grow large and impede movement when closely associated with the thoracic limbs. Radiographic signs include:
    - Homogeneously fat-opaque mass
    - Outward displacement of adjacent musculature, which remains well defined
    - Bulging (convex) skin margin
    - Possible displacement of adjacent ribs, which remain smooth and well defined
  - Neoplasms of the thoracic wall can cause aggressive bone lesions due to local extension to adjacent osseous structures, commonly with a sequential polyostotic distribution (Figure 8.55)
  - Soft tissue sarcomas arising from the body wall are common, particularly 'feline injection site sarcomas' (usually fibrosarcoma) although changes in vaccine practices to inoculate more distant sites are leading to reduced occurrence in the body wall. Infiltrative lipomas and liposarcomas are rare and aggressive; these neoplasms can extend between muscular layers of the thoracic wall and into the thoracic cavity. Peripheral nerve sheath tumours can extend from the cervical or thoracic vertebral bodies into the mediastinum and/or axillary region. Haemangiosarcomas can occur in the body wall or paravertebral musculature and are commonly poorly defined due to haemorrhage. Other masses rarely arise from paravertebral musculature but occasionally rhabdomyosarcoma can create a craniodorsal mediastinal mass (Figure 8.56)
  - Radiographic signs:
    - Soft tissue mass-like tumour that silhouettes the margins of body wall or paravertebral musculature
    - Mass may be variable in opacity, usually primarily soft tissue with smaller amounts of fat, particularly with infiltrative lipoma
    - May cause convexity to the skin margin and extend into the thoracic cavity
    - Lysis and periosteal reaction of multiple adjacent ribs
    - Any part of the rib can be affected
  - Pleural neoplasms (most commonly mesothelioma) can produce an aggressive periosteal reaction across multiple ribs and be difficult to differentiate from other neoplasms. Cross-sectional imaging (e.g. CT, ultrasonography) may be needed to see pleural nodules along the internal margin of the body wall.
- Osteochondroma is a benign, cartilage-capped exostosis usually arising at the metaphysis of bones undergoing endochondral ossification. Multiple cartilaginous exostosis (MCE) is a form of skeletal dysplasia characterized by multiple osteochondromas in long bones, vertebrae and ribs. MCE causes proliferative non-malignant masses that have overlapping radiographic features with benign and malignant bone neoplasms (see Chapter 7). The cause is incompletely understood but is most likely due to growth disturbance leading to abnormal chondrocyte migration and heterotopic ossification. A recent report described a genetic mutation in a litter of American Staffordshire terriers, suggesting a hereditary component (Friedenberg *et al.*, 2018). Lesions are

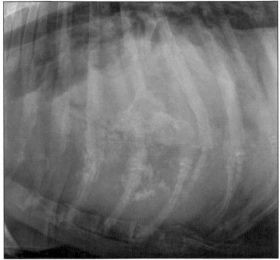

8.55 Lateral thoracic radiograph of a dog with locally extensive polyostotic aggressive bone lesions involving multiple sequential ribs, due to a large malignant body wall neoplasm that extends into the thoracic cavity, displacing and compressing the cardiopulmonary structures.

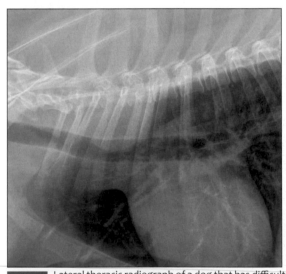

8.56 Lateral thoracic radiograph of a dog that has difficulty swallowing due to a longus colli rhabdomyosarcoma. In the dorsal part of the cranial mediastinum, immediately ventral to the vertebral column, the neoplasm forms a round soft tissue mass-like tumour that summates with the dorsal aspect of the trachea. Bone involvement is not detected. See also Figure 8.58.

commonly identified in young, growing dogs, and masses cease growing at skeletal maturity. MCE in cats has also been reported. Malignant transformation to osteosarcoma or chondrosarcoma is possible.
- Clinical signs are related to lesion location: neurological deficits can occur secondary to vertebral lesions causing extradural spinal cord compression, large tumours can impede cardiopulmonary efforts.
- Radiographic findings include:
  - Highly proliferative, usually expansile lesions arising from osteochondral junctions (i.e. physes, metaphyses and costochondral junctions)
  - Lesions are solitary monostotic with osteochondroma and polyostotic asymmetrical with MCE
  - Margin definition indicates activity; poorly defined margins are active.

- Alternative imaging modalities:
  - Radiographs commonly underestimate tumour extent
  - Ultrasonography:
    - Useful for differentiating individual soft tissue lesions that silhouette radiographically
    - Particularly useful in identifying thoracic wall and pleural masses in cases of substantial body wall swelling and/or pleural fluid
    - Provides information about the character of soft tissue masses, particularly fluid cavities in abscesses, and may help in identifying foreign material
    - Aids in sampling masses of the body wall and pleural cavity (Figure 8.57)
  - CT can be very helpful for:
    - Global assessment
    - Assessing tumour extent for surgical resection and radiation treatment planning (Figure 8.58)
    - Assessment of involvement of other thoracic organs
    - Detection of lung metastases too small to see radiographically

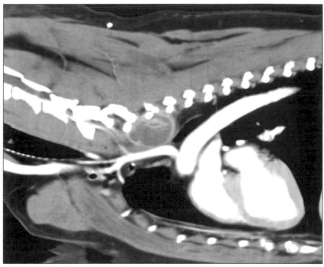

8.58 Sagittal cervicothoracic CT image of the same dog as in Figure 8.56. The longus colli mass, which is less discernible on the initial radiograph, is confirmed by contrast-enhanced CT obtained for radiation therapy planning.

- MRI is the best modality to assess spinal cord and/or nerve root compression by mass lesions. Some tumours only cause signal changes in bone due to alterations in fat and/or fluid content and cannot be identified by any other modality
- Bone scintigraphy may be used for detection of subtle active lesions or assessment of the number and location of skeletal metastases
- Contrast studies: fistulography and sinography may be used to explore the extension of sinuses and connections of fistulous tracts.

Metabolic bone disease
Calcium and phosphorus imbalance

Calcium and phosphorous imbalance can be caused by primary hyperparathyroidism, secondary hyperparathyroidism or vitamin D deficiency. Primary hyperparathyroidism is most often caused by a parathyroid adenoma and is common in middle-aged to older dogs and cats, with Keeshonds over-represented. Secondary hyperparathyroidism may be due to chronic renal insufficiency (most commonly in older animals) or due to nutritional imbalances, primarily with diets high in phosphorous and/or low in calcium (most commonly in juvenile patients fed all-meat diets). In growing animals, the physes are most severely affected because calcium is necessary for endochondral ossification. Other endocrinopathies, such as hyperthyroidism, can alter calcium homeostasis and dogs with hyperadrenocorticism can have secondary hyperparathyroidism, a proposed mechanism leading to calcinosis cutis. Radiographic findings include (Figure 8.59):

- Generalized osteopenia with thin cortices and coarse trabecular bone
- In growing animals, wide physes, lucencies in metaphyses
- Bone deformity, angular limb deformity and/or folding fractures (often dorsally located in ribs)
- Stippled mineral opacity along skin margin/within subcutaneous fat layer (calcinosis cutis).

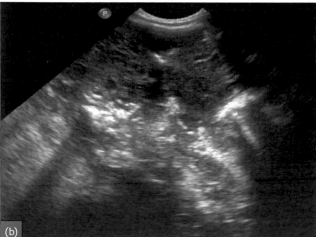

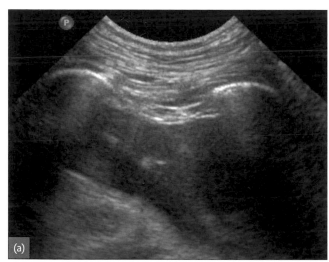

8.57 Thoracic ultrasound images of a dog with an extensive body wall neoplasm that has pleural extension. The transducer was placed on the costal region. (a) Normal ribs are observed. (b) The neoplasm forms a mass-like tumour in the body wall and causes severe rib lysis and periosteal proliferation. Normal ribs have smooth, concave, hyperechoic margins whereas the mass is characterized by disorganized mineral and soft tissue.

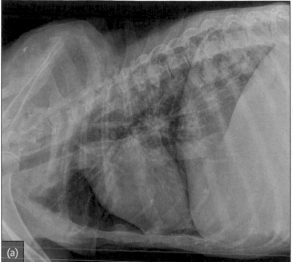

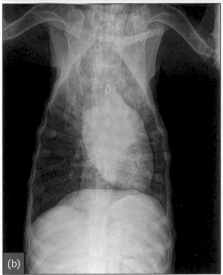

8.59 (a) Lateral and (b) VD thoracic radiographs of a dog with multiple endocrinopathies leading to diffuse osteopenia, pathological fractures and severe narrowing of the intervertebral disc spaces.

swelling of multiple limbs. The distal limb long bones, particularly metacarpal and metatarsal bones, are most commonly and severely affected; the ribs, scapulae and pelvic bones are less commonly affected. HO is reversible with removal/treatment of the inciting cause. The pathogenesis is incompletely understood but most likely related to increased peripheral blood flow leading to bone spicule formation; proposed causes include vasodilation due to circulating toxins, parasympathetic stimulation and growth factors (e.g. vascular endothelial growth factor (VEGF) or platelet-derived growth factor (PDGF)) promoting peripheral vascularization. Radiographic findings include:

- Subtle continuous periosteal reaction on multiple ribs and vertebrae
- Periosteal reaction along humeri and scapulae (Figure 8.60)
- Thoracic mass, usually pulmonary
- Occasionally, pleural disease.

Hypertrophic osteodystrophy ('metaphyseal osteopathy')

Hypertrophic osteodystrophy (HOD) most commonly affects the metaphyseal regions of long bones in the appendicular skeleton in young, growing, large- and giant-breed dogs, most commonly Great Danes. Clinical signs are often mild and self-limiting but can be severe, associated with multisystemic illness, and lead to crippling deformities. HOD causes necrosis with suppurative inflammation of the physes, and periosteal proliferation, fibrosis and/or subperiosteal haemorrhage may be seen histologically. Heritability has been demonstrated in several breeds, with strong inheritance documented in multiple litters of Weimaraners. Radiographic lesions are most seen in the metaphyses of long bones in the distal limbs. Common signs include wide metaphyses due to periosteal new bone formation and lucent bands in metaphyses

Juvenile osteomalacia ('rickets')

Diffuse softening and weakening of bone due to vitamin D deficiency is rare in animals (usually a nutritional deficiency, but abnormal vitamin D metabolism is possible). The condition occurs mostly in immature animals and may lead to growth reduction and skeletal deformities. During radiography, the classic signs are diffuse osteopenia with wide physes and flaring of the metaphyses. The latter may produce bony prominences and when this occurs at the costochondral junctions, the collection of bony prominences can be seen during thoracic radiography and resembles the beads of a Catholic rosary ('rachitic rosary').

Hypertrophic osteopathy

Hypertrophic osteopathy (HO) is an acquired condition caused by a variety of thoracic and abdominal abnormalities but is commonly a paraneoplastic syndrome secondary to primary or metastatic pulmonary neoplasia. HO has been reported in cases of abdominal neoplasia, infectious disease (e.g. heartworm, *Spirocerca lupi*), and congenital abnormalities like right-to-left shunting patent ductus arteriosus. HO is characterized by bilaterally symmetrical diffuse diaphyseal periosteal proliferation without osteolysis. The signs are typically seen in the appendicular skeleton and occasionally the axial skeleton (especially during CT). Patients typically present with pain, lameness and/or

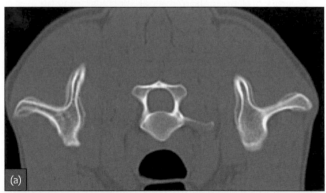

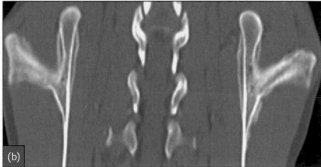

8.60 (a) Transverse and (b) dorsal CT images of the scapular regions of a dog with hypertrophic osteopathy secondary to a thoracic mass (not shown). Both scapulae have bilaterally symmetrical, smooth, continuous periosteal proliferation.

(often parallel to the physis). The radius, ulna and tibia are commonly affected, but similar lesions can occasionally be seen on thoracic radiographs in the proximal humeri and ribs. Progressive circumferential periosteal proliferation typically occurs in chronic cases.

Degenerative lesions

Intervertebral disc degeneration

Intervertebral disc degeneration is common in dogs and occurs with or without disc herniation; intervertebral disc degeneration and trauma are the two most common factors leading to disc herniation. In dogs, disc herniation that occurs in association with disc degeneration has two common clinical presentations and consequently potentially different treatment plans. Hansen Type I disc herniation tends to occur in chondrodystrophic dogs of any age and is typically associated with an acute disc herniation through a complete annular fissure. Hansen Type II disc herniation tends to occur in older non-chondrodystrophic dogs as a chronic disc herniation with gradual displacement into the vertebral canal. Classically, the difference between groups was attributed to the type of disc degeneration (chondroid *versus* fibrinoid) but, due to similar histopathological abnormalities in both groups, the disc degeneration is often simply referred to as chondroid metaplasia. Radiographic findings of disc degeneration may include:

- No radiographic abnormality: MRI is more sensitive for detecting early disc degeneration
- Narrowing of the intervertebral disc spaces, intervertebral foramina and/or synovial joints. This may be more severe when there is actual herniation rather than just tissue loss and desiccation
- Sclerosis and/or erosions of adjacent vertebral endplates
- Spondylosis deformans (see below)
- Mineral within the intervertebral disc space. When there is disc herniation, the calcified disc may be observed extending dorsally to summate with the vertebral canal or intervertebral foramina (Figure 8.61)
- Cross-sectional imaging or myelography is required for surgical planning when herniation is present (Figure 8.62)
- Non-mineralized intervertebral disc displacements may be seen on CT and MRI scans (Figure 8.63).

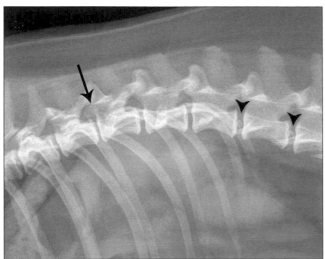

8.61 Lateral back radiograph of a Dachshund with a calcified T11–T12 intervertebral disc that has herniated dorsally and summates with the intervertebral foramen (arrowed), and several non-displaced calcified discs (arrowheads).

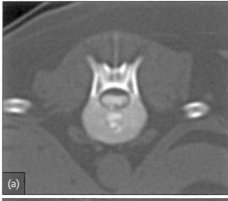

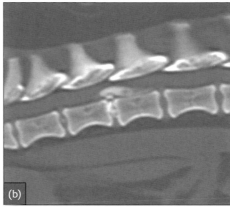

8.62 (a) Transverse and (b) sagittal back CT images of a dog with intervertebral disc herniation. CT allows for image reconstruction in multiple planes, is more accurate than radiography at identifying disc herniation and more precise for describing the location of displaced disc material, which is necessary for surgical planning. CT is especially helpful when the displaced disc is calcified. MRI is also excellent for evaluating intervertebral disc disease.

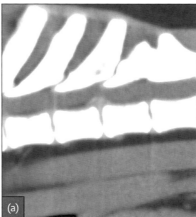

8.63 Sagittal back CT images of a dog with intervertebral disc herniation. Images obtained using (a) a soft tissue and (b) a bone window. CT can provide information about non-mineralized intervertebral disc herniation. There is a difference in conspicuity of the displaced disc material in the two images.

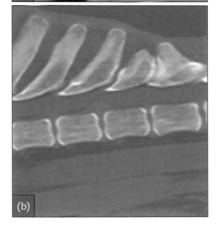

Spondylosis deformans

Spondylosis deformans is a very common enthesopathy of the ventral part of the vertebra (i.e. the vertebral body) and occurs where the annulus fibrosus attaches to the vertebral body. Spondylosis deformans is nearly always clinically silent, but new bone formation that encroaches on an intervertebral foramen may produce spinal nerve compression due to foraminal stenosis. Spondylosis is more common in middle-aged to older large-breed dogs, with German Shepherd Dogs and Boxers predisposed. Radiographic signs include:

- Well defined, smooth, osseous proliferation extending from the vertebral endplates and bridging the intervertebral disc spaces. The bridging may be partial or complete (Figure 8.64)
- Associated intervertebral disc spaces may be normal in width and opacity
- Signs of intervertebral disc degeneration may be present (see above, Figure 8.65)
- The most common sites are junctions of vertebral segments (e.g. cervicothoracic, thoracolumbar)
- One or more sites may be affected. Multiple affected sites may be contiguous or sporadic.

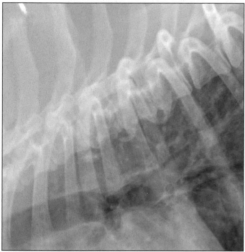

8.64 Lateral back radiograph of a dog with incidental/minor consequence spondylosis deformans, characterized as a smooth, well defined enthesopathy bridging intervertebral disc spaces. The enthesopathy occurs where the annulus fibrosus attaches to the apposing vertebral bodies.

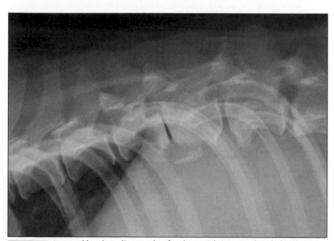

8.65 Lateral back radiograph of a dog with incompletely bridging spondylosis deformans and intradiscal vacuum phenomenon, indicative of intervertebral disc degeneration.

Vertebral osteoarthrosis

The articular process joints are synovial joints and therefore can develop degenerative joint disease (DJD) that affects the articular cartilage and subchondral bone. This form of DJD is common in dogs and may be clinically silent or associated with pain or neurological deficits. Myelography or MRI is necessary to demonstrate extradural spinal cord compression. Radiographic signs include:

- Periarticular osteophytes arising from the articular processes
- Subchondral sclerosis of articular processes
- Narrowing of articular process joint spaces.

Disseminated idiopathic skeletal hyperostosis

Disseminated idiopathic skeletal hyperostosis (DISH) is a rare systemic non-inflammatory disease characterized by extensive enthesopathy of the axial skeleton and, less commonly, appendicular skeleton. The term and description were originally borrowed from human medicine but are increasingly recognized in veterinary species, particularly large-breed dogs. DISH is most often asymptomatic and prevalence increases with age. The criteria for defining DISH are variable but it is generally characterized by continuous enthesopathy along the ventral longitudinal ligament of the vertebral column of 3–4 adjacent vertebral bodies in the absence of severe intervertebral disc degeneration, sacroiliac lesions or vertebral ankylosis. One study found vertebral osteoarthrosis to be common in dogs with DISH (Morgan and Stavenborn, 1991), suggesting dorsal vertebral abnormalities as part of the definition, but this is not universally accepted (De Decker and Volk, 2014; Wessman, 2014). DISH has also been described with intervertebral disc degeneration (particularly at adjacent, non-affected discs), spinal nerve compression and vertebral fractures. Adding to the confusion, spondylosis deformans occurs concurrently in approximately 70% of dogs with DISH, although some authors suggest some clinical importance in differentiating these processes. Radiographic signs include (Figure 8.66):

- Smooth, well defined, continuous bone bridging several vertebral bodies and sparing intervertebral endplates
- Lack of intervertebral disc degeneration at affected sites
- Signs of intervertebral disc degeneration at adjacent sites
- Lumbar vertebral column most affected (in contrast to spondylosis deformans).

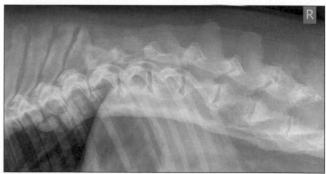

8.66 Lateral back radiograph of a dog with continuous flowing bone across more than four intervertebral disc spaces (consistent with a diagnosis of disseminated idiopathic skeletal hyperostosis) as well as signs of vertebral osteoarthrosis, worse at L2–L3 and L3–L4.

Alternative imaging modalities

Given the prevalence of degenerative vertebral lesions in asymptomatic dogs (particularly in older large-breed dogs), overlap in radiographic descriptions and prevalence of concomitant lesions, myelography or cross-sectional imaging are often necessary to determine clinical relevance. MRI is the best overall modality for assessing spinal cord and nerve roots for signs of compression, swelling and/or degeneration. Complete descriptions of cross-sectional findings are beyond the scope of this text (see the BSAVA Manual of Canine and Feline Neurology).

Diseases of the diaphragm

Altered radiographic appearance of the diaphragm may be due to technical or pathological factors that shift the location of the diaphragm (e.g. phase of respiratory cycle, lung collapse), or abnormalities in adjacent structures (e.g. lungs, peritoneal cavity) that partially or completely efface the cranial border of the diaphragm. Common conditions that alter the diaphragmatic appearance but do not involve the diaphragm include:

- Reduced lung volume shifts the diaphragm cranially, either regionally or diffusely
    - Atelectasis (common). Non-pathological conditions associated with sedation/general anaesthesia, recumbency and exhalation should be differentiated from pathological causes of lung collapse such as obstructive atelectasis due to foreign body, mucus plug or neoplasm
    - Lung lobectomy
- Pulmonary hyperinflation moves the diaphragm caudally
    - Obstructive air trapping (common, e.g. feline asthma)
        - Tenting, which is caused by attachment of the diaphragm to the ribs, may be observed, especially in asthmatic cats
    - Compensatory
- Conditions that produce border effacement:
    - Lung consolidation (e.g. non-cardiogenic or cardiogenic pulmonary oedema, haemorrhage, caudal or accessory lung lobe mass (Figure 8.67))
    - Pleural fluid (e.g. chylous fluid, haemorrhage, transudate (Figure 8.68))
    - Peritoneal fluid (especially ventrally, where the caudal border may normally be contrasted by falciform fat)
- Conditions that contrast with the caudal diaphragmatic margin:
    - Obesity
    - Pneumoperitoneum (Figure 8.69): postoperative, gastrointestinal rupture (e.g. mass, ulcer, foreign body), body wall penetrating wound, rupture of abscess or organ infected with gas-producing organisms (e.g. cholecystitis, pyometra)
    - Pneumoretroperitoneum: extension from pneumomediastinum
- Other conditions that may secondarily alter the appearance of the diaphragm:
    - Thoracic wall trauma (e.g. rib fractures, body wall swelling)
    - Vertebral malformations (e.g. scoliosis)
    - Body wall masses (e.g. rib neoplasm, abscess)
    - Cranial abdominal masses
    - Gastric dilatation (e.g. gastric dilatation with volvulus)
    - Pleural fibrosis, adhesions.

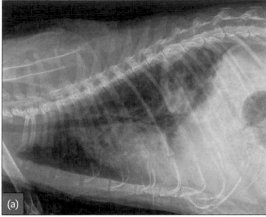
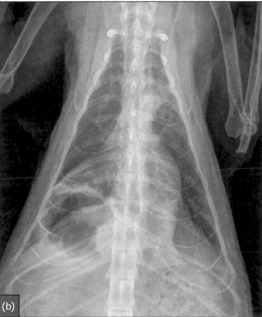

8.67 (a) Lateral and (b) VD thoracic radiographs of a cat with a solitary cavitated pulmonary mass. (a) The mass partially summates with the diaphragm, signifying its pulmonary origin. (b) The mass produces border effacement with the cranial margin of the diaphragm and could be mistaken for a diaphragmatic mass or abscess.

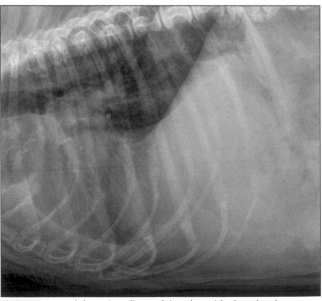

8.68 Lateral thoracic radiograph in a dog with pleural and peritoneal ('bicavitary') fluid, which causes border effacement of the ventral half of the diaphragm.

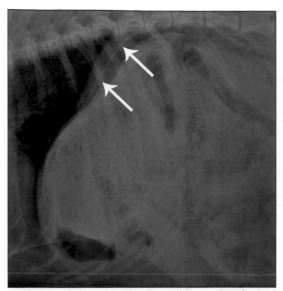

8.69 Right lateral trunk radiograph centred on the diaphragm of a dog with pneumoperitoneum caused by rupture of a large hepatic abscess. The caudal margin of the diaphragm is variably contrasted by a large amount of peritoneal gas. The left diaphragmatic crus is contrasted by gas between the diaphragm and stomach/emphysematous liver (arrowed). The border of the right diaphragmatic crus is effaced by the liver (i.e. normal). The cupula (ventral dome) of the diaphragm is partially contrasted by gas between the diaphragm and liver abscess.

Primary diseases of the diaphragm are rarer and commonly due to traumatic rupture or abnormal development with herniation of abdominal content. Less frequently, masses or functional diseases that alter diaphragmatic motion may be observed.

- Primary diaphragmatic abnormalities:
  - Diaphragmatic hernia (common)
    - Traumatic (diaphragmatic rupture)
    - Developmental (congenital or acquired)
  - Diaphragmatic eventration (rare)
  - Space-occupying lesions (rare): neoplasms, abscesses, granulomas
  - Muscular dystrophy (exceedingly rare)
  - Dynamic dysfunction.

Diaphragmatic hernias

A hernia is the displacement of tissues or organs through a boundary that normally holds the structures in place. To herniate means to protrude through an abnormal body opening. Any defect in the diaphragm with displacement of abdominal tissue or viscera through the defect and into the thoracic cavity is generally referred to as a diaphragmatic hernia. It should be noted, however, that the diaphragm does not herniate when there is a diaphragmatic hernia. Diaphragmatic hernias are further classified as true when the herniated contents are contained within a serosal ('hernia') sac. Otherwise, they are classified as false. Diaphragmatic defects, ruptures or rents that allow abdominal viscera to herniate are usually due to abnormal development or trauma. Other factors (e.g. changes in thoracic or abdominal pressures) may influence whether there is herniation (*versus* just a defect) and the severity of herniation. Herniated contents may be reducible or fixed (incarcerated) and may become strangulated. Herniated portions of the gastrointestinal tract may obstruct intraluminal flow.

Traumatic diaphragmatic hernia

Traumatic disruption of the diaphragm is termed diaphragmatic rupture and is most commonly caused by vehicular trauma. The rupture allows abdominal viscera to herniate into the pleural cavity. When abdominal viscera pass through the rupture, the hernia is false due to the absence of a serosal sac surrounding the herniated viscera. The diaphragm typically ruptures ventrally, in the weaker muscular portion, due to sudden severe increased abdominal pressure. The size of the diaphragmatic defect (or rent) and extent of organ displacement is variable. The liver is the most frequently displaced organ, but displacement of small intestine, gallbladder, stomach, spleen and falciform or omental fat is common. Displacement of the colon, pancreas and kidneys is also possible. Tachypnoea and dyspnoea are the most frequently reported clinical signs, although severity and type of clinical signs are related to the degree of lung compression and compliance. Other clinical signs (e.g. vomiting) may relate to injury of the herniated contents (e.g. strangulation, obstruction). Gastric prolapse is a surgical emergency because bloating leads to vascular compromise and can quickly become life-threatening.

- Radiography: orthogonal thoracic radiographs should be obtained. DV views are preferred to VD views, given the predominance of ventrally located tears and the desire to minimize respiratory compromise due to lung compression. In patients with severe respiratory distress, a lateral thoracic radiograph should be obtained using a horizontal beam with the animal in ventral recumbency, rather than the standard lateral view using a vertically oriented X-ray beam (see Chapter 1). Abdominal radiography is useful to assess for displacement of abdominal contents. Surgical diaphragmatic herniorrhaphy is the treatment of choice and intervention within 24 hours after trauma is generally associated with a good prognosis (approximately 80% survival). Poor prognostic indicators include concurrent orthopaedic injuries, oxygen dependence and prolonged surgical/anaesthetic times. Surgical repair more than 2 weeks after trauma has similar mortality rates but commonly requires organ resection. In addition, surgeries may be complicated due to adhesions. Radiographic signs may be subtle or obvious and include (Sullivan and Lee, 1989):
- Displacement of abdominal contents cranial to the diaphragm
  - The stomach and intestines are easier to identify when the lumens contain gas, ingesta, or faeces (Figure 8.70)
  - Herniated falciform and omental fat may be differentiated by their opacity (fat opacity)
- Inability to delineate the complete diaphragmatic border (differentiate from normal variations) due to the displaced content in the rent or the presence of pleural fluid (Figure 8.71)
- Border effacement of the cardiac silhouette, especially ventrally, laterally or both
- Dorsal displacement of the cardiac silhouette or trachea
- Pleural fluid
- Mediastinal shift/lung collapse
- Abdominal abnormalities
  - Small liver or falciform fat, suggestive of cranial displacement
  - Inability to detect expected content like the spleen or kidneys

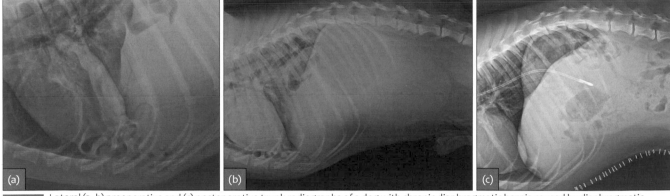

8.70 Lateral (a, b) preoperative and (c) postoperative trunk radiographs of a dog with chronic diaphragmatic hernia caused by diaphragmatic rupture. (a, b) Preoperatively, there is border effacement of portions of the diaphragm (cranial margin) due to intestinal herniation into the thoracic cavity. There is also severe gastric enlargement due to gastrointestinal obstruction. (c) Postoperatively, the cranial border of the diaphragm is well defined and contrasted by pulmonary gas (i.e. normal).

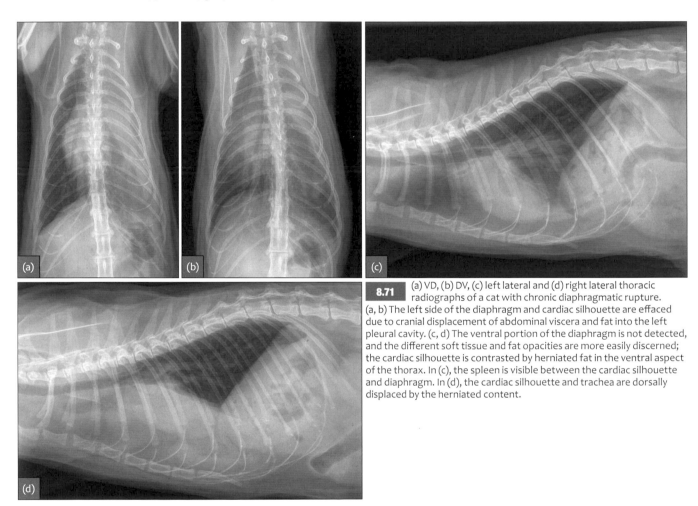

8.71 (a) VD, (b) DV, (c) left lateral and (d) right lateral thoracic radiographs of a cat with chronic diaphragmatic rupture. (a, b) The left side of the diaphragm and cardiac silhouette are effaced due to cranial displacement of abdominal viscera and fat into the left pleural cavity. (c, d) The ventral portion of the diaphragm is not detected, and the different soft tissue and fat opacities are more easily discerned; the cardiac silhouette is contrasted by herniated fat in the ventral aspect of the thorax. In (c), the spleen is visible between the cardiac silhouette and diaphragm. In (d), the cardiac silhouette and trachea are dorsally displaced by the herniated content.

- Concurrent thoracic trauma: rib fractures, body wall swelling, pneumothorax, lung contusions and appendicular skeleton fractures.
- Ultrasonography (Spattini *et al.*, 2003): point-of-care ultrasonography (e.g. abdominal or thoracic focused assessment with sonography for trauma (aFAST or tFAST)) is commonly used to rapidly assess patients for thoracic and abdominal trauma and can easily identify organ displacement in the thorax (Figure 8.72) and disruption of the diaphragmatic contour. This is especially important when radiography fails to determine whether there is a diaphragmatic hernia because of a large volume of pleural fluid, or pleural and peritoneal fluid. Mirror image artefact may produce spurious signs of abdominal content being displaced cranial to the diaphragm (Figure 8.73) but awareness of this artefact and how to identify it can reduce misdiagnosis.
- CT is the best overall imaging modality for patient assessment and surgical planning, especially when radiographic findings are subtle (Figure 8.74), there are multiple abnormalities, history is confusing and ultrasonography is unavailable or inconclusive. Availability of CT may be limited to specialist practices.
- Contrast radiographic techniques are adjunctive to survey radiographs but often are unnecessary or have been superseded by ultrasonography and CT.

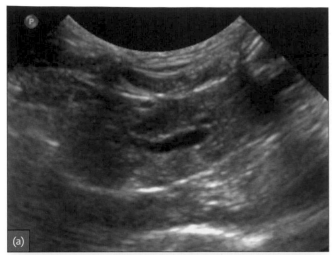

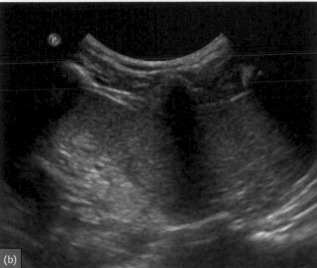

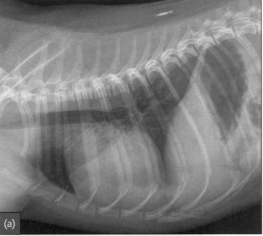

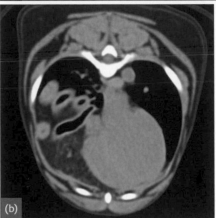

8.72 Thoracic ultrasound images of the same cat as in Figure 8.71, confirming diaphragmatic rupture by identifying herniation of (a) the pancreas and (b) the spleen within the thorax. Shadowing artefacts from the ribs can also be seen.

8.74 (a) Lateral thoracic radiograph and (b) non-contrast-enhanced thoracic CT image of a dog with a diaphragmatic hernia and unknown history of trauma. (a) The signs of diaphragmatic hernia are subtle and additional testing is needed. Herniated fat in the caudoventral aspect of the thorax produces a vague increased opacity with a distinct oblique cranial border that summates with the heart and lungs. In addition, the cranial border of the diaphragm is defined. (b) CT reveals that fat and small intestine have herniated through a rent in the diaphragm and are in the right pleural cavity adjacent to the heart.

- When the gastrointestinal tract cannot be identified based on normal shape (e.g. a tubular structure) or lumen contents (e.g. gas, granular material), then positive gastrointestinal contrast studies may be performed to determine the location of the stomach and intestines. These studies involve oral administration of contrast material (barium or iodinated). Barium is contraindicated in cases of suspected oesophageal or gastrointestinal rupture.
- Peritoneography using either iodinated contrast medium or gas has been described (Stickle, 1984). Inability to delineate the entire caudal border of the diaphragm, or detecting contrast medium in the pleural cavity, is a positive test result for diaphragmatic rupture. The former sign is more accurate because adhesions or abdominal content wedged in the rent may prevent contrast medium from passing through the diaphragm. False-negative results are also possible when pleural or peritoneal fluid dilutes the contrast medium such that it is undetectable.

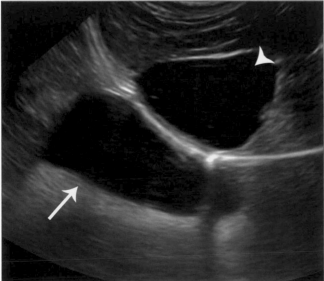

8.73 Ultrasound image of the liver, gallbladder and diaphragm of a dog. In the upper right part of the image (near field), the normal liver, gallbladder (arrowhead), and diaphragm can be identified. The diaphragm is the curvilinear hyperechoic line. In the bottom left part of the image, the liver and gallbladder are artefactually duplicated and displayed in the far field as a mirror image (arrowed).

Developmental diaphragmatic hernia

Diaphragmatic hernias can result from defects caused by abnormal development including diaphragmatic fusion and hiatal formation. In addition, these defects may be made worse by trauma or altered thoracic pressure. As with diaphragmatic hernias caused by traumatic rupture, the clinical signs are primarily based on severity of content displacement and tissue compromise. Congenital diaphragmatic hernias are often identified in juvenile patients with no history of trauma but can be found incidentally in older patients. In dogs and cats, PPDH and hiatal hernias are the most common and important. In contrast to traumatic rupture of the diaphragm and PPDH, most developmental diaphragmatic hernias tend to be located dorsally.

Peritoneopericardial diaphragmatic hernia: The pathogenesis of PPDH is incompletely understood. PPDH is often associated with other congenital malformations, most commonly other midline hernias (e.g. umbilical) and sternal anomalies. Clinical signs are related to abdominal organ displacement and dysfunction and/or cardiopulmonary compromise. Dogs more commonly present with gastrointestinal signs and cats more commonly present with respiratory signs. However, PPDH is often clinically silent and an incidental finding, particularly if only falciform fat herniation is present. The liver, gallbladder and small intestine are the most frequently herniated organs. Cardiovascular compromise is possible and reduced heart sounds are a common clinical examination finding. Acute presentation at a young or old age is possible with organ strangulation or small bowel obstruction. Abdominal radiographs may be helpful to identify organ displacement by determining whether there is a lack of organs within the abdominal cavity. Surgical reduction is the treatment of choice, commonly reducing or eliminating clinical signs, and is associated with low complication rates although adhesions are possible. Radiographic findings may be subtle or obvious and include:

- Mild to severe enlargement of the cardiac silhouette (Figure 8.75)
- Heterogeneous opacity of the cardiac silhouette with fat (due to falciform and/or omentum herniation) or tubular gas, mixed opacity ingesta and/or faeces (due to gastrointestinal herniation)
- Loss of diaphragmatic margin, ventrally on lateral views and midline on DV and VD views
- Dorsal displacement of the trachea and/or caudal vena cava
- Dorsal peritoneopericardial mesothelial remnant sign, which is a linear soft tissue opacity associated with the dorsal margin of the sac, has been described summating with the region of the caudal vena cava on lateral radiographs in cats (Berry *et al.*, 1990)
- Cranial displacement of the gastric axis, indicative of hepatic displacement
- Inability to identify organs within the abdomen, particularly the liver and intestine
- Other midline defects including pectus excavatum, split or absent sternebrae, and umbilical or other body wall defects.

Alternative imaging modalities:

- Ultrasonography is an excellent modality to differentiate causes of radiographic enlargement of the cardiac silhouette. Ultrasonography readily identifies abdominal organs adjacent to the heart and allows for assessment of cardiac function
- CT may be beneficial for evaluation when radiographic signs are subtle (Figure 8.76) and for surgical planning, particularly if concurrent cardiovascular abnormalities are present
- Contrast studies have been described but are uncommonly utilized.

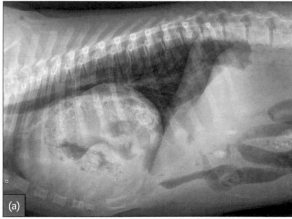

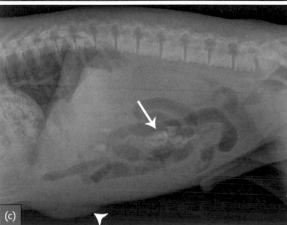

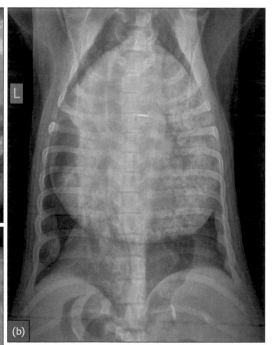

8.75 (a) Lateral and (b) VD thoracic, and (c) lateral abdominal radiographs of a juvenile dog with vomiting associated with PPDH. The cardiac silhouette is severely enlarged, globoid, and has a heterogeneous opacity due to abnormally located abdominal content, primarily intestines. In addition, the cranioventral margin of the diaphragm is effaced on all views and in the midline in (b). (c) There is reduced abdominal content and the small intestine is enlarged, consistent with obstruction of the small bowel. There is an incidental umbilical hernia (arrowhead) that is of minor consequence. The granular tubular material (arrowed) may be faeces in the colon or foreign material in the small intestine.

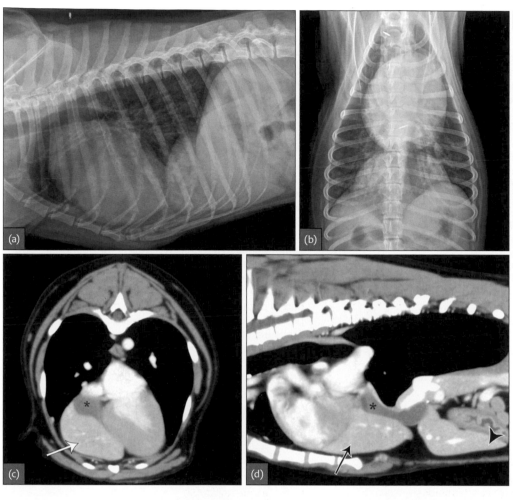

8.76 (a) Lateral and (b) VD thoracic radiographs, and (c) transverse and (d) sagittal contrast enhanced thoracic CT images (soft tissue window) of a 9-year-old dog with nasal discharge. (a, b) Thoracic radiography was performed to test for pulmonary metastasis, which was negative, and incidentally the diaphragmatic contour was noted to be lobular cranioventrally and in the midline. (c, d) During CT, the abnormal diaphragmatic contour was attributed to congenital PPDH. The liver and gallbladder (∗) are in the right ventral aspect of the pericardial sac. The portion of liver within the thorax (arrowed) and the portion of the liver in the abdomen (arrowhead) have normal and comparable contrast enhancement, indicating no vascular compromise.

Hiatal hernia: Hiatal hernia is defined as cranial displacement of abdominal organs through the oesophageal hiatus into the caudal mediastinum. The stomach is commonly displaced. Four types of hiatal hernia have been described in humans, dogs and cats:

- Type 1: dynamic gastro-oesophageal displacement (sliding hernia)
- Type 2: paraoesophageal displacement of the gastric fundus with the gastro-oesophageal junction remaining in its normal position
- Type 3: combination of types 1 and 2
- Type 4: herniation of abdominal organs other than the stomach (e.g. spleen, colon, small intestine).

Type 1 is the most common type in both dogs and cats. Shar Peis, Pugs and Bulldogs are predisposed. Dogs with congenital hiatal hernia can present with signs as early as 8 weeks of age, around the time of weaning. Most cats are older than 3 years of age at the time of diagnosis and commonly have concurrent illness (usually respiratory). Hiatal hernias can be congenital or acquired. Acquired hiatal hernia can occur secondary to trauma, tetanus infection, severe upper airway obstruction, brachycephalic airway syndrome or laryngeal paralysis. Hiatal hernia is poorly understood and may be due to interrelated factors but is typically due to secondary diaphragmatic muscle laxity, enlargement of the oesophageal hiatus and/or stretching of the phrenico-oesophageal ligament.

Mild cases may be asymptomatic. Clinical signs of hiatal hernia are primarily attributed to failure of the caudal ('lower') oesophageal sphincter mechanism leading to gastric reflux. Hiatal hernia becomes a self-perpetuating problem because gastric reflux leads to inflammation, further reducing lower oesophageal sphincter competence. Further reflux causes oesophagitis, reducing oesophageal motility and clearance of reflux. Eventually, megaoesophagus develops, worsening clinical signs and predisposing patients to aspiration pneumonia. Concurrent congenital megaoesophagus is also possible. Most dogs present with regurgitation. In contrast, cats present with non-specific gastrointestinal signs including vomiting, weight loss and anorexia; gagging and regurgitation are rare. Comorbidities are common and often related to upper or lower airway obstruction.

Medical and surgical management are described with variable success rates often related to underlying or secondary lesions. Medical management primarily aims to reduce oesophagitis and improve motility as well as treat any identified underlying diseases, such as airway inflammation. Surgery to treat the underlying causes, such as correction of brachycephalic airway lesions (e.g. elongated soft palate, stenotic nares) may be sufficient to eliminate hiatal hernia. However, in refractory cases, surgical intervention may include gastropexy or oesophagopexy (to physically anchor the stomach or oesophagus) and/or phrenoplasty to reduce the size of the oesophageal hiatus. Early surgical intervention in juvenile patients has been reported to have good outcomes with resolution of clinical signs. However, dogs may not improve after surgical intervention.

Severe clinical consequences of hiatal hernia have been reported, such as post-hepatic obstruction of the caudal vena cava and haemothorax secondary to gastric vasculature rupture. Type 4 is the most severe and is generally a surgical emergency. Megaoesophagus and hiatal hernia also rarely occur after surgical repair of diaphragmatic rupture but are usually transient and respond to prokinetics and nutritional support.

Radiographic signs include:

- A caudal mediastinal mass due to cranial displacement of the stomach into the caudal mediastinum; the stomach is usually identified by luminal gas
- A midline mass, consistent with a caudal mediastinal location, on DV or VD views
- Variable gastric displacement between views (intermittent, 'sliding'); displacement is most common on the left lateral view (Figure 8.77)
- Segmental oesophageal gas or diffuse oesophageal enlargement
- Secondary aspiration pneumonia
- Lesions associated with underlying causes, such as thick airways or hypoplastic trachea.

Dynamic disease processes can be difficult to diagnose with standard radiography. Since most hiatal hernias in dogs and cats are sliding hiatal hernias, multimodal diagnosis is commonly necessary. For example, in a recent study of 31 cats, fewer than half of hiatal hernias

were identified on survey radiographs (Phillips *et al.*, 2019). Adjunctive imaging could include:

- Positive contrast oesophagography using fluoroscopy to identify dynamic displacement of the gastro-oesophageal junction cranial to the diaphragm as well as oesophageal reflux and dysmotility
- Ultrasonography: the ultrasonographic appearance of the canine and feline abdominal portion of the oesophagus and cardia has been described but is limited by user experience and gastric contents, primarily gas. However, with appropriate patient preparation, caudal oesophageal and cardiac abnormalities can be identified, including masses and cranial displacement of the oesophagus in cases of sliding hiatal hernia
- CT can also be used in diagnosis and is an overall excellent modality to assess the thorax (Figure 8.78). It is more sensitive than radiography for pulmonary and bronchial lesions, providing additional information about underlying disease processes
- Endoscopy: this is useful to evaluate for oesophagitis and to obtain biopsies. Endoscopic evaluation performed during transient increases in abdominal pressure, such as elevating the pelvis relative the thorax (Trendelenberg position) or manually compressing the abdomen, causes gastric displacement in patients with brachycephalic airway syndrome and gastrointestinal

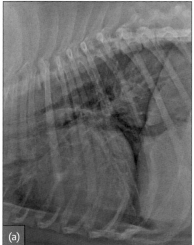
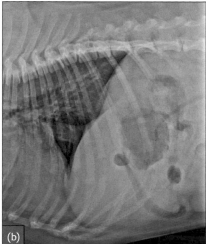
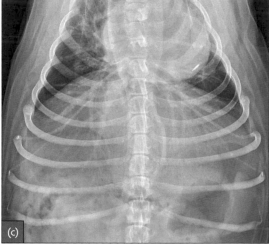

8.77 (a) Left lateral, (b) right lateral and (c) DV thoracic radiographs of a Bulldog with a sliding hiatal hernia (type 1). (a) Caudodorsal to the heart and summating with the caudal mediastinum, there is a focal soft tissue opacity with a cranially convex margin. In addition, the oesophageal lumen contains a small amount of gas dorsal to the cardiac silhouette. The soft tissue opacity was attributed to herniation of the stomach through the oesophageal hiatus. (b, c) The hernia was considered sliding or intermittent because the same opacity was not observed on the other views.

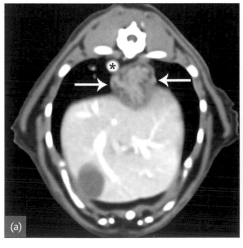
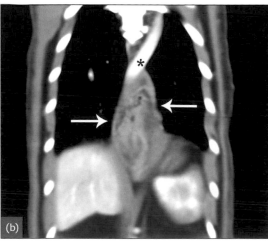

8.78 (a) Transverse and (b) dorsal contrast-enhanced thoracic CT images (soft tissue window) of a cat with a hiatal hernia identified by the intra-thoracic location of the stomach (arrowed). The stomach is in the dorsal aspect of the caudal mediastinum and to the left of the aorta. The herniated stomach also displaces the aorta (*) to the right.

signs, leading to increased detection of sliding hiatal hernia. Importantly, such manipulations did not result in gastric displacement endoscopically in normal beagles (Broux *et al.*, 2018).

Miscellaneous diaphragmatic hernia: Several additional true hernias have been reported in the veterinary literature but are rare and typically limited to case reports. They include ventral diaphragmatic hernias, body wall hernias and herniation of abdominal organs through the aortic hiatus. Herniation into the mediastinal serous cavity is also possible.

Diaphragmatic eventration

Diaphragmatic eventration is an uncommon condition that refers to a permanent, regional, cranial displacement of the diaphragmatic contour that occurs without disruption of the diaphragm. In other words, there is no herniation of abdominal contents into the thoracic cavity (the diaphragm still provides a continuous boundary). The affected portion of the diaphragm may be extremely thin and replaced by connective tissue. Unless the affected segment of the diaphragm is small, this condition may appear similar to hemiparalysis of the diaphragm due to unilateral phrenic nerve paralysis.

Diaphragmatic masses

Masses of the diaphragm are very rare in dogs and cats. Abscesses of the diaphragm can occur, usually secondary to penetrating foreign material, particularly grass awns migrating from the lungs. Neoplasms are possible and can be primary or metastatic. Mesothelioma and metastatic carcinomas can create multiple nodules or masses. Peripheral nerve sheath tumours of the phrenic nerve have been described. A mass due to increased muscular thickness has been described in a dog with muscular dystrophy (Bedu *et al.*, 2012; see 'Muscular dystrophy', below). Radiographic signs include:

- Diaphragmatic asymmetry
- A mass with broad-based surface contact with the diaphragm margin; the opacity of the mass may vary (e.g. soft tissue, soft tissue and gas, fat)
- Displacement of the adjacent lung margin
- Pleural fluid, which can obscure nodules and masses.

Pulmonary masses, diaphragmatic hernia, diaphragmatic eventration and diaphragmatic masses can be mistaken for one another.

Muscular dystrophy

Muscular dystrophy is a group of rare hereditary myopathies that have been described in humans, dogs and cats (Figure 8.79). Most muscular dystrophies are due to mutation in dystrophin, a protein found in skeletal and cardiac muscle, that leads to dysfunctional protein regeneration and progressive muscular replacement by fat and connective tissue. Muscular dystrophy has been described in multiple dog breeds and the Golden Retriever is a model organism for Duchenne, the most common form of muscular dystrophy in humans. Clinical signs include poor growth, generalized muscle atrophy, weakness, exercise intolerance, respiratory difficulties and collapse. Prognosis is considered guarded to poor, with death usually due to respiratory failure and/or euthanasia due to repeated episodes of aspiration pneumonia.

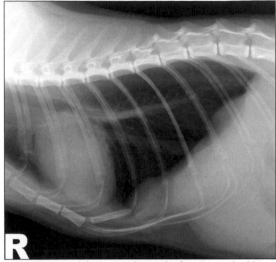

8.79 Lateral thoracic radiograph of an 18-month-old Domestic Shorthaired cat with muscular dystrophy, demonstrating an undulating diaphragm and mild cardiomegaly.

However, dogs have been reported to survive for longer than 7 years, suggesting heterogeneity of mutations as seen in humans. Radiographic findings are best described in Golden Retrievers, are variable over time with disease progression and most commonly include:

- Flat and/or scalloped diaphragm margin
- Lung hyperinflation: flat diaphragm, extension of the lungs cranial to the thoracic inlet and caudal to the costal arch, dorsal displacement of the cardiac silhouette, 'barrel chest' shape
- Hiatal hernia
- Displacement of the cranial portion of the sternum ('cranial pectus excavatum'), likely indicative of pulmonary hyperinflation
- Diaphragmatic asymmetry
- Bronchopneumonia
- Megaoesophagus.

Dynamic dysfunction

Phrenic nerve dysfunction, causing diaphragmatic paralysis, can be unilateral or bilateral, and temporary or permanent. Unilateral paralysis of the diaphragm is often clinically silent and difficult to diagnose; however, dyspnoea may develop during exercise. Bilateral paralysis often causes clinical signs, which can be severe. Phrenic nerve disfunction may be caused by trauma (Vignoli *et al.*, 2002), thoracic surgery, compression or degeneration of the phrenic nerve, congenital or infectious myopathies or inflammation (e.g. secondary to pneumonia), or may be idiopathic.

Due to neurological dysfunction, diaphragm motion is the opposite of normal: the diaphragm moves cranially during inhalation and caudally during exhalation, referred to as 'paradoxical motion.' Diaphragmatic paralysis should be differentiated from other causes of paradoxical respiratory motion, primarily flail chest and flail sternum (see 'Traumatic fractures' and 'Pectus excavatum', above). Conservative management is warranted because spontaneous resolution is reported in cases of known or suspected trauma.

Orthogonal radiographs centred on the diaphragm should be obtained during inhalation and exhalation. Obtaining radiographs in both lateral recumbencies can also be helpful. Radiographic findings include:

- Diaphragmatic asymmetry: cranial displacement of one diaphragmatic crus, asymmetry of costophrenic angle position, unilateral lung hypoinflation, asymmetry of intercostal spaces
- Cranial displacement of the same diaphragmatic crus in both right lateral and left lateral recumbency indicates unilateral dysfunction (Figure 8.80)
- Bilateral cranial displacement in all recumbencies
- Paradoxical motion during paired inhalation and exhalation radiographs.

Timing of radiographs for inhalation and exhalation can be challenging, particularly with panting or hyperventilation. Also, particularly in patients with bilateral nerve paralysis, abdominal muscular contractions can simulate diaphragmatic motion. Interestingly, a canine research study found that unilateral phrenic nerve resection reduced expansion of both lungs and led to bilaterally increased intercostal muscle activity to compensate for reduced diaphragm movement. Thus, phrenic nerve dysfunction is complex and dynamic imaging is often needed to reach a clinical diagnosis.

- Fluoroscopy: allows simultaneous evaluation of both crura and the cupula during the respiratory cycle. Unequal movement of the diaphragmatic crura in right lateral recumbency indicates unilateral paralysis. Absent or minimal bilateral motion (less than ½ length of T8 excursion between inhalation and exhalation) indicates bilateral dysfunction.
- Ultrasonography: only allows unilateral sequential evaluation of diaphragmatic motion but is less influenced by abdominal motion than fluoroscopy. With the transducer applied to the abdomen and the diaphragm margin visible deep to the liver, in normal respiration there is movement toward the transducer during inhalation and away from the transducer during exhalation. M-mode is best suited for dynamic studies and can assess normal excursion, reduced excursion and paradoxical motion (Figure 8.81). In normal dogs, the lower limit of diaphragm excursion is estimated to be 3 mm bilaterally with less than 50% difference between sides.

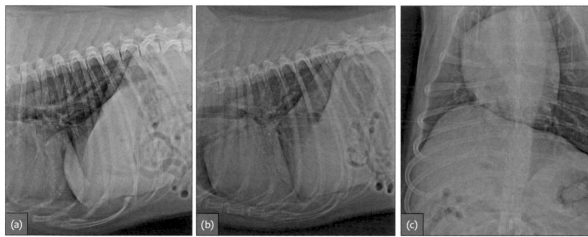

8.80 (a) Left lateral, (b) right lateral and (c) VD thoracic radiographs of a dog with right phrenic nerve paralysis, indicated by cranial displacement of the right diaphragmatic crus on all views.

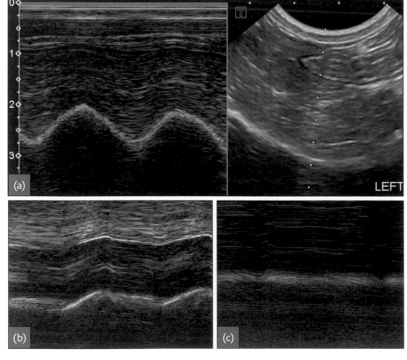

8.81 M-mode ultrasound images of the left diaphragmatic crus using a transabdominal approach. (a) Normal diaphragmatic motion is depicted. (b) Poor and (c) absent diaphragmatic motion are demonstrated, due to phrenic nerve dysfunction.

References and further reading

Allett B and Hecht S (2016) Magnetic resonance imaging findings in the spine of six dogs diagnosed with lymphoma. *Veterinary Radiology & Ultrasound* **57**, 154–161

Bainoo OJ, Lewis S and White RA (2002) Primary thoracic wall tumours of mesenchymal origin in dogs: a retrospective study of 46 cases. *Veterinary Record* **150**, 335–339

Bedu A-S, Labruyère JJ, Thibaud JL *et al.* (2012) Age-related thoracic radiographic changes in golden and labrador retriever muscular dystrophy. *Veterinary Radiology & Ultrasound* **53**, 492–500

Berry CR, Gaschen FP and Ackerman N (1992) Radiographic and ultrasonographic features of hypertrophic feline muscular dystrophy in two cats. *Veterinary Radiology & Ultrasound* **33**, 357–364

Berry CR, Koblik PD and Ticer JW (1990) Dorsal peritoneopericardial mesothelial remnant as an aid to the diagnosis of feline congenital diaphragmatic hernia. *Veterinary Radiology* **31**, 239–245

Bertram S, ter Haar G and De Decker S (2018) Caudal articular process dysplasia of thoracic vertebrae in neurologically normal French bulldogs, English bulldogs, and Pugs: Prevalence and characteristics. *Veterinary Radiology & Ultrasound* **59**, 396–404

Biller DS, Johnson GC, Birchard SJ and Fingland RB (1987) Aneurysmal bone cyst in a rib of a cat. *Journal of the American Veterinary Medical Association* **190**, 1193–1195

Bright RM, Sackman JE, DeNovo C and Toal C (1990) Hiatal hernia in the dog and cat: a retrospective study of 16 cases. *Journal of Small Animal Practice* **31**, 244–250

Broux O, Clercx C, Etienne A-L *et al.* (2018) Effects of manipulations to detect sliding hiatal hernia in dogs with brachycephalic airway obstructive syndrome. *Veterinary Surgery* **47**, 243–251

Burnie AG, Simpson JW and Corcoran BM (1989) Gastro-oesophageal reflux and hiatus hernia associated with laryngeal paralysis in a dog. *Journal of Small Animal Practice* **30**, 414–416

Caporn TM and Read RR (1996) Osteochondromatosis of the cervical spine causing compressive myelopathy in a dog. *Journal of Small Animal Practice* **37**, 133–137

De Decker S and Volk HA (2014) Dorsal vertebral column abnormalities in dogs with disseminated idiopathic skeletal hyperostosis (DISH). *Veterinary Record* **174**, 632–632

Dennis R (1993) Radiographic diagnosis of rib lesions in dogs and cats. *Veterinary Annual* **33**, 173–192

Feeney DA, Johnston GR, Grindem CB *et al.* (1982) Malignant neoplasia of canine ribs: clinical, radiographic and pathologic findings. *Journal of the American Veterinary Medical Association* **180**, 927–933

Forrest LJ and Thrall DE (1994) Bone scintigraphy for metastasis detection in canine osteosarcoma. *Veterinary Radiology & Ultrasound* **35**, 124–130

Fossum TW, Boudrieau RJ and Hobson HP (1989) Pectus excavatum in eight dogs and six cats. *Journal of the American Animal Hospital Association* **25**, 595–605

Fowler JD (1998) Thoracic cage defects. In: *BSAVA Manual of Cardiorespiratory Medicine and Surgery*, ed. V Luis Fuentes and S Swift, pp. 353–358. BSAVA Publications, Gloucester

Friedenberg SG, Vansteenkiste D, Yost O *et al.* (2018) A de novo mutation in the EXT2 gene associated with osteochondromatosis in a litter of American Staffordshire Terriers. *Journal of Veterinary Internal Medicine* **32**, 986–992

Grandage J (1974) The radiology of the dog's diaphragm. *Journal of Small Animal Practice* **15**, 1–17

Hammer AS, Weeren FR, Weisbrode SE and Padgett SL (1995) Prognostic factors in dogs with osteosarcomas of the flat or irregular bones. *Journal of the American Animal Hospital Association* **31**, 321–326

Hardie EM, Clary EM, Kornegay JN *et al.* (1998) Abnormalities of the thoracic bellows: stress fractures of the ribs and hiatal hernia. *Journal of Veterinary Internal Medicine* **12**, 279–287

Haskins ME, Aguirre GD, Jezyk PF, Desnick RJ and Patterson DF (1983) The pathology of the feline model of mucopolysaccharidosis I. *The American Journal of Pathology* **112**, 27–36

Herati RS, Knox VW, O'Donnell P *et al.* (2008) Radiographic evaluation of bones and joints in mucopolysaccharidosis I and VII dogs after neonatal gene therapy. *Molecular Genetics and Metabolism* **95**, 142–151

Heyman SJ, Diefenderfer DL, Goldschmidt MH and Newton CD (1992) Canine axial skeletal osteosarcoma. A retrospective study of 116 cases (1986 to 1989). *Veterinary Surgery* **21**, 304–310

Hornyak L. (1999) Malformation of the processus xiphoideus in two breed cats. *Kleintierpraxis* **44**, 370–378

Jankowski MK, Steyn PF, Lana S *et al.* (2003) Nuclear scanning with 99mTc-HDP for the initial evaluation of osseous metastasis in canine osteosarcoma. *Veterinary and Comparative Oncology* **1**, 152–158

Kraje BJ, Kraje AC, Rohrbach BW *et al.* (2000) Intrathoracic and concurrent orthopedic injury associated with traumatic rib fracture in cats: 75 cases (1980–1998). *Journal of the American Veterinary Medical Association* **216**, 51–54

Kramers P, Flückiger MA, Rahn BA and Cordey J (1988) Osteopetrosis in cats. *Journal of Small Animal Practice* **29**, 153–164

Kyöstilä K, Lappalainen AK and Lohi H (2013) Canine chondrodysplasia caused by a truncating mutation in collagen-binding integrin alpha subunit 10. *PLoS ONE* **8**, e75621

Lamb CR (2004) Radiology corner: loss of the diaphragmatic line as a sign of ruptured diaphragm. *Veterinary Radiology & Ultrasound* **45**, 305–306

Langley-Hobbs SJ, Carmichael S, Lamb CR, Bjornson AP and Day MJ (1997) Polyostotic lymphoma in a young dog: a case report and literature review. *Journal of Small Animal Practice* **38**, 412–416

Lodzinska J, Culshaw G, Hall JL, Schwarz T and Liuti T (2018) CT diagnosis of intermittent type IV paraoesophageal hernia in a dog. *Veterinary Records Case Reports* **6**, e000692

Montgomery RD, Henderson RA, Powers RD *et al.* (1993) Retrospective study of 26 primary tumors of the osseous thoracic wall in dogs. *Journal of the American Animal Hospital Association* **29**, 68–72

Moon S, Park S, Lee S, Cheon B and Choi J (2017) Fluoroscopic evaluation of diaphragmatic excursion during spontaneous breathing in healthy Beagles. *American Journal of Veterinary Research* **78**, 1043–1048

Morgan JP and Stavenborn M (1991) Disseminated idiopathic skeletal hyperostosis (DISH) in a dog. *Veterinary Radiology* **32**, 65–70

Phillips H, Corrie J, Engel DM *et al.* (2019) Clinical findings, diagnostic test results, and treatment outcome in cats with hiatal hernia: 31 cases (1995–2018). *Journal of Veterinary Internal Medicine* **33**, 1970–1976

Pirkey-Ehrhart N, Withrow SJ, Straw RC *et al.* (1995) Primary rib tumors in 54 dogs. *Journal of the American Animal Hospital Association* **31**, 65–69

Platt SR, Olby NJ and Beltran E (2024) *BSAVA Manual of Canine and Feline Neurology, 5th edn.* BSAVA Publications, Gloucester [in production]

Ponder KP, O'Malley TM, Wang P *et al.* (2012) Neonatal gene therapy with a gamma retroviral vector in mucopolysaccharidosis VI cats. *Molecular Therapy* **20**, 898–907

Pratschke KM, Hughes JML, Skelly C and Bellenger CR (1998) Hiatal herniation as a complication of chronic diaphragmatic herniation. *Journal of Small Animal Practice* **39**, 33–38

Spattini G, Rossi F, Vignoli M and Lamb CR (2003) Use of ultrasound to diagnose diaphragmatic rupture in dogs and cats. *Veterinary Radiology & Ultrasound* **44**, 226–230

Spellacy E, Shull RM, Constantopoulos G and Neufeld EF (1983) A canine model of human alpha-L-iduronidase deficiency. *Proceedings of the National Academy of Sciences* **80**, 6091–6095

Stickle RL (1984) Positive-contrast celiography (peritoneography) for the diagnosis of diaphragmatic hernia in dogs and cats. *Journal of the American Veterinary Medical Association* **185**, 295–298

Störk CK, Hamaide AJ, Schwedes C *et al.* (2003) Hemiurothorax following diaphragmatic hernia and kidney prolapse in a cat. *Journal of Feline Medicine and Surgery* **5**, 91–96

Sullivan M and Lee R (1989) Radiological features of 80 cases of diaphragmatic rupture. *Journal of Small Animal Practice* **30**, 561–566

Suter PF (1984) *Thoracic Radiography. A Text Atlas of Thoracic Diseases of the Dog and Cat.* Peter F. Suter, Wettswill

Vignoli M, Toniato M, Rossi F *et al.* (2002) Transient post-traumatic hemidiaphragmatic paralysis in two cats. *Journal of Small Animal Practice* **39**, 312–316

Vollmerhaus B, Roos H, Matis U, Veith G and Tassani-Prell M (1999) The specific anatomy and function of the thorax of the domestic cat. *Tierärztliche Praxis Ausgabe K, Kleintiere/Heimtiere* **27**, 365–370

Wessmann A (2014) Disseminated idiopathic skeletal hyperostosis: diagnostic criteria and clinical significance. *Veterinary Record* **174**, 630–631

Chapter 9

The heart and great vessels

Joanna Dukes-McEwan

Imaging anatomy

Basic cardiac anatomy

The heart is the largest mediastinal organ and its anatomy is complex. The heart develops from paired endocardial tubes that arise from splanchnic mesoderm. These gradually fuse and undergo elongation, various dilatations and constrictions, and finally partition into chambers to form the heart. A full description of the embryonic origin of the heart is beyond the scope of this chapter, but a good understanding of the embryology of cardiovascular development will improve understanding of congenital heart disease (an overview is provided as relevant for some of the congenital heart diseases; see later).

Partitioning of the heart results in four chambers (right and left atria and right and left ventricles) and two great arteries (the aorta and pulmonic trunk).

- Blood enters the right atrium (RA) from the cranial and caudal venae cavae and the coronary sinus.
- Blood leaves the right ventricle (RV) via the pulmonic trunk.
- Blood enters the left atrium (LA) from the pulmonary veins.
- Blood leaves the left ventricle (LV) via the aorta.

Valves divide the chambers. Each valve has a fibrous annulus and a number of cusps or leaflets. The atria are separated from the ventricles by atrioventricular valves: the mitral valve on the left and the tricuspid valve on the right. Both atrioventricular valves have two cusps and the term 'tricuspid' is a misnomer derived from human terminology. The ventricles are separated from the major arteries by semilunar valves, the aortic on the left and the pulmonic on the right. Both of these have three cusps.

The four chambers of the heart are encased within the pericardium (pericardial sac). There are two layers forming the pericardium:

- The fibrous pericardium: a strong external layer
- The serous pericardium: a thin lining that covers the heart. This is divided into parietal and visceral layers and there is a small amount of lubricating fluid between these layers (in the pericardial cavity).

The heart itself is supplied with blood by the coronary arteries. The left and right coronary arteries arise from the root of the aorta. Venous drainage is via the coronary veins and the coronary sinus.

Radiographic cardiac anatomy

Cardiac radiographic anatomy and normal position within the thorax is best assessed from a dorsoventral (DV) and a right lateral view. These positions keep the heart within its normal central position, maintained by the left-sided caudal mediastinal reflection.

The heart dominates a thoracic radiograph as it is the largest single soft tissue opacity in the thorax. It sits within the mediastinum from approximately the third to the sixth intercostal space. The larger, more dorsal part of the heart is known as the base, and the smaller, more ventral (sternal) part is known as the apex.

In the lateral view, the apex is formed by the interventricular septum (IVS) and apical LV. The heart lies at an angle within the thorax (easily seen on the lateral view) with the apex positioned more caudally than the base. The apex usually points towards the left on DV and ventrodorsal (VD) views. Variation in the location of the apex on DV and VD views may be extrinsic (e.g. due to alteration in lung volume) or intrinsic (a congenital malpositioning of the heart). The latter may be an incidental finding of minor importance or associated with other pathological abnormalities (e.g. situs inversus in Kartagener's syndrome) (Figures 9.1 and 9.2). In situations of left heart enlargement, the apex may also be shifted to the right.

The actual outline of the heart is not seen on a radiograph. Instead, the term cardiac silhouette is used to include the heart, pericardium, pericardial contents (such as fat and a small amount of fluid) and the origin of the aorta and pulmonic trunk. This is in contrast to an echocardiographic examination where the heart, origin of the major vessels, pericardium and pericardial contents are seen as separate structures. The outline of the cardiac silhouette is smooth, and details such as the coronary grooves and the separation of atria from the ventricles are not seen. The coronary arteries and veins are also not seen radiographically. However, it is possible to infer the location of the major chambers on a radiograph and to identify pathological changes in their size to some extent (see below).

The central and ventral margins of the cardiac silhouette are easily outlined on a radiograph as these areas are surrounded by contrasting air in the lungs. It is not possible to outline the margins of the heart in the area of the heart base as the surrounding soft tissues, i.e. the major blood vessels (aorta, pulmonic trunk and pulmonary veins) and lymph nodes, have the same radiographic opacity. It is often difficult radiographically to appreciate changes and

	Levoposition	Dextroposition	Dextroversion	Levocardia	Dextrocardia
Cause	Normal	Displacement or congenital malposition	Congenital malposition	Congenital malposition	Congenital malposition
Location of viscera	Situs solitus	Situs solitus	Situs solitus	Partial situs inversus	Total situs inversus
Image					
Description	Normal situation in dogs and cats. The heart is located slightly to the left and the apex points towards the left	Normal variant. The apex is positioned more towards the right than normal. May be extrinsic (e.g. due to mediastinal shift) or intrinsic (actual embryological abnormality)	Congenital abnormality where the heart is positioned in the right side of the thorax. Dextroversion also means that the heart is 'twisted' with the LV lying in the correct left-sided position but lying anterior to the RV	Heart is positioned on the left side of the thorax. Mirror image arrangement of the abdominal viscera	Heart is positioned on the right side of the thorax. Mirror image arrangement of the thoracic and abdominal viscera. The most important of the positional abnormalities. Other congenital cardiac abnormalities may be present. May be seen as part of Kartagener's syndrome along with bronchiectasis and recurrent sinusitis

Definitions:

- Dextrocardia – location of the heart in the right side of the thorax, the apex pointing towards the right. The cardiac chambers are reversed
- Dextroposition – displacement towards the right
- Dextroversion – version (turning) to the right. In terms of the heart, dextroversion means the location of the heart in the right thorax, the LV lying in the correct position on the left but lying cranial to the RV
- Levocardia – location of the heart in the left side of the thorax, the apex pointing towards the left
- Levoposition – displacement towards the left
- Situs inversus – the thoracic and abdominal viscera are reversed (i.e. a mirror image of the normal arrangement)
- Situs solitus – the thoracic and abdominal viscera are in a normal location

There is some controversy over the exact definitions but those listed above are most commonly accepted

9.1 Cardiac position as seen on a DV radiograph. Variation in position may be a normal variant or a congenital abnormality. Some of the reported congenital abnormalities are included; many other variants are possible. Ao = aorta; Ap = apex; ST = stomach.
(Line diagrams adapted from Suter (1984) with permission)

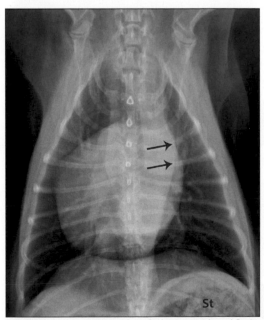

9.2 Dextroposition identified as an incidental finding in a dog. The cardiac silhouette and apex are located to the right of the median plane and there is no evidence to suggest that this is associated with a mediastinal shift. Note the aorta (arrowed) and stomach (St) are on the left; there is no suggestion of a situs inversus in this dog.

pathology in this region; ultrasonography and computed tomography (CT) are useful alternative imaging modalities.

Many factors alter the appearance of a normal cardiac silhouette on a radiograph and this is a major source of misdiagnosis and confusion in thoracic radiography. These include tremendous variation with canine breed as well as variation with respiratory phase, age, body condition and radiographic view (see below).

Identifying the cardiac chambers

The internal chambers of the heart and the lumens of the great vessels can only be visualized on a radiograph with the administration of positive contrast media (see Chapter 1). This is known as angiocardiography. However, it is possible to use the location of the borders of the various chambers to assess cardiac or great vessel enlargement on plain radiographs.

Normal angiocardiograms are very useful in understanding the location of the chambers within the shadow of the cardiac silhouette (Figures 9.3 and 9.4). These have been used to formulate diagrams showing the radiographic location of the cardiac chambers (Figures 9.5 and 9.6). The presence of pericardial effusion usually precludes the evaluation of changes in specific cardiac chambers.

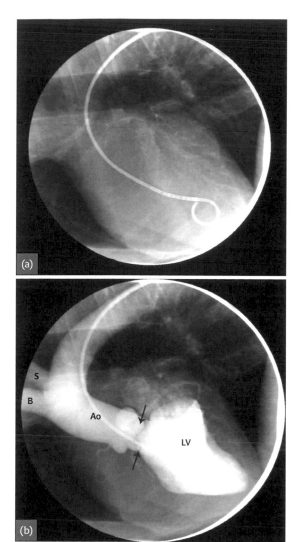

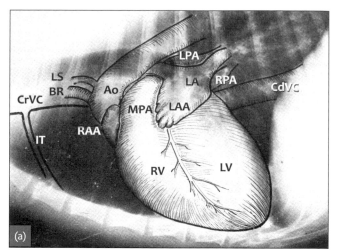

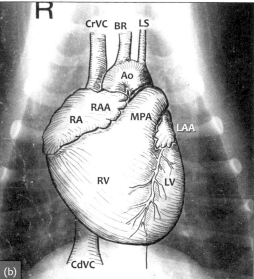

9.3 Left ventricular angiocardiograms of a 5-year-old Golden Retriever. (a) The catheter has been placed into the LV via the femoral artery and aorta ready for the contrast medium injection. (b) Positive contrast medium fills the LV, ascending aorta (Ao), brachiocephalic trunk (B) and left subclavian artery (S), and surrounds the aortic valves (arrowed).

(Courtesy of J. Buchanan)

9.5 Location of the cardiac chambers on thoracic radiographs of a dog. (a) Lateral view. (b) VD view. Ao = aortic arch; BR = brachiocephalic trunk; CdVC = caudal vena cava; CrVC = cranial vena cava; IT = internal thoracic arteries and veins; LAA = left atrial appendage; LPA = left pulmonary artery; LS = left subclavian artery; MPA = pulmonic trunk; RAA = right atrial appendage; RPA = right pulmonary artery.

(Reproduced from Suter (1984) with permission)

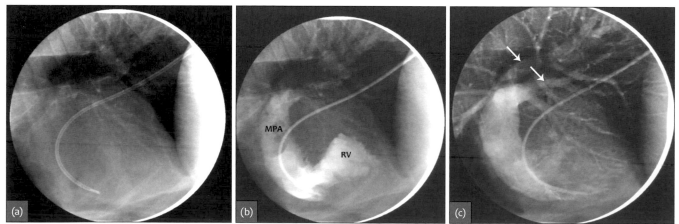

9.4 Right ventricular angiocardiograms of the same dog as in Figure 9.3. (a) The catheter has been placed into the RV via the caudal vena cava ready for the contrast medium injection. (b) Positive contrast medium is present within the RV and has started to enter the right ventricular outflow tract and pulmonic trunk (MPA). (c) The contrast medium has now reached the left and right pulmonary arteries (arrowed) and the smaller pulmonary arterial branches in the lungs.

(Courtesy of J. Buchanan)

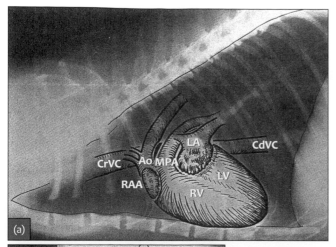

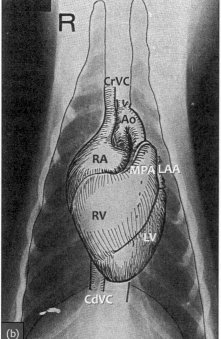

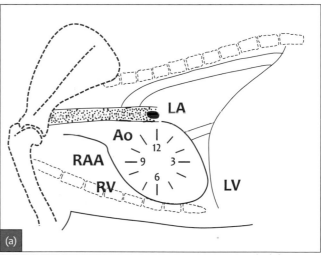

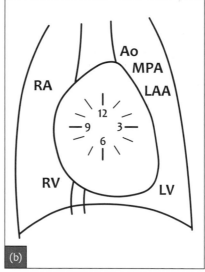

• The dorsal and caudodorsal borders of the LA do not have distinct outlines on the lateral view as the pulmonary veins enter in this area and the right pulmonary artery also overlaps this region.

Clock face analogy

A clock face analogy has been used to identify specific chamber locations on a radiograph. The clock numbers are used to indicate the approximate position of the chambers and great vessels (Figure 9.7).

9.7 Clock face analogy identifying location of cardiac chambers. (a) Lateral view. (b) DV view. Ao = aortic arch; LAA = left atrial appendage; MPA = pulmonic trunk; RAA = right atrial appendage.
(Reproduced from Dennis *et al.* (2001) with permission)

9.6 Location of the cardiac chambers on thoracic radiographs of a cat. (a) Lateral view. (b) VD view. Ao = aortic arch; CdVC = caudal vena cava; CrVC = cranial vena cava; LAA = left atrial appendage; MPA = pulmonic trunk; RAA = right atrial appendage.
(Reproduced from Suter (1984) with permission)

Some basic rules help in the assessment of cardiac chambers:

• In the dog, the LV and LA are located on the left and caudal aspect of the heart; the RV and RA are located on the right and cranial aspect of the heart
• The position of the cardiac apex can be used to separate the right and left sides of the heart
• The RV is cranial to the apex on the lateral view and is to the right on DV and VD views. The LV is caudodorsal to the apex on the lateral view and is to the left of the apex on DV and VD views
• The exact apical point can be difficult to determine due to the variation in cardiac position. This can sometimes make evaluation of left- versus right-sided enlargement difficult
• The two atria are located dorsal to the level of the caudal vena cava (CdVC) on the lateral view and are mainly on the cranial aspect of the cardiac silhouette on DV and VD views; the LA is more caudal

Lateral view		
12–2	o'clock:	left atrium
2–5	o'clock:	left ventricle
5–9	o'clock:	right ventricle
9–10	o'clock:	pulmonic trunk and right atrial appendage
10–11	o'clock:	aortic arch

Dorsoventral view		
11–1	o'clock:	aortic arch
1–2	o'clock:	pulmonic trunk
2.30–3	o'clock:	left atrial appendage (LAA)
2–5	o'clock:	left ventricle
5–9	o'clock:	right ventricle
9–11	o'clock:	right atrium

Species differences

Dogs

- The cardiac apex points more to the left on DV and VD views.
- The LAA is located at 2.30–3 o'clock on DV and VD views.
- When the LA is enlarged it summates with the rest of the cardiac silhouette in the 5–7 o'clock position (between the principal bronchi) on DV and VD views.

Cats

- The apex is more variable but usually closer to the midline.
- The LA and LAA are located at 1–2 o'clock on these views and the pulmonic trunk may be cranial to this or not seen at all.
- The more cranial location of the LA may make it difficult to see on the lateral view.
- When the LA is enlarged it is located more cranially at the 1–2 o'clock position. This explains the so-called 'valentine heart shape' seen only in the cat and created by left atrial enlargement with or without concurrent right atrial enlargement.

Factors affecting cardiac size and appearance

Many factors can alter the appearance of the normal heart on a radiograph. It is important to be aware of the influence of these factors to avoid the misdiagnosis of normal anatomical variation as disease. These include breed, pericardial fat, age, body position, respiratory phase and stage of the cardiac cycle.

Species differences

- The normal canine heart shows substantial breed-associated variations in size and shape. The normal feline heart is generally unaffected by breed (Figure 9.8).
- Variation in cardiac shape and size with body position is an important consideration in the dog. Generally size and shape alteration with body position are negligible in the cat.

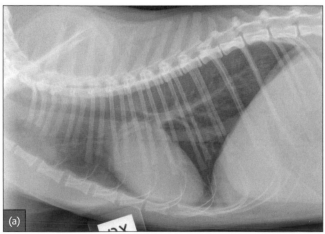

9.8 (a) Lateral radiograph of a cat with a normal cardiac silhouette. The cardiac silhouette is ovoid. Alteration in cardiac shape is useful in radiographic diagnosis of cardiac disease in the cat. (continues)

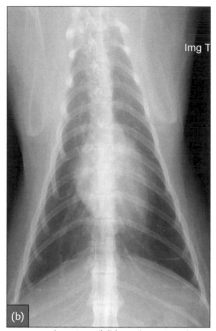

9.8 (continued) (b) DV thoracic radiograph of a cat with a normal cardiac silhouette. The cardiac silhouette is ovoid. Alteration in cardiac shape is useful in radiographic diagnosis of cardiac disease in the cat.

Breed

The canine heart varies tremendously between different dog breeds; breed-associated conformational variation is the single most important cause of variation in the normal canine cardiac silhouette. A basic outline of these differences is shown in Figures 9.9 and 9.10; however, there are many more variations. A good understanding of these differences is paramount to cardiac assessment in thoracic radiography. It may be useful to build up a collection of normal thoracic radiographs of different breeds for easy reference.

Pericardial fat

An incorrect diagnosis of cardiomegaly is often made in animals with a large amount of pericardial fat. Pericardial fat contributes to the overall size of the cardiac silhouette,

Thorax type	Lateral view	Dorsoventral view
Wide shallow (e.g. Dachshund, Shi-Tzu, Boston Terrier, Bulldog)	Shorter rounder cardiac silhouette at a large inclination to the vertebral column. Cardiac silhouette has a long contact area with the sternum (mimicking right-sided cardiomegaly)	Rounded right and left ventricular borders. Apex is usually well to the left of the median plane
Deep narrow (e.g. Greyhound, Afghan Hound, Whippet)	Long oval heart with a vertical position in the thorax (almost perpendicular to the vertebral column)	Almost circular cardiac silhouette due to upright position of heart in thorax. Apex is close to median plane
Intermediate (e.g. German Shepherd Dog, Labrador Retriever)	Heart appears ovoid or lop-sided egg-shaped	Heart appears similar to lateral view. Apex is usually slightly to the left of the median plane

9.9 Variation in the appearance of the cardiac silhouette with thoracic shape in dogs.

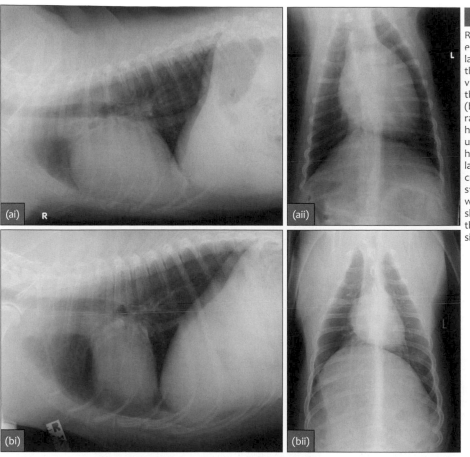

9.10 (ai) Right lateral and (aii) DV thoracic radiographs from a Golden Retriever with a normal heart confirmed by echocardiography. The lateral view shows a large amount of sternal contact (common in the breed and conformation type), but the DV view excludes right-sided cardiomegaly and the cardiac silhouette is within normal limits. (bi) Right lateral and (bii) DV thoracic radiographs from a Dobermann with a normal heart confirmed by echocardiography. As is usual for the Dobermann's conformation, the heart is vertical within the thorax on the lateral view, and therefore appears small craniocaudally on the DV view with the apex still left-sided. Volume depletion can be seen, with a slightly small cardiac silhouette and slender CdVC. Pericardial fat is also visible on the lateral view, ventral to the cardiac silhouette.

however it is often possible to identify the presence of fat on careful inspection. Pericardial fat has a lower opacity compared with the heart and often the cardiac margin is not as sharp (Figure 9.10bi). The latter is due to the gradual change in opacity from soft tissue (heart) to fat to air-filled lung, rather than the sharp soft tissue–air interface seen in thinner animals. Altering radiographic technique may also assist in identification of pericardial fat.

In the cat, pericardial fat is seen better on DV and VD, rather than lateral, radiographs. Pericardial fat should be suspected if a large amount of falciform or subcutaneous fat is present and may be seen as a characteristic triangular corner on the right cranial margin of the cardiac silhouette on DV and VD views (Figure 9.11).

Age

Young dogs appear to have large hearts. This is, in part, due to the relatively small size of the thoracic cavity. Thus, it is particularly important to take into account shape changes as well as overall cardiac size in younger animals.

About 40% of cats over 10 years old have a cranially sloping cardiac silhouette with increased sternal contact (Figure 9.12). The reason for this is poorly understood and no association with increased cardiac size has been found. It is considered likely to be associated with age-related changes in thoracic conformation.

Body position

Variation in body position will cause variations in the appearance of the cardiac silhouette due to the effects of gravity. Consistency in the radiographic technique is

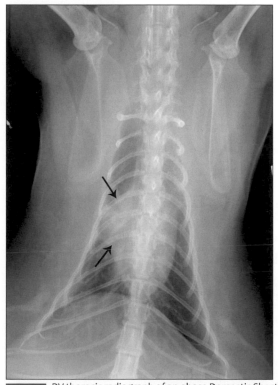

9.11 DV thoracic radiograph of an obese Domestic Shorthaired cat. The cardiac silhouette has an unusual shape due to border effacement with a triangular soft tissue opacity on the right side (arrowed). A CT examination confirmed the lung was within normal limits and the opacity was due to a large amount of pericardial fat (even though it has a soft tissue opacity). This appearance should not be confused with pathology.

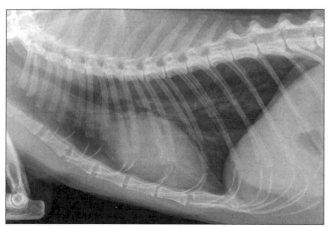

9.12 Left lateral thoracic radiograph of a clinically normal 12-year-old cat. In about 40% of older cats the heart has a more horizontal, cranially sloping position.

important in assessment of sequential radiographs and helps to avoid misinterpretation. Right lateral and DV radiographs are generally acquired for radiographic assessment of cardiac disease (see Chapter 1).

Regardless of view, the cardiac silhouette is always slightly larger than the heart itself due to the effects of magnification. In deep-chested dogs, the cardiac silhouette may be more noticeably magnified on VD views because it is further from the detector than on DV views. Specific changes in the appearance of the canine cardiac silhouette on different radiographic views are given in Figure 9.13.

Right lateral
• Cardiac silhouette shape and position of apex are more consistent • May have a longer sternal contact area than on left lateral view
Left lateral
• Cardiac silhouette is more rounded • Apex may be displaced slightly dorsally from the sternum
Dorsoventral
• Cardiac silhouette shape and position of apex are more consistent • Cardiac silhouette is more oval • The apex is more to the left on DV views
Ventrodorsal
• Cardiac silhouette is more elongated • Apex may be more in the midline • May see bulge in position of pulmonic trunk

9.13 Variation in the appearance of the cardiac silhouette with body position.

Respiratory phase

Expiratory radiographs create a false impression of cardiomegaly as the overall thoracic size is decreased, while the cardiac size stays the same (for examples of inspiratory and expiratory radiographs, see Chapter 12). Sternal contact increases at expiration which exacerbates the impression of cardiomegaly; there is also a small but real increase in cardiac size during expiration.

At expiration the cardiac silhouette can be more difficult to outline cranially due to adjacent mediastinal fat and caudally due to overlapping of the diaphragm. In addition, loss of air content in the lung tissue contacting the cardiac silhouette creates a surrounding hazy indistinct zone.

The effects of all of these changes are exaggerated in older, obese and shallow-breathing dogs.

Cardiac cycle

Variations due to cardiac cycle seldom cause major changes or radiographic misinterpretation (see Chapter 1). They are most easily seen in large-breed dogs and dogs with a slow heart rate.

Most radiographs are exposed during ventricular diastole simply because it is longer in duration than systole. Near the end of ventricular systole the atrial borders can be rounded and bulging, and the ventricles may appear as slightly smaller with a narrow 'V' instead of 'U' shape (Figure 9.14). On DV and VD views the pulmonic trunk can be more prominent in systole. One report suggested that there was less alteration in shape due to cardiac cycle on the VD view than the DV view in cats. A fluoroscopic study has shown the cardiac cycle does impact on vertebral heart score and cardiothoracic ratio measurements (Brown *et al.*, 2020).

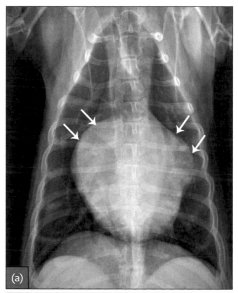

(a)

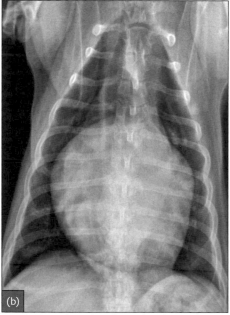

(b)

9.14 VD thoracic radiographs of a Cavalier King Charles Spaniel with cardiomegaly, obtained at different phases of the cardiac cycle. Note the difference in the appearance of the heart. (a) Systole: the ventricles are smaller and the atria are dilated (arrowed). (b) Diastole: the entire heart is rounded and the atrial bulges are not as prominent. The changes in this dog are also exacerbated by slight differences in respiratory phase.

Measuring the cardiac silhouette

It is important to be able to assess cardiac size radiographically and many techniques have evolved in order to do this. Note that radiographs are often inaccurate in the assessment of heart size and identification of specific chamber enlargement. Ultrasonography remains the gold standard for chamber size assessment (see Chapter 2).

Guidelines for cardiac size

Various methods for quantifying normal heart size have been reported. These techniques have many limitations and should only be used in combination with a good understanding of the normal sources of variation in the cardiac silhouette. A good general principle is that the heart should be considered radiographically normal unless there is an obvious change in size or shape. Note also that a radiographically normal heart by no means excludes cardiac disease. The cardiac silhouette is more likely to be abnormal in disease associated with left-sided volume overload.

Canine cardiac size: rules of thumb

- The cardiac length (apex to base) should be approximately 70% of the dorsal to ventral distance of the thoracic cavity on a lateral view.
- The craniocaudal width should be between 2.5 (deep-chested dogs) and 3.5 (round-chested dogs) intercostal spaces on a lateral view.
- Cardiac width is usually 60–65% of the thoracic width on a DV view and no more than two-thirds of the thoracic width on a VD view.

Feline cardiac size: rules of thumb

- The cardiac silhouette should be no wider than 2.5 intercostal spaces on a lateral view.
- The maximal width should be approximately the same as the distance between the cranial border of the fifth rib and the caudal border of the seventh rib on a lateral view.

Vertebral heart score

A novel system of cardiac measurement was proposed by Buchanan and Bücheler in 1995, which aimed to circumvent the limitations in other methods attributable to inherent breed variation in cardiac size. It is called the vertebral (or Buchanan) heart score (or sum or size) (VHS). In this technique, using either a left or right lateral view, the cardiac long axis is measured from the ventral margin of the left principal bronchus to the most ventral contour of the cardiac apex and the maximal cardiac short axis in the central third region of the cardiac silhouette, perpendicular to the long axis, is measured. The left principal bronchus is located slightly ventral to the right principal bronchus and is better visible on a left lateral view. Each measurement is then transposed against the thoracic vertebral column from the cranial endplate of the fourth thoracic vertebra. Vertebral bodies are counted, and the sum gives the VHS (Figures 9.15 and 9.16).

The VHS is useful for those new to evaluating cardiac size on radiographs and also for the sequential assessment of cardiac size on repeat radiographs of the same animal. It has not been proven to be superior to subjective assessment. The suggested mean value for dogs in the original

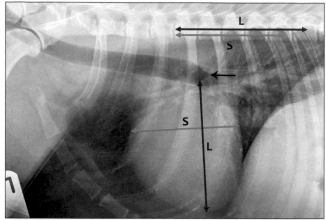

9.15 Technique to perform a VHS on a left lateral thoracic radiograph of a 6-year-old Labrador Retriever. First draw the long axis of the heart (L), connecting the ventral margin of the left stem bronchus at the carina with the ventral contour of the cardiac apex. Then draw the maximal short axis (S) of the dorsal third of the heart (at or above the level of the caudal vena cava) perpendicular to the long axis. Transpose both measurements on to the vertebral column, starting at the cranial endplate of the 4th thoracic vertebra. Count and add the number of vertebrae covered by both measurements. In this example L = 5.6 vertebrae and S = 4.6 vertebrae, giving the dog a VHS of 10.2 vertebrae, which is within the normal range for the breed (10.2–11.4). Both lateral views can be used for the VHS, but on the left lateral view, the left principal bronchus is more ventral than the right principal bronchus (arrowed), making it easier to determine the dorsal landmark for the L measurement.

How to perform a vertebral heart score

1. Take a well-positioned lateral thoracic radiograph.
2. Measure the distance between the ventral aspect of the carina and cardiac apex (length).
   - This can be with electronic callipers, a ruler or simply by marking the two points on the edge of a piece of paper.
3. Take a second measurement, perpendicular to the first at the widest part of the cardiac silhouette (usually corresponding to ventral border of caudal vena cava) (width).
4. From the cranial border of T4, transpose the initial length measurement (from step 2) caudally along the vertebral bodies. Count vertebral bodies, estimating to nearest 0.1 of a vertebra. Record v1 (number of vertebral bodies).
5. From the cranial border of T4, transpose the second width measurement (from step 3) caudally along the vertebral bodies. Count vertebral bodies, estimating to nearest 0.1 of a vertebra. Record v2 (number of vertebral bodies).
6. Add the two figures (v1 + v2) to get the VHS.

Normal vertebral heart score

Dog breed-specific values

Australian Cattle Dog: 10.5 ± 0.5 v
Beagle: 10.3 ± 0.4 v
Boston Terrier: 11.7 ± 1.4 v
Boxer: 11.6 ± 0.8 v
Bulldog: 12.7 ± 1.7 v
Cavalier King Charles Spaniel: 10.6 ± 0.5 v
Chihuahua: 10.0 ± 0.6 v
Dachshund: 9.7 ± 0.5 v
Dobermann: 10.0 ± 0.6 v
German Shepherd Dog: 9.7 ± 0.7 v
Greyhound: 10.5 ± 0.1 v
Labrador Retriever: 10.8 ± 0.6 v
Lhasa Apso: 9.6 ± 0.8 v
Norwich Terrier: 10.6 ± 0.6 v
Pomeranian: 10.5 ± 0.9 v
Pug: 10.7 ± 0.9 v
Rottweiler: 9.8 ± 0.1 v
Whippet: 11.0 ± 0.5 v
Yorkshire Terrier: 9.7 ± 0.5 v or 9.9 ± 0.6 v (data from two sources)

9.16 How to perform a VHS and normal values (mean ± standard deviation) for some dog breeds, puppies and cats.
T4 = fourth thoracic vertebra; v = vertebrae. (continues) ▶
(Data from Lamb *et al.* (2001), Bavegems *et al.* (2005), Marin *et al.* (2007), Kraetschmer *et al.* (2008), Jepsen-Grant *et al.* (2013), Luciani *et al.* (2019), Taylor CJ *et al.* (2020) and Puccinelli *et al.* (2021))

Normal vertebral heart score *continued*		
Puppies		
8.5–10.5 v		
Cats		
7.5 ± 0.3 v on a lateral view (The cardiac width on a DV or VD view is 3.4 ± 0.25 v if measured perpendicular to the long axis)		

9.16 (continued) How to perform a VHS and normal values (mean ± standard deviation) for some dog breeds, puppies and cats. T4 = fourth thoracic vertebra; v = vertebrae.

(Data from Lamb *et al.* (2001), Bavegems *et al.* (2005), Marin *et al.* (2007), Kraetschmer *et al.* (2008), Jepsen-Grant *et al.* (2013), Luciani *et al.* (2019), Taylor CJ *et al.* (2020) and Puccinelli *et al.* (2021))

multibreed study was 9.7 ± 0.5 vertebrae (range 8.5–10.5 vertebrae). However, considerable breed variation exists even in the VHS, and later studies have established breed-specific reference intervals (Lamb *et al.*, 2001; Jepsen-Grant *et al.*, 2013) (Figure 9.16). Note, the presence of thoracic vertebral anomalies will confound use of this measurement. Dogs with a higher body condition score may have a higher VHS (likely reflecting pericardial fat).

Artificial intelligence (see Chapter 6) may be used in the future for calculation of VHS or assessment of the cardiac silhouette (Burti *et al.*, 2020).

Vertebral left atrial size

Recently, measurement of the cardiac silhouette has attempted to quantify the severity of left atrial enlargement in dogs by using the vertebral left atrial size (VLAS), performed as follows (Figure 9.17):

1. Measure a line from the ventral border of the carina to the caudal border of the cardiac silhouette where the LA intersects with the dorsal margin of the CdVC.
2. Transpose this line to the same measurement used for VHS, starting at the cranial border of the fourth thoracic vertebra.
3. Count vertebral bodies, to the nearest 0.1 v.
   - Normal values are 1.4–2.2 v.

This appears to be clinically useful in assessing LA enlargement in various stages of myxomatous mitral valve disease (MMVD) (Malcolm *et al.*, 2018; Vezzosi *et al.*, 2020).

Trachea and carina position

The location of the trachea and carina can be useful in assessing cardiac size and chamber enlargement (Figure 9.18). On a lateral radiograph, the trachea diverges from the thoracic vertebral column. The angle of divergence is fairly standard amongst cat breeds but shows variation between dog breeds. The greatest angle is seen in deep-chested dogs, whereas in shallow-chested breeds the trachea may be almost parallel to the vertebral column. This should not be erroneously interpreted as representing cardiac enlargement. The caudal trachea is normally parallel to the sternum, and assessing this alignment may be preferable to assessing the vertebral–tracheal angle to assess for changes in height of the cardiac silhouette in the lateral view.

Just cranial to the tracheal bifurcation there is a normal ventral bend in the trachea (Figure 9.19). This is often lost in animals with left-sided cardiac enlargement; however, it may not be evident in normal dogs of shallow, round-chested breeds.

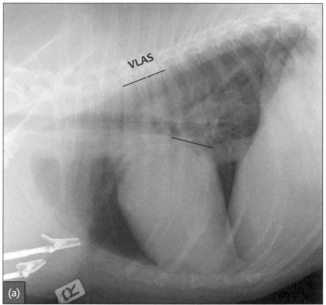

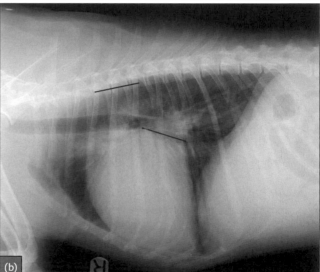

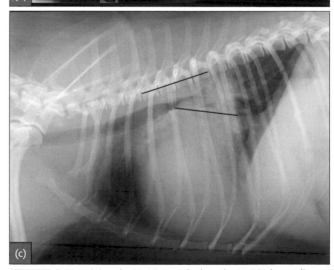

9.17 Determining the VLAS. To calculate the VLAS, draw a line from the carina to the caudal vena cava and compare the length of that line to the vertebral column. See text for measurement details. (a) Lateral thoracic radiograph of a normal Boxer with a VLAS of approximately 2.2. (b) Lateral thoracic radiograph of an Airedale Terrier with stage B2 myxomatous mitral valve disease (MMVD) and a VLAS of approximately 2.6. (c) Lateral thoracic radiograph of a Jack Russell Terrier with advanced MMVD with congestive heart failure and a VLAS of 4.

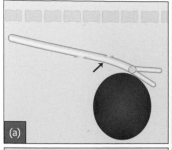
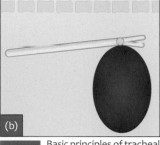
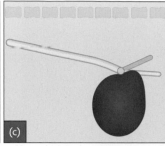
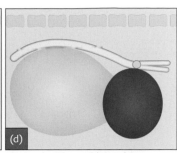
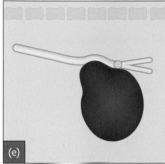

9.18 Basic principles of tracheal and bronchial displacement on lateral radiographs. The positions of the trachea, carina and principal bronchi can be very useful to assess cardiac chamber enlargement. Note that there is also variation in tracheal position between different dog breeds. (a) Normal. The trachea and principal bronchi have a gentle ventral divergence from the thoracic vertebral column. Note the slight ventral concavity (arrowed) in the trachea just cranial to the carina. (b) Left ventricular enlargement in isolation. When it is enlarged, the LV displaces the entire trachea dorsally and there is loss of the normal ventral bend cranial to the carina. (c) Left atrial enlargement in isolation. The LA creates a triangular or wedge-shaped soft tissue opacity at the caudal border of the cardiac silhouette and pushes the left principal bronchus (shown in dark blue) dorsally. (d) Cranial mediastinal mass. A cranial mediastinal mass (shown in pink) can elevate the trachea cranial to the carina anywhere along its length. Depending on the size and location of the mass, this may be focal elevation or, more commonly, elevation of the entire thoracic trachea with a pivotal point of the elevation over the mass. The cardiac size will be normal. (e) Right atrial enlargement or right atrial mass in isolation. It is very rare to see severe focal right atrial enlargement. An enlarged RA can focally dorsally deviate the trachea cranial to the carina (note that a heart base mass can also elevate the trachea in this position but usually has a different appearance on DV and VD views; see 'Cardiac neoplasia', below).

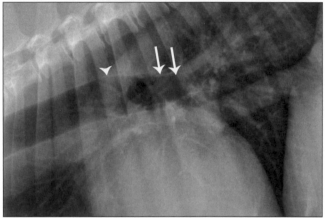

9.19 Close-up of a lateral thoracic radiograph of a dog demonstrating the normal appearance of the caudal trachea. Note the normal ventral bend (arrowhead) cranial to the carina, and the two principal bronchi almost level with one another (arrows point to their dorsal margins).

The carina should be located at the fourth or fifth intercostal space. The round radiolucent ring-like structures extending out from the trachea are cross-sectional views of either the left or the right principal bronchus (see Chapter 10). On DV and VD views the angle between the left and right principal bronchi is around 60 degrees at the bifurcation. The principal bronchi should create an inverted V shape on these views (Figure 9.20).

Pericardial fat stripe

It can be difficult to assess cardiac size when pleural effusion is present. Fat present between the fibrous pericardium and the pericardial mediastinal pleura may remain visible on the lateral view in animals with pleural effusion. This is known as the pericardial fat stripe and may aid radiographic assessment of the heart in animals with pleural fluid (Figure 9.21).

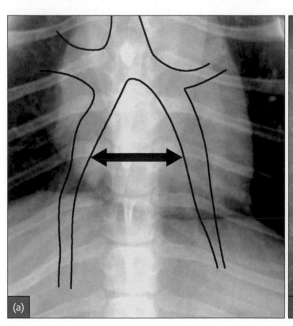

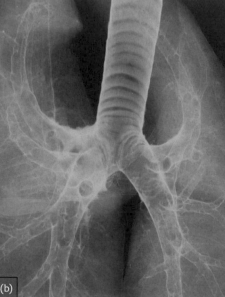

9.20 (a) Close-up of a DV thoracic radiograph of a normal dog at the level of the heart. The bronchial tree is outlined. The angle between the left and right principal bronchi (arrowed) should be about 60 degrees and form an upside-down V shape. This does vary somewhat with breed, but an increased angle or splayed appearance ('cowboy legs' sign) suggests left atrial or tracheobronchial lymph node enlargement. (b) Postmortem bronchogram showing the normal angle between the principal bronchi.
(Courtesy of B. Hopper)

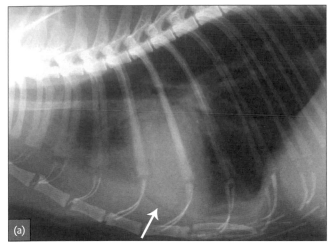

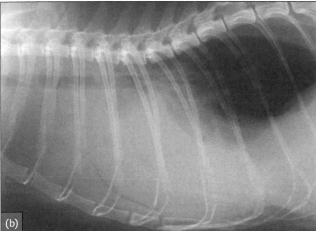

9.21 (a) Lateral thoracic radiograph of a cat with a small volume of pleural fluid associated with feline leukaemia virus infection. A narrow radiolucent line is visible in a position compatible with the cranial aspect of the heart (arrowed). Together with the position of the trachea and the caudal aspect of the cardiac silhouette, this line has the effect of completing a cardiac silhouette of normal appearance. (b) Lateral thoracic radiograph of a different cat with a larger volume of pleural fluid. In this instance, the position and size of the pericardial fat stripe, relative to the position of the trachea, suggests enlargement of the cardiac silhouette. Ultrasonography subsequently confirmed marked hypertrophic cardiomyopathy (and ruled out a mediastinal mass).
(Reproduced from Lamb (2000) with permission)

Normal major vessel physiological and radiographic anatomy

Aorta

The aorta is divided into three sections:

- The ascending aorta: short and arises from the cranial aspect of the heart. Has the same orientation as the LV
- The aortic arch: short and curves caudally. Gives rise to the brachiocephalic trunk and left subclavian artery
- The descending aorta: long and can be divided into thoracic and abdominal portions.

The aortic isthmus is the junction of the ascending aorta and the aortic arch. The ascending aorta contributes to the cranial heart base area and cannot be seen clearly due to border effacement with nearby structures (see Figure 9.3). The aortic arch and descending aorta are identified on lateral, DV and VD views (Figure 9.22). In the normal animal, the left border of the descending aorta is identified on DV and VD views.

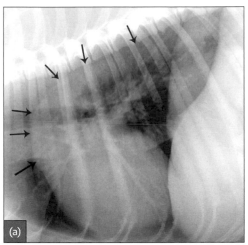

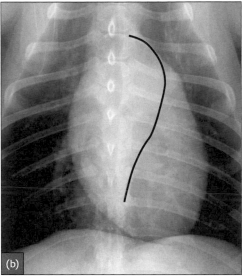

9.22 (a) Lateral and (b) DV thoracic radiographs of a dog showing the normal location and appearance of the aorta (arrowed in (a); black line in (b)).

The aortic diameter is similar to the height of adjacent vertebral bodies; aortic size does not alter in association with hypovolaemia or volume overload (unlike the CdVC).

A focal bulge in the aorta (sometimes also referred to as an elongated, redundant or tortuous aorta) at the aortic isthmus may be seen in a proportion of older cats (Figure 9.23). One study found that this was present in 28% of cats over 10 years of age.

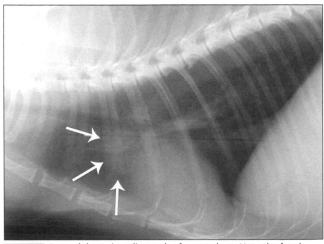

9.23 Lateral thoracic radiograph of an aged cat. Note the focal bulge in the aorta (arrowed).

Caudal vena cava

The CdVC receives blood from the abdomen, pelvis and hindlimbs. The final abdominal tributaries are the hepatic and phrenic veins. The CdVC enters the thorax by crossing the diaphragm on the right side within the plica venae cavae. It then traverses between the accessory and right caudal lung lobes to enter the RA dorsal to the inlet of the coronary sinus. It lies in close association with the right phrenic nerve.

The majority of the intrathoracic CdVC is easily seen on radiographs (Figure 9.24). On the lateral view, the CdVC typically extends cranioventrally from the diaphragm, crosses the caudal half of the right ventricular border and can often be seen overlapping the cardiac silhouette for a short distance. On DV and VD views, it is seen to the right of the median plane between the caudal right border of the heart and the diaphragm. On fully inspiratory or inflated lateral radiographs, the ventral border of the CdVC may be poorly defined because of the overlying accessory lung lobe.

The diameter of the CdVC is highly variable due to variations in intrathoracic pressure with respiration and stage of the cardiac cycle. It may also vary in pathological conditions such as right-sided heart disease, hypovolaemia or CdVC obstructive conditions (e.g. caval syndrome, masses; see 'Acquired vascular disease', below). Enlargement of the CdVC is more likely to suggest right-sided heart disease in the dog when:

- The CdVC:Ao ratio is >1.5 (strongly suggestive of right-sided heart abnormality)
- The CdVC:VL ratio is >1.3
- The CdVC:R4 ratio is >3.5.

Where Ao = aortic diameter, CdVC = the greatest diameter of the CdVC not overlapping the heart or diaphragm, R4 = diameter of the right fourth thoracic rib just ventral to the vertebral column and VL = the length of the thoracic vertebra over the tracheal bifurcation. CdVC:Ao should be interpreted with caution; considerable overlap has been shown in normal animals and those with right-sided heart disease.

Cranial vena cava

The cranial vena cava (CrVC) receives blood from the head, neck, thoracic wall and thoracic limbs. The axillary veins, together with the internal and external jugular veins, converge to form the right and left brachiocephalic veins. These then unite to create the CrVC, which continues into the cranial mediastinum and receives the costocervical and internal thoracic veins, as well as the azygos vein just cranial to the RA. Finally, the CrVC empties into the RA.

The CrVC is not seen as an individual structure on a radiograph unless a pneumomediastinum is present. Its ventral border is seen in the cranial mediastinum on the lateral view.

Azygos vein

The azygos vein forms from the first lumbar veins and passes through the aortic hiatus into the thorax. It then receives intercostal, subcostal, oesophageal and broncho-oesophageal veins and terminates in the CrVC outside the pericardium. It is not seen on a radiograph unless a severe pneumomediastinum is present or it is markedly enlarged. It then appears as a wavy vessel immediately ventral to the thoracic vertebral column, receiving tributaries from every intervertebral space (Figure 9.25). It may rarely be seen in very deep-chested, narrow breeds, such as the Greyhound, in the absence of a pneumomediastinum. In dogs and cats, the azygos vein is normally located to the right and dorsal to the descending aorta and enters the CrVC outside of the pericardium (right azygos type).

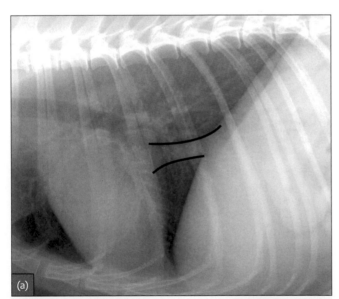
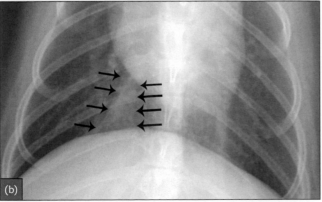

9.24 Close-ups of (a) lateral and (b) DV thoracic radiographs of a dog showing the normal size and location of the CdVC (lines in (a); arrows in (b)).

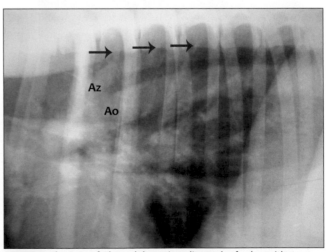

9.25 Close-up of a lateral thoracic radiograph of a dog with a severe pneumomediastinum after trauma. The azygos vein (Az) is visible as a narrow tube of soft tissue opacity ventral to the vertebral column and dorsal to the aorta (Ao), connecting with vessels from each intercostal space (arrowed).

Thoracic duct

The thoracic duct is the cranial continuation of the cisterna chyli and originates between the diaphragmatic crura. It has a variable course within the thorax but usually runs cranially along the right dorsal border of the descending aorta and the left border of the azygos vein. Cranial to the heart, the thoracic duct moves to the left and ventrally, along the surface of the left longus colli muscle. Its termination is variable, but it usually enters the CrVC or left jugular vein at the level of the thoracic inlet. The thoracic duct receives the left and right tracheal (jugular) trunks at the thoracic inlet for lymphatic drainage of the head and neck.

The thoracic duct is not seen on radiographs. It can be identified using radiographic or CT lymphangiography or on heavily T2-weighted magnetic resonance images.

Pulmonic trunk

The pulmonic trunk arises from the pulmonic valve and arches dorsally and caudally. It splits into right and left pulmonary arteries immediately caudal to the level of the aortic root. These then form further branches within the left and right lungs. The ligamentum arteriosum (the ductus arteriosus in fetal life) arises near the origin of the left pulmonary artery and joins with the aorta.

The pulmonic trunk is usually not seen on a lateral radiograph as it summates with the cardiac silhouette. On occasion it may be identified as a round soft tissue opacity located immediately ventral to the carina and it should not be confused with a nodule in this location (see Figure 9.41). An enlarged pulmonic trunk may overlie the ventral aspect of the trachea (pulmonic cap; see Figure 9.61). The left and right branches may be radiographically identified on the lateral view. The left branch runs slightly more cranial and also dorsal to the right branch. The pulmonic trunk contributes to the cranial left cardiac silhouette on DV and VD views (Figure 9.26). It appears more prominent during systole and on the VD view, compared with the DV view. This should not be interpreted as pathology. The left and right pulmonary arteries initially summate with on the heart, but further along their course they are seen as tubular soft tissue structures coursing caudo-laterally in association with the lateral aspects of the principal bronchi.

Cranial lobar pulmonary arteries and veins

Useful tip

To remember the location of the pulmonary veins compared with the arteries use the rhyme:

'Veins are ventral and central'

(i.e. veins are ventral to arteries on the lateral view and central (medial) to the arteries on the VD view).

The pulmonary arteries and veins in the cranial lung lobes can be seen on the lateral view with the arteries dorsal to the veins (Figure 9.27). They are best separated on the left lateral view. Arteries follow the bronchial tree closely, but veins are not as closely associated with the bronchi. Arteries are often slightly curved and often better defined compared with veins. Normally, the artery and vein of each pair are approximately the same size.

Various rules exist for the measurement of cranial lobar vessel size on the lateral view (see below), but a good general rule of thumb is that no cranial lobar vessel should be wider than the narrowest part of the third or fourth rib where it crosses the rib.

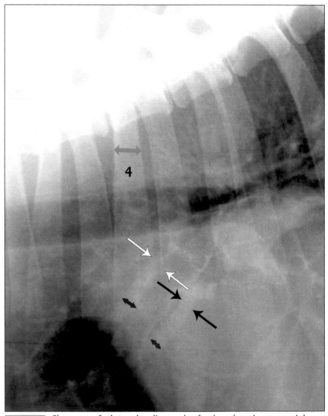

9.26 VD thoracic radiograph of a normal dog. The pulmonic trunk appears as a small focal bulge at the 1–2 o'clock location (arrowed). This can be a normal finding on a VD view, or when an exposure is made during systole, and should not be interpreted as disease.

9.27 Close-up of a lateral radiograph of a dog showing a cranial lobar pulmonary artery (white arrows) and vein (black arrows). At the point where they cross the third or fourth rib (blue arrow), these vessels (red arrows) should be no wider than the narrowest part of the rib.

Rules for cranial lobar pulmonary vascular size in the dog and cat (lateral radiographs)

Dog
The cranial lobar pulmonary vessels should be approximately the same size. The ratio of the diameter of the artery or vein to that of the proximal third of the fourth rib, at the level of the fourth intercostal space, is 0.73 (± 0.24) with a 95% confidence interval of 0.26–1.2.

These vessels should be considered enlarged when more than 1.2 times greater in diameter than the proximal third of the fourth rib at the fourth intercostal space.

Alternatively, the cranial lobar pulmonary arteries should not be greater in diameter than the proximal third of the third rib on the lateral radiograph.

Cat
The diameter of the right cranial lobar artery should be 0.5–1.0 times that of the proximal third of the fourth rib (mean artery:rib of 0.70), when measured at the level of the fourth rib. The cranial lobe veins should be 0.2 cm (± 0.03 cm) in diameter at the same point.

Rules for caudal lobar pulmonary vascular size in the dog and cat (DV radiographs)
The pulmonary artery and vein of each caudal lobe should be similar in size.

The diameter of the artery or vein should be no greater than that of the ninth rib where they cross (anecdotal).

In the cat, a cut-off for pulmonary arterial enlargement of a diameter 1.6 times that of the ninth rib has been suggested in assessment for heartworm disease.

Caudal lobar pulmonary arteries and veins

On DV and VD views, the caudal pulmonary arteries are located lateral to the veins and can be traced cranially towards the pulmonic trunk (Figure 9.28). Caudal lobar pulmonary arteries and veins are more easily identified on the DV view due to the presence of surrounding aerated lung, angle of the X-ray beam relative to the diaphragm, and the effects of magnification. The veins are medially located and run towards the LA, which is located centrally in the cardiac silhouette between the principal bronchi.

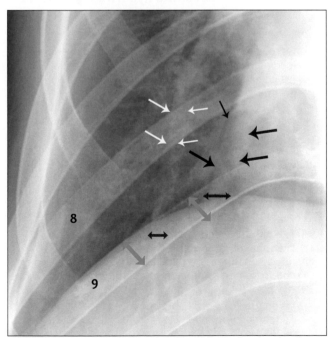

9.28 Close-up of a DV thoracic radiograph of a dog showing the right caudal lobar pulmonary artery (white arrows) and vein (black arrows) as they cross the eighth and ninth ribs. The vessels are measured where they cross the ninth rib. Blue arrows = rib measurements; red arrows = vessel measurements.

Interpretative principles

Thoracic radiographs are extremely useful in the evaluation of animals with cardiovascular disease. However, radiography and echocardiography are complementary techniques and it is important to understand the benefits and limitations of both imaging modalities in the assessment of cardiac disease.

In simple terms, echocardiography is far more accurate than radiography in identifying chamber enlargement and other structural abnormalities. Echocardiography also provides vital functional information that cannot be obtained radiographically. However, radiographs remain indispensable in the evaluation of pulmonary vascular and parenchymal changes secondary to heart disease. For example, a radiograph will quickly reveal evidence of pulmonary venous congestion and/or cardiogenic pulmonary oedema in left-sided failure, or pleural effusion in right-sided or biventricular failure. Thoracic radiographs are also extremely valuable in monitoring the progress of therapy in heart failure.

Chapter 2 provides further information on echocardiographic technique and some normal echocardiographic measurements.

This section covers the radiographic features of specific cardiac chamber and major vessel enlargement, and the evaluation of congestive heart failure (CHF). It is important to have a good knowledge of cardiac anatomy, physiology and pathophysiology when approaching a thoracic radiograph for the evaluation of cardiac disease. It should be remembered that radiographic changes do not show the disease itself, but rather the haemodynamic consequences of the condition. Additional radiographic findings in certain cardiac conditions are described with the specific acquired or congenital heart diseases in later parts of this chapter.

Microcardia
Radiographic features

- The cardiac silhouette is narrow and pointed on the lateral view (Figure 9.29) and narrow on DV and VD views.
- The apex may lose contact with the sternum.
- There may be small pulmonary arteries and veins.
- The lung fields may be hyperlucent (without hyperinflation) depending on the cause of the microcardia.
- The CdVC may be narrow.

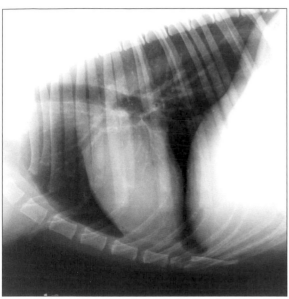

9.29 Lateral thoracic radiograph of a dog with Addison's disease (hypoadrenocorticism). The dog has microcardia. Note the narrow pointed appearance of the cardiac silhouette.

Differential diagnoses

- Hypovolaemia: shock, dehydration. The lungs are underperfused and the CdVC may be small (Figure 9.30).
- Addison's disease (hypoadrenocorticism). The heart is physically smaller due to chronic electrolyte abnormalities with or without hypovolaemia and shock in an acute Addisonian crisis.
- Emaciation.
- Atrophic myopathies.
- Artefact: causes include pneumothorax, deep-chested dogs, deep inspiration or pulmonary hyperinflation.

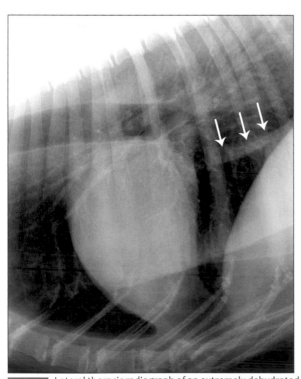

9.30 Lateral thoracic radiograph of an extremely dehydrated dog. The CdVC is narrow (arrowed), the lungs are hyperlucent, and the cardiac silhouette is small and pointed.

Normal radiographic cardiac size

Some cardiac diseases may not produce any apparent radiographic changes. Examples include:

- Endocarditis
- Concentric ventricular hypertrophy:
    - Aortic stenosis (if no post-stenotic dilatation)
    - Hypertrophic cardiomyopathy (HCM) (preclinical)
    - Pulmonic stenosis (when mild and no post-stenotic dilatation)
- Other myocardial disease:
    - Acute myocardial failure
    - Early or mild myocarditis
    - Myocardial neoplasia
- Acute ruptured chordae tendinae
- Small atrial septal defect (ASD), ventricular septal defect (VSD) or patent ductus arteriosus (PDA)
- Some types of pericardial disease:
    - Constrictive pericarditis
    - Acute traumatic haemopericardium
- Arrhythmias
- Overzealous use of diuretic therapy in heart disease with CHF.

Cardiac chamber enlargement

The limitations of radiography for the evaluation of each specific cardiac chamber are discussed above (see 'Identifying the cardiac chambers', above). Often, more than one chamber will be enlarged and this will complicate interpretation of changes in the cardiac silhouette. Artefactual chamber and major vessel enlargement will be seen on poorly positioned radiographs and the utmost care should be taken in obtaining perfectly straight views.

In the following section, the DV view is described rather than the VD view, as the former is more commonly obtained to assess cardiac cases.

Concentric and eccentric hypertrophy: what is the difference?

Ventricular hypertrophy may occur in response to:

- Increased systolic pressure (a pressure overload) leading to concentric hypertrophy: the ventricular wall gets thicker and the lumen size remains normal (or reduced)
- Increased diastolic pressure and volume (a volume overload) leading to eccentric hypertrophy (also known as dilatation): the ventricular wall remains a normal size and the lumen size increases. Initially, the proportion of wall thickness and chamber diameter remains preserved (compensatory eccentric hypertrophy) but later the wall may appear relatively thin compared with the chamber diameter (maladaptive remodelling).

The different types of hypertrophy have implications for radiographic interpretation. Only changes that affect the outline of the cardiac silhouette can be appreciated radiographically·

- Concentric hypertrophy can be extremely difficult to recognize on a radiograph
- Eccentric hypertrophy is more easily seen as it reflects volume overload.

Note that, in contrast to the ventricles, only the atria usually show dilatation (no evident hypertrophy) in cardiac disease.

Right atrium

Right atrial enlargement is very uncommon in isolation and is also difficult to see radiographically unless it is severe (Figure 9.31).

Lateral view:
- Focal bulge on cranial aspect of cardiac silhouette just ventral to the terminal trachea (cranial to the carina).
- May push the trachea dorsally at this point if large enough or if a right atrial mass is present.
- May merge with an enlarged RV.

Dorsoventral view:
- Bulge in cardiac silhouette at 9–11 o'clock.
- May merge with an enlarged RV.

Right ventricle

Right ventricular enlargement is commonly overdiagnosed during thoracic radiography. This is partly because the shallow-chested conformation of many dog breeds can mimic certain features of right-sided cardiomegaly (such as increased sternal contact). Great care must be taken to differentiate breed-specific variation from true right-sided cardiac enlargement. It is very important to evaluate the two orthogonal views before confirming increased sternal contact is due to right ventricular enlargement (Figure 9.32). If accompanied by left-sided changes and right atrial enlargement, it may be difficult to identify right ventricular enlargement as a single entity.

Lateral view: To evaluate the size of the RV, a line can be drawn from the carina to the cardiac apex; approximately two-thirds of the cardiac silhouette should lie cranial to this line and one-third caudal to it. An increased cranial component (e.g. four-fifths cranial and one-fifth caudal to the line) suggests right-sided enlargement. Rotation of the cardiac apex caudodorsally away from the sternum (i.e. pointing more towards the liver than the sternum; apex tipping) is a sensitive sign of right ventricular enlargement but is not always present. Right ventricular (or atrial) enlargement may displace the trachea dorsally over the heart base and cranial to the carina, but the trachea will still maintain its normal terminal ventral bend (unlike in left ventricular enlargement; see Figure 9.18).

Other findings with RV enlargement include widening of the cardiac silhouette (non-specific) and increased cardiosternal contact (non-specific and not very useful – do not rely on this in isolation).

Dorsoventral view: This is often more reliable than the lateral view for evaluation of right-sided enlargement. Findings include:

- Increased size of the cardiac silhouette on the right side of the thorax
- Reduced distance between the right cardiac border and the right thoracic wall
- A typical 'reversed D' shape
- On occasion, the apex may be pushed towards the left, creating a false impression of left-sided cardiomegaly.

Left atrium

Radiography is very useful in identifying left atrial enlargement and is generally sensitive for moderate to severe dilatation (Figures 9.33 and 9.34).

Lateral view:
Dogs:
- Elevation (with or without compression) of the left principal bronchus (seen as a separation of the two principal bronchi) (see also Chapter 10).
- Loss of the normal gentle cranial curvature of the caudal margin of the cardiac silhouette. Instead, the caudodorsal margin of the cardiac silhouette becomes straight and then eventually triangular, forming a left atrial 'tent' or 'wedge'.
- Increased height of the caudodorsal border of the heart.
- Enlarged pulmonary veins may be seen entering the LA as indistinct nodular opacities in this region.

Cats:
- The LA is situated more cranially than in dogs and it is harder to identify on the lateral view.

Dorsoventral view:
Dogs:
- The enlarged LA is projected over the cardiac silhouette at the 5–7 o'clock position (between the principal bronchi). This results in divergence (or splaying) of the principal bronchi (also known as the

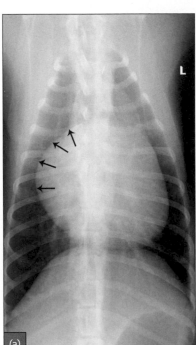

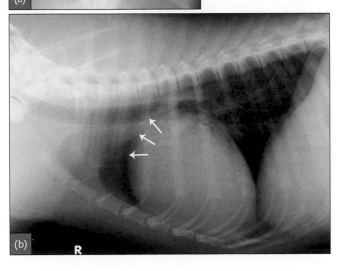

9.31 (a) DV and (b) right lateral thoracic radiographs of a 7-month-old Old English Sheepdog with tricuspid dysplasia. Right atrial enlargement can be seen on both views (arrowed). The RV is also volume overloaded with this condition, which affects the cardiac silhouette. (a) The DV view shows slight rotation, so the cranial mediastinum is projected to the left side.

'cowboy legs' sign). This must be differentiated from enlargement of the middle tracheobronchial lymph node, which will produce divergence of the principal bronchi on DV and VD views but will push them ventrally on a lateral view (see Chapter 10).

- A large LA may also create a 'double density' or more correctly, 'double opacity' sign on this view. This is the presence of two differing soft tissue opacities between the principal bronchi. This results from the enlarged atrium summating with the ventricle and producing more attenuation of the X-ray beam.
- An enlarged LAA may be seen at the 2.30–3 o'clock position.

Cats:

- The more cranial location means that an enlarged LA and LAA are seen at the left cranial border of the cardiac silhouette (even as cranial as the 1–2 o'clock position).

- A severely enlarged LA will bulge towards the left and can cause a shift of the cardiac apex to the right. Right atrial enlargement may also be present, or the LA may be so enlarged that the interatrial septum and right atrial wall are pushed rightwards. This can create the appearance of a 'valentine heart' shaped cardiac silhouette (Figure 9.35).

Left ventricle

Left ventricular enlargement due to eccentric hypertrophy is usually easily recognized on radiographs, whereas enlargement due to concentric hypertrophy is difficult to identify. This is important as animals with severe left-sided concentric hypertrophy (e.g. aortic stenosis) may have radiographically normal cardiac silhouettes.

Left ventricular enlargement is often accompanied by left atrial enlargement (see Figures 9.33 and 9.34). It may also be accompanied by right-sided changes.

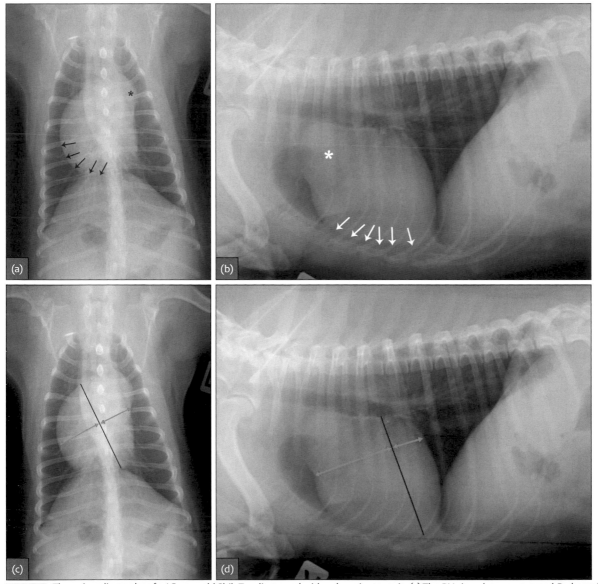

9.32 Thoracic radiographs of a 1.5-year-old Shih Tzu diagnosed with pulmonic stenosis. (a) The DV view shows a reversed-D-shaped cardiac silhouette, typical of right ventricular enlargement (arrowed). (b) The lateral view shows increased sternal contact with pericardial fat confirming mild apex tipping, consistent with right ventricular enlargement and concentric hypertrophy (arrowed). Both views show an enlarged pulmonic trunk (∗). The lateral view is rotated, but still of diagnostic quality. (c) On the DV view, a line is drawn through the cardiac silhouette from the right side of the mediastinum to the cardiac apex; the right:left ratio of the cardiac silhouette is >1:1, consistent with right heart enlargement (normal is approximately 1:1). (d) On the lateral view, a line is drawn from the carina to the apex; the cranial:caudal ratio of the cardiac silhouette is >2:1, consistent with right heart enlargement (normal is approximately 2:1).

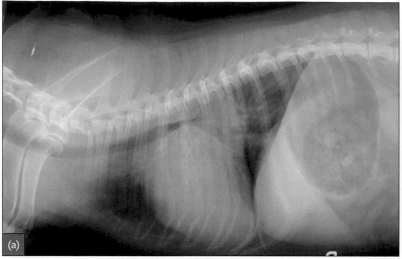

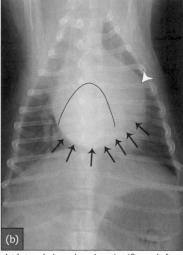

9.33 Thoracic radiographs of a Lancashire Heeler with advanced MMVD and CHF. (a) Right lateral view showing significant left atrial enlargement tenting from the caudodorsal border of the cardiac silhouette (green shading). There is marked tracheal elevation; concurrent left ventricular enlargement contributes to the increased height of the cardiac silhouette. The principal bronchi are divided by the left atrial enlargement, elevating the left caudal lobar bronchus by a greater extent than the right bronchus. (b) DV view. The lateral deviation of the caudal lobar bronchi giving the cowboy leg sign is seen (black line = medial walls). The double opacity sign is evident (arrowed), showing the enlarged LA as a positive summation shadow on the cardiac silhouette. The LA extends to the LAA, projecting beyond the cardiac silhouette at 2–3 o'clock (arrowhead).

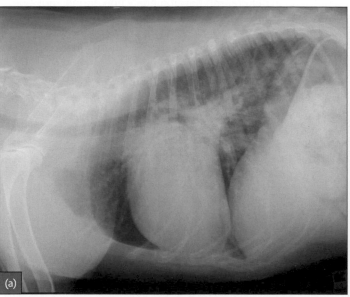

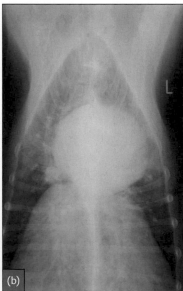

9.34 (a) Lateral and (b) DV thoracic radiographs of a Dobermann with dilated cardiomyopathy and CHF. Note that left atrial enlargement is often the most prominent feature of the cardiac silhouette in this breed. Because of the very vertical heart in the normal Dobermann, left atrial enlargement can result in the LA being the most caudal part of the cardiac silhouette; as evident on the DV view. (a) The lateral view shows tracheal elevation and left atrial tenting. (b) This is difficult to see on the DV view as the left ventricular apex summates with the LA.

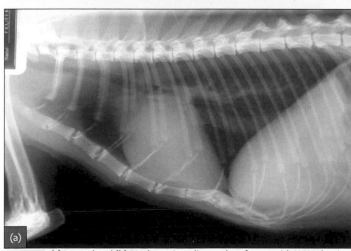

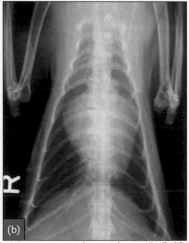

9.35 (a) Lateral and (b) DV thoracic radiographs of a cat with HCM that is receiving treatment for CHF (controlled). (a) The lateral view does not clearly identify the left atrial enlargement. There is increased sternal contact, but echocardiography showed only left ventricular enlargement (concentric hypertrophy) and no right heart enlargement. (b) The DV view shows apparent biatrial enlargement, resulting in the 'valentine heart' shaped cardiac silhouette. Echocardiography did not identify right atrial enlargement; marked left atrial enlargement can result in the interatrial septum and right atrial wall being displaced to the right.

Lateral view:

- Tracheal elevation (of the entire trachea and with loss of the normal terminal ventral bend) (Figure 9.36).
- The caudal cardiac border becomes straighter (see Figures 9.33, 9.34 and 9.36) or, less commonly, rounder than usual.

Dorsoventral view:

- Increased length of cardiac silhouette.
- Other signs are not as reliable.
- The cardiac apex may be more displaced into the left hemithorax or may sometimes be shifted to the right (Figure 9.36a).
- The apex becomes rounder.

Generalized cardiomegaly

The entire cardiac silhouette may appear enlarged in many diseases and this is called generalized cardiomegaly. It is difficult (and usually inaccurate) to detect mild generalized cardiomegaly unless previous radiographs are available from the same animal. A moderate to severe generalized cardiomegaly is seen as an increase in width and height on the lateral view, and width and length on DV views (Figure 9.37). The cardiac silhouette may also appear more generally rounded than usual. Care should be taken to try and distinguish generalized cardiomegaly from pericardial effusion (see below).

Pericardial enlargement

Any increase in pericardial content or thickness can create the appearance of generalized, rounded (or globoid) enlargement of the cardiac silhouette. The most common cause is the presence of pericardial effusion (see 'Pericardial disease', below).

Pericardial effusion can be distinguished from generalized cardiomegaly using:

- Ultrasonography (quick, accurate and extremely easy to perform for this distinction). Effusion will be apparent as an anechoic area peripheral to the heart
- Radiographs (not nearly as reliable and not recommended):
  - The border of the cardiac silhouette is sharp in pericardial effusion, compared with a blurry border in generalized cardiomegaly (the normal movement blur of the beating heart is not recognized when it is encased in a fluid-filled pericardial cavity) (Figure 9.38)

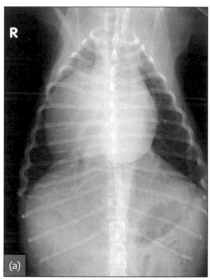

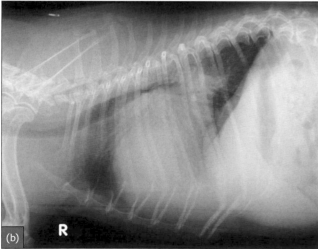

9.36 Thoracic radiographs of a Cavalier King Charles Spaniel that is receiving treatment for advanced MMVD and CHF. (a) The DV view shows the left ventricular apex is shifted to the right, which is associated with left ventricular enlargement. The very enlarged LA can be seen, resulting in double opacity, and the caudal lobar bronchi can be seen as a cowboy leg appearance. (b) The lateral view shows a very tall cardiac silhouette, resulting in severe dorsal displacement of the caudal trachea. This is due to both left atrial and left ventricular enlargement.

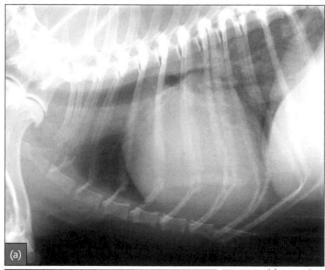

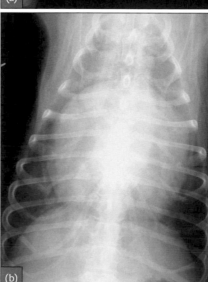

9.37 (a) Lateral and (b) DV thoracic radiographs of a middle-aged crossbreed dog with generalized cardiomegaly, secondary to MMVD.

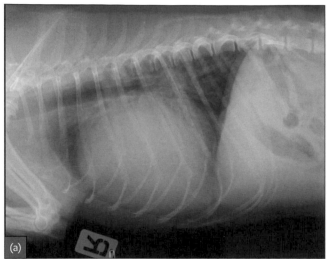

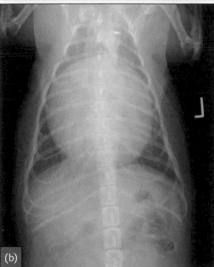

9.38 Thoracic radiographs of a 12-year-old terrier cross with a long-standing heart murmur that suffered an episode of collapse and then presented in cardiogenic shock. Both the (a) lateral and (b) DV views show a globoid cardiac silhouette with a static outline (most evident on the DV view). The dog had advanced MMVD but no overt CHF. Pericardial effusion was present and was believed to be due to a left atrial tear, as the LA was very dilated on echocardiography. The LA can be seen on the lateral view. Most cases of pericardial effusion do not show any radiographic evidence of specific chamber enlargement, but when the LA is very dilated (as detected by echocardiography), left atrial rupture must be considered as a cause.

- The cardiac silhouette often appears almost spherical on lateral, DV and VD views
- No individual specific chamber enlargement is usually recognized in pericardial effusion (except in cases of left atrial rupture; Figure 9.38). This is also often the case for generalized cardiomegaly, by definition
- The lungs may be underperfused due to the effects of tamponade (may see pulmonary venous distension in generalized cardiomegaly)
- In cases of slowly accumulating pericardial effusion, there may be clinical and radiographic evidence of right-sided heart failure (but this may also be present with generalized heart disease)
- In cats, pericardial effusion is commonly mild, in which case the cardiac silhouette resembles a normal canine cardiac silhouette (see Figure 9.167c).

Changes in the major vessels
Aorta
Entire aortic arch enlarged:
- Seen as a focal bulge on the cranial aspect of the heart on the lateral view.
- Seen as widening of the caudal part of the cranial mediastinum on the DV view.
- Possible causes:
  - Subaortic stenosis (or, less commonly, valvular stenosis) resulting in turbulence and post-stenotic dilatation (Figure 9.39)
  - Age-related change in the cat (see Figure 9.23).

Enlarged descending part of the aortic arch:
- Usually only seen on the DV view as a focal bulge when the left lateral border of the aorta is traced from caudal to cranial.
- May be seen as a bulge at the classic 11–1 o'clock location on the DV view and an apparent elongation of the cardiac silhouette.
- Possible causes: PDA (see Figure 9.50c) or reverse PDA (rPDA) (see Figure 9.54).

Other aortic enlargements or abnormalities:
- Aortic aneurysm:
  - Secondary to *Spirocerca lupi* infestation (see Chapter 10)
  - Dissecting aortic aneurysms have been reported in dogs and cats
  - Ductus aneurysm or ductus diverticulum.
- Marfan-like syndrome leads to pronounced dilatation of the aortic root and aortic arch (see 'Vascular abnormalities' below; see Figure 9.115) (Lenz *et al.*, 2015).
- Coarctation of the aorta with post-stenotic dilatation (see 'Vascular abnormalities' below; see Figure 9.114).
- Redundant aorta:
  - Aged cats
  - Brachycephalic dogs
  - Congenital hypothyroidism.
  Abnormal location:
  - Situs inversus
  - Vascular ring anomalies (most commonly persistent right aortic arch).
- Calcification or mineralization of the aorta:
  - Incidental non-significant aortic mineralization in dogs (more common in older dogs and Rottweilers) (Figure 9.40)

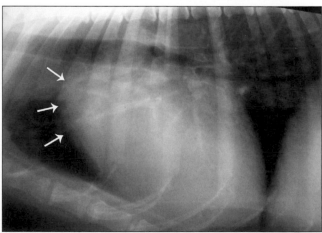

9.39 Lateral thoracic radiograph of a dog with subaortic stenosis. The entire aortic arch is enlarged (arrowed). This was confirmed on the DV view.

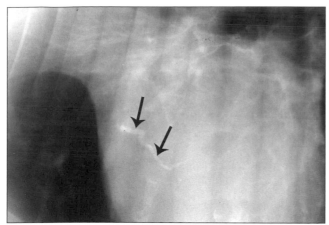

9.40 Incidental aortic calcification identified on a lateral thoracic radiograph of a 10-year-old Weimaraner. The calcification is seen as a wavy opaque line over the cranial border of the cardiac silhouette (arrowed).

- Primary or secondary hyperparathyroidism
- Hypervitaminosis D
- Lymphoma
- Hyperadrenocorticism
- *S. lupi* infestation
- Arteriosclerosis.
- Aortic body tumour (see 'Cardiac neoplasia', below).

Caudal vena cava

The normal size of the CdVC is described above (see 'Imaging anatomy'). Caution should be used when diagnosing changes in CdVC size on a radiograph. Caval size varies markedly with respiratory and cardiac cycle and thoracic and abdominal pressures. Changes in caval size should not be diagnosed from a single radiograph. A genuine alteration in size will be seen on repeated radiographs.

Wide caudal vena cava:

- Right-sided CHF.
- Cardiac tamponade.
- Constrictive pericarditis.
- Obstruction of the CdVC from the level of the hepatic veins to the level of the RA (Budd–Chiari-like syndrome):
  - Thrombosis
  - Caval syndrome associated with heartworm disease
  - Compression or invasion of the cava by tumours or other masses (see Figure 9.189)
  - Trauma-induced stricture
  - Fibrosis
  - Diaphragmatic hernia
  - Congenital cardiac (e.g. cor triatriatum dexter) or caval (e.g. membranous obstruction) anomalies.

Narrow caudal vena cava:

- Shock.
- Hypovolaemia (see Figure 9.30).
- Addison's disease (hypoadrenocorticism).
- Artefactual (pulmonary hyperinflation).

Mineralized caudal vena cava: This is rare. Causes include:

- Mineralized masses (see Figure 9.189)
- Other dystrophic mineralization
- Metastatic mineralization (e.g. hyperadrenocorticism, secondary hyperparathyroidism).

Segmental aplasia of the caudal vena cava: This is a rare congenital anomaly where part of the CdVC is missing and blood returns to the heart via the azygos vein. A markedly enlarged azygos vein will be identified. The azygos vein can be on the right or the left side of the aorta.

Persistent left cranial vena cava: This is relatively common and only really of significance when performing cardiac catheterization or thoracic surgery. The left CrVC persists from fetal life and drains into the coronary sinus. It is not identified on plain radiographs but can be suspected based on echocardiography with a dilated coronary sinus (see Figures 9.116 and 9.117 and 'Congenital vascular disease', below).

Pulmonic trunk

Dilatation of the pulmonic trunk is difficult to detect on the lateral view due to superimposition over the cardiac silhouette. The DV view will show an enlarged pulmonic trunk as a bulge at the 1–2 o'clock position.

Enlarged pulmonic trunk segment:

- Pulmonic stenosis: post-stenotic dilatation (Figure 9.41; see Figures 9.32 and 9.61).

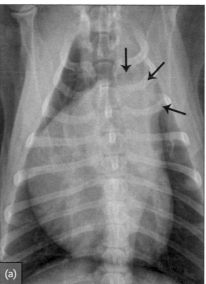

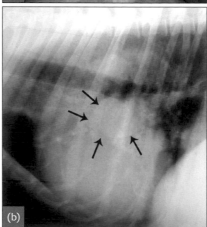

9.41 (a) DV and (b) lateral thoracic radiographs of a dog with pulmonic stenosis and heartworm disease. (a) The enlarged pulmonic trunk can be seen as a bulge at the 1–2 o'clock position (arrowed). (b) The pulmonic trunk may mimic a nodule on the lateral radiograph when an end-on view is obtained (arrowed). This may occasionally occur in normal dogs or, as in this case, when the pulmonic trunk is enlarged. The lateral radiograph is slightly rotated.

- Increased circulating volume due to PDA, ASD or VSD (see Figure 9.50).
- Pulmonary hypertension.
- Severe heartworm disease or angiostrongylosis.
- Artefactual:
  - VD position
  - Systole
  - Positional rotation.

Pulmonary arteries and veins

Methods of assessing pulmonary artery and vein size are described above. Examples of pulmonary arterial and venous enlargement are shown in Figure 9.42. Figure 9.43 gives differential diagnoses for variations in pulmonary vascular size.

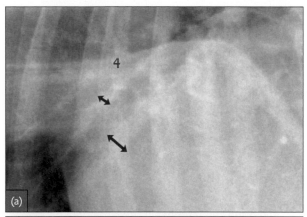

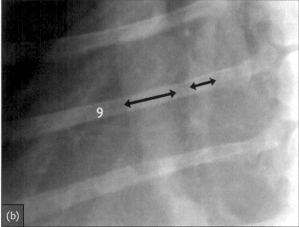

9.42 Pulmonary arterial and venous enlargement. The pulmonary artery and vein measurements are shown by arrows and the rib number is also shown. (a) Moderately enlarged cranial lobar pulmonary veins on a close-up of a lateral radiograph of a dog with heart failure. (b) Severely enlarged right caudal lobar pulmonary artery on a DV view of a dog with heartworm disease.

Small pulmonary arteries and veins
• Dehydration
• Shock
• Hypoadrenocorticism
• Positive pressure ventilation (and other causes of pulmonary hyperinflation)
• Pericardial effusion with tamponade
• Constrictive pericarditis
• Severe pulmonic stenosis
• Right-to-left shunts (tetralogy of Fallot, reverse PDA)
• Focal due to pulmonary thromboembolism

9.43 Differential diagnoses for variations in pulmonary blood vessel size. (continues)

Large pulmonary arteries
• Pulmonary hypertension
• Pulmonary thromboembolism
• Heartworm disease
• Left-to-right shunts (PDA, VSD, ASD)
• Angiostrongylosis (but often not a feature)
• Peripheral arteriovenous fistula

Large pulmonary veins
• Congestive left heart failure
• In right-to-left shunts the veins may appear larger as the arteries are small

Large pulmonary arteries and veins
• Left heart failure
• Left-to-right shunts (PDA, VSD, ASD)
• Excessive intravenous fluid administration

9.43 (continued) Differential diagnoses for variations in pulmonary blood vessel size.

Heart failure

Heart failure can be defined in many ways. One definition is that heart failure is the end result of severe heart disease and is a clinical syndrome, resulting in systolic and/or diastolic dysfunction severe enough to overwhelm the cardiovascular system's compensatory mechanisms. Forward heart failure is usually not evident from radiographs (hypotension and signs of poor cardiac output are present). Backwards heart failure is CHF and this can be subdivided into:

- Left-sided CHF
- Right-sided CHF
- Biventricular CHF.

Radiographic examination provides an invaluable insight into the presence and severity of CHF.

Radiographic features of left-sided congestive heart failure in the dog

Depending on severity of presentation or treatment prior to obtaining the radiographs, overt signs of CHF are inferred if the following triad of signs is identified:

- Left atrial enlargement is normally present (rare exception: acute rupture of chordae tendinae)
- Pulmonary venous congestion (can resolve with prior diuretic treatment)
- Cardiogenic pulmonary oedema. A pulmonary infiltrate is inferred as being cardiogenic pulmonary oedema in the presence of the other two signs. In the dog, it is predominantly caudodorsal or perihilar on the lateral view and may be worse in the right lung field on the DV view (Figures 9.44 and 9.45).

Cardiogenic pulmonary oedema can vary in severity depending on clinical signs on presentation (e.g. mild tachypnoea to severe dyspnoea) and prior treatment with diuretics before obtaining the radiographs (although radiographic changes often lag behind clinical responses to treatment).

Signs of cardiogenic pulmonary oedema can be identified within the lungs:

- Progresses from faint interstitial infiltrate or ground-glass opacity (Figure 9.45) to severe lung consolidation (alveolar pattern) (see Figure 9.44)

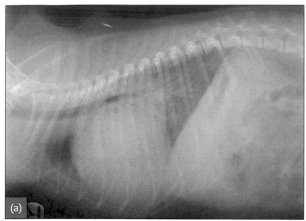

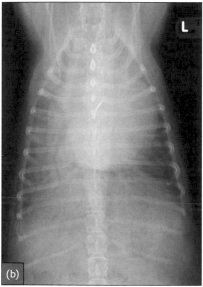

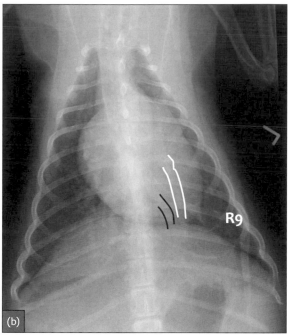

9.45 (continued) Thoracic radiographs of a Cocker Spaniel with dilated cardiomyopathy, following initial diuretic treatment. (b) The DV view confirms mainly left-sided cardiomegaly. The caudal lobar pulmonary arteries and veins are both increased in size compared with the ninth rib (R9) as they cross it (the left-sided vessels are more easily assessed). White lines = pulmonary artery; black lines = pulmonary vein.

- Usually first seen in the perihilar region on the lateral view and often symmetrical, though the right caudal lobe is also often a predilection site (seen on the DV view; see Figure 9.44)
- Usually extends from a central to a more peripheral, especially caudodorsal, location.

Since cardiogenic pulmonary oedema is a consequence of pulmonary capillary hypertension, with hydrostatic pressures pushing fluid into the interstitial space in the lungs, there is always an interstitial component. As the pulmonary oedema worsens, the pressures push fluid into the airspaces (alveoli) causing progressive pulmonary parenchymal opacification. However, cardiogenic pulmonary oedema never gives a solely alveolar pattern.

Note that severe left-sided heart disease must also be present to make the diagnosis of left-sided heart failure. Non-cardiogenic pulmonary oedema may mimic the radiographic appearance (see Chapter 12) in the absence of left atrial enlargement. One complicating situation is that of acute-onset heart failure, such as secondary to ruptured chordae tendinae. In this situation, substantial left-sided cardiomegaly may not be present. Echocardiographic examination will provide an accurate diagnosis.

Radiographic features of left-sided congestive heart failure in the cat

- Cardiogenic pulmonary oedema (Figures 9.46 and 9.47; see also Chapter 12). May appear similar to that in the dog or may appear as patchy unevenly distributed parenchymal opacification throughout the lung fields. The variable appearance of cardiogenic oedema in the cat makes diagnosis harder.
- Pleural effusion. In cats, pleural effusion may be seen in left-sided heart failure. This is poorly understood but is thought to be due to an anatomical variation in visceral pleural drainage.

9.44 Thoracic radiographs of a Jack Russell Terrier with advanced MMVD and left-sided CHF. (a) The lateral view shows marked, mainly left-sided cardiomegaly with tracheal elevation. The caudodorsal border of the cardiac silhouette cannot be easily seen because of the presence of a parenchymal opacification (mixed interstitial–alveolar pulmonary infiltrate). (b) The DV view shows generalized cardiomegaly and reveals that the parenchymal opacification is mainly right sided and consolidated (alveolar pattern) with air bronchograms. The pulmonary vasculature cannot be reliably assessed from either view because of the lung pattern.

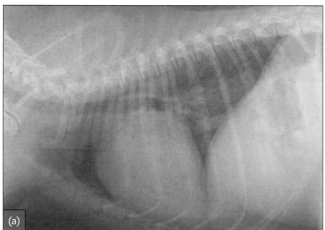

9.45 Thoracic radiographs of a Cocker Spaniel with dilated cardiomyopathy, following initial diuretic treatment. (a) The right lateral view shows generalized cardiomegaly and a mild residual interstitial lung pattern, which is mainly perihilar. The cranial lobar pulmonary vessels are within normal limits. (continues) ▶

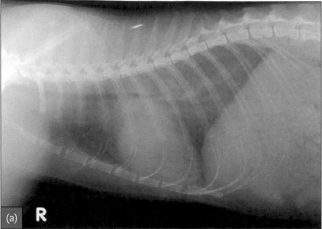

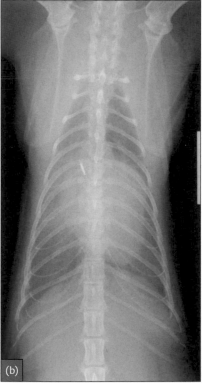

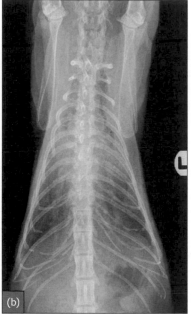

9.46 (a) Lateral and (b) DV thoracic radiographs of a cat with HCM and left-sided CHF. Both views show a patchy interstitial pattern. (b) The DV view shows the beginnings of an alveolar pattern in the right lung.

9.47 (continued) Thoracic radiographs obtained 24 hours after drainage of a pleural effusion in a cat with end-stage cardiomyopathy and severe left-sided CHF. (b) On the DV view, this makes it difficult to define the cardiac silhouette.

Radiographic features of right-sided congestive heart failure in the dog and cat

- Pleural effusion, typically bilateral (Figure 9.48):
  - Note that right-sided heart failure is a rare cause of pleural effusion in the cat
  - Pleural effusion in both dogs and cats is usually caused by a combination of both left- and right-sided failure
  - It is important to identify severe right-sided cardiac disease in order to attribute a pleural effusion to right-sided heart failure.
- Wide CdVC; see previous comments on CdVC size.
- Hepatomegaly.
- Ascites (peritoneal effusion). Pleural fluid without concurrent ascites is rarely due to heart failure.

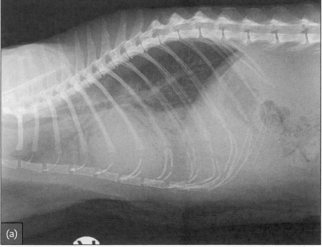

9.47 Thoracic radiographs obtained 24 hours after drainage of a pleural effusion in a cat with end-stage cardiomyopathy and severe left-sided CHF. (a) The lateral view shows severe ventral lung consolidation (alveolar pattern) with air bronchograms and partial border effacement of the cardiac silhouette and diaphragm. (continues) ▶

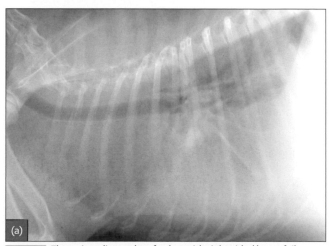

9.48 Thoracic radiographs of a dog with right-sided heart failure. (a) Lateral view. A large volume of pleural effusion is present, obscuring the cardiac silhouette. The dog also has ascites and an enlarged liver (not seen on these radiographs). It is not possible to identify the cause of the effusion from these radiographs and further work-up would be required to confirm right-sided heart failure. (continues) ▶

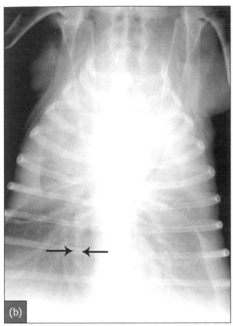

9.48 (continued) Thoracic radiographs of a dog with right-sided heart failure. (b) DV view. A large volume of pleural effusion is present, obscuring the cardiac silhouette. The dog also has ascites and an enlarged liver (not seen on these radiographs). An enlarged right pulmonary caudal lobar vein (arrowed) suggests that pulmonary venous congestion may also be present due to left-sided heart disease. It is not possible to identify the cause of the effusion from these radiographs and further work-up would be required to confirm right-sided heart failure.

Pericardial effusion can cause right-sided CHF. However, pericardial effusion may also result from right-sided or biventricular CHF, although this rarely results in cardiac tamponade. CHF is the most common cause of pericardial effusions in the cat.

Congenital cardiac disease

Congenital heart disease is relatively common in both dogs and cats, with estimates of 0.13% and 0.14% in a shelter population of mixed-breed dogs and cats, respectively (Schrope, 2015), increasing to over 20% of a specialist veterinary hospital population (Oliveira *et al.*, 2011), which includes predominantly pedigree animals. Most congenital heart diseases that are diagnosed are simple, single defects. More than one defect or complex defects can occur, but it is likely that a severely affected animal within a litter will die prior to any veterinary evaluation. The breed predisposition apparent for several congenital heart defects and high prevalence in certain breeds, suggests a possible inherited component for some conditions and breeding from affected animals should be avoided.

Dogs and cats with congenital heart defects are most commonly identified at primary health and vaccination checks because of the detection of a heart murmur. Puppies and kittens may also have innocent murmurs, which are typically low grade, left basilar, localized and systolic. These normally decrease in intensity and disappear by the time the animal is 5–6 months of age, so a watchful monitoring approach can be adopted. However, any loud systolic murmurs, continuous murmurs or systolic–diastolic murmurs should be promptly investigated. Other animals may present with one or more clinical signs including stunting, failure to thrive, exercise intolerance, collapse or signs of CHF.

Congenital heart defects represent embryonic abnormalities, so some understanding of normal development is important in making a diagnosis, but this is beyond the scope of this chapter. Even more importantly, appreciation of the pathophysiological abnormalities of specific congenital heart defects is required to understand the echocardiographic approach to making a diagnosis. Most conditions can be diagnosed by transthoracic Doppler echocardiography, but additional investigations such as radiology, transoesophageal echocardiography and selective angiocardiography are complementary. Figure 9.49 gives an overview of the echocardiographic appearance, differential diagnoses and confirmation of diagnosis of congenital defects. Thoracic radiographs may also reflect the consequences of congenital heart disease, especially those resulting in volume overload. Radiological findings are usually not specific for a particular condition.

> ## Practical tips
>
> - A systematic approach to echocardiography is essential. One defect may be obvious, but it is important to search for additional defects that may be present.
> - The echocardiographer must be skilled to diagnose more complex congenital disease and have a full understanding of the pathophysiological process of each condition.

Patent ductus arteriosus

PDA is one of the most common congenital cardiac diseases in dogs. Breed predispositions are reported, which may vary between continents but include Bichons Frises, Border Collies and their crosses, Chihuahuas, Corgis, German Shepherd Dogs, Maltese, Newfoundlands, Poodles, Pomeranians and Shetland Sheepdogs. Bitches are more affected than dogs. Cats are also affected but the condition is less common than in dogs and there is no sex predisposition.

The ductus arteriosus is an important part of normal fetal circulation. In the fetus, this blood vessel extends from the pulmonic trunk, near its bifuration into the left and right pulmonary arteries, to the descending aorta and allows oxygenated blood from the placenta to bypass the lungs and travel back into the systemic circulation. After birth, pulmonary vascular resistance falls, systemic vascular resistance increases with loss of the placenta, and flow in the ductus reverses. The ductus then closes by constriction of smooth muscle within its wall, brought about by increased arterial oxygen tension that inhibits local prostaglandin release. The ductus is usually closed by 7–10 days after birth. It remains in the adult as the ligamentum arteriosum.

PDA results from failure of normal closure of the ductus arteriosus, resulting in a shunting vessel between the descending aorta and the pulmonic trunk. In dogs, this is associated with incomplete smooth muscle around the ductus and the presence of elastic tissue which does not permit the ductus to close (Buchanan, 2001). Since the aortic pressure is much higher than the pulmonary arterial pressure throughout the cardiac cycle, there is aortic to pulmonary shunting through systole and diastole (giving rise to the continuous heart murmur in the most common, left-to-right shunting, PDA). The morphology of the ductus is best visualized by angiography. It is important to evaluate

2D echocardiographic/M-mode appearance	Differential diagnoses	Features
Left atrial and left ventricular volume overload (dilated chambers, eccentric left ventricular hypertrophy)	PDA	Often dilated pulmonic trunk. Colour flow Doppler shows continuous, high velocity turbulent flow entering the pulmonic trunk via the ductus from the descending aorta
	VSD	May be able to see the defect using echocardiography, unless very small. Colour flow Doppler and spectral Doppler show flow entering the RV (inflow part) or RVOT. There may or may not be evidence of volume overload in the RV
	Mitral valve dysplasia	Mitral valve apparatus appears abnormal. Mitral regurgitation evident on Doppler (possibly with mitral stenosis, uncommon)
Left ventricular pressure overload (left ventricular concentric hypertrophy)	Aortic/subaortic stenosis	Abnormalities of the LVOT and/or aortic valves may be evident unless disease is very mild. Increased aortic velocity with a significant increase in velocity between the LVOT prior to obstruction and the aorta
	Dynamic LVOT obstruction, which may be associated with SAM of the mitral valve septal leaflet	Abnormal mitral valve leaflets, especially long septal leaflets, are consistent with mitral dysplasia. SAM is confirmed from 2D, mitral M-mode and colour flow Doppler studies. The main differential is HOCM; this is rare in dogs and common in cats
Right atrial and right ventricular volume overload	Tricuspid dysplasia	Abnormalities of the tricuspid valve apparatus. Tricuspid regurgitation. Tricuspid stenosis (very rare)
	ASD (left-to-right shunting)	This may result in mild volume overload of the right heart. May be visualized on echocardiography or may see transatrial septal flow on colour flow Doppler studies
Right ventricular pressure overload (right ventricular concentric hypertrophy, evidence of flattening of IVS and abnormal septal motion)	Pulmonic stenosis	May be valvular (most common), supravalvular or subvalvular; abnormality may be visualized on echocardiography. Increased velocity, turbulent flow beyond obstruction in pulmonic trunk. May have post-stenotic dilatation of pulmonic trunk
	Infundibular pulmonic stenosis of the RVOT or double-chambered RV	May see fibromuscular ridge within RVOT, with colour flow Doppler confirming it as the site of obstruction
	Pulmonary hypertension	Pulmonary hypertension may complicate congenital heart disease, especially shunting defects most commonly associated with left-to-right shunts (e.g. VSD, PDA, ASD). Increased right-sided pressure or pulmonary arterial pressure may reduce, balance or even reverse left-to-right shunts (Eisenmenger's syndrome). Pulmonary pressures may be estimated (in absence of pulmonic stenosis) by Doppler studies, and echocontrast studies may confirm right-to-left shunting
	Tetralogy of Fallot	Pulmonic stenosis is part of this complex congenital heart defect. The pulmonic trunk may be hypoplastic. Increased right ventricular pressure results in right-to-left shunting across the VSD
Abnormal atrium (left, right or both)	Endocardial cushion defect	Low (septum primum) atrial septal defect. May also have VSD and, typically, mitral and tricuspid regurgitation (clefted atrioventricular valves). Pulmonary hypertension is common
	Cor triatriatum dexter	RA split into two compartments, one high pressure (usually receiving caudal vena caval flow) and the other normal pressure (usually receiving cranial vena cava flow). The membrane may be perforate but offers high resistance within the atrium
	Cor triatriatum sinister (or supravalvular mitral stenosis)	Membrane separating the LA, similar to that seen in cor triatriatum dexter. High pressure and low pressure compartments, with high velocity flow crossing the membrane

9.49 Echocardiographic features resulting from pathophysiology of congenital heart lesions and differential diagnosis of causal conditions. HOCM = hypertrophic obstructive cardiomyopathy; LVOT = left ventricular outflow tract; RVOT = right ventricular outflow tract; SAM = systolic anterior motion.

morphology prior to considering the optimal method of closure, especially for cardiac catheterization techniques such as use of the Amplatz canine duct occluder (ACDO). The Miller classification includes three main types of PDA morphology, but subsequent reports indicate that more unusual morphologies are also possible.

- Type I: gradually tapers from the aorta to the pulmonic trunk.
- Type II: abrupt narrowing prior to the pulmonic trunk:
  - IIA: PDA is near parallel walled prior to the abrupt narrowing
  - IIB: PDA gradually narrows like a cone, prior to more abrupt narrowing before insertion into the pulmonic trunk.

- Type III: cylindrical or tubular ductus without significant narrowing. This type is most commonly associated with pulmonary hypertension (Eisenmenger's syndrome); this can be associated with right-to-left shunting if pulmonary arterial pressure is sufficiently high to exceed systemic pressures – an rPDA.

Left-to-right shunting patent ductus arteriosus

Clinically, a left-to-right shunting PDA is characterized by a continuous heart murmur that is louder in systole than diastole and heard over the left heart base. Typically, it is very loud, and associated with a precordial thrill. The pulse quality is bounding due to a large systolic–diastolic pulse pressure, reflecting run-off of systemic blood flow across the PDA.

Most animals are asymptomatic when the murmur is discovered. Others will present with left-sided CHF. This congenital heart defect can be completely resolved by closure of the PDA, which is strongly recommended. Closure can be by surgical ligation or device closure, such as with an ACDO.

Radiography: Radiographic findings include (Figure 9.50):

- Lateral view:
  - Classically, left-sided enlargement is present, but generalized cardiomegaly may be seen
  - Prominent aortic arch
  - Prominent LA
  - Left ventricular enlargement, leading to straightening of the caudal margin of the heart
  - Vascular lung pattern with increased number and size of both the pulmonary arteries and veins; peripherally located pulmonary blood vessels are visible due to enlargement (the vascular pattern is due to increased blood flow to the lung, caused by the left-to-right shunt and termed pulmonary overcirculation)
  - Eventually, signs of left-sided heart failure with pulmonary oedema
- DV view:
  - Elongated cardiac silhouette; possible apical shift with marked left ventricular enlargement
  - Prominence of the aortic arch, pulmonic trunk and LAA at 12–1, 1–2 and 2–3 o'clock, respectively: this 'triple knuckle' finding has been reported to be pathognomonic for PDA but is only present in around 20% of cases
  - Occasionally, an aortic bulge ('ductus bump') may be seen near the level of the ductus. This is caused by the abrupt narrowing of the descending aorta beyond the level of the origin of the ductus
  - Enlarged LA with splayed principal bronchi with or without double opacity sign
  - Increased vascular lung pattern
  - Eventually, signs of left-sided heart failure.

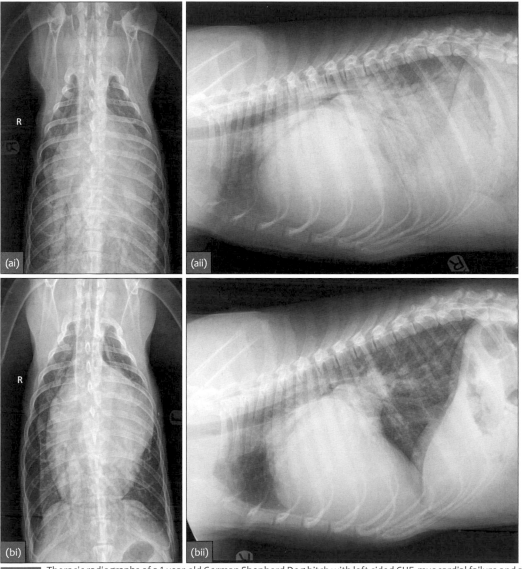

9.50 Thoracic radiographs of a 1-year-old German Shepherd Dog bitch with left-sided CHF, myocardial failure and atrial fibrillation, subsequently diagnosed with a PDA. (ai) DV and (aii) right lateral views obtained at presentation. The dog was severely dyspnoeic and radiographs showed severe, generalized cardiomegaly, especially affecting the left side. There is a mixed interstitial and alveolar lung pattern, most marked in the perihilar and caudodorsal lung fields, consistent with cardiogenic pulmonary oedema. Pulmonary vasculature is difficult to assess given the lung pattern, but the left caudal lobar artery is enlarged. (bi) DV and (bii) right lateral views of the same dog after receiving CHF medication for three days, with almost complete resolution of the lung pattern. There is severe left atrial and left ventricular enlargement, and the aortic arch, pulmonic trunk and LAA are all prominent, giving the 'triple knuckle' appearance between 1 and 3 o'clock on the DV view. The right caudal lobar pulmonary artery is enlarged on the DV view and the cranial lobar vessels, especially the pulmonary vein, are enlarged on the lateral view. (continues) ▶

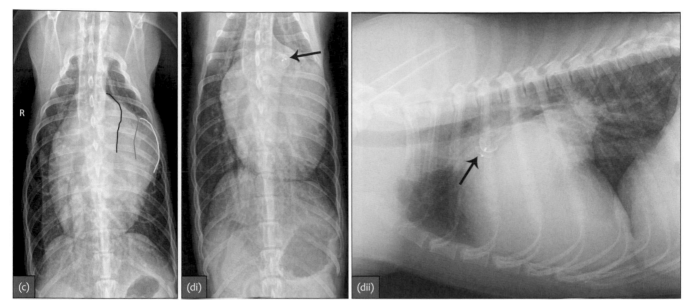

9.50 (continued) Thoracic radiographs of a 1-year-old German Shepherd Dog bitch with left-sided CHF, myocardial failure and atrial fibrillation, subsequently diagnosed with a PDA. (c) Same image as (bi), with the aorta marked in red, pulmonic trunk in blue and LAA in yellow to illustrate the triple knuckle appearance between 1 and 3 o'clock. (di) DV and (dii) right lateral views of the same dog on day 12, following placement of an ACDO (arrowed) to close the PDA. This was placed using cardiac catheterization of the descending aorta via the right femoral artery.

Echocardiography: Ultrasonography is useful both for confirmation of diagnosis and to evaluate the consequences of the PDA on cardiac function.

The ductus itself can be seen from either the right parasternal short-axis or left parasternal cranial window optimizing the pulmonic trunk (Figure 9.51ai). Colour flow Doppler shows continuous flow from the ductus into the pulmonic trunk (Figure 9.51aii). Spectral Doppler (continuous wave) confirms the continuous PDA flow, which is of high velocity (peak >4.5 m/s) if pulmonary arterial pressure is normal (Figure 9.51b). In some cases, the ductus is not well visualized on transthoracic echocardiograms but may be visualized with transoesophageal echocardiography (Figure 9.52). Transoesophageal echocardiography can be used to guide interventional procedures to close the PDA via cardiac catheterization and can help reduce radiation exposure time.

PDA results in pulmonary overcirculation and increased return to the left heart, so echocardiography may show evidence of left-sided volume overload. The following Doppler echocardiographic features are therefore common in cases of PDA:

- Left atrial dilatation
- Left ventricular dilatation (eccentric hypertrophy)
- Stretching of the mitral annulus may result in mitral regurgitation
- Systolic function is initially normal, but myocardial failure may be evident (e.g. increased systolic diameter or increased end-systolic volume index (ESVI))
- The pulmonic trunk may be subjectively dilated (greater in diameter than the aortic annulus). In some cases, the visible aorta may also be subjectively dilated
- With a significant left-sided volume overload, aortic velocities may be increased and it may be difficult to exclude concurrent aortic stenosis until assessment following PDA closure.

Care should be taken to distinguish PDA from similar congenital abnormalities, such as an aortopulmonary window (which usually results in Eisenmenger's syndrome) or an anomalous systemic-to-pulmonary trunk shunt. These conditions are very rare and are beyond the scope of this manual.

Angiocardiography: This is essential if the minimally invasive cardiac catheterization approach to PDA closure is planned. It is performed by selective catheterization of the aorta, usually via a femoral artery approach. A pigtail catheter is preferred, which is positioned in the aorta dorsal to or near the likely PDA location. Contrast medium is injected and the angiocardiogram recorded for subsequent review. Size markers, either on the pigtail catheter or a sizing catheter within the oesophagus, are required to correct for magnification prior to determining PDA measurements.

- With left-to-right shunting, contrast medium is seen in the aorta and the pulmonic trunk and its branches immediately after injection.
- The PDA should be identified (Figure 9.53). However, if there is significant dilatation of the great vessels and contrast opacification of these, it can be difficult to identify a small PDA.

Right-to-left shunting patent ductus arteriosus

Occasionally, right-to-left shunting occurs through a PDA due to high pulmonary vascular resistance. This is thought to occur because the non-tapering tubular shape of the ductus in these animals permits aortic pressures to be transmitted to the pulmonary arterial system. The resulting extreme increase in pulmonary perfusion eventually leads to intimal arteriolar damage and muscular proliferation, causing marked pulmonary arterial hypertension and reversed flow through the ductus arteriosus (Eisenmenger's syndrome). This change has been shown to usually occur in the first few weeks of life. The pulmonary vascular changes are poorly understood, but are known to be irreversible, thereby precluding surgical treatment for this condition.

The anomaly is quite different in presentation to a left-to-right shunting PDA. Clinical signs include fatigue, shortness of breath and weakness. No murmur or only a soft systolic murmur is heard on auscultation and a loud or split second heart sound may be detected. Differential cyanosis may be seen with normal pink cranial mucous membranes but cyanotic caudal mucous membranes, due

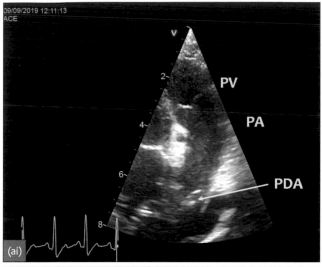

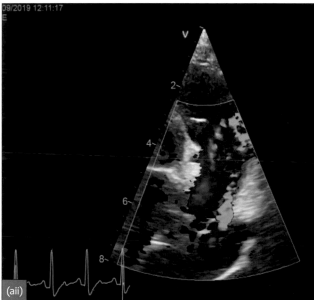

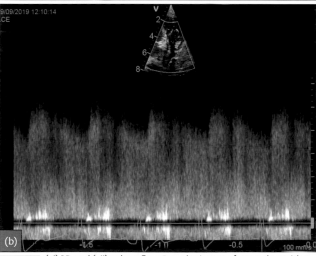

9.51 (ai) 2D and (aii) colour flow Doppler images from a dog with a PDA. This is a cranial left parasternal view optimizing alignment with the pulmonic trunk (PA), beyond the pulmonic valves (PV). The PDA can be seen entering the pulmonic trunk prior to its bifurcation. (aii) The colour flow Doppler shows laminar flow in the ductus (red) which becomes turbulent after crossing the narrow pulmonary ostium of the PDA and flowing into the pulmonic trunk. This is a systolic frame, so pulmonary outflow can also be seen (blue). (b) Continuous wave Doppler of PDA flow, with the cursor aligned with flow. High-velocity flow is consistent with a normal aorta–pulmonic trunk pressure gradient (excluding significant pulmonary hypertension).

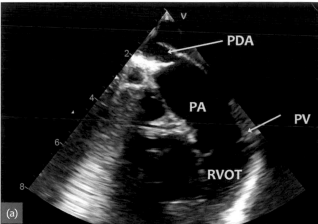

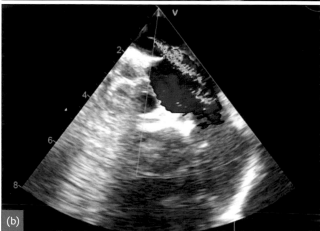

9.52 (a) 2D and (b) colour flow Doppler intraprocedural transoesophageal echocardiographic images, prior to placement of an ACDO to close a left-to-right shunting PDA. The PDA narrows to a pulmonary ostium as flow enters the distal pulmonic trunk (PA). Flow in the PA during systole is red, as it is travelling towards the probe, from the right ventricular outflow tract (RVOT). PV = pulmonic valves.

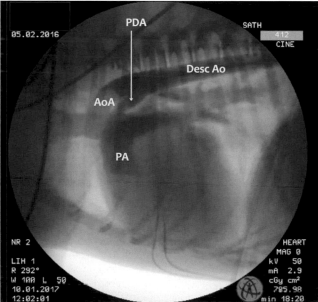

9.53 Still frame from a video-recorded angiocardiogram in a dog with a PDA. The pigtail catheter, delivered via the femoral artery, is in the descending aorta (Desc Ao), although it cannot easily be seen once the aorta is opacified with contrast material. Its pigtail tip is positioned near the PDA, so contrast material can be seen within the PDA and opacifying the pulmonic trunk (PA) and left and right pulmonary arteries. There is minimal contrast enhancement of the aortic arch (AoA). The morphology is consistent with a type IIB PDA. This study preceded subsequent ACDO closure of the ductus.

to the fact that the PDA originates downstream from the brachiocephalic trunk and left subclavian artery. This may only be apparent after exertion. Affected dogs may show pelvic limb weakness or collapse. The animal may bo poly cythaemic, which may result in neurological signs.

Radiography: Radiographic findings (Figure 9.54) include:

- Right heart enlargement on both lateral and DV views
- Dilatation of the pulmonic trunk (seen best on the DV view)
- A 'ductus bump' or aortic bulge may be seen on the DV view
- Lobar pulmonary arteries may be increased in size, reflecting pulmonary arterial hypertension
- In other cases, the lungs may appear relatively hypovascular.

Doppler echocardiography: Echocardiographic findings include:

- Enlarged pulmonic trunk
- Concentric hypertrophy of the RV and flattening of the IVS, reflecting right ventricular pressure overload due to pulmonary hypertension (Figure 9.55)
- A wide tube-like ductus may be identified and

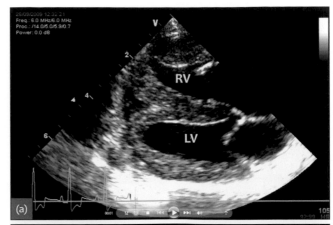

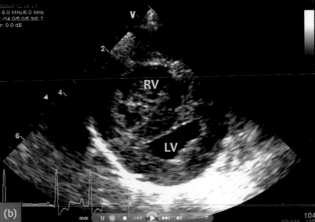

9.55 (a) Right parasternal long-axis four-chamber view and (b) short-axis view at the level of the papillary muscle in the same Border Terrier as in Figure 9.54. There is marked concentric hypertrophy of the RV resulting in flattening of the IVS. The pulmonic trunk was dilated with no evidence of pulmonic stenosis. Bidirectional flow was evident in a tubular ductus.

bidirectional flow may be seen in colour flow or spectral Doppler studies, confirming right-to-left shunting (Figure 9.56)

- Evidence of pulmonary hypertension (tricuspid or pulmonic insufficiency jets, with increased pressure gradients suggesting pulmonary hypertension).

Contrast echocardiography: This is extremely useful in confirming the right-to-left shunt and is easy to perform. Intracardiac shunts (ASD or VSD) should first be excluded. Agitated sterile saline (possibly mixed with colloid) is injected into a cephalic or saphenous vein. The descending aorta is observed for bubbles confirming shunting from the pulmonic trunk across the ductus to the descending aorta; this is best seen in the caudal abdomen, ventral to the vertebral column.

Angiocardiography:

- This is rarely indicated since closure of a PDA is contraindicated with right-to-left shunting (as it will worsen pulmonary hypertension). However, it may be performed if echocardiography or contrast echocardiography findings do not confirm the diagnosis.
- Right-to-left shunting can be demonstrated by an injection of contrast medium in the RV or pulmonic trunk. The contrast medium shunts from the pulmonic trunk to the descending aorta through the wide ductus (Figure 9.57).
- Pulmonary arteries may be normal or tortuous.

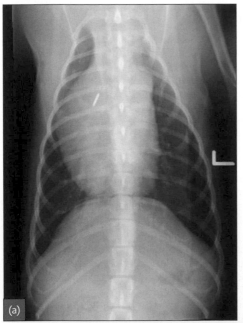

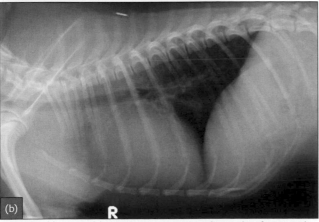

9.54 (a) DV and (b) right lateral thoracic radiographs of a 9-month-old male Border Terrier with an rPDA associated with pulmonary hypertension. The right heart is enlarged. An aortic bulge ('ductus bump') is evident on the DV view. The lung field is hypovascular.

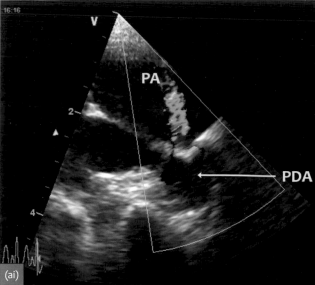

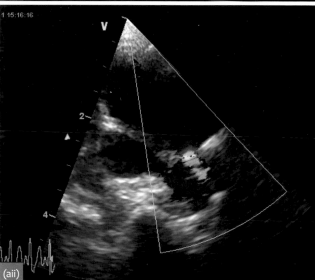

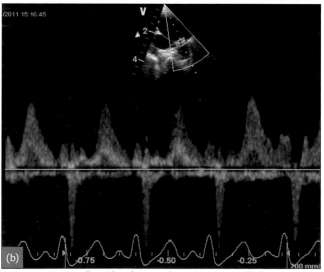

9.56 Toy Poodle with pulmonary hypertension and bidirectional flow across the PDA. (a) Cranial left parasternal view of the pulmonic trunk and PDA in (ai) a diastolic frame showing some left-to-right flow and (aii) a systolic frame showing right-to-left flow across the ductus. (b) Spectral Doppler study of the PDA flow. The brief right-to-left flow (below baseline) and more prolonged left-to-right flow during diastole (above baseline) confirms bidirectional shunting and similar pulmonary arterial and systemic pressures (the PDA velocities are low). PA = pulmonic trunk.

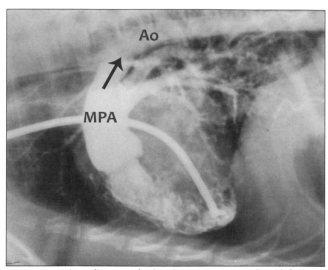

9.57 Angiocardiogram of a dog demonstrating a right-to-left shunt through a PDA in a case where significant pulmonary hypertension was present. The contrast medium was injected in the RV, and the aorta (Ao) is opacified at the same time as the pulmonic trunk (MPA). The region of the PDA is indicated by the arrow.
(Courtesy of J. Buchanan)

Pulmonic stenosis

Pulmonic stenosis encompasses any obstruction of blood flow from the RV to the pulmonic trunk. The prevalence is higher in Bulldogs, Beagles, Boxers, Chihuahuas, Cocker Spaniels, French Bulldogs, Schnauzers and all terriers. Pulmonic stenosis is a rare condition in cats. The condition usually occurs in isolation but on occasion other cardiac anomalies such as tricuspid dysplasia, ASD, patent foramen ovale or VSD may be present.

The stenosis may occur at different levels:

- Valvular stenosis (most common form): a variety of anomalies may occur and these have been subdivided into type A and type B (Bussadori et al., 2000)
  - Type A valves can be thickened, but the main pathology is fusion of the valve cusps, which leads to systolic doming and a diastolic windsock appearance on echocardiography (Figure 9.58). The pulmonic valve annulus and the pulmonic trunk are normal in diameter (similar to aortic annulus diameter) but there may be post-stenotic dilatation of the pulmonic trunk, often resulting in a pulmonary cap, and the lobar pulmonary arteries are often also dilated
  - Type B valves are very thickened and dysplastic. The valve annulus or regions of the pulmonic trunk may be hypoplastic. This is common in French Bulldogs. A fibrous ring may also be present below the valve
  - Note that some cases have a mixture of features of type A and B
- Supravalvular stenosis (rare): This can be seen in French Bulldogs (Chetboul et al., 2018) and Giant Schnauzers
  - During echocardiography, specifically during systole, the fused valve leaflet tips of a type A stenosis may give the impression of concurrent supravalvular stenosis
- Subvalvular stenosis (less common):
  - Subvalvular stenosis can be due to a fibrous ring beneath the valve, usually in association with type B valvular stenosis

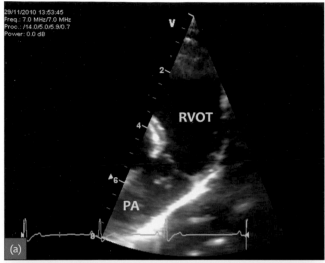

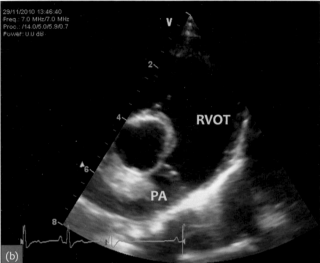

9.58 Labrador Retriever with type A valvular pulmonic stenosis. Right parasternal short-axis views optimizing the right ventricular outflow tract (RVOT) to plumonic trunk (PA). The pulmonic valve leaflets are thick and fused. (a) 'windsock' appearance during diastole. (b) domed appearance during systole.

- A specific form of this occurs in Bulldogs and Boxers due to an anomalous origin of the left coronary artery. Many variations are possible, but most commonly the left and right coronary arteries branch from a single large coronary artery that arises from the right aortic sinus of Valsalva and wraps around the right ventricular outflow tract (RVOT) (Figure 9.59). In some cases, this is the sole cause of the obstruction; in other cases, there is valvular stenosis as well, but awareness of aberrant coronary artery encirclement of the pulmonic trunk is vital (Figure 9.60). These cases usually cannot be treated with balloon valvuloplasty
- A similar condition with an obstructive lesion within the RVOT results in similar pathophysiology to pulmonic stenosis. Conditions include double-chambered RV or infundibular stenosis. Golden Retrievers are over-represented.

It is important to fully evaluate the anatomy and possible presence of coronary artery anomalies prior to making decisions about treatment or intervention. This may require a combination of echocardiography (Figure 9.60) and other imaging modalities such as angiocardiography and CT (see below).

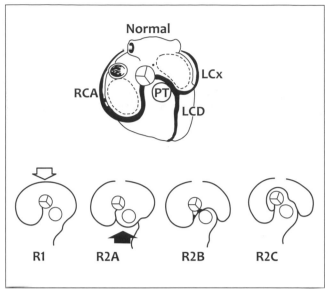

9.59 Normal coronary artery distribution in dogs and humans, and common patterns of single right coronary artery in the latter. In the type R1 pattern, the right coronary artery (RCA) continues as a single vessel and crosses the caudal crux of the atrioventricular sulcus (open arrow), then continues as the left circumflex (LCx) and left caudal descending (LCD) arteries. In type 2 patterns, the single vessel branches shortly after leaving the aorta. Sub-classifications are made depending on whether the crossing vessel (solid arrow) passes cranial to the pulmonic trunk (PT) (R2A), between the aorta and pulmonic trunk (R2B) or caudal to the aorta (R2C).
(Reproduced from Buchanan (1990) with permission)

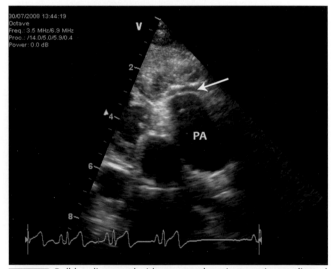

9.60 Bulldog diagnosed with severe pulmonic stenosis complicated by an aberrant coronary artery. Cranial left parasternal view optimized for the large, single coronary artery (arrowed) that encircles the RVOT immediately below the pulmonic valves, which were also abnormal (not shown). Oblique view of the pulmonic trunk (PA).

The stenosis leads to a pressure overload and concentric hypertrophy of the RV. This in turn leads to decreased right ventricular diastolic compliance, ventricular filling impairment and increased right atrial pressure. Tricuspid regurgitation may result and further increases right atrial pressure leading to eventual right-sided heart failure. Depending on severity, the right ventricular pressure overload compromises the left ventricular filling and function (seen as LV underfilling, flattened IVS, abnormal or paradoxical motion of the IVS).

The animal is usually asymptomatic at the time of diagnosis and pulmonic stenosis is usually detected by the presence of a left basilar systolic murmur that radiates dorsally. Dogs with severe disease may be exercise intolerant or have syncopal episodes on exertion. Right-sided CHF may develop if functional or concomitant tricuspid insufficiency (tricuspid dysplasia) is present.

Therapy for the condition includes both medical and surgical options and the appropriate choice depends on the severity of the stenosis and the clinical status of the animal. The condition should be monitored over time as some dogs can gradually develop more severe obstructions. In addition, some dogs may suffer restenosis over time following successful balloon valvuloplasty.

Radiography

Radiographic findings are more likely to be evident in moderate or severe cases of pulmonic stenosis. These include:

- Right-sided cardiomegaly:
  - Increased sternal contact on the lateral view (moderate) (Figure 9.61a)
  - Rounding of the heart with reversed D shape on the DV view (moderate) (Figure 9.61b)

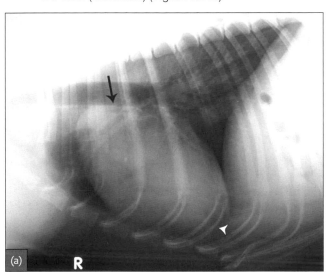

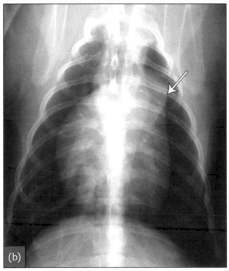

9.61 (a) Right lateral and (b) DV thoracic radiographs of a Labrador Retriever cross with pulmonic stenosis. The increased sternal contact and 'reversed D' on the DV view support right ventricular enlargement. The apex tipping on the lateral view (arrowhead) supports right ventricular hypertrophy pushing the left ventricular apex dorsally. The post-stenotic dilatation of the pulmonic trunk (arrowed) is shown as a 'pulmonic cap' overlying the ventral trachea on the lateral view, and as a 1–2 o'clock bulge on the DV view.

- Apex tipping reflects right ventricular hypertrophy pushing the left ventricular apex off the sternum on the lateral view (Figure 9.61)
- Prominence of the pulmonic trunk (post-stenotic dilatation). This is best seen on the DV view (between 1 and 2 o'clock) (Figure 9.61)
- In a minority of dogs, the dilated post-stenotic pulmonic trunk segment summates with the caudal trachea on the lateral view. This has been termed the 'pulmonic cap' (Figure 9.61)
- In very severe cases, pulmonary hyperlucency and small pulmonary vessels may be seen
- There may be signs of right-sided heart failure: right ventricular and atrial enlargement, enlarged CdVC, hepatomegaly, ascites and pleural effusion.

Doppler echocardiography

Echocardiography is ideal to non-invasively confirm the diagnosis and to grade the severity of the stenosis. Findings include:

- Concentric hypertrophy of the RV secondary to pressure overload. Seen as a thickening of the right ventricular free wall (RVFW) that can approach or exceed the thickness of the left ventricular free wall (LVFW) (Figure 9.62)
- Prominent right ventricular papillary muscles
- Flattening of the IVS due to the increased right ventricular pressure (Figure 9.62). On M-mode images, paradoxical motion of the septum may be seen (Figure 9.63)

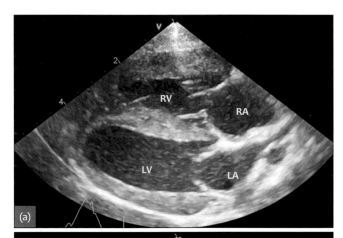

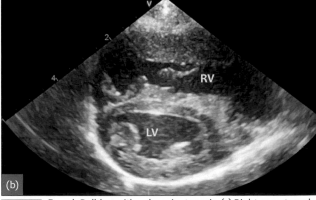

9.62 French Bulldog with pulmonic stenosis. (a) Right parasternal long-axis four-chamber view and (b) short-axis view at the level of the papillary muscles. Both views show an enlarged right heart, with concentric hypertrophy of the right ventricular wall (thicker than the LVFW). The pressure overload in the RV has resulted in flattening of the IVS, apparent in both views.

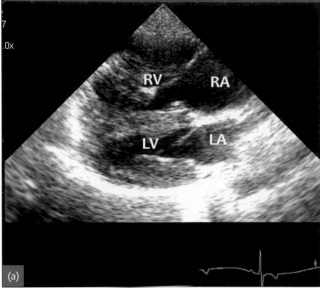

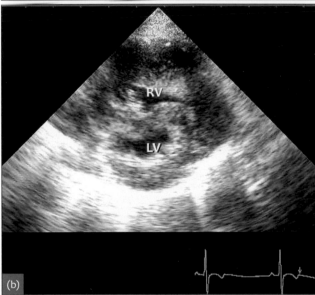

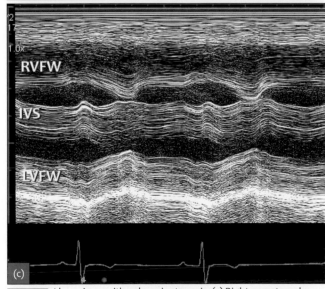

9.63 Lhasa Apso with pulmonic stenosis. (a) Right parasternal long-axis four-chamber view. Note the right ventricular hypertrophy and the right atrial enlargement. (b) Right parasternal short-axis view at the level of the papillary muscles. The RVFW is severely thickened and the IVS is flattened. (c) M-mode echocardiogram acquired from the level shown in (b). Paradoxical motion of the IVS is present.
(© J. Dukes-McEwan)

- Abnormal pulmonic valve (see Figure 9.58):
  - Thickened, often hyperechoic
  - In type A, fused valve leaflets, with doming during systole and windsock appearance in diastole (see Figure 9.58)
  - In type B, very thickened, hyperechoic, dysplastic valve leaflets
- Concurrent subvalvular or supravalvular lesions (Figure 9.64)
- Post-stenotic dilatation of the pulmonic trunk distal to the valve (mainly type A)
- Possible right atrial dilatation (and occasionally right ventricular dilatation if myocardial dysfunction develops)
- Double-chambered RV or infundibular stenosis can be regarded as a form of subvalvular pulmonic stenosis (Minors *et al.*, 2006). During 2D echocardiography, a discrete fibromuscular ridge (infundibular stenosis) or complex muscular obstruction (double-chambered RV) may be seen (usually best visualized with the right parasternal short-axis view, optimizing the RVOT) (Figure 9.65).

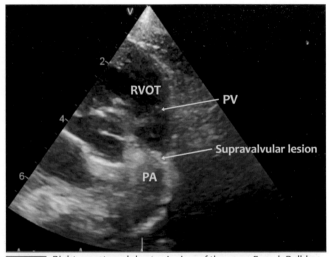

9.64 Right parasternal short-axis view of the same French Bulldog as in Figure 9.62, optimizing the RVOT and pulmonic trunk (PA). The pulmonic valves (PV) were thickened and dysplastic, but the greatest site of obstruction was a supravalvular lesion.

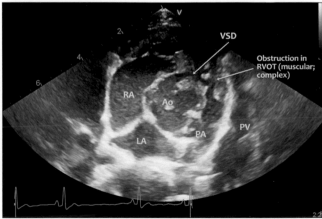

9.65 A young Chow Chow with a double-chambered RV. Right parasternal short-axis view showing the RA, RVOT, pulmonic valves (PV) and pulmonic trunk (PA). This case showed a complex muscular obstruction in the RVOT. This separated the inflow part of the RV (high pressure; associated with concentric right ventricular hypertrophy) from a lower pressure chamber of the RVOT between the obstruction and the pulmonic valve. This lesion resulted in RVOT obstruction. In addition, there was a VSD with right-to-left shunting across it. The aorta (Ao) is wide, and the pulmonic trunk is relatively small in comparison.

Colour flow and spectral Doppler findings include:

- Colour flow Doppler can show the site of obstruction with onset of turbulence in the RVOT or pulmonic trunk (Figure 9.66). If there is dynamic RVOT obstruction, colour variance will be evident before the pulmonic valve
- Increased RVOT–pulmonic trunk velocity (continuous wave Doppler required to record high-velocity signals) (Figure 9.67)
- From the peak velocity, the pressure gradient between the RVOT and pulmonic trunk can be estimated using the modified Bernoulli equation (see Chapter 2). The criteria for classification of the severity of pulmonic stenosis are given by the following pressure gradients:
  - Mild: <50 mmHg
  - Moderate: 50–80 mmHg
  - Severe: >80 mmHg. Such animals are likely to develop right-sided heart failure early and are candidates for balloon valvuloplasty
- From continuous wave envelopes of pulmonic velocity, evidence of dynamic RVOT obstruction can be seen with an internal envelope of late accelerating, lower velocity flow (Figure 9.67)

- Pulmonic insufficiency (pulmonic valve regurgitation due to incomplete valve closure) is also commonly recognized, especially with dysplastic valves (type B)
- Tricuspid regurgitation is common as a consequence of the altered right ventricular loading and geometry. This may result in right atrial enlargement and increased risk for development of right-sided CHF
- Long-standing pulmonic stenosis may result in eventual right ventricular systolic dysfunction (can be assessed by tricuspid annular plane systolic excursion). This may result in decreased pulmonic pressure gradient, which is a poor prognostic finding.

Angiocardiography

This is not usually required for diagnosis but is indicated prior to surgical intervention. Diagnosis can be established after selective catheterization of the RV or RVOT using a jugular approach.

- Stenosis is visible at the level of the valve or the infundibulum, or at the subvalvular level (muscular hypertrophy, creating a filling defect in the RVOT) (Figures 9.68a and 9.69).
- Post-stenotic dilatation of the pulmonic trunk can be identified (see Figure 9.68).

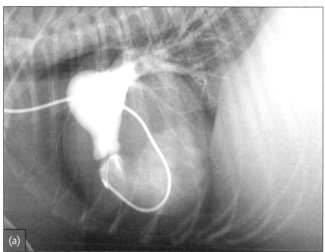

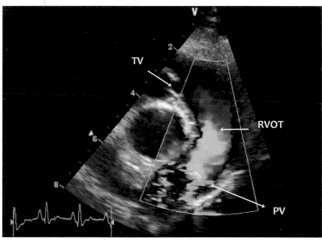

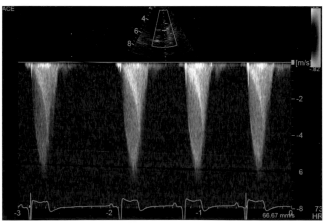

9.66 Cocker Spaniel with valvular pulmonic stenosis (type A). Cranial right parasternal short-axis view with colour flow Doppler showing normal laminar flow in the RVOT, which suddenly develops colour variance reflecting turbulent flow with increased velocity beyond the pulmonic valves (PV) in the pulmonic trunk. TV = tricuspid valve.

9.67 French Bulldog with pulmonic stenosis. Continuous wave Doppler obtained from a cranial right parasternal view optimized for the RVOT and pulmonic trunk. Peak velocity is over 6 m/s, consistent with very severe pulmonic stenosis. There is also a late-accelerating envelope, which corresponds to concurrent dynamic RVOT obstruction as a consequence of severe right ventricular hypertrophy (an indication for beta-blockers).

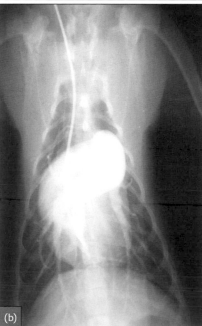

9.68 Angiocardiograms after injection of contrast medium in the RV of a West Highland White Terrier with pulmonic stenosis. Both views show a catheter and fair to good opacification of the RV, RVOT, pulmonic trunk and pulmonary arteries. (a) On the lateral view, there is a clear narrowing at the level of the infundibulum as well as post-stenotic dilatation of the pulmonic trunk. (b) The VD view shows post-stenotic dilatation of the pulmonic trunk.
(Courtesy of J. Buchanan)

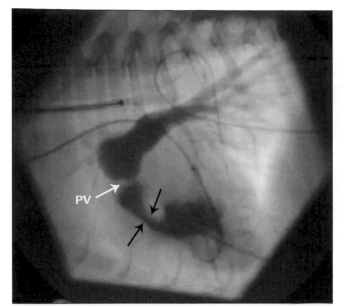

9.69 Still frame right-sided angiocardiogram of a Bulldog with pulmonic stenosis. Cranial is to the right of the image. Catheterization of the right side of the heart was performed via the right jugular vein. A pigtail catheter delivered contrast into the right ventricular apex. Very thick pulmonic valves (PV) can be seen, with little contrast filling at the level of the valves, suggestive of severe narrowing. The severe right ventricular hypertrophy is seen as soft tissue between the contrast material in the RV and the cranioventral border of the cardiac silhouette. There also appears to be some dynamic RVOT obstruction (between the two black arrows). The pulmonic trunk and lobar pulmonary arteries are dilated, consistent with post-stenotic dilatation.

- In cases of functional tricuspid insufficiency, regurgitation of contrast medium is seen from the RV to the RA.
- The pulmonary annulus can be measured from angiocardiograms, to determine required balloon diameter if balloon valvuloplasty is scheduled.
- In Bulldogs and Boxers, it is vital to search for an abnormal origin of the left coronary artery as an underlying cause of the stenosis (Figure 9.70; see Figure 9.59). The coronary arteries may be normal (Figure 9.70) or abnormal (Figure 9.71). An aortic root angiogram is usually obtained (rather than selective coronary angiograms). Alternatively, the aortic root and coronary arteries could be examined in the late levophase after a right ventricular injection of contrast medium, but coronary arteries are often indistinct at this time. In affected animals, a single coronary artery is seen wrapping around the RVOT and a right coronary artery branches from this single artery a few millimetres from its aortic origin (Figure 9.71).

Computed tomography

Thoracic CT is not required to make the diagnosis of pulmonic stenosis. However, electrocardiogram-gated CT angiography during the arterial phase can document coronary artery anatomy after a peripheral venous injection of contrast material, saving time and operator radiation exposure compared with selective aortic root angiography with fluoroscopy (Laborda-Vidal *et al.*, 2016). R2A is the most common coronary abnormality and is characterized by a single right coronary artery with left branches encircling the pulmonic trunk or RVOT (Figure 9.72). Multiplanar reconstructions can also evaluate the anatomy of the RVOT, pulmonic valves and pulmonic trunk (Figure 9.73), especially in cases with multiple sites of stenosis.

Aortic stenosis

Aortic stenosis is a common congenital heart defect most likely to be diagnosed in large breeds of dog. Predisposed breeds include Boxers, Dogues de Bordeaux, Bull Terriers, German Shepherd Dogs, Golden Retrievers, Newfoundlands and Rottweilers. There can be a range of severity in affected dogs, from mild to severe. Concurrent congenital defects may also be identified (e.g. mitral valve dysplasia, commonly in Bull Terriers). Cats may also be affected, although it is an uncommon diagnosis in this species and uniformly severe when it occurs.

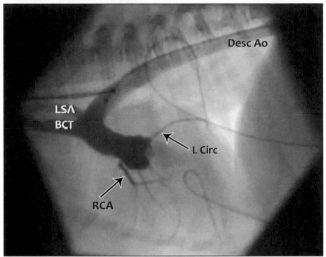

9.70 Still frame aortic root angiogram from the same dog as in Figure 9.69, with pulmonic stenosis but normal coronary arteries. Cranial is to right of the image. The aortic root has been catheterized via a femoral artery. The pigtail catheter is at the level of the aortic valves. There is contrast enhancement of the aortic root, brachiocephalic trunk (BCT), left subclavian artery (LSA), right coronary artery (RCA) and left circumflex branch (L Circ) of the left coronary artery. The sequence of contrast enhancement confirmed that both coronary arteries arose independently from the aortic root. There is mild blushing of contrast in the LV (aortic regurgitation caused by the presence of the catheter). A temperature probe in the oesophagus and leads associated with transthoracic defibrillation/pacing patches can also be seen. Desc Ao = descending aorta.

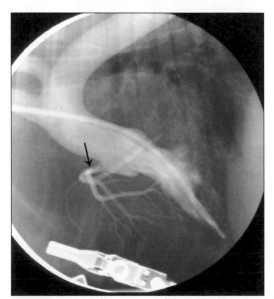

9.71 Angiocardiogram in a Bulldog with pulmonic stenosis. The contrast medium was injected in the left ventricular outflow tract to opacify the aorta and the coronary arteries. A single coronary artery (arrowed) is seen, which then branches into right and left coronary arteries.
(Courtesy of J. Buchanan)

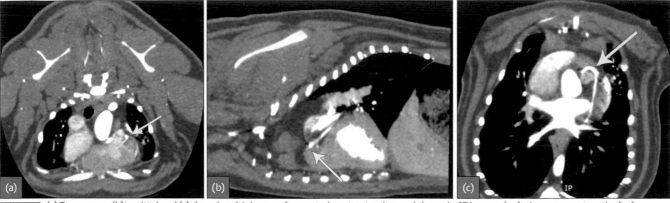

9.72 (a) Transverse, (b) sagittal and (c) dorsal multiplanar reformatted contrast-enhanced thoracic CT images (soft tissue reconstruction) of a Bulldog with confirmed valvular pulmonic stenosis. The aberrant course of the left coronary artery (arrowed) cranial to the pulmonic trunk (prior to branching into paraconal interventricular and left circumflex branches) is consistent with an R2A coronary artery abnormality.
(Courtesy of Will Humphreys, University of Liverpool)

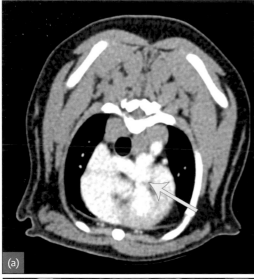

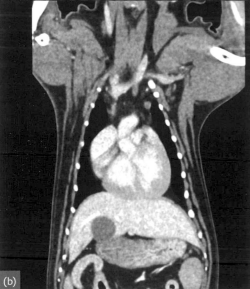

9.73 (a) Transverse and (b) dorsal reformatted contrast-enhanced thoracic CT images (soft tissue reconstruction) of a 10-month-old French Bulldog with supravalvular pulmonic stenosis (the pulmonic valve did not appear to be contributing to the obstruction). The focal circumferential narrowing and interruption of the contrast column within the pulmonic trunk (arrowed) is consistent with pulmonic stenosis or segmental hypoplasia of the pulmonic trunk. The coronary artery anatomy in this dog was within normal limits. (continues)
(Courtesy of Will Humphreys, University of Liverpool)

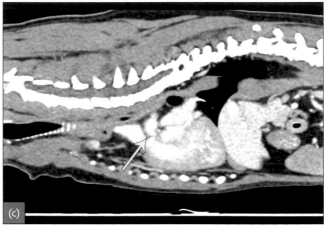

9.73 (continued) (c) Sagittal multiplanar reformatted contrast-enhanced thoracic CT images (soft tissue reconstruction) of a 10-month-old French Bulldog with supravalvular pulmonic stenosis (the pulmonic valve did not appear to be contributing to the obstruction). The focal circumferential narrowing and interruption of the contrast column within the pulmonic trunk (arrowed) is consistent with pulmonic stenosis or segmental hypoplasia of the pulmonic trunk. The coronary artery anatomy in this dog was within normal limits.
(Courtesy of Will Humphreys, University of Liverpool)

Mostly, aortic stenosis is a subvalvular lesion that results in obstruction to left ventricular ejection (subaortic stenosis). Valvular and very rare supravalvular lesions have also been described.

Although it is defined as a congenital heart disease, dogs with subaortic stenosis have progressive disease as they grow. For this reason, predisposed breeds should not be screened for aortic stenosis until over 12 months of age (although the diagnosis can be achieved in puppies with loud heart murmurs or clinical signs prior to this). It has been proposed that an abnormal (reduced) aortoseptal angle is present in some breeds (Boxers, Dogues de Bordeaux, Golden Retrievers), which results in turbulent flow in the left ventricular outflow tract (LVOT). This in turn results in focal hypertrophy or a fibroblastic response which causes or exacerbates the subvalvular lesion (Belanger et al., 2014). In some dogs, the aortic valves may also appear thickened, but this is likely to be a secondary change as a consequence of high-velocity turbulent flow crossing the aortic valves. Aortic regurgitation may also be evident. The subvalvular lesions of aortic stenosis range in severity from distinct nodules to a ridge or a circumferential ring of fibromuscular tissue in the LVOT. In very mild disease, it may not be possible to see these lesions on 2D echocardiography, but the increased velocity and turbulent blood flow is recognized. This LVOT obstruction results in pressure overload of the LV and, therefore, concentric left ventricular hypertrophy in more severe cases. In mild cases, left ventricular chamber and wall thicknesses may remain within the reference interval for the breed and weight of dog. Images of the ascending aorta or aortic arch may show a post-stenotic dilatation. Some breeds (e.g. Boxers, Bull Terriers) may have narrow aortas compared with other breeds of similar size.

Dogs with severe subaortic stenosis are at risk of syncopal episodes on exertion, or sudden death, often associated with myocardial ischaemia and malignant ventricular arrhythmias. Those with advanced disease may develop myocardial failure with a subsequent decrease in aortic velocities. Development of CHF is possible, especially if there is concurrent mitral regurgitation. Dogs with subaortic stenosis are also at increased risk of developing infective endocarditis. Dogs with mild disease may never show clinical signs.

Although interventional procedures including cutting balloons followed by high pressure balloon valvulopasty have been described, these procedures have not been proven to prolong life and carry a high risk of morbidity or mortality. Severe aortic stenosis cases are mainly managed with beta blockers, which have a myocardial protectant and antiarrhythmic effect.

Radiography

Radiography is often unremarkable in mild cases and in cases where there is no post-stenotic dilatation of the aorta. In many cases, the left ventricular concentric hypertrophy does not affect the cardiac silhouette. Changes may be seen in more severe cases and/or cases with mitral regurgitation (e.g. concurrent mitral valve dysplasia).

- Lateral view (Figure 9.74a):
  - Elongated cardiac silhouette, with dorsally displaced trachea and carina and straightened caudal margin of the heart due to left ventricular enlargement
  - Prominent ascending aorta and aortic arch (post-stenotic dilatation)
  - Occasional mild left atrial enlargement (if severe, suggests concurrent mitral regurgitation)
  - In cases with left-sided heart failure: left atrial dilatation, pulmonary venous congestion and pulmonary oedema.
- DV view (Figure 9.74b):
  - Rounding of the left contour of the heart
  - Aortic bulge at the 11–1 o'clock position
  - There may be left atrial enlargement (see 'Left atrium', above)
  - In cases with left-sided heart failure: left atrial dilatation, pulmonary venous congestion and pulmonary oedema.

Doppler echocardiography

It can be extremely difficult to detect mild aortic stenosis with standard 2D echocardiography. Changes may be subtle or may not be seen, and chamber sizes and wall thicknesses can be within reference limits.

The diagnosis relies on Doppler evidence of increased aortic velocity and turbulent flow (spectral dispersion of pulsed wave spectral signal or colour variance) beyond the site of obstruction. While cut-offs for normal aortic velocity

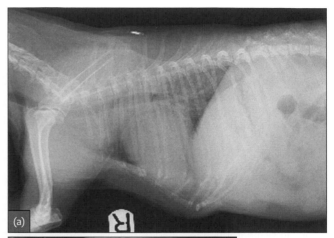

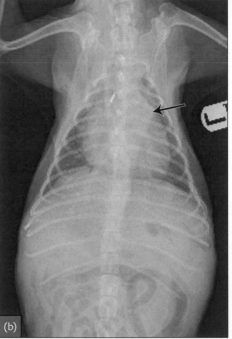

9.74 (a) Right lateral and (b) DV thoracic radiographs of an 11-year-old neutered Yorkshire Terrier bitch with stage B2 MMVD and concurrent mild valvular aortic stenosis. The aortic arch is prominent on the DV view (arrowed) and was dilated during echocardiography. The dog also had hyperadrenocorticism and systemic hypertension, which may contribute to the changes in the cardiac silhouette.

have been suggested (Bussadori *et al.*, 2000), there is an overlap between normal dogs and those with aortic stenosis for the following reasons:

- Dogs that are stressed or excited during echocardiography have increased stroke volume in response to catecholamines, which increases aortic velocity
- In dogs with marked sinus arrhythmia, aortic velocity will be higher following a pause than during periods of faster heart rate; mean, rather than peak, velocity should be recorded over a large number (>5) of cardiac cycles in dogs with variable heart rates
- Breeds that may have a narrow aorta (e.g. Boxers, Bull Terriers) may have increased velocity of aortic flow without aortic stenosis
- If the cursor is not parallel to flow, aortic velocities will be underestimated and may be erroneously considered acceptable in a dog with aortic stenosis

- In dogs with severe aortic stenosis that develop subsequent myocardial failure, aortic velocity will decrease and severity of disease will be underestimated.

Some dogs screened for the presence of aortic stenosis prior to breeding may therefore be labelled as 'equivocal' with aortic velocities in the grey area but no conclusive other documentation to confirm aortic stenosis.
2D echocardiographic findings include:

- Moderate to severe cases:
  - Left ventricular concentric hypertrophy with increased LVFW and IVS thickness (Figure 9.75)
  - Hyperechoic ridge or circumferential ring of hyperechoic tissue in the region of the LVOT (Figures 9.76–9.78)
  - In some dogs, a reduced aortoseptal angle can be seen (see Figure 9.76c)
  - Post-stenotic dilatation of the ascending aorta (see Figure 9.76a).
- Severe cases involve the above findings and:
  - Hyperechoic papillary muscles and endocardial surface due to areas of myocardial ischaemia and subsequent fibrosis (see Figure 9.75)
  - If there is mitral regurgitation, left atrial enlargement may be observed
  - Myocardial dysfunction may occur (Figure 9.79a), which may be associated with a decrease in aortic velocity (Figure 9.79b).

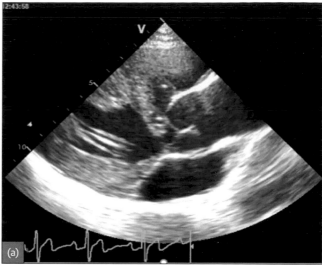

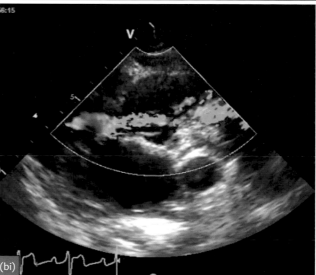

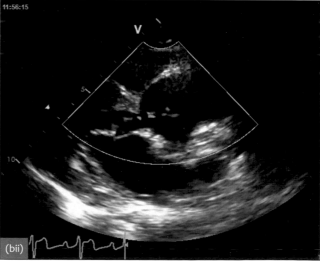

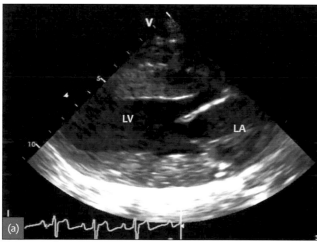

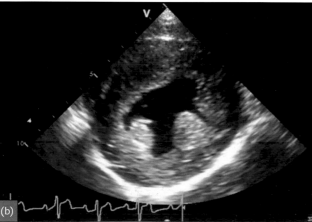

9.75 Newfoundland with subaortic stenosis. (a) Right parasternal long-axis four-chamber view and (b) short-axis view (diastolic frames). There is concentric left ventricular hypertrophy with hyperechoic papillary muscles and subendomyocardium. The increased echogenicity is consistent with myocardial ischaemia or fibrosis.

9.76 The same Newfoundland as in Figure 9.75. (a) Right parasternal long-axis five-chamber view, which shows the aorta. There is a marked subvalvular muscular ridge from the basal septum, resulting in subvalvular aortic stenosis. The aortic valve leaflets look thick in this diastolic frame, but a systolic frame showed that they opened normally and the apparent increased valve thickness may be a secondary change in response to turbulent high-velocity flow. Post-stenotic dilatation of the ascending aorta is apparent. (b) Colour flow Doppler superimposed on a 2D image similar to (a). (bi) In systole, the turbulent flow can be seen to occur at the site of the subvalvular ridge. (bii) In diastole, aortic regurgitation can be seen. Ao = aorta. (continues) ▶

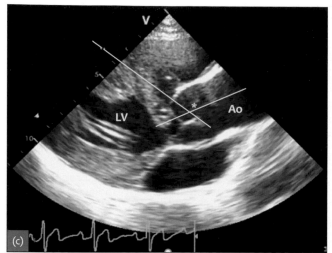

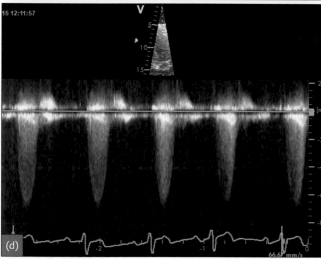

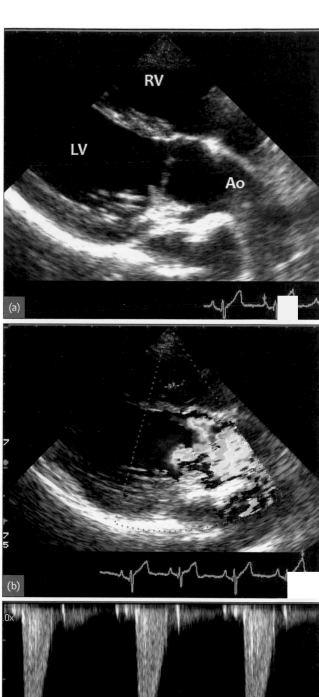

9.76 (continued) The same Newfoundland as in Figure 9.75. (c) This right parasternal five-chamber view shows a steep angle between the longitudinal line of the IVS and the line of the aorta. Reduced aortoseptal angle (∗) has been implicated in postnatal (acquired) changes in the subvalvular region worsening or causing subvalvular obstruction. (d) Continuous wave Doppler from a subcostal view aligned with left ventricular outflow tract and aortic flow. Peak velocity is over 6 m/s, which corresponds to an LV–Ao pressure gradient exceeding 144 mmHg (severe stenosis). Ao = aorta.

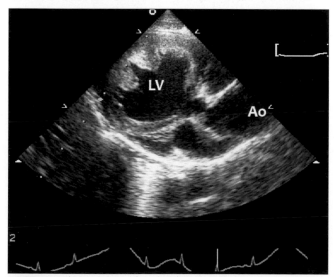

9.77 Right parasternal five-chamber view of a Maine Coon cat with valvular and supravalvular aortic stenosis. Two focal regions of narrowing are identified in the LVOT and there is dilatation of the post-stenotic aorta (Ao).

(© J. Dukes-McEwan)

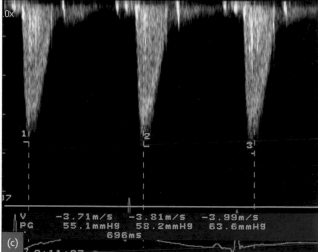

9.78 German Shepherd Dog with subvalvular aortic stenosis. (a) Right parasternal five-chamber view. Note the prominent ridge in close proximity to and just below the aortic valve. The aortoseptal angle does not appear reduced in this dog. (b) Right parasternal five-chamber view, showing a colour Doppler map of the aortic outflow during systole. Note the turbulent flow within the aorta due to the stenosis. (c) Continuous wave Doppler trace from the aorta obtained from a subcostal position. A maximal aortic velocity of 3.99 m/s was recorded. Ao = aorta.

(© J. Dukes-McEwan)

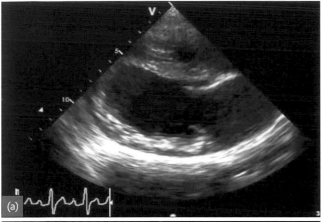

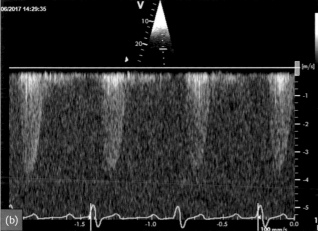

9.79 The same Newfoundland as in Figures 9.75 and 9.76. These images were obtained 2 years later, when the dog was developing myocardial failure. (a) Note the more rounded, dilated LV. The LA was also dilated and mitral regurgitation had developed. The LV walls are no longer subjectively concentrically hypertrophied, and there are focal hyperechoic regions within the myocardium (possible fibrosis). (b) Subcostal continuous wave Doppler. Aortic velocity has reduced from over 6 m/s to less than 4 m/s, reflecting the myocardial dysfunction.

Colour flow and spectral Doppler findings: The colour flow and spectral Doppler echocardiographic findings help confirm the diagnosis. It is critical to align the transducer parallel to aortic flow; the subcostal view optimizes alignment with aortic flow in most dogs but is not usually effective in cats. Whichever view optimizes parallel alignment with flow (subcostal, left apical five-chamber or three-chamber) and gives the highest velocities should be documented, and the mean velocity of a number of cardiac cycles should be recorded. Imaging at depth (using the subcostal view especially in large or giant-breed dogs) and recording high velocities usually requires continuous wave Doppler. It should be appreciated that this is not specific for the actual site or sites of the obstruction, and it can be useful to 'walk' a pulsed wave sample volume across from the LVOT into the aorta to identify the site of sudden step-up of velocity. A step-up of over 0.5 m/s has been suggested to indicate mild stenosis, and much higher step-ups are evident in moderate or severe stenosis.

- Aortic velocities above 1.7 m/s (or 2.0 m/s in Boxers) are likely to be abnormal, especially if supported by lesions evident on 2D echocardiography or a significant step-up in velocity (see Figures 9.76ad and 9.78bc).
- Spectral Doppler envelopes of pulsed wave Doppler (only possible in mild disease) no longer show laminar flow but show spectral dispersion consistent with turbulent flow.

- Colour flow Doppler shows colour variance from the site of obstruction into the aorta (see Figures 9.76b and 9.78b).
- Note also that conditions of excitement and stress will increase the velocity, and myocardial failure will reduce it (see Figures 9.76d and 9.79b).
- Dogs with severe aortic stenosis without compensatory left ventricular concentric hypertrophy or those who develop myocardial failure can be described as having afterload mismatch and are likely to decompensate more quickly.
- Calculation of the pressure gradient across the stenosis (using the maximal aortic velocity) may be used for grading severity and estimating prognosis:
  - Dogs with a maximal pressure gradient of <50 mmHg and minimal ventricular hypertrophy are more likely to lead normal lives
  - Dogs with a maximal pressure gradient of >125 mmHg are very likely to develop serious complications or die suddenly.
- Mitral inflow studies may show increased velocity of the A wave during diastole (decreased E:A ratio) due to impaired relaxation of the hypertrophied LV.
- Functional mitral regurgitation might be present in severe cases and those with concurrent mitral valve dysplasia. When present, it usually has a higher velocity than normal due to increased left ventricular pressure (and hence increased pressure gradient between the LV and the LA).

Angiocardiography

Angiocardiography is rarely indicated as a diagnosis and estimation of severity can be gained by Doppler echocardiography. In the rare situation where a cardiac interventional procedure is being contemplated, it may be performed.

- Subaortic stenosis is demonstrated by a left ventricular injection of contrast medium, which can be introduced via the carotid artery or femoral artery.
- Narrowing of the outflow tract is usually obvious on the lateral view (Figure 9.80).
- Varying degrees of post-stenotic dilatation of the ascending aorta can be identified: in a normal dog, the ascending aorta is widest at the level of the aortic sinuses (sinus of Valsalva). This widened base, formed by the aortic sinuses, is also called the aortic bulb.

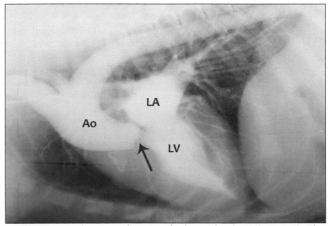

9.80 Lateral angiocardiogram of a dog with subaortic stenosis. The contrast medium was injected in the RA and this is the levophase of the study, 7 seconds after injection of the contrast medium. There is clear narrowing of the subaortic region (arrowed) and mild post-stenotic dilatation of the aorta (Ao). Some degree of concentric hypertrophy of the LV can also be seen on this view. (Courtesy of J. Buchanan)

Ventricular septal defect

VSD is a fairly common congenital disorder in dogs and one of the most common congenital heart defects in cats. Predisposed breeds include Cocker Spaniels and West Highland White Terriers. VSD is known to have a genetic basis in the Keeshond with malformations of the conotruncal septum.

Anomalous development of any part of the ventricular septal components may lead to a VSD. These may be further classified depending on which part of the ventricular septum is affected:

- Most commonly, the defect is high in the perimembranous ventricular septum, so the left side is located proximal to the aortic valves and the right side is in the inflow part of the tricuspid valve, beneath the septal leaflet
- In other cases, with conotruncal abnormalities, the right ventricular side is distal to the crista terminalis and extends into the outflow part of the RV (supracristal defects)
- Rarely, muscular defects in the IVS are present
- May be part of an atrioventricular canal defect (endocardial cushion defect; associated with septum primum ASDs).

Animals with a VSD may present in a number of ways, but most commonly with an asymptomatic murmur. Since the left ventricular pressure during systole is substantially higher than right ventricular pressure, a VSD normally results in systolic left-to-right shunting across the defect. This is at high velocity for small defects, where the LV–RV pressure gradient is preserved. This is called a restrictive VSD and is associated with loud murmurs, typically loudest cranially on the right side and more caudally on the left side ('diagonal murmur'). These animals usually have a normal lifespan and activity level.

Larger VSDs offer less resistance to flow and a significant volume of blood can pass across them. This blood will enter the pulmonary circulation from the RV and return to the left side of the heart (pulmonary overcirculation may be evident on radiographs), so there will be evidence of left-sided volume overload on echocardiography. Despite the left-to-right shunting, most of the VSD flow leaves the RVOT, so the RV often does not appear to be volume overloaded. The increased volume of blood crossing the pulmonic valve can result in 'relative pulmonic stenosis' and a left basilar murmur. These animals may develop left-sided CHF.

Animals with large VSDs with marked pulmonary overcirculation may develop pulmonary arterial hypertension (Eisenmenger's syndrome). Pulmonary hypertension will increase pressure load on the RV, and increased right ventricular pressures will reduce the pressure gradient between the LV and RV, so flow will have lower velocity if it is still left-to-right (producing quieter murmurs). Very high RV pressure, close to or exceeding LV pressure, will result in bidirectional or right-to-left shunting across the VSD. Animals will be clinically severely affected, including having cyanosis of all mucous membranes.

Some animals will have other concurrent congenital defects in association with a VSD.

Radiography

Radiographic findings include:

- Small defects: thoracic radiographs can be normal
- Larger defects: left atrial and left ventricular enlargement with or without increased vascular pattern in the lungs (Figure 9.81)

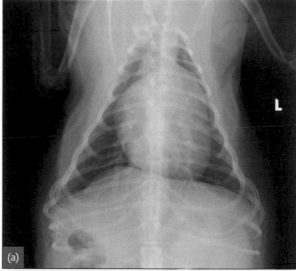

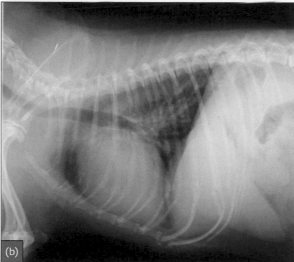

9.81 Thoracic radiographs obtained from an 11-year-old Cocker Spaniel with an asymptomatic restrictive VSD. There is mild generalized cardiomegaly. (a) The DV view shows enlargement of the left caudal lobar pulmonary artery and vein. (b) The lateral view shows increased vascularity in the caudodorsal lung field. These findings are consistent with pulmonary overcirculation.

- In cases with left-sided CHF: pulmonary oedema
- In cases with biventricular heart failure: pulmonary oedema, pleural and peritoneal effusion
- Varying degrees of right ventricular and pulmonic trunk enlargement are also possible, depending on the level and size of the defect
- Pulmonic trunk enlargement and an underperfused lung periphery suggests pulmonary hypertension or concurrent pulmonic stenosis and shunt reversal (right-to-left).

Doppler echocardiography

- The VSD is best imaged from the right parasternal long-axis five-chamber view, examining the perimembranous basal septum between the aortic and tricuspid valve leaflets. Very small defects may be difficult to image in 2D, but colour flow Doppler identifies flow across the obstruction (Figures 9.82ab and 9.83). If the VSD can be imaged from a cranial short-axis view, just beneath the aortic valve leaflets, it is possible to identify whether the VSD enters the inflow or outflow part of the LV (see Figure 9.82b).

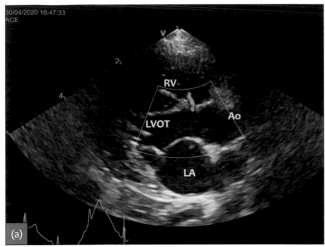

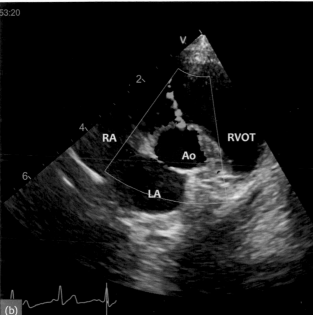

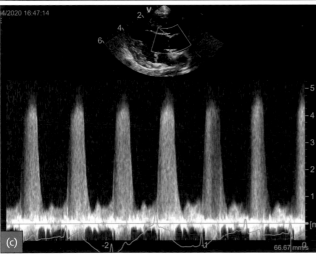

9.82 French Bulldog puppy diagnosed with a restrictive VSD and a peritoneopericardial diaphragmatic hernia (not shown). (a) Right parasternal long-axis five-chamber view showing the turbulent colour flow jet crossing the perimembranous part of the IVS, just below the aortic valve leaflets, into the inflow part of the RV, just below the tricuspid valve leaflets. (b) Right parasternal short-axis view confirming the VSD flow is into the inflow part of the RV. (c) Spectral Doppler with continuous wave cursor placed parallel to flow, from the right parasternal five-chamber view. Velocity is high, at over 4.5 m/s, reflecting a normal expected pressure gradient between the LV and RV of over 81 mmHg. This is, therefore, a restrictive VSD. Ao = aorta.

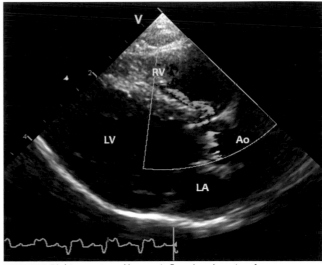

9.83 Right parasternal long-axis five-chamber view from an 8-month-old male British Shorthaired cat, with colour flow Doppler showing VSD flow crossing the perimembranous IVS into the RV. Although both ventricles appear volume overloaded, this cat was asymptomatic at the time. Ao = aorta.

- Spectral Doppler (continuous wave as there is high-velocity flow) confirms left-to-right shunting (see Figure 9.82c). From peak velocity of the VSD flow, the pressure gradient between the LV and RV can be estimated using the modified Bernoulli equation. Small VSDs with a flow velocity of >4.5 m/s and no evidence of significant left-sided remodelling have a good prognosis. These are known as restrictive VSDs.
- With larger left-to-right shunting VSDs, significant left-sided volume overload is evident, with left ventricular eccentric remodelling (Figure 9.84ab). VSD flow should still be at high velocity in the absence of pulmonary hypertension (Figure 9.84c). Evidence of left-sided volume overload indicates risk of developing left-sided CHF. The right heart might not show evidence of volume overload if VSD flow goes straight out of the RVOT.
- Increased volume of blood crossing a normal pulmonic valve can lead to turbulent and increased velocity flow (Figure 9.84de). This may result in a murmur of relative pulmonic stenosis (left heart base). This must be distinguished from true pulmonic stenosis.
- The close proximity of the VSD to the aortic valve may result in aortic regurgitation. It is important to check for this, as it may result in increased volume (and pressure) load on the LV. The right coronary cusp of the aortic valve can sometimes be dragged back into the VSD during diastole. It is also possible that the tricuspid valve septal leaflet may be affected.
- VSDs can sometimes close spontaneously; serial examinations may confirm this.

Eisenmenger's syndrome:

- Eisenmenger's syndrome occurs when chronic overcirculation of the pulmonary vasculature results in pulmonary hypertension. It is not clear whether the increased pulmonary vascular resistance is reactive or present from birth in dogs (retained fetal type vasculature).

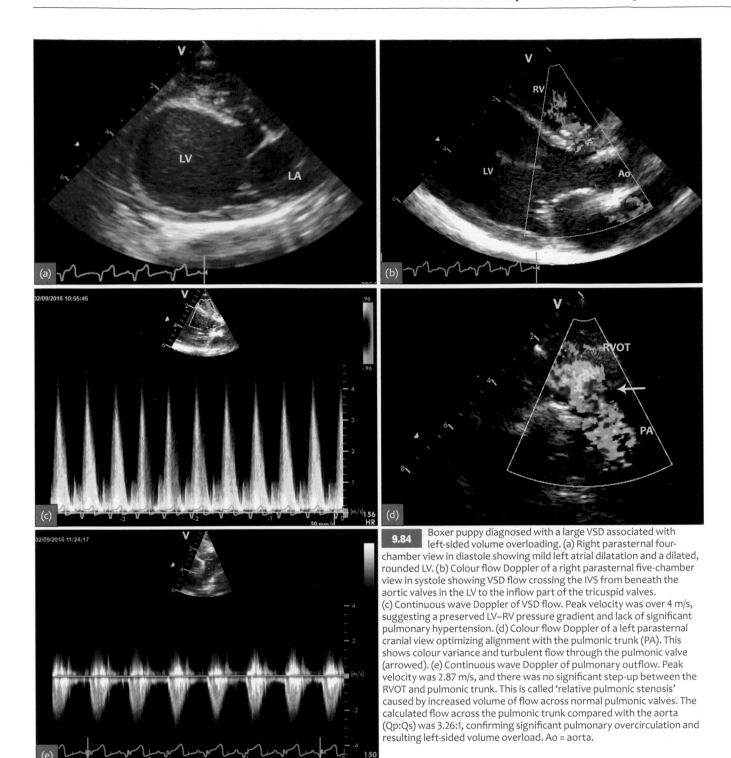

9.84 Boxer puppy diagnosed with a large VSD associated with left-sided volume overloading. (a) Right parasternal four-chamber view in diastole showing mild left atrial dilatation and a dilated, rounded LV. (b) Colour flow Doppler of a right parasternal five-chamber view in systole showing VSD flow crossing the IVS from beneath the aortic valves in the LV to the inflow part of the tricuspid valves. (c) Continuous wave Doppler of VSD flow. Peak velocity was over 4 m/s, suggesting a preserved LV–RV pressure gradient and lack of significant pulmonary hypertension. (d) Colour flow Doppler of a left parasternal cranial view optimizing alignment with the pulmonic trunk (PA). This shows colour variance and turbulent flow through the pulmonic valve (arrowed). (e) Continuous wave Doppler of pulmonary outflow. Peak velocity was 2.87 m/s, and there was no significant step-up between the RVOT and pulmonic trunk. This is called 'relative pulmonic stenosis' caused by increased volume of flow across normal pulmonic valves. The calculated flow across the pulmonic trunk compared with the aorta (Qp:Qs) was 3.26:1, confirming significant pulmonary overcirculation and resulting left-sided volume overload. Ao = aorta.

- If there is significant pulmonary hypertension associated with Eisenmenger's syndrome, concentric right ventricular hypertrophy (possibly with RV dilatation) will be evident, associated with flattening of the IVS. This is usually associated with large and therefore easily imageable and measurable VSDs (Figure 9.85ab).
- With pressure overload of the RV, concurrent pulmonic stenosis must be excluded before presuming this is due to pulmonary hypertension. If there is any tricuspid regurgitation or pulmonic regurgitation, pulmonary arterial systolic and diastolic pressures can be estimated using the modified Bernoulli equation.

- Increased RV pressure means that the LV–RV pressure gradient is reduced, which means a left-to-right shunting VSD will be at reduced velocity. If RV pressure is sufficiently high, bidirectional shunting (Figure 9.85cd) or even solely right-to-left shunting VSD flow can be documented.

Contrast echocardiography: Right-to-left shunts can be assessed using an ultrasound bubble study: the heart is examined from a right parasternal long-axis five-chamber view while an intravenous injection of agitated saline (possibly mixed with colloid) is made. Contrast material (bubbles) normally enters only the right heart.

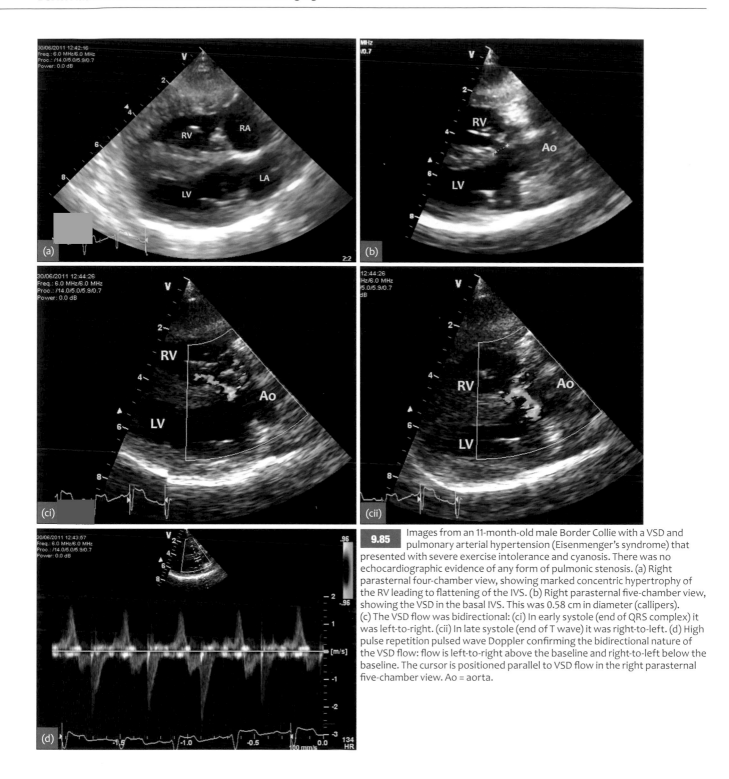

9.85 Images from an 11-month-old male Border Collie with a VSD and pulmonary arterial hypertension (Eisenmenger's syndrome) that presented with severe exercise intolerance and cyanosis. There was no echocardiographic evidence of any form of pulmonic stenosis. (a) Right parasternal four-chamber view, showing marked concentric hypertrophy of the RV leading to flattening of the IVS. (b) Right parasternal five-chamber view, showing the VSD in the basal IVS. This was 0.58 cm in diameter (callipers). (c) The VSD flow was bidirectional: (ci) In early systole (end of QRS complex) it was left-to-right. (cii) In late systole (end of T wave) it was right-to-left. (d) High pulse repetition pulsed wave Doppler confirming the bidirectional nature of the VSD flow: flow is left-to-right above the baseline and right-to-left below the baseline. The cursor is positioned parallel to VSD flow in the right parasternal five-chamber view. Ao = aorta.

If any appears in the LV, crossing the VSD, some right-to-left shunting is confirmed. However, note that this is rarely required, since colour flow Doppler is normally confirmatory.

Angiocardiography

VSDs with left-to-right shunts are best demonstrated by injection of contrast medium in the LV (Figure 9.86):

- The left ventricular opening is usually high in the ventricular septum, in the outflow tract just below the aortic valve

- The right ventricular opening is usually just under the cranial part of the septal leaflet of the tricuspid valve
- Shunting usually occurs only in systole, as the pressure gradient between both ventricles is almost absent in diastole.

VSDs with right-to-left shunts secondary to pulmonary hypertension (Eisenmenger's syndrome) are best demonstrated by injection of contrast medium in the RV; there is evidence of passage of contrast medium into the LV immediately after the injection into the RV and simultaneous opacification of the aorta and pulmonic trunk. This condition can be difficult to differentiate from tetralogy of Fallot.

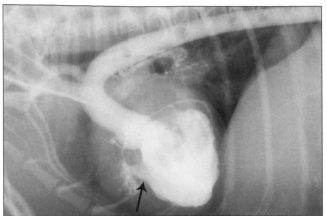

9.86 Lateral angiocardiogram of a 2-year-old German Shepherd Dog with a VSD. The contrast medium was injected in the LV and shunting can be seen from the LV to the RV through a membranous VSD (arrowed). There is also eccentric hypertrophy of the LV and apparent dilatation of the LA.
(Courtesy of J. Buchanan)

Atrial septal defect

ASDs are uncommon congenital abnormalities in dogs. Breeds at risk include the Boxer, German Shepherd Dog, Old English Sheepdog and Samoyed. They may be seen as concurrent defects in animals with other congenital heart disease. They are also infrequently seen in cats (mostly as part of endocardial cushion defects).

ASDs can occur at three main locations:

- In the middle of the interatrial septum (most common). These are ostium secundum ASDs and vary in size. This might be an incidental finding of minor importance, or it may result in right atrial and ventricular volume overload and pulmonary overcirculation, if sufficiently large
  - Another mid-atrial septal 'defect' is a patent foramen ovale. Strictly speaking, there is no actual defect; the two components of the interatrial septum, the septum primum on the left side and septum secundum on the right side, would be functionally closed unless the pressure in the RA is increased, when the two components of the septum are pushed apart to allow right-to-left flow (as in the fetus)
- High in the atrial septum, near the entrance of the pulmonary veins. These are sinus venosus ASDs and are very rare
- At the base of the septum. These are either ostium primum defects or endocardial cushion defects and are also known as atrioventricular canal defects. Various types of endocardial cushion defects exist and they are often accompanied by abnormal atrioventricular valve development. These defects are usually large and are more commonly reported in cats. A complete endocardial cushion defect comprises a large ASD in the lower atrial septum, a high VSD and fusion of the septal leaflets of the two atrioventricular valves. This results in a communication between all four cardiac chambers and is also known as an atrioventricular valve canal defect. An incomplete defect occurs in the absence of a VSD.

Most ASDs are associated with left-to-right shunting, unless there is a reason for reversal of the flow such as increased right atrial pressure (pulmonic or tricuspid valve malformation or pulmonary hypertension).

The shunting occurs predominantly during diastole. Large defects result in significant left-to-right shunting with right atrial dilatation, dilatation with eccentric hypertrophy of the RV and pulmonary overcirculation. However, because of the low pressure difference between the left and right atria, it is unusual to identify a significant volume overload.

If left atrial enlargement is identified then the examiner should look for an additional defect, such as an endocardial cushion defect with mitral regurgitation. These animals may develop left-sided or bilateral heart failure.

Shunt reversal may occur in certain conditions, when right ventricular pressure is increased, such as pulmonic stenosis or pulmonary hypertension (Eisenmenger's syndrome).

Most ASDs are not clinically significant and treatment is usually not necessary.

Radiography

Radiographs are often normal, though findings may include:

- Right-sided cardiomegaly: dilatation of the RV with or without dilatation of the RA (Figures 9.87 and 9.88)
- There may be enlarged pulmonary arteries or evidence of pulmonary overcirculation (Figure 9.88)
- Left atrial enlargement may be seen, especially with some endocardial cushion defects.

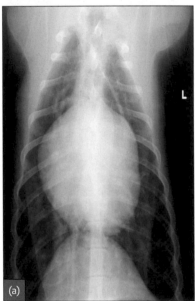

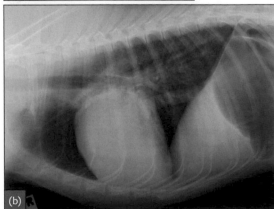

9.87 (a) DV and (b) lateral thoracic radiographs of a 2-year-old male German Shepherd Dog diagnosed with an ASD. There is mild cardiomegaly, which appears to be predominantly right sided, with increased sternal contact on the lateral view and a prominent right atrial region on the DV view. Pulmonary vasculature is within normal limits.

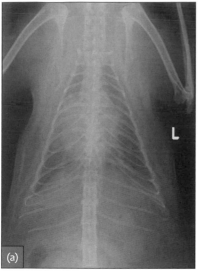

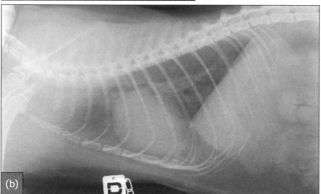

9.88 (a) DV and (b) lateral thoracic radiographs of a 5-year-old Persian cat, diagnosed by echocardiography with a partial atrioventricular canal (endocardial cushion) defect with a septum primum ASD and mitral and tricuspid regurgitation. The cat had moderate pulmonary hypertension. There is a moderate diffuse unstructured parenchymal opacification of both lungs likely highlighted by obesity and poor lung inflation. The cardiac silhouette is enlarged with a VHS of roughly 10, without specific chamber enlargement. The pulmonary veins and arteries are moderately enlarged. The cat was reported to be asymptomatic; it was referred for assessment as its congenital heart murmur had become louder.

Doppler echocardiography

ASDs can be identified at various locations as listed above. They are best seen using the right parasternal long-axis four-chamber view. However, it is important to be aware that, dependent on ultrasound beam orientation, the thin nature of the septum may result in the false appearance of a defect (e.g. echo dropout in the region of the fossa ovalis). Colour flow Doppler studies must be used for confirmation of flow crossing the defect. It is important to assess the interatrial septum systematically, as small defects can be easily overlooked (Chetboul *et al.*, 2006). Flow associated with ASDs may be easier to appreciate if the colour Nyquist limit is turned low (e.g. 50 cm/s). The colour flow is typically from the LA to the LV (i.e. red on the right parasternal views) (Figures 9.89 and 9.90).

Other evidence of significant right-sided volume overload includes:

- Right atrial dilatation
- Right ventricular dilatation with eccentric hypertrophy.

Occasionally, there is increased velocity of the blood flow through the pulmonic valve, due to an increased volume of flow through a normal valve, associated with

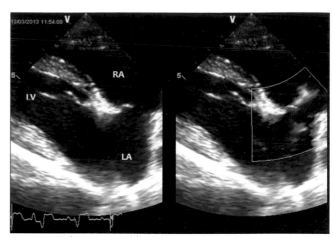

9.89 Right parasternal four-chamber view of the same dog as in Figure 9.86. Dual image showing defect in mid-atrial septum in 2D (left) and superimposed colour flow Doppler (right) showing left-to-right flow. Location is consistent with an ostium secundum ASD. The right heart is prominent, consistent with volume overload associated with the left-to-right shunting.

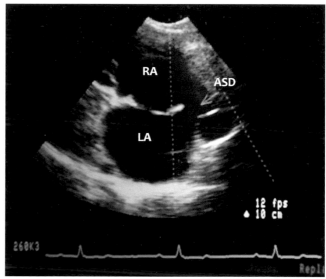

9.90 Right parasternal long-axis four-chamber view of a Boxer with a very high defect in the interatrial septum, resulting in left-to-right flow. This is consistent with a sinus venosus defect.
(© J. Dukes-McEwan)

left-to-right shunting. This can be identified as a murmur of relative pulmonic stenosis on clinical examination. There may also be evidence of additional defects (e.g. mitral regurgitation and tricuspid regurgitation in some endocardial cushion defects). Causes include:

- Ostium secundum defect with right-sided volume overload (see Figure 9.89)
- Sinus venosus defect (high ASD) (Figure 9.90)
- Ostium primum defect (low ASD) with an endocardial cushion defect (Figure 9.91). Animals with endocardial cushion defects also have mitral and tricuspid regurgitation due to cletted atrioventricular valves, as a consequence of the development anomaly of the endocardial cushions, and sometimes have VSDs
- Patent foramen ovale. The two components of the atrial septum, the septum primum and septum secundum, are separated by right-to-left flow, associated with any condition which increases the right atrial pressure. Flow is from low in the septum on the right atrial side to more dorsally on the left atrial side (Figure 9.92).

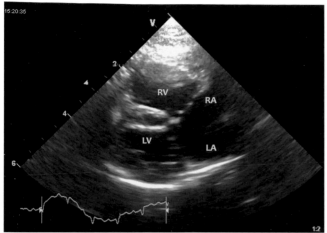

9.91 Right parasternal long-axis four-chamber view of the same cat as in Figure 9.88. The atrioventricular valves are abnormal, both on the same plane, which is consistent with atrioventricular valve dysplasia. There is virtually no evidence of an interatrial septum (except very dorsally in the atrium). These findings are consistent with an ostium primum ASD and, together, the findings are consistent with an endocardial cushion defect. The right heart is dilated and shows concentric hypertrophy of the RVFW; the cat was confirmed to have mild pulmonary hypertension.

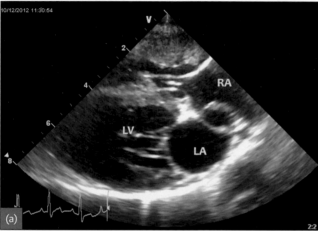

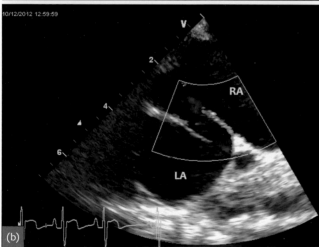

9.92 7-month-old male Cocker Spaniel that was diagnosed with both a double-chambered RV and pulmonic stenosis with a hypoplastic pulmonic trunk. (a) Right parasternal four-chamber view. Note the severe concentric hypertrophy of the right ventricular free wall. The interatrial septum appears to have two components. (b) Colour flow Doppler shows flow between the interatrial septum components and across the interatrial septum, from right-to-left (blue) during diastole, as a consequence of the increased right heart pressures. These findings are consistent with a patent foramen ovale (PFO).

Echocontrast ('bubble') study: In some cases, there may be uncertainty about whether there is a small ASD or a patent foramen ovale. In animals that have concurrent right sided congenital heart defects and where right-to-left shunting is suspected, a peripheral vein injection of agitated saline (possibly with colloid) will confirm right-to-left shunting by producing bubbles in the LA and LV.

Angiocardiography

Uncomplicated ASDs are demonstrated using left atrial injections of contrast medium. The study reveals abnormal shunting of the contrast material from the LA to the RA through the septal defect. In cyanotic animals, where right-to-left shunting is suspected, the septal defect can be demonstrated using a right atrial injection of contrast medium.

Mitral valve dysplasia

This condition is frequently encountered in dogs, especially Bull Terriers, Springer Spaniels, Great Danes, German Shepherd Dogs, Mastiffs, Golden Retrievers and Newfoundlands. Mitral valve dysplasia is one of the most common congenital cardiac defects in cats.

The disease encompasses any combination of malformed valve leaflet or cusps, abnormal chordae tendinae (short, absent or too long) and abnormal papillary muscles (fused, abnormally positioned). Concurrent cardiac abnormalities, such as subvalvular aortic stenosis, may be noted in dogs. Most commonly, the abnormality is associated with systolic mitral regurgitation. Valvular insufficiency leads to volume overloading and left atrial and ventricular dilatation. Left-sided CHF may eventually result. Mitral stenosis can also occur, especially in the Bull Terrier but also other terrier breeds.

Animals may be asymptomatic or may present with exercise intolerance or even left-sided heart failure. A holosystolic murmur will be heard over the left apex (or left sternal border in cats). The prognosis is variable and influenced by the presence of heart failure. For cases of mitral valve dysplasia with mitral regurgitation alone, pathophysiology and management is very similar to that for MMVD (see 'Myxomatous mitral valve disease', below).

Radiography

Radiographic changes are very similar to those of acquired MMVD in dogs, but are also seen in cats:

- Left atrial and left ventricular enlargement (Figure 9.93)
- Pulmonary venous congestion
- At the stage of left-sided CHF: cardiogenic pulmonary oedema (Figure 9.93) (± pleural effusion in cats)
- Mitral stenosis should be considered when a markedly enlarged atrium is not accompanied by changes in the ventricle.

Doppler echocardiography

Echocardiographic findings of mitral valve dysplasia with isolated mitral regurgitation include:

- Left atrial and left ventricular dilatation with LV eccentric hypertrophy (Figure 9.94a)
- Abnormal mitral apparatus:
  - Malformed valve leaflet or cusps (thickened, hyperechoic)
  - Abnormal motion of the mitral leaflets: may appear rigid, show a lack of complete diastolic opening

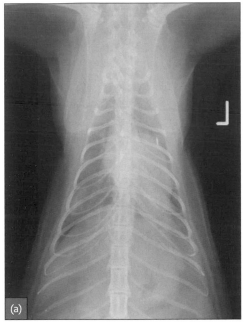

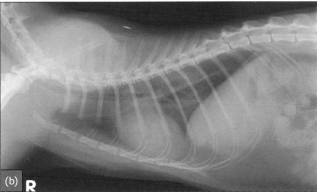

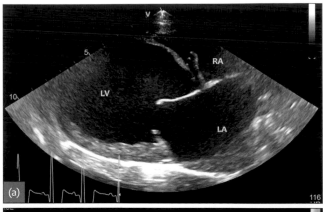

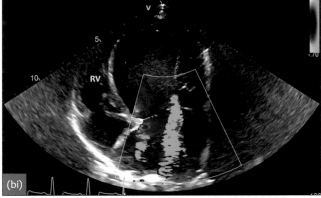

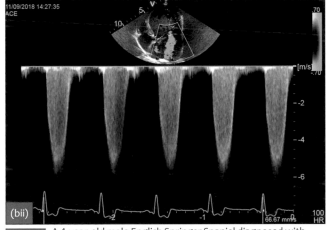

9.93 (a) DV and (b) right lateral thoracic radiographs from a 2-year-old neutered female Toyger cat with dyspnoea and initial response to diuretic treatment that was subsequently diagnosed with mitral valve dysplasia and subaortic stenosis. The radiographs show left-sided cardiomegaly and a diffuse, patchy interstitial lung pattern consistent with pulmonary oedema.

leading to 'hockey stick' appearance (Figure 9.94a), and failure to close during systole to the level of the mitral annulus – i.e. they appear tethered during both diastole and systole
- One of the mitral valve leaflets may be abnormally long or short (Figure 9.95)
- Hyperechoic chordae tendinae, which can be short, absent or too long
- Abnormal papillary muscles (fused or abnormally positioned) (Figure 9.96)
- Colour flow Doppler confirms the presence of mitral regurgitation in most cases (see Figures 9.94bi and 9.95b). Continuous wave Doppler of the mitral regurgitant jet allows estimation of the left ventricular to left atrial pressure gradient (see Figure 9.94bii)
- Systolic function is preserved initially, with an increased fractional shortening and ejection fraction reflecting the reduced afterload associated with severe mitral regurgitation. Myocardial failure can develop later (increased M-mode LV systolic diameter or ESVI)
- Transmitral flow pattern may be normal or show evidence of significant mitral regurgitation with increased E wave velocity, increased left-sided filling pressures or restrictive diastolic dysfunction (mitral E:A ratio >2).

9.94 A 4-year-old male English Springer Spaniel diagnosed with mitral valve dysplasia and being treated for left-sided CHF. (a) Right parasternal four-chamber view. There is marked left atrial and left ventricular dilatation with eccentric hypertrophy. The mitral valve does not open fully, with a 'hockey stick' appearance to the anterior leaflets and a relatively immobile posterior leaflet. In addition, the mitral valve did not close to the level of the mitral annulus during systole, although this finding can be attributed to the altered geometry of the LV affecting the mitral valve apparatus. (bi) Left apical four-chamber view confirming mitral regurgitation on colour flow Doppler. (bii) Continuous wave Doppler of mitral regurgitation.

The less common cases of mitral valve dysplasia with mitral stenosis (with or without mitral regurgitation) may show the following additional features:

- Very abnormal mitral valve motion, showing little diastolic opening
  - Marked 'hockey stick' appearance on 2D views
  - Mitral valve M-mode shows reduced excursion of the anterior leaflet and the posterior leaflet motion may be minimal, or show movement towards the IVS rather than the posterior wall; i.e. it is dragged by the anterior leaflet (Figure 9.97a)

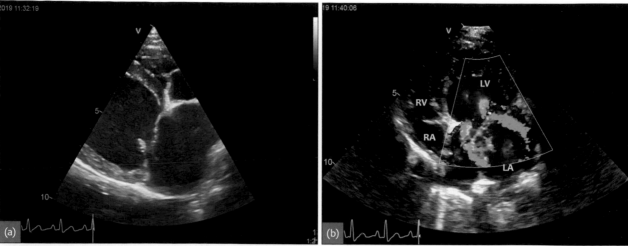

9.95 A 2-year-old French Bulldog known to have a heart murmur but investigated only after developing left-sided CHF and subsequently diagnosed with mitral valve dysplasia with severe mitral regurgitation. (a) Right parasternal long-axis four-chamber view during ventricular systole. The mitral valve is abnormal, with a very long anterior leaflet and relatively immobile, short posterior leaflet. The anterior leaflet prolapses and overlaps the posterior leaflet. (b) Left apical four-chamber view with colour flow Doppler confirming an eccentric jet of mitral regurgitation coursing around the LA (coandal effect).

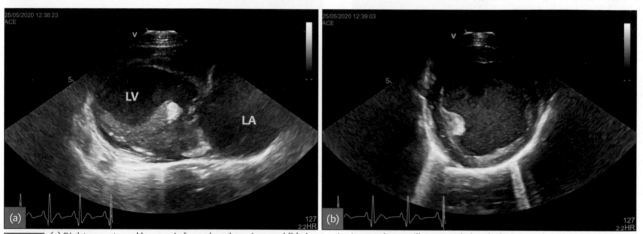

9.96 (a) Right parasternal long-axis four-chamber view and (b) short-axis view at the papillary muscle level of a 3-month-old male Old English Sheepdog with mitral valve dysplasia and left-sided CHF. There was a single papillary muscle, which was large, with a well demarcated hyperechoic tip, attached to short chordae on both mitral valve leaflets. There is also a small pericardial effusion.

- Colour flow Doppler shows aliasing or colour variance indicating turbulent flow during normal diastolic left ventricular filling (Figure 9.97b)
- Spectral Doppler of diastolic transmitral flow shows increased E and A wave velocities. The E wave velocity shows increased deceleration time (increased pressure half-time). The mitral A wave velocity is higher than the mitral E wave velocity, indicating increased dependence on atrial contraction to achieve ventricular filling (Figure 9.97c).

In dogs, a dysplastic and abnormally long anterior mitral valve leaflet may be affected by systolic anterior motion (SAM) during left ventricular ejection. This results in dynamic obstruction of the LVOT and also mitral regurgitation. If there is significant dynamic LVOT obstruction, there will be a pressure overload on the LV and concentric left ventricular hypertrophy may result. The SAM and dynamic LVOT obstruction may be persistent or intermittent. Young animals and terrier breeds are over-represented. Some young animals may show resolution as they grow. Echocardiographic features include:

- Confirmation of SAM from 2D or mitral M-mode studies (Figure 9.98ab)
- Colour flow Doppler shows that the SAM results in dynamic LVOT obstruction with or without an eccentric jet of mitral regurgitation
- Spectral Doppler (continuous wave or pulsed wave) with the sample volume placed in the LVOT at the site of colour variance shows increased LVOT velocity, with a biphasic acceleration (scimitar shape) (Figure 9.98c). The LVOT velocity reflects the severity of the pressure gradient between the LV and the aorta (aortic stenosis must be excluded).
- Concentric left ventricular hypertrophy can be seen with persistent and severe dynamic LVOT obstruction (Figure 9.98a).

The main differential diagnosis is hypertrophic obstructive cardiomyopathy (HOCM), but this is very rare in dogs and the mitral valve leaflets may be obviously thickened or dysplastic.

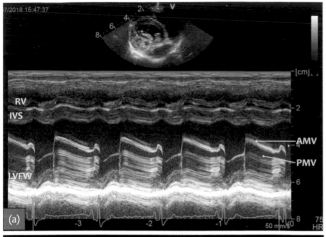

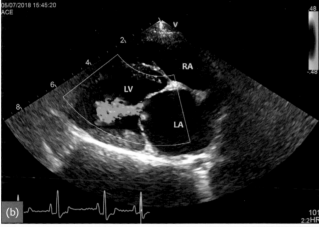

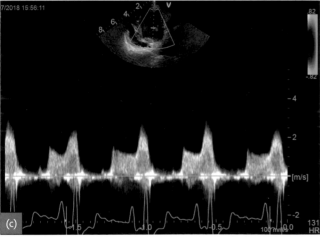

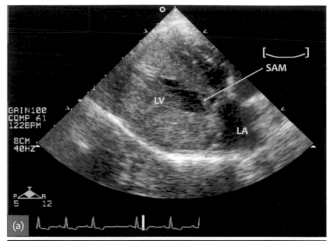

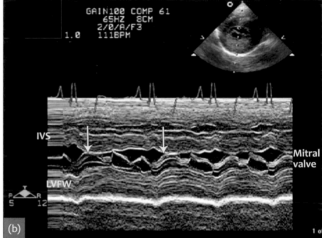

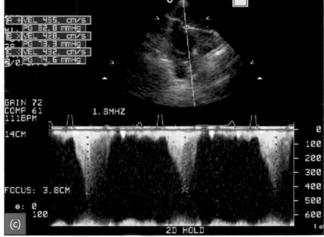

9.97 A 4-year-old Welsh Terrier with evidence of left-sided cardiomegaly on CT, but no clinical signs referable to cardiac disease. No heart murmur was detected. (a) M-mode at mitral valve level showing abnormal mitral valve motion. The anterior leaflet (AMV) moves towards the IVS with restricted excursion and shows delayed partial closure during diastasis prior to atrial contraction (reduced EF slope). The most striking finding is that the posterior leaflet (PMV) does not move in the opposite direction towards the LVFW, but is tethered to the AMV, so its movement parallels that of the AMV. The valve is thick and the M-mode confirms incomplete opening. (b) Right parasternal four-chamber view during late diastole (associated with atrial contraction). The mitral valve leaflets did not open completely, appearing tethered and with a 'hockey stick' appearance. The colour flow Doppler shows colour variance of transmitral flow on the ventricular side of the mitral valve. (c) Left apical four-chamber view continuous wave Doppler of transmitral flow, showing increased E and A wave velocities, with the A wave higher than the E wave (E:A ratio <1) indicating dependence on atrial contraction to achieve ventricular filling. The E wave shows slow deceleration, so the A wave starts before the E wave is completed. These findings are all consistent with mitral stenosis. This case did not have mitral regurgitation.

9.98 A 2-year-old male Border Terrier following a syncopal episode. (a) Right parasternal four-chamber view, showing marked concentric left ventricular hypertrophy but subjectively normal left atrial size. The anterior mitral valve leaflet appeared slightly thick and elongated, and during systole this was pushed into the left ventricular outflow tract. This resulted in dynamic left ventricular outflow tract obstruction and mild mitral regurgitation. (b) M-mode at the level of the mitral valve showing normal E and A peaks of the anterior leaflet during diastole, but also opening of the anterior leaflet during systole, confirming SAM (arrowed) of this anterior mitral valve leaflet. (c) Subcostal view with continuous wave Doppler confirming significant dynamic left ventricular outflow tract obstruction, with scimitar envelope, resulting from biphasic acceleration of left ventricular outflow. In a cat, these changes could be due to hypertrophic obstructive cardiomyopathy. In dogs, it is more common that they are associated with mitral valve dysplasia, especially with elongated anterior mitral valve leaflets. The SAM results in dynamic left ventricular outflow tract obstruction and the concentric left ventricular hypertrophy is likely secondary to this.

Angiocardiography

This is rarely indicated for diagnosis of mitral valve dysplasia. Mitral regurgitation is demonstrated by left ventricular injection of contrast medium. Prominent left atrial dilatation accompanied by left ventricular dilatation will usually be identified. Mitral stenosis is best demonstrated using a left atrial injection of contrast medium (performed by transseptal puncture) but is certainly difficult to recognize.

Tricuspid valve dysplasia

This condition is mostly observed in dogs, with larger breeds such as Labrador Retrievers most commonly affected. In Labrador Retrievers, familial disease and a genetic basis to the disease have been confirmed. The condition is also seen in cats.

Tricuspid valve dysplasia is characterized by malformed tricuspid leaflets, chordae tendinae and/or papillary muscles. This is most commonly associated with tricuspid regurgitation, which results in severe volume overload of the RA and RV. Rarely, tricuspid stenosis may occur. Additional congenital cardiac anomalies, such as pulmonic stenosis or ASD, may be present.

Ebstein's anomaly is a rare form of tricuspid valve dysplasia. In this condition, the base of the cusps of the abnormal tricuspid valve are displaced into the ventricle and part of the RV is therefore 'atrialized'. It should be remembered that the tricuspid valve is more apically positioned than the mitral annulus in normal animals. Criteria for the diagnosis of Ebstein's anomaly in dogs have been proposed (Chetboul *et al.*, 2020).

Clinical signs are usually not apparent early on in the condition. A holosystolic murmur will be identified over the tricuspid valve region, but this is often low grade, reflected by the normally low pressure gradient between the RV and RA. Eventually, right-sided heart failure may result (e.g. hepatomegaly, ascites and distension of the jugular veins).

Radiography

Radiographic findings reflect the right-sided volume overload and include:

- Right ventricular and right atrial enlargement (Figure 9.99)
- A marked apex shift to the left is often noted
- The cardiac enlargement can be substantial and the cardiac silhouette may almost appear globoid
- Tricuspid stenosis should be considered when the atrium is markedly enlarged but not accompanied by changes in the ventricle
- There may be enlargement of the CdVC
- Hepatomegaly and ascites, resulting in increased opacity, poor abdominal serosal contrast and abdominal distension when there is overt right-sided CHF.

Doppler echocardiography

Echocardiographic findings include:

- Marked right atrial dilatation (Figure 9.100ab)
- Right ventricular dilatation (unless the valve is stenotic) (Figure 9.100ab)
- Abnormal papillary muscles (may find a large fused papillary muscle instead of the small discrete muscles)

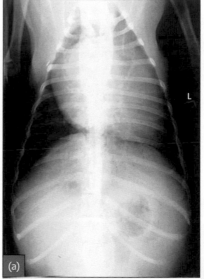

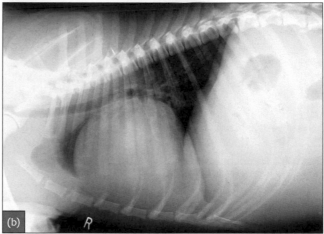

9.99 (a) DV and (b) right lateral thoracic radiographs of a 10-month-old male Boxer with right-sided CHF. Ascites is confirmed by abdominal distension and poor abdominal serosal contrast. There is marked right ventricular and right atrial enlargement.

- Abnormal conformation of the tricuspid valve (Figure 9.100ab)
  - Hyperechoic leaflets and chordae tendinae
  - Decreased motion of the tricuspid leaflets
  - Decreased separation from the RVFW and/or IVS (tethered appearance)
  - Apical implantation of the tricuspid valves with a seemingly reduced right ventricular chamber and a seemingly enlarged RA (right ventricular 'atrialization' – Ebstein's anomaly)
- Colour flow Doppler confirms presence of tricuspid regurgitation (Figure 9.100c)
- Continuous wave spectral Doppler aligned with tricuspid regurgitation will give the peak velocity of the tricuspid regurgitation (Figure 9.100d). The pressure gradient between the RV and RA can be determined (usually <30 mmHg; may be reduced in right-sided CHF reflecting increased right atrial pressure)
- If the tricuspid regurgitation velocity is increased, concurrent congenital defects such as pulmonic stenosis need to be excluded (Figure 9.100d). If excluded, an increase in tricuspid regurgitation velocity would suggest pulmonary hypertension
- In the presence of tricuspid stenosis, the transtricuspid diastolic velocities will be increased, and early diastolic velocity is slow to decelerate.

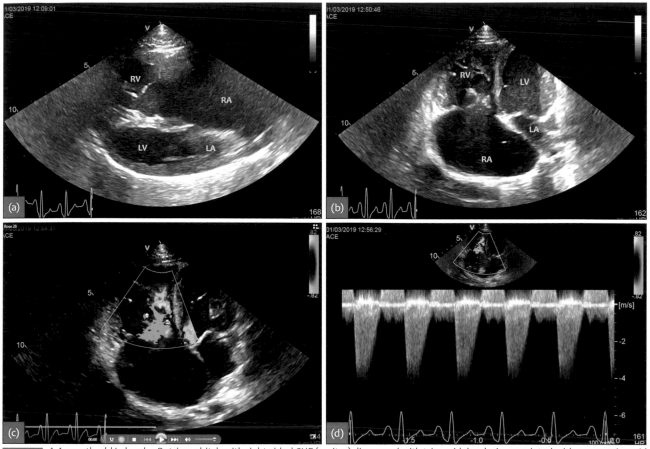

9.100 A 4-month-old Labrador Retriever bitch with right-sided CHF (ascites) diagnosed with tricuspid dysplasia associated with severe tricuspid regurgitation, and mild aortic stenosis and pulmonic stenosis. (a) Right parasternal long-axis four-chamber view. There is severe right atrial and right ventricular dilatation. The mural tricuspid valve leaflet is directly attached to a papillary muscle and is tethered. The septal leaflet is very short and immobile. (b) The left apical four-chamber view confirms severe right atrial and right ventricular dilatation and abnormal tricuspid valve leaflets, which appear apically displaced. This systolic frame confirms poor coaptation between both tricuspid valve leaflets. (c) Colour flow Doppler of the left apical four-chamber view; systolic frame confirming tricuspid regurgitation. (d) Continuous wave Doppler of the tricuspid regurgitation jet. Peak velocity is increased (nearly 4 m/s) because of the concurrent mild pulmonic stenosis.

Angiocardiography

Contrast studies are not very useful in the diagnosis and/or management of tricuspid valve malformations. They can demonstrate right atrial and right ventricular enlargement. Tricuspid regurgitation can be demonstrated by a right ventricular injection of contrast medium. If there is tricuspid stenosis, balloon valvuloplasty may be attempted with fluoroscopy used to guide the procedure.

Tetralogy of Fallot

Tetralogy of Fallot is a complex congenital disorder, resulting from a failure of the conotruncal septum to align properly at the embryonic stage. The Keeshond and Bulldog are predisposed and the condition is also seen in cats. Tetralogy of Fallot is the most common cause of cyanotic cardiac disease in young animals.

The disease is characterized by four features:

- Pulmonic stenosis leading to right ventricular outflow obstruction (pulmonic trunk hypoplasia or atresia may also be present)
- Secondary right ventricular concentric hypertrophy
- A supracristal VSD, which enters the RV in the RVOT but is located beneath the aortic valve leaflets on the left ventricular side
- Dextroposition of the aorta (rightward positioning or overriding aorta).

The right ventricular outflow obstruction results in right ventricular pressure overload. Increased right ventricular pressure leads to shunting of blood from the right side to the left via the VSD. Deoxygenated blood mixes with left-sided oxygenated blood and hypoxaemia results. The LA and LV are small and the pulmonary arteries and veins are underperfused. The bronchial arteries increase the systemic collateral circulation that they provide to the lungs.

Animals present with exercise intolerance, failure to grow, shortness of breath, syncope, cyanosis and secondary polycythaemia. Note that since shunting occurs at the level of the ventricles the cyanosis is generalized and not differential as in rPDA. Medical and surgical treatment options exist and the prognosis is variable.

Radiography

Radiographic findings include:

- The overall size of the heart is usually small to normal
- Right ventricular enlargement may be apparent (Figure 9.101). This may result in tipping of the left ventricular apex off the sternum (lateral view), consistent with severe right ventricular hypertrophy
- The overriding of the aorta and dilated aorta may result in a prominent aorta or aortic bulge
- The pulmonic trunk is not enlarged with pulmonary artery hypoplasia; there is no post-stenotic dilatation

- Hypovascularity of the lungs may be identified as hyperlucent lung fields and decreased size of the pulmonary lobar vessels (Figure 9.101)
- The lungs are often hyperinflated, contributing to the hypolucent appearance.

Doppler echocardiography

Echocardiographic findings include:

- Right ventricular concentric hypertrophy
- High and often large VSD
- Aorta 'overriding' the IVS. The aorta is dextroposed (Figure 9.102a)
- Pulmonic stenosis. The pulmonic trunk is usually hypoplastic (Figure 9.102b) or atretic (no post-stenotic dilatation evident)
- Reduced dimensions of the LA and LV; reflecting the pressure overload of the RV and underfilling
- If right ventricular pressure exceeds left ventricular pressure, there is right-to-left flow evident on colour flow and spectral Doppler interrogating the VSD flow (Figure 9.103)

- With a very dextroposed aorta, flow from the RV can enter the aorta, rather than going into the LV across the VSD (see Figure 9.102c)
- Colour flow and spectral Doppler confirms the pulmonic stenosis.

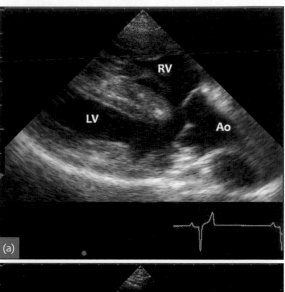

(a)

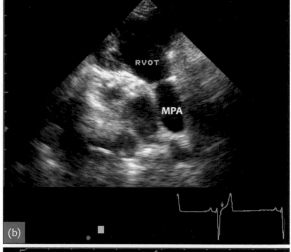

(b)

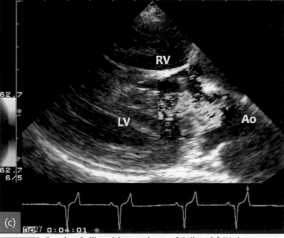

(c)

9.102 Border Collie with tetralogy of Fallot. (a) Right parasternal long-axis five-chamber view. The aorta (Ao) is overriding or dextroposed and a high VSD is present. (b) Right parasternal short-axis view obtained at the level of the heart base and optimized for the RVOT. The pulmonic valve is stenotic and the valves are thickened and echogenic. The pulmonic trunk (MPA) is hypoplastic. (c) Right parasternal long-axis five-chamber view with colour Doppler. Blood is shunting from right-to-left across the VSD.

(© J. Dukes-McEwan)

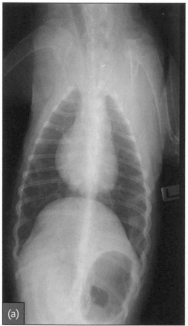

(a)

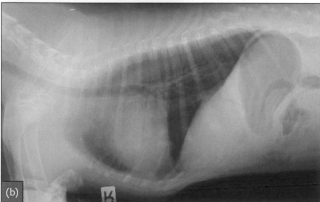

(b)

9.101 (a) DV and (b) lateral thoracic radiographs of a 5-month-old male Airedale Terrier with stunted growth, severe exercise intolerance and cyanosis due to tetralogy of Fallot. There is no generalized cardiomegaly, but there is evidence of right ventricular enlargement resulting in slight apex tipping on the lateral view. The aortic arch is prominent on both the lateral and the DV view. The lungs appear hyperinflated and relatively hypovascular.

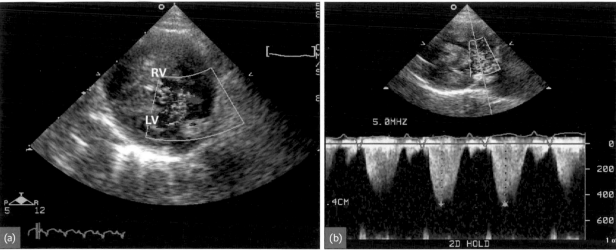

9.103 Domestic Shorthaired cat with tetralogy of Fallot. (a) A high VSD is evident on the right parasternal short-axis view and the colour flow map documents the right-to-left flow. (b) Continuous wave Doppler shows the right-to-left flow across the septal defect.
(© J. Dukes-McEwan)

Angiocardiography

Angiocardiography can be useful to confirm the diagnosis but is usually unnecessary if echocardiography is carefully performed. However, in severely symptomatic, hypoxaemic animals with hyperinflation of the lungs, lung interference may compromise use of standard echocardiographic windows.

It can be difficult to differentiate a tetralogy of Fallot from a VSD with reversed shunt direction (right-to-left) secondary to pulmonary hypertension (Eisenmenger's syndrome):

- In both cases, after a right ventricular injection of contrast medium, there will be simultaneous opacification of the pulmonic trunk and ascending aorta
- In tetralogy of Fallot, narrowing or hypoplasia of the pulmonic trunk should be looked for (Figure 9.104). This will assist in differentiation from a reversed VSD (in which the RVOT, pulmonic trunk and its branches appear normal in size and will fill up with contrast medium)
- Note that pulmonic stenosis in combination with an isolated right-to-left shunting VSD can be extremely difficult to differentiate from tetralogy of Fallot in all imaging studies.

Cor triatriatum abnormalities

Cor triatriatum is a rare congenital defect that manifests as a partitioned RA (cor triatriatum dexter (CTD)) or even less commonly, a partitioned LA (cor triatriatum sinister (CTS)).

Cor triatriatum dexter

- The condition is rare but well documented in dogs. It is extremely rare in cats.
- CTD is caused by failure of the right sinus venosus valve to regress during embryogenesis.
- A membrane develops within the RA, affecting systemic venous return to the RA and compartmentalizing the RA into high and low pressure parts.
- Most commonly, the CdVC and sometimes the coronary sinus enters the high pressure part, but the CrVC enters the low pressure part of the RA, above the tricuspid valve. The membrane is usually perforate, permitting some flow but offering high resistance to flow from the distal (caudal) to more proximal (cranial) right atrial chambers.
- Affected animals present with caudal signs of right-sided CHF (e.g. ascites). This can mimic other conditions obstructing caudal vena caval flow (Budd–Chiari-like syndrome). A heart murmur is not usually detected (unless there is a concurrent congenital defect).

Radiography: Radiographic findings include:

- Marked dilatation of the RA, creating a bulge with soft tissue opacity between 9 and 11 o'clock on DV and lateral views (Figure 9.105)
- Dilatation of the CdVC
- There may be hepatomegaly, abdominal distension and peritoneal effusion (right-sided heart failure) (Figure 9.105).

9.104 Lateral angiocardiogram of a dog with tetralogy of Fallot. The contrast medium was injected in the RV. There is narrowing of the pulmonic trunk (MPA) at the infundibular level (arrowed) and there is simultaneous opacification of the pulmonic trunk and the aorta (Ao), which means that there is a right-to-left shunt.
(Courtesy of J. Buchanan)

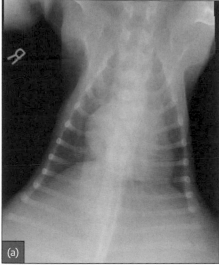

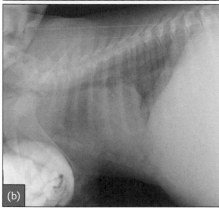

9.105 (a) DV and (b) right lateral thoracic radiographs of an 11-week-old male Golden Retriever with severe ascites, imperforate CTD, patent foramen ovale and double-chambered RV. The DV view shows right heart enlargement, especially the RA. Both views confirm ascites and the DV view shows distension of the CdVC.

Doppler echocardiography: Echocardiographic findings in CTD include:

- The RA has two compartments; the high pressure caudal compartment often appears rounded and the CdVC and coronary sinus usually enter this part (Figure 9.106)
- Colour flow Doppler should show flow across the membrane into the cranial (low pressure) RA if the membrane is perforate
- Turbulent venous inflow can be seen through the membrane using spectral Doppler studies
- Sometimes, the high pressure caudal chamber results in a patent foramen ovale, so colour flow Doppler will show flow from this into the LA
- Right atrial dilatation without other obvious changes
- A thin membrane in the caudal RA, dividing the atrium into a larger cranial compartment and a smaller caudal compartment
- The caudal compartment includes the entrance of the CdVC, which is distended
- An echocardiographic contrast study with peripheral injections of agitated saline (possibly with colloid) into a caudal peripheral vein shows the high pressure chamber receives caudal blood flow with the arrival of contrast material. Contrast studies will also confirm presence of a patent foramen ovale if the LA shows presence of contrast.

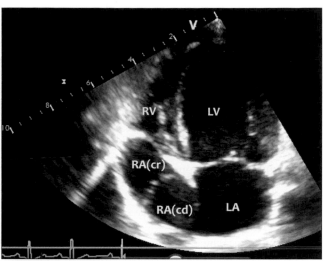

9.106 A 6-month-old Boxer bitch that presented with ascites. This left apical four-chamber view shows that the RA is in two compartments: a high pressure caudal compartment (RA(cd)) and a low pressure cranial compartment (RA(cr)) above the tricuspid valve.

Angiocardiography: In an animal with typical CTD, injection of contrast medium in the CdVC might reveal an obstruction to venous return at the level of the RA, with saccular dilatation of the caudal RA (Figure 9.107).

Cor triatriatum sinister

- CTS is very rare and was originally thought to only occur in cats but it has recently been described in dogs.
- CTS is caused by an abnormal connection of the LA with the pulmonary veins.
- A membrane separates the LA into a high pressure distal part (receiving the pulmonary veins) and a lower pressure part above the mitral valve. This membrane may be perforate, and the degree of resistance it offers will result in pulmonary venous congestion and, commonly, left-sided CHF.

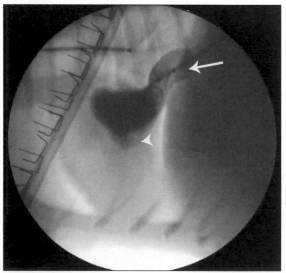

9.107 Lateral angiocardiogram of a 6-month-old Boxer bitch with ascites due to CTD (same dog as in Figure 9.106). Angiocardiography was performed during a fluoroscopic study prior to intervention (balloon dilation of the perforated CTD membrane) with a pigtail catheter in the CdVC (arrowed). The dog is also lying on an echotable to facilitate intraprocedural transthoracic echocardiography (edge of cut-out with staples seen to left of image). The caudal RA is very dilated, as is the CdVC, and some contrast shows retrograde flow into a dilated coronary sinus (arrowhead). In this frame, contrast cannot yet be seen in the cranial RA or RV.

- Note that supravalvular mitral stenosis closely resembles CTS. The only difference is the level of the obstructing membrane. In supravalvular mitral stenosis the obstruction is distal to the foramen ovale and LAA and the LAA will be dilated. In CTS the obstruction is proximal to the foramen ovale and the LAA is therefore downstream and does not enlarge.

Radiography: Radiographic findings include:
- Left atrial dilatation
- Pulmonary venous congestion
- There may be cardiogenic pulmonary oedema (left-sided congestive heart failure).

Doppler echocardiography:
- Echocardiography can provide the diagnosis of CTS.
- A visible partition of the LA is seen. It is perforate but gives high resistance.
- Colour flow and spectral Doppler confirms diastolic high-velocity turbulent flow crossing the membrane (Figure 9.108).
- The location of this membrane and whether or not the LAA is dilated distinguishes supravalvular mitral stenosis (LAA in high pressure chamber) from true CTS (LAA distal to the obstruction so not dilated).
- CTS may be identified in the presence of other congenital heart disease (Figure 9.109).
- Perforations in the dividing membrane are occasionally identified.

Angiocardiography: Selective angiocardiography is difficult as the dividing membrane in the LA makes it difficult to opacify the entire LA. Non-selective angiocardiography at the late phase (levophase) can provide more information, revealing that the large soft tissue opacity corresponds to a saccular dilatation of the LA, which will occasionally appear bilobed (Figure 9.110).

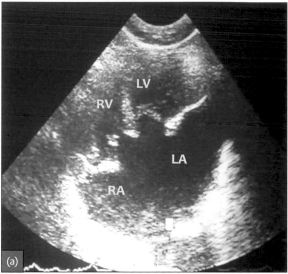

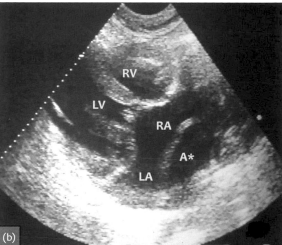

9.109 Cat with an endocardial cushion defect and an unusual cor triatriatum. (a) Left apical four-chamber view. Large confluent atrial and ventral septal defects are evident. (b) Right parasternal long-axis view. The ASD can be seen and an additional thin dividing membrane is evident within the common atrium, creating an extra chamber (A*). This was considered to be CTS; however, the decision as to whether the lesion is left- or right-sided is difficult when a common atrium is present. (© J. Dukes-McEwan)

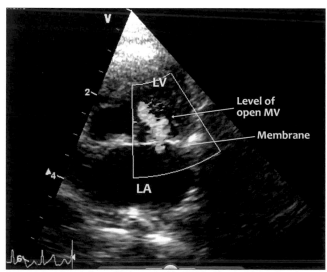

9.108 A Ragdoll cat diagnosed with CTS. Left apical four-chamber view showing a very dilated LA and subjectively distended pulmonary veins. There is a membrane proximal to the mitral valve, with high-velocity turbulent flow crossing it. The mitral valve (MV) leaflets are open normally during diastole. This lesion is just proximal to the mitral valve. The LAA cannot be assessed from this image; a dilated LAA suggests the cat is more likely to have supravalvular mitral stenosis (SVMS). However, CTS and SVMS are very similar in pathophysiology.

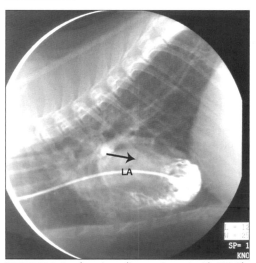

9.110 Lateral angiocardiogram in a cat with CTS. The contrast medium was injected in the RV after catheterization of the jugular vein. A levophase image is presented, where the contrast medium has reached the LA. The LA is enlarged and a linear filling defect is visible in its lumen, corresponding to the dividing membrane (arrowed). (Courtesy of J. Buchanan)

Congenital vascular disease

Vascular ring and other anomalies

A vascular ring anomaly results from abnormal embryonic development of the primordial aortic arches (aortic arch III, IV or VI) around the embryonic pharynx. This developmental anomaly results in a vascular ring around the trachea and oesophagus, leading to postnatal constriction of the thoracic oesophagus and development of a secondary segmental enlargement of the oesophagus cranial to the heart base (see also Chapter 10). Dogs and cats are affected. German Shepherd Dogs and Irish Setters are predisposed to this condition.

A spectrum of abnormalities may be encountered, the most common are:

- Persistence of the right fourth aortic arch (PRAA) with a left-sided ligamentum arteriosum (most common anomaly) and/or a retro-oesophageal left subclavian artery
- Double aortic arches
- Normal fourth aortic arch with retro-oesophageal (aberrant) right subclavian artery (usually not a major problem from a clinical standpoint)
- Anomalous right subclavian artery arising from the aortic arch.

Rarely, a PDA is associated with a vascular ring anomaly.

Radiography

Radiographic findings include:

- If the vascular ring anomaly has entrapped the oesophagus, then segmental oesophageal dilatation may be seen cranial to the heart base. Oesophagography may occasionally be required to identify this
- The lumen of the enlarged oesophagus may have a soft tissue or heterogenous granular opacity depending on what was ingested. General ventral displacement of the trachea may be seen (Figure 9.111)
- There may be a cranioventral lung consolidation (alveolar pattern) if aspiration pneumonia has occurred
- Moderate or marked focal leftward curvature of the trachea near the cranial border of the heart on DV or VD radiographs is a reliable sign of PRAA in young dogs with consistent clinical signs (as opposed to the right-sided tracheal curvature seen in normal animals)
- In cases of PRAA, the leftward margin of the descending aorta is not visible on DV views
- If a well defined, normal left descending aortic margin is clearly identified on the DV or VD view, a less common vascular ring anomaly may be suspected. CT angiography is warranted in such cases to confirm the diagnosis, the specific type of vascular ring anomaly, and plan the best surgical approach.

Oesophagography: Oesophageal contrast studies show accumulation of the contrast medium in a distended oesophagus cranial to the heart base and abrupt tapering at the level of the sixth pair of ribs (Figure 9.112). Occasionally, the oesophageal dilatation is generalized and these cases carry the worst prognosis.

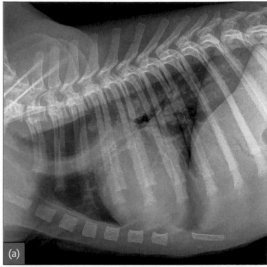
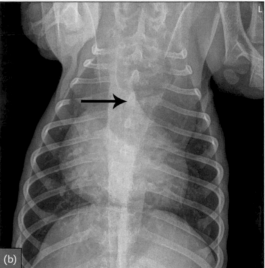

9.111 (a) Left lateral and (b) DV thoracic radiographs of a 2-month-old intact crossbreed bitch with regurgitation and thin body condition due to a vascular ring anomaly. The oesophagus is severely segmentally enlarged (orange) cranial to the heart base, causing ventral tracheal deviation (yellow). The most common type of vascular ring anomaly is a PRAA with a persistent left ligamentum arteriosum. Based on the focal tracheal deviation to the left (arrowed), this dog has a PRAA. The ligamentum arteriosum cannot be seen with this type of study.

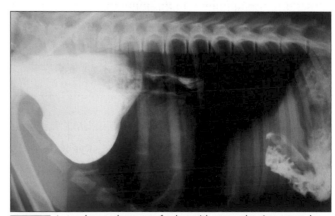

9.112 Lateral oesophagram of a dog with a vascular ring anomaly associated with a PRAA, after oral administration of barium sulphate. There is accumulation of the contrast medium in a distended oesophagus cranial to the heart base and abrupt tapering at the level of the heart base.
(Courtesy of J. Buchanan)

Computed tomography angiography

CT angiography with multiplanar reconstruction is useful to diagnose different vascular ring anomalies. The arterial phase following an intravenous injection of contrast medium can identify vascular ring anomalies. If the vascular ring is completed by a left ligamentum arteriosum (in addtition to the PRAA), then a full contrast-enhanced ring will not be observed as there is no blood flow through the ligamentum arteriosum. A full ring may be seen with a PRAA and a PDA or 'double aortic arch' (Figure 9.113).

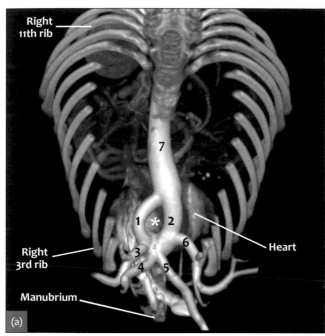

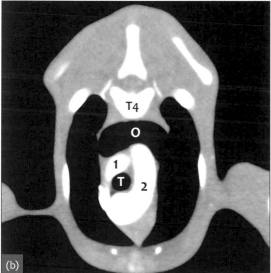

9.113 Thoracic CT angiograms of a 14-week-old neutered crossbreed bitch with regurgitation and thin body condition. (a) Craniodorsal aspect, 3D volume rendered image. (b) Transverse CT image (arterial phase; soft tissue window) acquired at the level of the fourth thoracic vertebra (T4). Thoracic radiography performed by the referring veterinary surgeon showed segmental oesophageal enlargement cranial to the heart base. The clinical signs and segmental oesophageal enlargement were attributed to a congenital developmental vascular ring anomaly (∗) formed by left and right aortic arches (double aortic arches). The ring encircles the trachea and oesophagus, the latter of which is enlarged cranial to the ring. Surgery was performed to ligate and transect the right aortic arch. The dog recovered well and was discharged. 1 = right aortic arch; 2 = left aortic arch; 3 = right subclavian artery; 4 = right common carotid artery; 5 = left common carotid artery; 6 = left subclavian artery; 7 = descending aorta; O = oesophagus; T = trachea.

Angiocardiography

This is not usually necessary. An adequate presurgical diagnosis of vascular ring constriction of the oesophagus can be made with thoracic radiographs, barium studies of the oesophagus or CT angiography to examine the vascular anatomy at the heart base and associated thoracic structures.

It may be valuable to identify animals that have a normal left fourth aortic arch but abnormal formation of the right fourth and/or right sixth aortic arch: in these cases a right thoracotomy is the best surgical approach as opposed to the more common left approach.

A left ventricular injection of contrast medium is usually performed:

- PRAA is more consistently demonstrated on DV views, where the opacified aortic arch can be seen coursing to the right of the trachea
- A retro-oesophageal left subclavian artery can be demonstrated on lateral views as it courses cranially from its origin dorsally and to the left of the aorta at about the level where the thoracic aorta begins to run parallel to the vertebral column. The persistent left subclavian artery compresses the oesophagus dorsally when it begins running ventral to the thoracic inlet
- An anomalous right subclavian artery can be seen crossing dorsally over the cranial mediastinal oesophagus, potentially causing oesophageal constriction.

Aortic coarctation

Aortic coarctation is a very rare condition in dogs and even rarer in cats. The disease consists of a narrowing of the aortic lumen that usually occurs at the aortic isthmus, the segment of the aorta between the origin of the left subclavian artery and the insertion of the ductus arteriosus.

It is believed to be due to spreading of the specialized contractile ductal tissue into the aorta to form a sling around it, which after birth becomes part of an obstructive curtain of tissue. The narrowing is responsible for obstruction to the flow into the descending aorta and aneurysmal dilatation of the aorta caudal to the obstruction. The narrowing process takes weeks to develop, which leaves time for the LV to adjust to the increased pressure load and for collateral circulation to develop; this is why there are often no clinical signs associated with the disease.

Radiography

Radiographic findings are non-specific:

- An exaggerated and enlarged aortic arch is visible, creating a soft tissue opacity bulging out from the mediastinum into the left cranial thorax
- The trachea can be displaced ventrally (lateral view) and to the right (DV or VD view) by the soft tissue opacity
- Notching of the ribs (small indentation surrounded by fine rim of sclerotic bone) is highly suggestive of aortic coarctation in humans and has also been reported in dogs. It occurs due to enlargement of the intercostal arteries. These carry collateral circulation in a retrograde direction from both the costocervical trunk and internal thoracic arteries to supply the caudal aorta.

Angiocardiography

Cardiac catheterization and aortography are indicated to accurately localize the site of obstruction, determine the length of the coarctation and identify associated malformations (Figure 9.114).

CT angiography

CT angiography will also show the site and severity of coarctation (Cuddy *et al.*, 2013).

Echocardiography

Echocardiography does not allow the diagnosis of aortic coarctation, though transoesophageal echocardiography might be helpful. Echocardiography can rule out the presence of associated congenital heart defects.

Marfan-like syndrome

Marfan syndrome in humans is a connective tissue disorder with a genetic basis. The aortic root and aortic arch are often massively dilated, and this can result in severe aortic regurgitation.

There have been sporadic reports suggesting a similar condition in dogs (Lenz *et al.*, 2015; Biasato *et al.*, 2018).

Angiography or CT angiography can confirm the dilatation of the aortic arch (Figure 9.115a). Marfan-like syndrome is suspected from echocardiography if there is a very dilated aortic root with significant aortic regurgitation (a diastolic murmur may be detected) (Figure 9.115b).

Persistent left cranial vena cava

Persistent left cranial vena cava (PLCrVC) is a congenital developmental venous vascular anomaly that does not have any functional significance or clinical relevance on its own. It is not uncommon and is usually an incidental finding. It can be associated with other congenital heart disease. It may be clinically important in the presence of cardiac disease if catheterization or other interventions are indicated, so it is important to be aware of the abnormality.

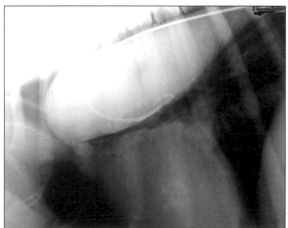

9.114 Lateral aortogram of a dog with aortic coarctation. Contrast medium was injected in the aortic arch after catheterization of the femoral artery. There is narrowing of the aorta caudal to the origin of the left subclavian artery, followed by marked dilatation of the aorta caudal to the stenosis. The catheter is seen curving around in the dilated portion of the aorta.
(Courtesy of M. Herrtage)

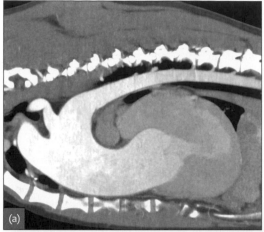

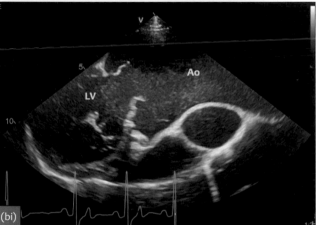

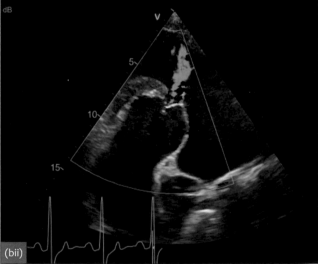

9.115 A 1-year old spaniel with Marfan-like syndrome. (a) Multiplanar reconstruction of a CT angiogram (sagittal image). There is severe dilatation of the aortic root. This affects the entire aortic arch, including the brachiocephalic and left subclavian arteries. Aortic regurgitation can also be noted. The descending aorta is within normal limits. (bi) Right parasternal long-axis five-chamber view showing the aortic valves and ascending aorta during systole. (bii) Colour flow Doppler from a left apical five-chamber view showing the aorta (Ao) and aortic regurgitation during diastole.

During embryonic development, there are two cranial venae cavae and the left normally regresses, leaving the right as the definitive CrVC, entering directly into the RA. If the left CrVC persists, it courses around the caudal part of the LA and empties into the coronary sinus. This results in a dilated coronary sinus.

Radiography

Plain radiography is generally unremarkable unless there is another congenital cardiovascular defect.

Echocardiography

The hallmark of a PLCrVC is identification of a dilated coronary sinus.

- A dilated coronary sinus can be seen coursing around the left atrioventricular groove, emptying into the RA, when this structure is optimized (Figure 9.116a).
- In a standard right parasternal long-axis four-chamber view, the dilated coronary sinus may be seen as an end-on vessel in the left atrioventricular groove, between the base of the LVFW and caudal part of the LA (Figure 9.116c). It may make it difficult to optimize left atrial diameter.
- The left apical view can also show the dilated coronary sinus crossing the left atrioventricular groove and entering the RA (Figure 9.116b).
- Colour flow Doppler confirms normal venous flow in this structure (usually superimposed on the right

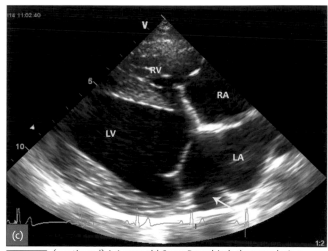

9.116 (continued) A 4-year-old Great Dane bitch that was being screened for dilated cardiomyopathy, with no clinically significant cardiac disease apparent at time of examination. A dilated coronary sinus was noted as an incidental finding. This is usually associated with a PLCrVC. (c) With a standard right parasternal long-axis four-chamber view, the dilated coronary sinus is often seen in short axis in the left atrioventricular groove (arrowed).

parasternal long-axis four-chamber view optimizing this structure).
- An echocontrast study can confirm the dilated coronary sinus is the result of a PLCrVC. Agitated saline (possibly with colloid) is injected into a left cephalic vein. If the coronary sinus is opacified, this confirms the PLCrVC. Note – some dogs may have both venae cavae, so the right-sided peripheral veins should not be used.

NB: A dilated coronary sinus can also be seen in situations with high right-sided pressures or right-sided CHF of any cause (see Figure 9.160)

Angiocardiography

Non-selective angiography can confirm the PLCrVC. This can be done via a left jugular catheter, with the animal positioned in a ventrodorsal position. Contrast material can be seen in the left CrVC, coursing caudally around the LA and passing cranially to enter the RA via the coronary sinus.

Computed tomography

Multiplanar reconstructed contrast CT (venous phase) can also confirm the presence of a PLCrVC (Figure 9.117).

Aberrant coronary arteries

See 'Pulmonic stenosis', above; see also Figures 9.59, 9.60 and 9.70–9.72.

Other vascular abnormalities

These are not uncommon and include aortopulmonic vascular malformation (aberrant bronchoesophageal artery), anomalous pulmonary venous return, caudal vena caval abnormalities and various types of portosystemic shunts, including oesophageal varix formation. However, they are beyond the remit of a thoracic imaging manual.

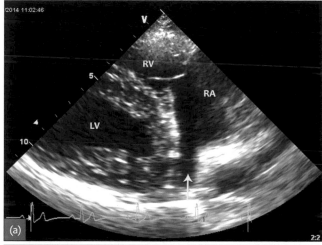

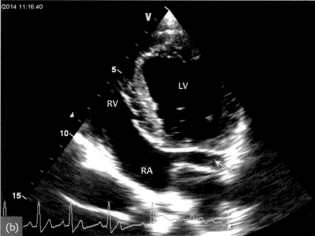

9.116 A 4-year-old Great Dane bitch that was being screened for dilated cardiomyopathy, with no clinically significant cardiac disease apparent at time of examination. A dilated coronary sinus was noted as an incidental finding. This is usually associated with a PLCrVC. (a) Right parasternal long-axis view showing the dilated coronary sinus, which courses around the left atrioventricular groove, opening into the RA (arrowed). (b) Left apical four-chamber view optimized for the dilated coronary sinus (arrowed), which can be seen opening into the RA. (continues) ▶

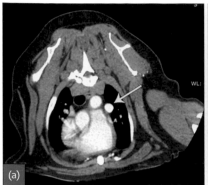 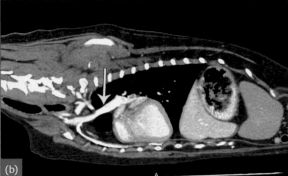 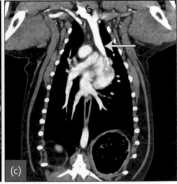

9.117 (a) Transverse, (b) sagittal and (c) dorsal multiplanar reformatted contrast-enhanced CT images (soft tissue reconstruction) of a PLCrVC (arrowed) in a dog.
(Courtesy of Will Humphreys, University of Liverpool)

Myocardial diseases

Cardiomyopathies are defined as diseases of the myocardium associated with cardiac dysfunction. They may be primary or secondary to another condition. In making a diagnosis of idiopathic cardiomyopathy, active exclusion of inflammatory, neoplastic, metabolic, endocrine, nutritional, pulmonary, systemic hypertensive, toxic and other conditions is required. Specific secondary cardiomyopathies may be subdivided according to their aetiology (e.g. hyperthyroid cardiomyopathy).

Idiopathic primary cardiomyopathies may be further subdivided according to their morphological (echocardiographic) appearance and dysfunction:

- Dilated cardiomyopathy (DCM)
- Arrhythmogenic right ventricular cardiomyopathy (ARVC)
- HCM
- Restrictive cardiomyopathy (RCM)
- Non-specific cardiomyopathy.

In humans, as an aetiological genetic basis to many of the cardiomyopathies is now known, the classification is moving away from an entirely morphological or functional classification (Arbustini *et al.*, 2013; McKenna *et al.*, 2017). In most veterinary cases of primary cardiomyopathies, the aetiology is unknown and so the morphological and functional classification is used. In cats, all forms of cardiomyopathy are seen, including non-specific cardiomyopathy, which does not neatly meet criteria of the other forms (Luis Fuentes *et al.*, 2020).

Canine myocardial disease
Dilated cardiomyopathy

A DCM phenotype (usually defined by echocardiography) can be seen secondary to a number of other conditions that should be actively excluded prior to making a diagnosis of primary or idiopathic DCM. These include tachyarrhythmias (tachycardia-induced cardiomyopathy (TICM)), nutritional causes (e.g. taurine deficiency in certain breeds such as American and English Cocker Spaniels, Golden Retrievers, Newfoundlands, and DCM associated with grain-free diets) and myocarditis, among others.

- DCM is characterized by left-sided or four-chamber dilatation and impaired left ventricular systolic function.

- DCM is a major cause of morbidity and mortality in various large and giant breeds of dog, including Deerhounds, Dobermanns, Great Danes, Irish Wolfhounds, Newfoundlands, St Bernards and spaniel breeds (Cocker and American Cocker, English Springer).
- Because of breed and familial predisposition, a genetic aetiology is most commonly suspected, but other potential causes of a DCM phenotype should be sought and excluded, including TICM and nutritional causes (e.g. grain-free diets, taurine deficiency).
- Presentation is usually associated with the onset of CHF with coughing or dyspnoea. Exercise intolerance may be marked. It may be associated with sustained or episodic tachyarrhythmias, such as atrial fibrillation or ventricular tachycardia, resulting in syncopal episodes.
- There is a long presymptomatic phase of this disease and the onset of CHF is merely the 'tip of the iceberg'. In Dobermanns, the PROTECT study showed that identification of preclinical or occult DCM is important, as treatment slows progression before development of CHF or death (Summerfield *et al.*, 2012). This may be true in other breeds.
- Clinical findings may be subtle. Arrhythmias, such as atrial fibrillation, may be present. A soft murmur may be detected, due to mitral regurgitation secondary to dilatation of the mitral annulus. Diastolic gallops may be detected in the decompensated animal.
- Imaging is essential to making the diagnosis of DCM. It demonstrates chamber dilatation and impaired systolic function. It also has an important role in excluding other cardiac conditions, which may secondarily result in CHF or poor output signs. Echocardiographic screening may be requested prior to breeding of a presymptomatic dog from a breed or family with DCM prevalence.

Radiography: Thoracic radiographs should be obtained for all dogs where left-sided CHF is suspected clinically or is imminent. Radiographs are very sensitive for documenting the volume load associated with left-sided CHF (pulmonary oedema). A caudodorsal to diffuse pulmonary infiltrate associated with left atrial enlargement and pulmonary venous congestion is consistent with cardiogenic pulmonary oedema (Figures 9.118 and 9.119).

In clinically symptomatic DCM, the cardiac silhouette is almost always abnormal. Possible findings include:

- Left atrial and ventricular enlargement
- Right atrial and ventricular enlargement

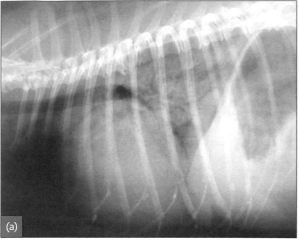

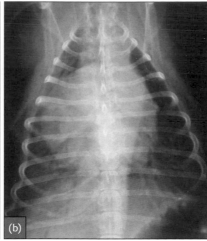

9.118 (a) Right lateral and (b) DV thoracic radiographs from a Cocker Spaniel with coughing and dyspnoea. There is generalized cardiomegaly with left atrial enlargement and pulmonary venous distension. There is a caudodorsal mixed interstitial–alveolar lung pattern, consistent with pulmonary oedema. Echocardiography confirmed that this dog had DCM resulting in the left-sided CHF.

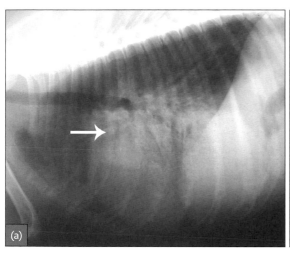

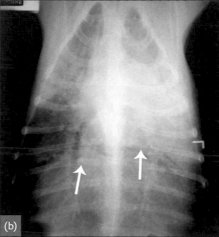

9.119 (a) Right lateral and (b) DV thoracic radiographs of a Dobermann with a history of several weeks coughing, recent syncopal episodes and then dyspnoea. DCM in the Dobermann is not associated with radiographic evidence of massive cardiomegaly, but there is left atrial and left ventricular enlargement. Note the pulmonary venous distension (arrowed) and the predominantly perihilar mixed interstitial and alveolar infiltrate.

- The cardiac silhouette may have a sharp 'static' outline with severe systolic function (loss of normal systolic–diastolic movement blur with each cardiac cycle). The concomitant presence of left atrial enlargement helps distinguish this from a pericardial effusion
- In left-sided congestive failure:
  - Triad of signs: LA enlargement, pulmonary venous distension and pulmonary opacification
  - The pulmonary opacification due to oedema in the lung parenchyma is normally predominantly perihilar or caudodorsal to diffuse. It may be interstitial or mixed interstitial–alveolar
- In right-sided congestive failure:
  - Evidence of abdominal effusion (ascites) in the cranial abdomen, with distension if there is a large volume
  - Distended CdVC
  - Pleural effusion
  - Note: in a dog with cardiomegaly presenting with predominantly right-sided CHF, pericardial effusion must be excluded. DCM normally presents with left-sided congestive failure
- There are breed variations. Many breeds show the typical, globular, cardiomegalic cardiac silhouette. Dobermanns may show a tall but not globular cardiac silhouette with significant left atrial enlargement (and features of left-sided CHF if present).

In presymptomatic (preclinical or 'occult') DCM, the lungs and pulmonary vasculature are usually unremarkable. The cardiac silhouette may or may not show signs of generalized cardiomegaly or specific chamber enlargement. Radiographs are not useful in screening for preclinical DCM, but they are useful in determining whether or not the dog is likely to show clinical signs in the near future (e.g. left atrial enlargement, pulmonary venous congestion).

Echocardiography (including Doppler studies): 2D and M-mode echocardiography are normally sufficient to make the diagnosis of DCM. However, since the stringent diagnosis of DCM requires the active exclusion of other congenital or acquired cardiac disease, colour flow and Doppler echocardiography are indicated. Furthermore, Doppler studies are required for identifying and classifying abnormalities in diastolic function, estimation of left-sided filling pressures and for demonstrating the presence of systolic function. Guidelines for the robust diagnosis of DCM have been proposed (Dukes-McEwan *et al.*, 2003) and, more recently, refined for Dobermanns (Wess *et al.*, 2017).

2D echocardiographic abnormalities in DCM typically include:

- Subjective findings include left ventricular dilatation with relatively thin walls and reduced systolic function (Figure 9.120a)

- A rounded rather than elliptical left ventricular chamber (Figure 9.120a) (increased sphericity), although it should be noted that the sphericity index has not been shown to be useful in screening for DCM (Holler and Wess, 2014). Sphericity index is calculated as LV diastolic length:LV diastolic width at chordae tendinae level (= M-mode left ventricular internal diameter at end-diastole (LVIDd))
- Increased left ventricular volume. Volumetric measurements from 2D echocardiographic images are superior to single dimensional M-mode images in assessing size and function of the LV. The left ventricular end-diastolic volume (EDV) and end-systolic volume (ESV) are calculated by Simpson's method of discs (See Chapter 2) or the length–area method (Figure 9.121) and then compared with breed-specific reference values if available
- The volume of the LV at the end of systole is inversely proportional to left ventricular systolic function. It is often indexed to the dog's body surface area (calculated from bodyweight). An increased ESVI compared with breed-specific reference ranges is evidence of systolic dysfunction. A commonly cited abnormal figure is >30 ml/m². However, many breeds have an ESVI higher than this (e.g. >55 ml/m² is abnormal in a Dobermann), so breed-specific reference ranges should be consulted where available (Figure 9.121)
- Simpson's derived ejection fraction is reduced (e.g. <40%) (Figure 9.121)
- The LA may be dilated in symptomatic dogs or dogs at risk of developing overt left-sided CHF
- The right-sided chambers may or may not be dilated.

M-mode echocardiographic abnormalities in DCM include:

- Increased LVIDd and left ventricular internal diameter at end-systole (LVIDs) compared with breed-based reference ranges where available or for bodyweight (allometric scaling) (Cornell *et al.*, 2004; Esser *et al.*, 2020)

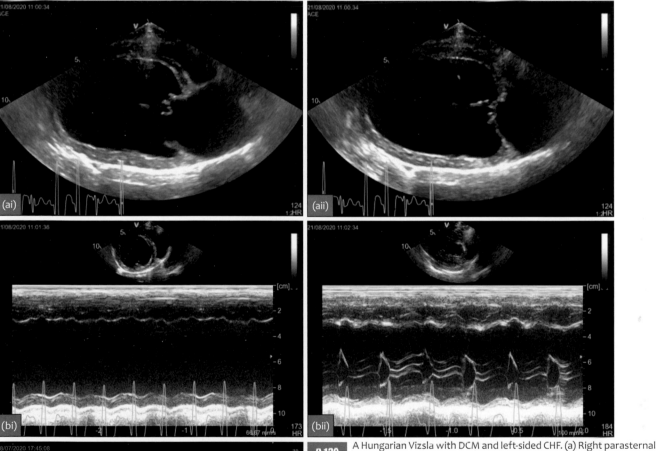

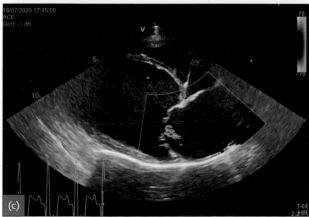

9.120 A Hungarian Vizsla with DCM and left-sided CHF. (a) Right parasternal long-axis four-chamber view in (ai) diastole and (aii) systole. There is very little difference in left ventricular area between diastole and systole because of severely impaired left ventricular systolic function. The LV is subjectively dilated and rounded, with relatively thin walls. The dog also has an arrhythmia. (bi) Left ventricular M-mode with the cursor positioned on the short-axis view, at the level of the chordae tendinae, bisecting the LV. There is markedly impaired LV systolic function. (bii) Mitral M-mode with the cursor positioned on the short-axis 'fish-mouth' view, showing the increased E point to septal separation. (c) Colour flow Doppler using a right parasternal long-axis four-chamber view showing mitral regurgitation, likely to be a consequence of stretch of the mitral annulus with the left ventricular and left atrial dilatation.

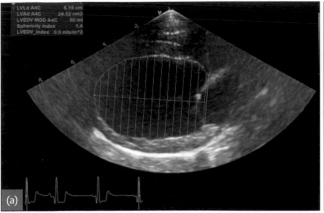
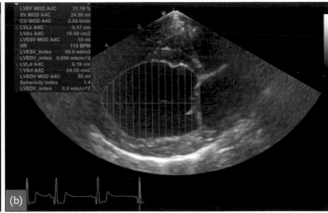

9.121 A Cocker Spaniel with DCM. Echocardiographic measurement of left ventricular volumes in (a) diastole and (b) systole by Simpson's method of discs. The EDV is 80 ml and the ESV is 55 ml. The calculated left ventricular ejection fraction was low at 31.2% and the left ventricular ESVI was increased at 90 ml/m². The sphericity index was also calculated from the diastolic left ventricular length and M-mode diastolic diameter: this was reduced at 1.4, confirming a rounded LV.

- Relative wall thickness (left ventricular free wall in diastole (LVFWd):LVIDd) is decreased
- Fractional shortening is reduced compared with breed-specific reference ranges (where available) or is <20%
- Increased mitral valve M-mode E-point to septal separation (EPSS) (see Figure 9.120b)
- Reduced aortic root systolic excursion on aortic M-modes, and possibly premature closure of the aortic valve
- Systolic time intervals: an M-mode aortic pre-ejection period (PEP):ejection time (ET) ratio of >0.4.

Findings with colour flow and spectral Doppler studies in DCM include:

- Colour flow Doppler may identify mitral and/or tricuspid regurgitation, without grossly abnormal valvular apparatus, due to stretch of the atrioventricular annuli (see Figure 9.120c)
- Mitral regurgitant velocity may be lower than normal, due to impaired left ventricular systolic function and/or increased left atrial pressures, giving a reduced systolic pressure gradient between the LV and LA. A mitral regurgitant velocity of <4 m/s is associated with poor prognosis
- Aortic velocity and velocity time integrals may be lower than normal, due to systolic dysfunction
- Aortic PEP:ET ratio may be increased (>0.4)
- The assessment of diastolic function is important to provide prognostic information. Dogs with a restrictive physiology have reduced survival
- Left-sided filling pressures can be estimated. A mitral E wave velocity:isovolumic relaxation time (IVRT) ratio (E:IVRT) of >1.8 is consistent with left-sided CHF in DCM (Schober et al., 2010).

If dogs are screened for preclinical DCM, various echocardiographic abnormalities may be identified, such as impaired systolic function prior to unequivocal evidence of left ventricular dilatation. Other cases may have enlargement of the LV with apparently preserved systolic function. Serial evaluation is required to confirm that these echocardiographic findings progress and therefore precede the development of DCM, and a scoring system has been proposed to monitor these cases. An increased left ventricular end-systolic (and/or end-diastolic) volume index may be the most sensitive 2D finding for diagnosing preclinical DCM (Wess et al., 2017).

Arrhythmogenic right ventricular cardiomyopathy

ARVC is most commonly recognized in Boxer dogs and was previously known as Boxer cardiomyopathy. However, it is also reported in the Bulldog and sporadically in other breeds. Echocardiographic findings in this condition can vary. Some affected dogs have malignant ventricular arrhythmias and minimal echocardiographic changes. Others may have subjective evidence of right heart enlargement (Figure 9.122), possibly predominantly affecting the RVOT (Bulldogs), sometimes with concurrent left ventricular systolic dysfunction. The right ventricular papillary muscles may also look dysplastic (Figure 9.122c). Others have a DCM phenotype on echocardiography and they may develop left and/or right-sided CHF.

Hypertrophic cardiomyopathy

HCM is rare in dogs, although it has been documented (Schober et al., 2022). Echocardiographic features are similar to those described in cats (see below). One unusual condition that may represent a form of HCM is dynamic LVOT obstruction, due to SAM of the anterior mitral valve leaflet (Figure 9.123). This has been described in young, growing dogs. They may outgrow this lesion. It must be distinguished from mitral valve dysplasia and subaortic stenosis.

Feline myocardial disease

Cats display a plethora of primary myocardial diseases (Luis Fuentes et al., 2020). Imaging, particularly Doppler echocardiography, plays a vital role in diagnosis. However, the phenotype observed at the time of assessment may not be fixed. HCM is by far the most common feline cardiomyopathy and the only one that may be identified during the preclinical phase of the disease (e.g. after detection of an asymptomatic heart murmur). Ancillary diagnostic techniques (e.g. blood pressure measurement, clinical pathology) are required to exclude conditions that may secondarily affect the myocardium.

Hypertrophic cardiomyopathy

HCM is the most common form of primary myocardial disease affecting cats. It is likely to be genetically transmitted as an acquired autosomal dominant trait (proven in Maine Coons and Ragdolls). It is characterized by concentric left ventricular hypertrophy, which may be focal,

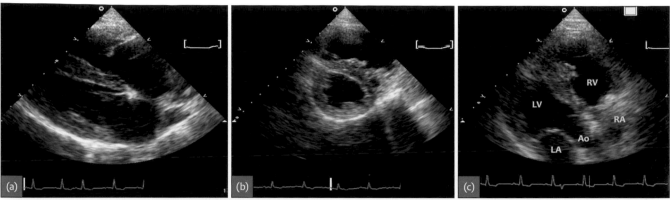

9.122 A Boxer with ARVC, collapse and ventricular tachycardia. The arrhythmia was treated. (a) The right parasternal long-axis and (b) short-axis views show dilatation of the RA and RV. (c) The apical sternal right parasternal view shows dysplastic papillary muscles in the RV apex. Ao = aorta.

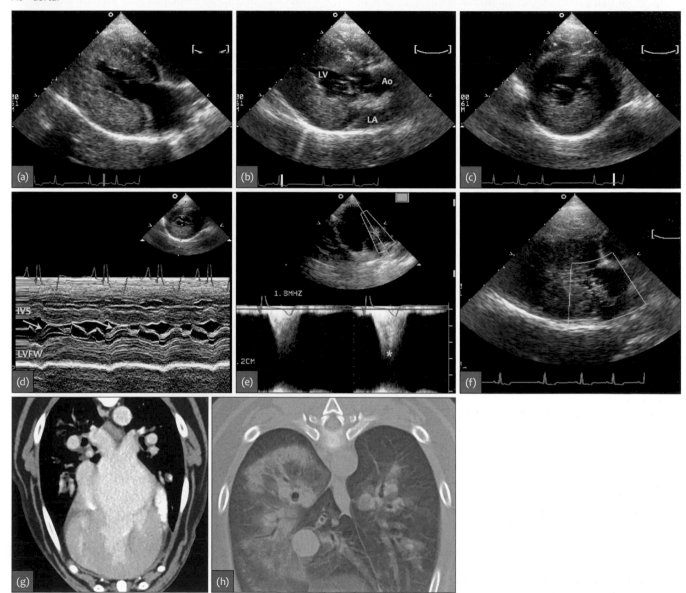

9.123 (a–f) A 2-year-old Border Terrier with frequent syncopal episodes when excited and a heart murmur due to HOCM. There is marked concentric hypertrophy of the LV, evident from (a) the right parasternal long-axis four-chamber view, (b) the five-chamber view and (c) the short-axis view. (b) The aortic valves, LVOT and ascending aorta are grossly normal. However, the mitral valve anterior leaflet is moving towards the basal septum (*) in this early systolic frame (endocardial thickening of the basal septum may be consistent with a 'kissing' lesion). (d) The presence of SAM of the anterior mitral valve leaflet (arrowed) is confirmed by the superior temporal resolution of M-mode at mitral valve level. SAM results in dynamic LVOT obstruction. (e) This can be documented from a left apical view. There is increased aortic outflow velocity with a biphasic acceleration slope (*). In this example, continuous wave Doppler shows aortic peak velocities to be >6 m/s. (f) SAM also results in mitral valve incompetence and colour flow Doppler typically shows an eccentric mitral regurgitation jet, coursing towards the posterior-lateral wall of the LA. (g–h) Transverse CT images of a 9-year-old Dalmatian with a cough. There is marked thickening of the left ventricular myocardium and reduced lumen, and dilatation of the left atrium as well as perivascular pulmonary oedema. HOCM with right and left congestive heart failure was confirmed using echocardiography. Ao = aorta.

regional, symmetrical or asymmetrical. The wall thickness:LV chamber diameter ratio (the relative wall thickness) is greatly increased. Papillary muscles are usually subjectively abnormal (elongated, hypertrophied, hyperechoic, sometimes asymmetrical changes). Evidence of diastolic dysfunction is documented by Doppler studies and this is manifested by progressive left atrial enlargement.

Symptomatic cats present with signs of left-sided CHF (dyspnoea due to pulmonary oedema) or with feline arterial thromboembolism (FATE). Left-sided CHF is often apparently sudden in onset and may be preceded by a stressful incident or fluid loading. There is also a reversible condition called transient myocardial thickening (TMT) that can occur following periods of stress in young cats, which can lead to CHF (Novo Matos *et al.*, 2018). At the time of initial presentation, TMT is indistinguishable from primary HCM. HCM has a long preclinical phase. Heart murmurs in affected cats may be detected fortuitously, which leads to an early diagnosis. Other cats may be diagnosed via echocardiographic screening schemes in breeds such as Bengals, Maine Coons, Persians, Ragdolls and Sphinxes.

Radiography: This is indicated in cats with clinical signs consistent with CHF to identify the haemodynamic consequences of diastolic dysfunction with evidence of increased left-sided filling pressures:

- Left atrial enlargement
- Pulmonary venous distension
- Pulmonary opacification, which may affect any region of the lungs and may be patchy, interstitial, alveolar or mixed. This is consistent with pulmonary oedema (Figure 9.124).

In asymptomatic HCM, there may be no gross radiographic evidence of cardiomegaly or specific chamber enlargement. In more advanced preclinical or symptomatic HCM, left atrial enlargement is evident. Radiographically, apparent biatrial enlargement may be documented. In most cases, echocardiography shows that the marked left atrial enlargement pushes the interatrial septum and the right atrial wall more to the right, giving the impression of biatrial enlargement on the cardiac silhouette. The apparent biatrial enlargement gives the classical 'valentine-shaped' heart on the DV view (Figure 9.124b). A pleural effusion may be present, associated with biventricular failure. Radiography does not differentiate between the various myocardial diseases.

Doppler echocardiography: This is the imaging modality of choice to distinguish between the various forms of myocardial disease. The following 2D and M-mode findings (Figure 9.125) are typical in HCM:

- Generalized or focal, symmetrical or asymmetrical hypertrophy, with diastolic wall thickness ≥6 mm (Figure 9.126). Be aware that weight-based reference ranges should be consulted for very small and very large cats (Häggström *et al.*, 2016)
- The left ventricular chamber diameter may be normal or small (Figure 9.126ab)
- Subjectively hypertrophied papillary muscles
- Left atrial size may be normal (Figure 9.127) or dilated (see Figures 9.126h and 9.128)
- Systolic function is normally preserved; fractional shortening can often be >45%, indicating a hyperkinetic LV, due to the low wall stress (see Figure 9.126e).

Hypertrophic obstructive cardiomyopathy: This term is reserved for the form of HCM where dynamic obstruction of the LVOT is documented by echocardiography. In human medicine, the term 'HCM with dynamic left ventricular outflow tract obstruction' is preferred, as it does not imply HOCM and HCM are separate entities. A simplified series of events leading to this finding includes:

- Turbulence of flow in the LVOT as blood travels around a basal septal bulge associated with the hypertrophy. This may be recognized as colour variance in the LVOT on colour flow Doppler
- This may result in abnormal motion of the anterior mitral valve leaflet, which is 'pushed' or 'sucked' into the LVOT during systole (SAM). This further narrows the LVOT (see Figure 9.126cd)
- The LVOT and aortic velocities may then be increased, with abnormal biphasic acceleration evident as a scimitar shape on spectral Doppler (Figure 9.129)
- The mitral valve is therefore incompetent and an eccentric jet of mitral regurgitation, coursing towards the posterior-lateral LA wall, is typically recorded by colour flow Doppler (see Figure 9.126d). The combination of colour variance associated with the dynamic LVOT obstruction and the mitral regurgitation gives a characteristic 'double jet' appearance on the right parasternal five-chamber view
- Other factors are almost certainly involved in SAM of the mitral valve, such as altered papillary muscle alignment and left ventricular geometry

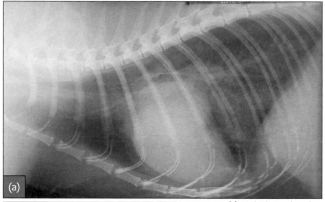
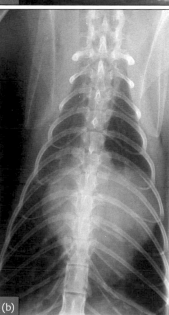

9.124 (a) Right lateral and (b) DV thoracic radiographs of a cat with apparently sudden onset left-sided CHF. There is marked left atrial enlargement and dilatation of the LAA, which results in the appearance of a 'valentine heart' on the DV view. The pulmonary arteries and veins are dilated (pulmonary hypertension may be secondary to left-sided heart failure in the cat). The pulmonary opacification associated with cardiogenic pulmonary oedema in the cat can be patchy and variable in distribution, as indicated here. This cat also has pericardial fat.

Measurement	Normal	HCM	RCM	DCM
IVSd	3.5–5.0 mm	≥6 mm	Normal or mild increase	Normal or reduced
LVFWd	3.5–4.5 mm	≥6 mm	Normal or mild increase	Normal or reduced
LVIDd	14–15 mm	Normal or reduced	Normal or mild increase	>16 mm
LVIDs	7.0–8.5 mm	Normal or reduced	Normal or mild increase	>9 mm
FS	30–50%	Normal or increased	Normal	<25%
Mitral M-mode	EPSS <2 mm	Normal EPSS ± SAM	Normal or mildly increased EPSS	Increased EPSS
Mitral E:A	>1<2	Impaired relaxation: <1. May be pseudonormal, or restrictive depending on stage of disease	Restrictive filling pattern: E>>A	Normal or restrictive, depending on stage of the disease
E deceleration time	60 ms	>65 ms	<55 ms	Normal or decreased
IVRT	55–60 ms	>60 ms	<55 ms	Normal or decreased
PVF S:D	<1 (unless aged cat)	>1	<<1	Low S (<0.2 m/s), S:D <<1
PVF Ar velocity	<0.2 m/s	Normal or increased	Normal, increased or decreased	Normal or decreased
PVF Ar duration: Mitral A duration	<1	Normal or >1, depending on stage of disease	>1 in cats with CHF	>1 in cats with CHF
PW–TDI (longitudinal velocities; IVS or LVFW)	E':A' ratio >1 (unless old cat)	E':A' ratio usually <1	E':A' ratio variable, usually low velocity E'	Low velocity S', E':A' ratio variable, usually low velocity E'

9.125 Typical echocardiographic findings in feline myocardial disease based on 2D and M-mode criteria and assessment of diastolic function. Ar = atrial reversal wave; FS = fractional shortening; IVSd = interventricular septum in diastole; PVF = pulmonary venous flow; PW–TDI = pulsed wave tissue Doppler imaging; S:D = systolic:diastolic velocity ratio.

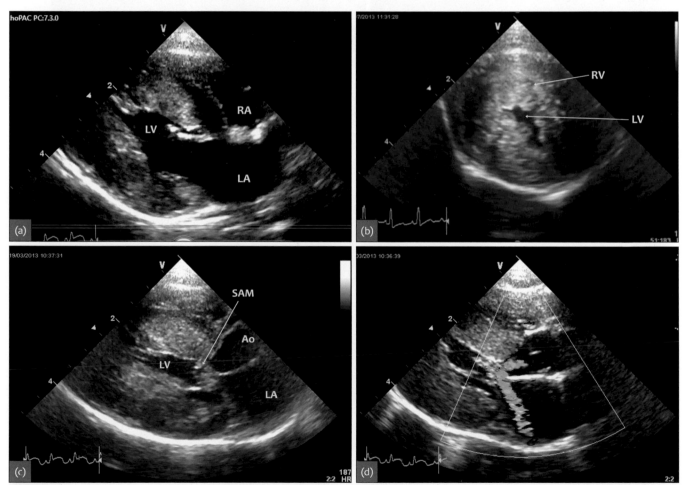

9.126 A young neutered male Domestic Shorthaired cat with HOCM. (a) Right parasternal long-axis four-chambered view in diastole showing concentric hypertrophy of the left ventricular wall (symmetrical in this case). (b) Right parasternal short-axis view confirming the severe left ventricular hypertrophy. In systole, there is obliteration of the left ventricular cavity. The right ventricular wall is also subjectively hypertrophied. (c) Right parasternal long-axis five-chamber view during systole. The anterior mitral valve leaflet moves towards the IVS during systole – this is SAM. This narrows the left ventricular outflow tract, causing dynamic obstruction to ejection, and also results in mitral regurgitation. (d) Colour flow Doppler superimposed on similar image to (c). This shows the 'double jet' typical of HOCM, with left ventricular outflow tract obstruction causing colour variance, and there is an eccentric jet of mitral regurgitation. Ao = aorta. (continues) ▶

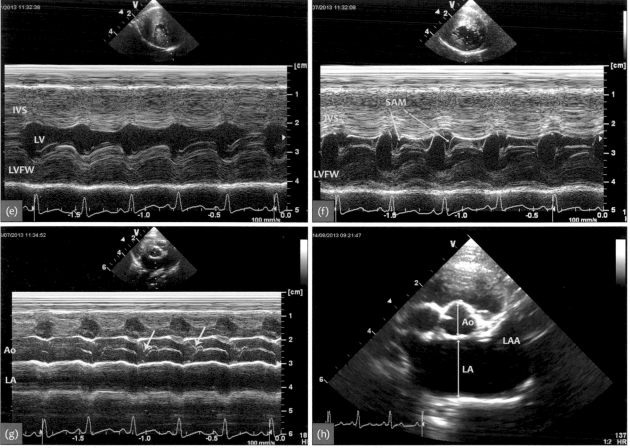

9.126 (continued) A young neutered male Domestic Shorthaired cat with HOCM. (e) Left ventricular M-mode with the cursor positioned from a short-axis view, bisecting the left ventricular cavity. With HCM, the M-mode typically has a cluttered appearance and it can be difficult to avoid the hypertrophied papillary muscles. (f) M-mode at the level of the mitral valve (cursor positioned from the short-axis 'fish-mouth' 2D view). The mitral valve anterior leaflet opens normally in diastole but demonstrates SAM. (g) M-mode at the level of the aortic valves. The M-mode cursor was positioned on a right parasternal short-axis of the heart base. The aortic valves partially close prematurely (arrowed). This is a consequence of SAM, which obstructs left ventricular outflow during systole. (h) Right parasternal short-axis view at the level of the aortic valve, optimizing the left atrial size. The LA is dilated, although the LAA appears dilated to a greater extent than the body of the LA. Ao = aorta.

- SAM can be confirmed by mitral M-mode (see Figure 9.126f). For machines with low frame rate, it can be difficult to appreciate the SAM in 2D, even when the colour flow appearance of the 'double jets' is typical. The superior temporal resolution of M-mode allows the SAM to be confirmed, provided the cursor is placed at the correct level of the mitral valve

- The dynamic LVOT obstruction can result in premature closure or mid-systolic partial closure then reopening of the aortic valves during systole. This is evident on aortic valve M-mode (see Figure 9.126g). It can produce a 'double-diamond' appearance during systole (Figure 9.130).

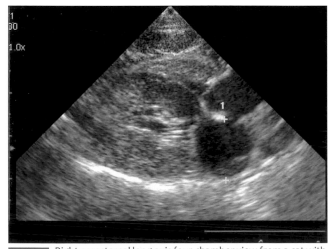

9.127 Right parasternal long-axis four-chamber view from a cat with HCM and normal left atrial diameter (14.4 mm) during ventricular systole; <16 mm is normal.

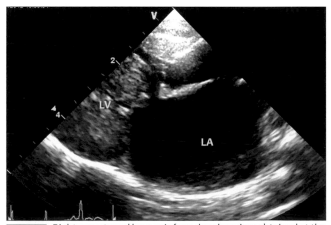

9.128 Right parasternal long-axis four-chamber view obtained at the end of ventricular systole (frame before the mitral valve opens) showing left atrial dilatation in a cat with HCM. The atrial septum is pushed to the right, and the atrium has a rounded appearance. The maximal diameter exceeds 16 mm, which confirms left atrial enlargement.

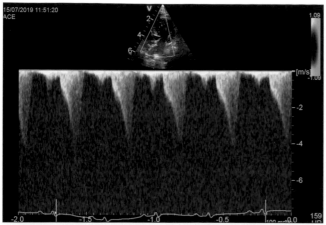

9.129 Continuous wave Doppler from a left apical five-chamber view of a cat with asymptomatic HOCM. The cursor is aligned with the colour variance in the left ventricular outflow tract, with dynamic left ventricular outflow tract obstruction due to SAM of the anterior mitral valve. The biphasic acceleration of the left ventricular outflow tract and aortic envelopes can be seen, with peak velocity just less than 4 m/s.

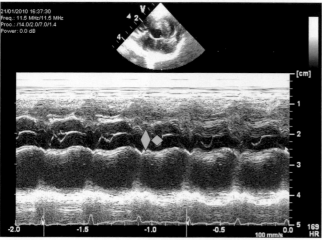

9.130 Aortic M-mode from an asymptomatic cat with HOCM, showing the mid-systolic closure and biphasic opening of the aortic valves during ejection typical of dynamic left ventricular outflow tract obstruction, producing a double-diamond appearance (superimposed in blue).

HOCM is frequently diagnosed in asymptomatic cats following the identification of a heart murmur. The murmur is due to mitral regurgitation and/or dynamic LVOT obstruction, and it may be variable depending upon how relaxed or stressed the cat is. It may not be possible to confirm SAM or dynamic LVOT obstruction (or the cause of the murmur) in a sedated or very relaxed cat during echocardiography.

Pulsed wave Doppler assessment of diastolic function:
Diastolic function can be classified by studies of:

- Transmitral flow
- Isovolumic relaxation time
- Pulmonary venous flow (PVF)
- Mitral flow propagation in LV
- Pulsed wave tissue Doppler imaging.

The typical findings in feline HCM at various stages of the disease are documented in Figure 9.131. The mitral inflow patterns are illustrated in Figures 9.132 and 9.133. Corresponding abnormalities in diastolic dysfunction are illustrated for IVRT (Figure 9.134) and PVF (Figure 9.135).

Restrictive cardiomyopathy

RCM is much less common than HCM in the cat. Although it is recognized as a specific entity in the species (Fox *et al.*, 2014), some cases may represent an end-stage of HCM, when the diastolic wall thickness is no longer increased (e.g. due to loss of cardiomyocytes and/or myocardial fibrosis). RCM is characterized by relatively normal wall thickness, left ventricular chamber size and systolic function, but marked left atrial enlargement. The pathophysiology is associated with reduced left ventricular compliance and diastolic dysfunction. With increased filling pressures, there is a restrictive filling pattern on mitral inflow (however, note that this diastolic abnormality is not specific for RCM).

A secondary cardiomyopathy (e.g. associated with hyperthyroidism) may present as RCM; as with any cardiomyopathy, primary or contributing causes should be actively excluded.

There are two main forms (Chetboul *et al.*, 2019):

- A myocardial form: the initiating factor is unknown and the endocardium appears normal (Fox *et al.*, 2014)
- An endomyocardial form: there is irregular endocardial thickening and bridging scars crossing the left ventricular cavity (Fox, 2004). This is associated with fibrosis and evidence for a preceding inflammatory condition is lacking (Kimura *et al.*, 2016). Oriental breeds (e.g. Siamese) may be predisposed.

A consequence of the marked left atrial enlargement may be arterial thromboembolism (ATE) and cats may present with severe clinical signs associated with this (FATE). See 'Acquired vascular disease', below, for further information on ATE. RCM is usually not detected until the cat presents with left-sided CHF or thromboembolic complications.

Condition	Mitral inflow	IVRT	PVF	PW–TDI (longitudinal IVS/LVFW velocities)
Asymptomatic HCM. Abnormal left ventricular relaxation	E:A <1, prolonged E deceleration time (>65 ms)	Long (>60 ms)	S>D, increased Ar velocity	E':A' ratio <1
Progressive increase in LA–LV pressure gradient (increased filling pressures), so E wave velocity increases and exceeds A: **pseudonormalization**	E:A >1, E deceleration time normal or prolonged	Long or normal	S>D, usually increased Ar velocity	E':A' ratio <1
With further disease progression, left atrial pressure increases further and the LV may become less compliant. Results in **restrictive physiology**	E:A >2, E deceleration time short (<55 ms)	Short (<55 ms)	Low S, increased D, Ar can be normal if atrial function preserved, or low velocity, prolonged Ar duration (> mitral A duration)	E':A' ratio variable, but usually low E' velocity

9.131 Criteria for the classification of diastolic abnormalities recognized in feline myocardial disease. Note the theoretical progression of disease as left atrial pressure and filling pressures increase and the LV becomes less compliant. Ar = atrial reversal wave; D = diastolic velocity; PW–TDI = pulsed wave tissue Doppler imaging; S = systolic velocity.

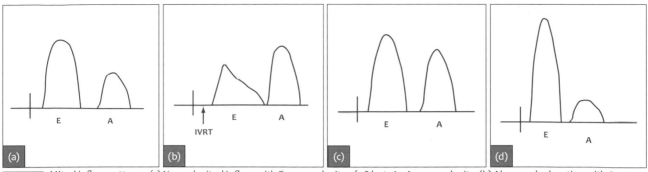

9.132 Mitral inflow patterns. (a) Normal mitral inflow with E wave velocity of <2 but >1 x A wave velocity. (b) Abnormal relaxation with A wave velocity >E wave velocity. As active relaxation (lusitropy) of the LV is compromised, E wave velocity is reduced and E wave deceleration time is prolonged. IVRT is prolonged. Atrial contraction is important to achieve ventricular filling. (c) With development of the disease, left atrial pressures increase and E wave velocity increases, giving a relatively normal E:A ratio again (pseudonormalization). (d) Further worsening of the disease, with high left atrial pressure and a stiff, poorly compliant LV, can result in a high E wave velocity, short E wave deceleration time and E:A velocity ratio of >2 (restrictive filling pattern).

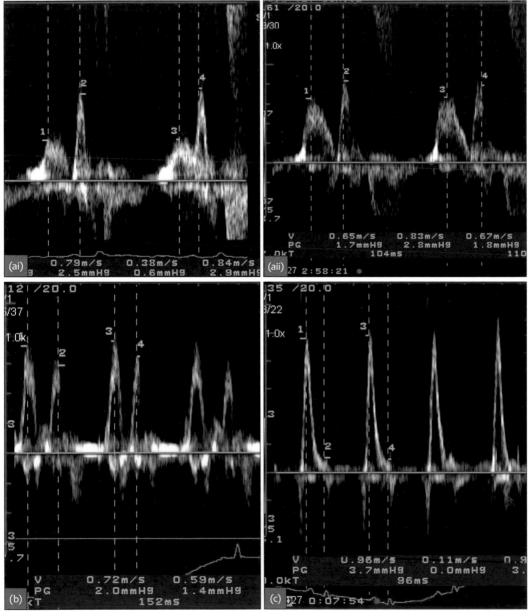

9.133 Pulsed wave Doppler echocardiograms showing mitral inflow patterns from cats with myocardial disease. (ai) A cat with HOCM that was presented for investigation of an asymptomatic heart murmur. Note the abnormal relaxation pattern (E<A; prolonged E deceleration time). (aii) Re-evaluation 6 months later. The cat was still asymptomatic but there is evidence of increased left atrial pressure; the E wave velocity is increased, although there is still E:A reversal and evidence of abnormal relaxation. (b) A cat with pseudonormalization. Note that although the left atrial pressures have increased, the abnormal relaxation is now masked, and other methods are required to document the diastolic dysfunction. (c) A cat with severe biventricular failure and RCM. A restrictive filling pattern with probable left atrial dysfunction is shown, with E much greater than A, low-velocity A wave and short E wave deceleration time.

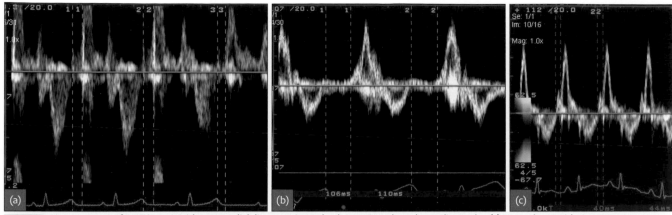

9.134 Measurement of IVRT in cats with myocardial disease using pulsed wave Doppler echocardiography. (a) Normal cat, with time measurement from aortic valve closure to onset of mitral flow. (b) A cat with abnormal relaxation time, showing increased IVRT (>65 ms). (c) A cat with a restrictive filling time, showing very short IVRT (<55 ms).

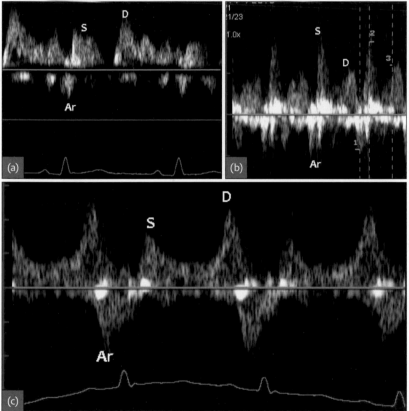

9.135 Assessment of PVF pattern in cats with myocardial disease using pulsed wave Doppler echocardiography. (a) Normal, middle-aged cat with D>S. (b) A cat with abnormal relaxation, with increased S wave (measurement 2) and lower D wave (measurement 3) velocity but increased velocity of the atrial reversal wave (Ar) (measurement 1). (c) A cat with a restrictive filling pattern, with normal atrial function (increased Ar). D wave velocity exceeds S, and D deceleration is rapid.

Radiography: This does not differentiate between the various myocardial diseases. In RCM, there is usually dramatic left atrial enlargement (which may appear to be consistent with biatrial enlargement), and echocardiography predominantly shows left atrial but occasional biatrial dilatation. Signs of left-sided CHF include pulmonary venous distension and a pulmonary opacification.

Doppler echocardiography: Echocardiographic findings include:

- Marked left atrial enlargement (Figure 9.136ab) and sometimes biatrial enlargement
- An organized thrombus may be apparent in the LA or LAA (Figures 9.136bc and 9.137)
- Spontaneous echocontrast of blood within the LA may be seen, giving the impression of swirling 'smoke'. This represents a prothrombotic state (see Figure 9.136c)
- The LV has relatively preserved systolic function, and relatively normal dimensions and wall thickness
- RCM is a disease of diastolic dysfunction. Detailed Doppler assessment of myocardial function is consistent with restrictive physiology (see Figures 9.125 and 9.131)
- In the endomyocardial form of RCM, bridging scars or adhesions may be seen crossing the left ventricular chamber and the endocardium may appear hyperechoic and irregularly thickened (see Figures 9.136d and 9.138a). These bridging scars may result in mid-ventricular obstruction (Figure 9.138b)
- In the myocardial form of RCM, the myocardium and endocardium echotexture appear unremarkable.

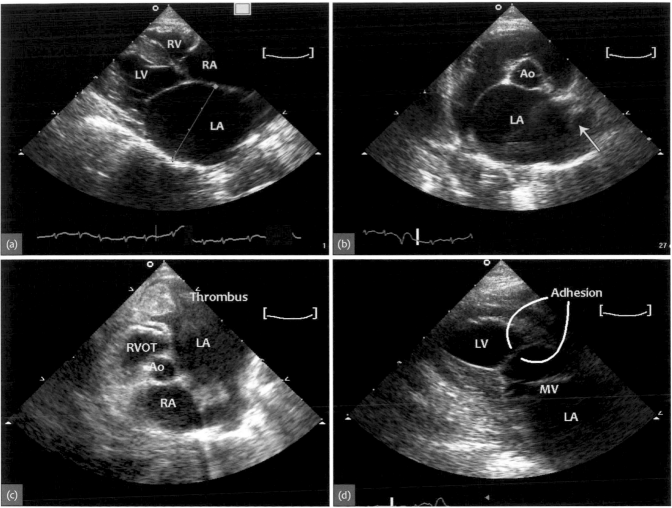

9.136 A cat with RCM. Marked left atrial enlargement is apparent on both (a) the right parasternal long-axis four-chamber view (33 mm diameter) and (b) the right parasternal short-axis view at the level of the aortic valves. (b) On the short-axis view, there is a poorly defined thrombus (arrowed) in the LAA with a real-time image showing spontaneous echocontrast in the LA. This cat had atrial fibrillation with occasional ventricular premature complexes. (c) A modified left parasternal cranial view, optimized for the LAA. The thrombus in the LAA can be seen with spontaneous echocontrast appearing as 'smoke', swirling in the junction of the LAA and LA. (d) right parasternal four-chamber view of the LV showing an irregular endocardium, particularly on the septum, and a probable adhesion crossing the LV chamber. Ao = aorta; MV = mitral valve.

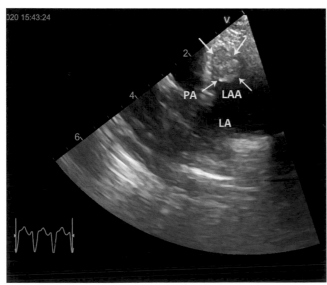

9.137 Cranial left parasternal view optimized for the LA and LAA in a Siamese cat with the endomyocardial form of restricted cardiomyopathy, with an organized thrombus (arrowed) within the LAA. PA = pulmonic trunk.

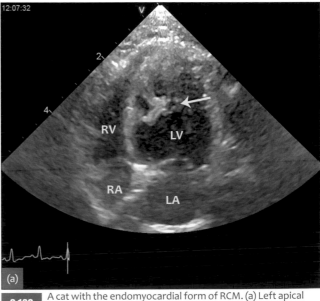

9.138 A cat with the endomyocardial form of RCM. (a) Left apical four-chamber view, showing a bridging scar crossing the LV (arrowed). (continues) ▶

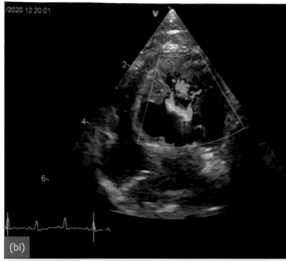

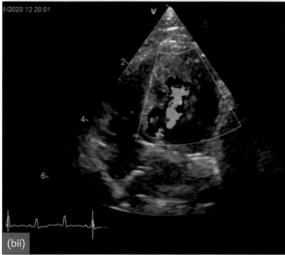

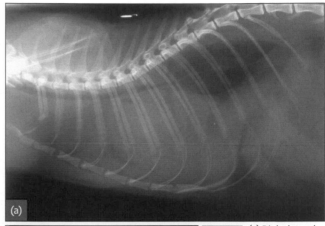

9.139 (a) Right lateral and (b) DV thoracic radiographs of a cat with DCM. There is a large-volume bilateral pleural effusion, masking detail of the cardiac silhouette and the lung fields. From the degree of tracheal elevation, the cardiac silhouette appears to have marked generalized enlargement.

9.138 (continues) A cat with the endomyocardial form of RCM. (b) Colour flow Doppler shows that the bridging scar is associated with turbulence in the mid-LV in both (bi) diastole and (bii) systole.

Dilated cardiomyopathy

DCM is now rarely diagnosed in the cat; it was one of the most common forms of feline myocardial disease prior to taurine deficiency being implicated in this disease in the late 1980s. The nutritional history of any cat diagnosed with this condition should be ascertained. DCM may be familial in certain breeds of cat, such as the Abyssinian.

Presymptomatic disease is not normally recognized. Cats usually present with severe, biventricular failure with cardiogenic shock. Therefore, they must be stabilized prior to carrying out diagnostic tests. Myocardial dysfunction and left ventricular dilatation may be an end-stage consequence of a variety of primary and secondary cardiomyopathies in the cat (e.g. HCM, hyperthyroid cardiomyopathy).

Radiography: Radiographic findings include:

* Affected cats often have a pleural effusion, so assessment of the lung fields and cardiac silhouette is compromised (Figure 9.139)
* Generalized cardiomegaly. The left ventricular apex may appear to be rounded.

Radiographic findings do not distinguish reliably between the various forms of myocardial disease.

Doppler echocardiography: Similar changes are described as listed for canine DCM:

* The LV is dilated in both diastole and systole and systolic function is impaired (see Figures 9.125 and 9.140). A left ventricular systolic diameter of >14 mm is abnormal and consistent with severe systolic dysfunction. Wall thickness is normal or reduced
* There may be mitral and/or tricuspid regurgitation, secondary to stretch of the atrioventricular annulus.

An example of a cat with myocardial dysfunction, secondary to untreated hyperthyroidism and possibly associated with myocardial infarction, is shown in Figure 9.141.

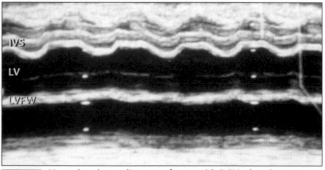

9.140 M-mode echocardiogram of a cat with DCM, showing a pleural effusion and marked hypokinesis, especially of the LVFW.

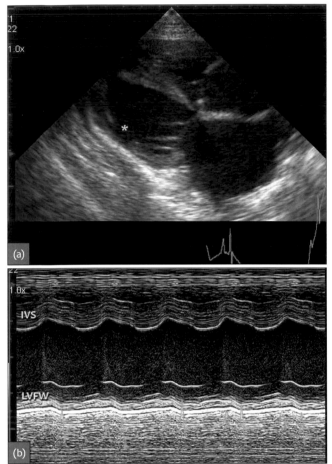

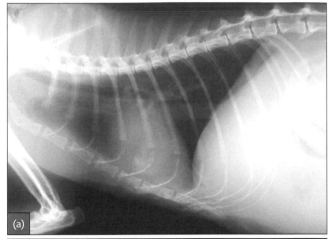

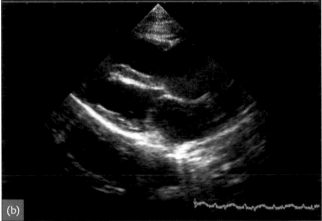

9.141 An elderly cat with untreated, probably long-standing, hyperthyroidism. (a) The right parasternal long-axis four-chamber view shows four-chamber dilatation. (b) In real time, the LV was hypokinetic, which is indicated on the M-mode view. Notice that the LVFW is not functioning on the M-mode, and the wall is thin. A segmental region of the thin posterior wall is shown in (a) (✱). This may correspond to a myocardial infarct (although post-mortem confirmation was not achieved in this cat).

9.142 A cat later confirmed to have ARVC. (a) Right lateral thoracic radiograph. There is right-sided heart enlargement, and ascites with a dilated CdVC supports right-sided CHF. (b) Right parasternal long-axis four-chamber view, indicating marked right atrial and right ventricular enlargement.

Arrhythmogenic right ventricular cardiomyopathy

Feline ARVC is relatively uncommon but more likely to occur in older cats. The disease is histopathologically characterized by fibrofatty replacement and infiltration in the myocardium, most pronounced in the RV (Fox *et al.*, 2000). Affected cats typically show marked right heart dilatation (right heart larger than the left heart, although left heart involvement can also be recognized). They may develop right-sided CHF (ascites) or biventricular congestive failure. Affected cats may have arrhythmias that may or may not cause associated clinical signs. Ventricular arrhythmias and atrial fibrillation have been reported but a proportion of feline ARVC cases may also develop third degree atrioventricular block.

Radiography: Radiographic findings include:

* Right heart enlargement or generalized cardiomegaly
* There may be radiographic evidence of right-sided CHF or biventricular failure; ascites in association with a dilated CdVC indicates that the abdominal effusion is associated with right-sided CHF (Figure 9.142a). Abdominal distension, pleural effusion or both may also be present
* There may or may not be radiographic evidence of left-sided CHF.

Doppler echocardiography: Echocardiographic findings include:

* There is marked right atrial and right ventricular dilatation (Figure 9.142b)
* Tricuspid regurgitation may be evident due to stretch of the tricuspid annulus (Figure 9.143a). ARVC must be distinguished from tricuspid dysplasia, which usually has an immature age of onset compared with the middle- or older-age onset of ARVC
* A feature of this condition may be evidence of dysplastic papillary muscles within the RV apex (the transducer needs to be moved far enough caudally and sternally to observe this feature from the right parasternal long-axis view)
* Variable changes affect the LV. In advanced disease, the LV also becomes dilated and hypokinetic (Figure 9.143).

Non-specific cardiomyopathy phenotype

A non-specific phenotype is a cardiomyopathy that does not meet the criteria to diagnose one of the other cardiomyopathies. This nomenclature is now preferred (Luis Fuentes *et al.*, 2020) to the historical name of unclassified cardiomyopathy, but it should be followed by a description of the echocardiographic abnormalities (Figure 9.144). This is likely to be a heterogeneous group. It may reflect an end-stage of other primary or secondary cardiomyopathies.

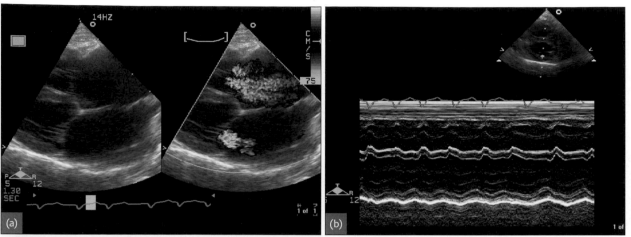

9.143 A cat with ARVC. (a) Right parasternal long-axis four-chamber view. Colour flow mapping indicates the presence of tricuspid and mitral regurgitation due to stretch of the atrioventricular annuli secondary to myocardial disease, although the RV is predominantly affected. (b) M-mode, showing dilatation of both ventricles and impaired left ventricular systolic function. This cat was in atrial fibrillation.

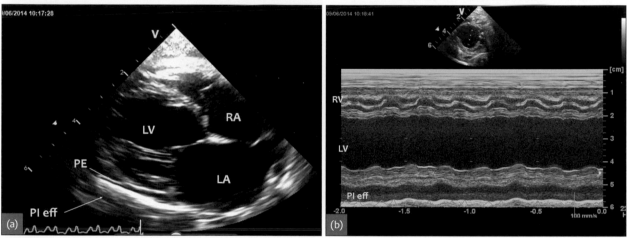

9.144 End-stage (non-specific) cardiomyopathy in a cat with biventricular CHF. Echocardiography follows thoracocentesis. (a) Right parasternal four-chamber view, showing residual pleural effusion (Pl eff), a trivial pericardial effusion (PE) and four-chamber dilatation. (b) Left ventricular M-mode indicating severely impaired left ventricular systolic function.

Secondary myocardial disease

The myocardium and myocardial function may be affected by various systemic diseases in dogs and cats. These include:

- Systemic hypertension
- Hyperthyroidism
- Hypothyroidism
- Chronic kidney disease
- Acromegaly
- Respiratory disease.

These may result in significant cardiac disease or CHF. Secondary cardiomyopathies may be called specific cardiomyopathies (Simpson *et al.*, 2009). Diagnostic tests other than imaging are required to make the diagnosis of a secondary myocardial disease.

Systemic causes of myocardial depression

In the presence of impaired systolic function, it should not be merely presumed that this represents, for example, a preclinical phase of DCM. The following conditions should be excluded:

- Tachyarrhythmia. An animal that is tachycardic (e.g. supraventricular tachycardia) may develop a phenotype similar to DCM (TICM or tachycardiomyopathy). Control of rate (and/or rhythm) should result in improved systolic function and reverse remodelling (i.e. change back towards more normal echocardiographic function and chamber sizes)
- Assessment of systolic function or chamber dimensions should not be carried out in the presence of a dysrhythmia, if possible. Altered electrical activation of the ventricles or abnormal rate can give misleading results
- Hypothyroidism. There have been several case reports of dogs with hypothyroidism and DCM, which have improvement in systolic function associated with thyroid supplementation. It is not clear that the association is cause and effect; many breeds show prevalence of both conditions. There is no association of DCM and hypothyroidism in Dobermanns (Beier *et al.*, 2015)
- Systemically ill animals may show myocardial depression, possibly associated with increased cytokine levels. They may also show spontaneous echocontrast in heart chambers with a severe inflammatory state (this may be a prothrombotic state) (Figure 9.145).

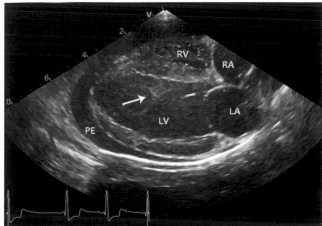

9.145 A whippet with steroid responsive meningoarteritis. Right parasternal four-chamber view, showing a small pericardial effusion and spontaneous echocontrast in the LV (arrowed). These changes are associated with an inflammatory state. Left ventricular systolic function was also impaired (not shown). PE = pericardial effusion.

Systemic hypertension

Systemic hypertension results in increased afterload (arterial resistance) on the LV; left ventricular pressure then increases to maintain cardiac output. To normalize wall stress, concentric left ventricular hypertrophy occurs. Therefore, the walls are thick and the left ventricular chamber may be proportionately small.

Systemic hypertension is normally believed to be secondary to a primary problem in animals. Essential hypertension is considered to be rare. Conditions that may result in hypertension include:

- Kidney disease (especially protein-losing nephropathies); chronic kidney disease
- Hyperthyroidism
- Hyperadrenocorticism
- Acromegaly
- Phaeochromocytoma
- Hyperaldosteronism (Conn's syndrome).

Note that some of these conditions are associated with factors that have a direct trophic effect on the myocardium, so not all changes are related to the hypertension.

Radiography: Thoracic radiographs may be unremarkable where there is concentric left ventricular hypertrophy alone in the absence of left atrial enlargement. If the underlying disease and hypertension leads to left-sided CHF, there will be left atrial enlargement, pulmonary venous distension and a pulmonary opacification consistent with pulmonary oedema.

Doppler echocardiography: 2D and M-mode echocardiographic findings are similar to those described for HCM (see above).

- Concentric hypertrophy of the LV (Figure 9.146).
- Abnormalities of relaxation may be apparent with gross hypertrophy.
- In older dogs, systemic hypertension may result in accelerated progression of degenerative valvular disease.
- Mitral regurgitation is often of high velocity (increased pressure gradient between the LV and LA).

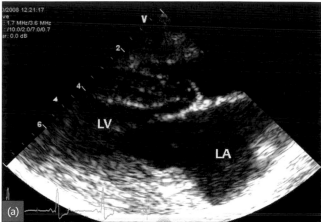

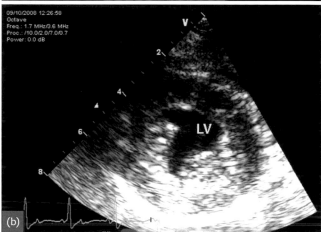

9.146 A Cocker Spaniel with myxomatous degenerative valvular disease with high-velocity mitral regurgitation, associated with systemic hypertension, which caused concentric left ventricular hypertrophy (aortic stenosis was excluded). (a) Right parasternal long-axis four-chamber view and (b) short-axis view at the level of the papillary muscles, showing mild left atrial dilatation and concentric hypertrophy of the LV.

Pulmonary hypertension (and cor pulmonale)

Pulmonary hypertension will increase afterload on the RV. Various conditions may result in pulmonary hypertension, and these have been categorized by the ACVIM consensus statement on pulmonary hypertension (Reinero *et al.*, 2020). It may be the consequence of increased pulmonary blood flow, increased pulmonary vascular resistance or increased pulmonary venous pressure.

- Type 1: pulmonary arterial hypertension. May be associated with cardiac shunts, drugs or toxins, or may be idiopathic. Pulmonary hypertension that is sufficiently severe to exceed systemic pressures in the presence of cardiac shunts may result in right-to-left shunting (Eisenmenger's syndrome) and hypoxaemia (e.g. rPDA, VSD, ASD; See 'Congenital cardiac disease', above).
- Type 2: pulmonary hypertension associated with left heart disease. Increasing left atrial pressure results in pulmonary venous hypertension leading to pulmonary arterial hypertension. This is the most common form recognized in dogs, especially with MMVD (see Figure 9.160).
- Type 3: pulmonary hypertension associated with respiratory disease or hypoxia. This includes brachycephalic conformation and severe lung conditions such as idiopathic pulmonary fibrosis.

- Type 4: pulmonary thromboembolism (PTE). Note that any reason for pulmonary hypertension may increase risk of pulmonary thrombosis in situ.
- Type 5: parasitic disease (e.g. *Dirofilaria immitis* or *Angiostrongylus vasorum* infestation).
- Type 6: unclear or multifactorial causes of pulmonary hypertension.

Pulmonary hypertension can also be divided into pre-capillary and post-capillary hypertension; the latter is usually associated with left heart disease and increased left-sided filling pressures (type 2) but could also be associated with pulmonary venous compression by mass lesions.

Cor pulmonale is the term given to right heart changes or development of right-sided CHF associated with primary respiratory disease (usually associated with pulmonary hypertension type 3).

Radiography: Radiographic findings include:

- Right heart enlargement (Figure 9.147)
- It may be possible to appreciate an enlarged pulmonic trunk or lobar pulmonary arteries, if changes are sufficiently severe (Figure 9.147)
- If pulmonary hypertension is associated with respiratory disease, abnormalities of the lung field should be apparent (Figure 9.147)
- Evidence of pulmonary vascular disease may include dilated, tortuous or 'pruned' appearance to the pulmonary arteries (particularly in heartworm disease) (Figure 9.148).

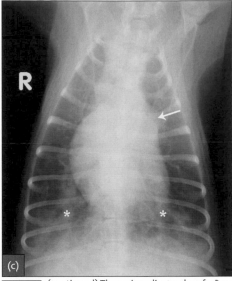

9.147 (continued) Thoracic radiographs of a 2-year-old neutered male mixed-breed dog subsequently diagnosed with angiostrongylosis and severe pulmonary arterial hypertension. All views show pulmonary opacification, which is predominantly peripheral, typical of angiostrongylosis. (c) The DV view shows a pulmonary knuckle (arrowed) and distended caudal lobar pulmonary arteries (*).

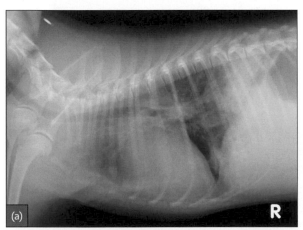

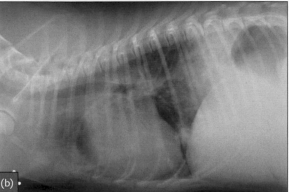

9.147 Thoracic radiographs of a 2-year-old neutered male mixed-breed dog subsequently diagnosed with angiostrongylosis and severe pulmonary arterial hypertension. All views show pulmonary opacification, which is predominantly peripheral, typical of angio-strongylosis. The (a) right and (b) left lateral views show increased sternal contact of the cardiac silhouette with apex tipping, consistent with right ventricular hypertrophy. (continues) ▶

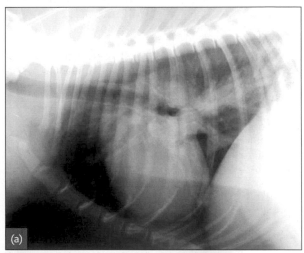

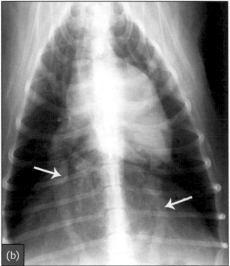

9.148 (a) Right lateral and (b) DV thoracic radiographs of a dog with *Dirofilaria immitis* (heartworm) infection. The pulmonary arteries are moderately dilated and tortuous (arrowed).
(Courtesy of M. Sullivan)

Doppler echocardiography:

- Pulmonary hypertension is associated with right ventricular enlargement. The RV is both dilated and concentrically hypertrophied (Figure 9.149ab).
- As RV pressure is increased, the IVS appears flattened (Figure 9.149ab), which may be most apparent on the right parasternal short-axis view. This may lead to the impression of underfilling of the left heart.
- Commonly, there is also right atrial enlargement (Figure 9.149a).
- The pulmonic trunk is frequently dilated (wider than the aortic diameter) (Figure 9.149c). The right parasternal four-chamber view optimizing the dorsal LA, to show the right pulmonary artery adjacent to the pulmonary vein entering the LA, reveals a dilated right pulmonary artery (greater in diameter than the corresponding vein) with reduced distensibility (Figure 9.149ac).
- A detailed Doppler echocardiographic examination, including intravenously administered echocontrast to demonstrate any right-to-left shunts, is indicated to actively exclude structural heart disease which may result in pulmonary hypertension.
- Tricuspid regurgitation (Figure 9.149d) and pulmonic insufficiency (Figure 9.149e) are commonly both present, whatever the cause of pulmonary hypertension.

- In the absence of pulmonic stenosis, the tricuspid regurgitant velocity can indicate, by the modified Bernoulli equation, the systolic pressure gradient between the RV and RA, and therefore the systolic pulmonic trunk pressure. Thus, a non-invasive determination of systolic pulmonary arterial pressure is possible (Figure 9.149d). A tricuspid regurgitation velocity of >3.4 m/s alone corresponds to a high probability of pulmonary hypertension (in the absence of pulmonic stenosis or RVOT obstruction). A tricuspid regurgitation velocity of >3.0 m/s in the presence of supporting anatomical features, such as dilated pulmonic trunk and right ventricular dilatation, also indicates a high probability of pulmonary hypertension (Reinero et al., 2020).
- In the presence of pulmonic regurgitation, the velocity of this jet indicates the diastolic pressure gradient between the pulmonic trunk and RV. Thus, non-invasive estimation of diastolic pulmonary arterial pressure is possible (Figure 9.149e).
- The spectral Doppler pulmonary flow envelopes can also be informative. With pulmonary hypertension, there is a steeper acceleration (more aortic-like). There may also be delayed deceleration and mid-systolic notching (Figure 9.149f).

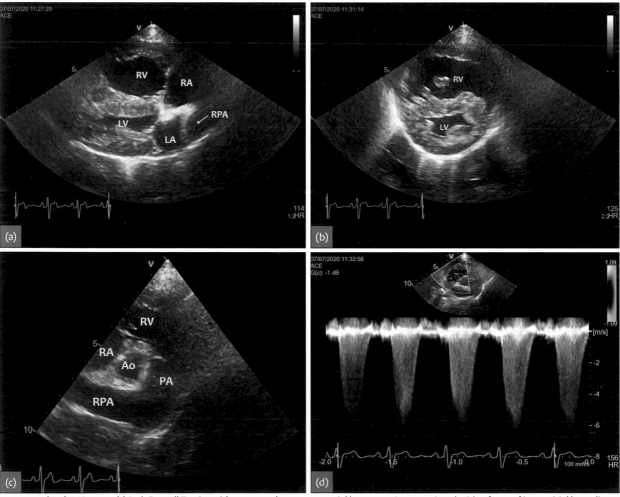

9.149 (a–e) A 10-year-old Jack Russell Terrier with severe pulmonary arterial hypertension associated with a form of interstitial lung disease (cause not identified). (a) Right parasternal long-axis four-chamber view, showing right heart dilatation, with hypertrophy of the RVFW and flattening of the IVS. The right pulmonary artery (RPA) dorsal to the LA is very dilated. (b) Short-axis view at ventricular level, confirming flattening of the IVS and underfilling of the LV due to pressure overload of the RV. (c) Right parasternal short-axis view, optimizing the pulmonic trunk (PA), which is very dilated compared with the aorta (Ao). The RPA is also very dilated. (d) Tricuspid regurgitation (optimized alignment from a right parasternal short-axis view). Peak velocity (TR Vmax) was 5.7 m/s (reference value <2.7 m/s) corresponding to an RV–RA pressure gradient (TR maxPG) of 130 mmHg (reference value <30 mmHg). In the absence of pulmonic stenosis, this reflects severe systolic pulmonary arterial hypertension. (continues) ▶

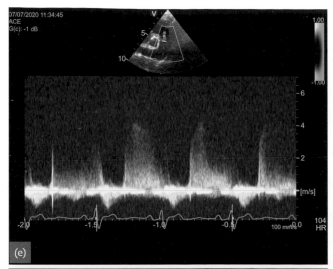

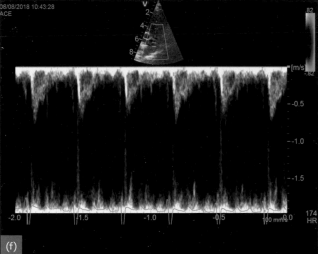

- The normal myocardial echotexture is disrupted. The myocardium may:
  - Appear diffusely hyperechoic
  - Show local hypoechoic regions
  - Have a general 'moth-eaten' appearance
- Both systolic and diastolic dysfunction may be evident as a consequence of the infiltrate.

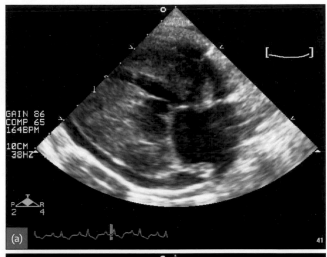

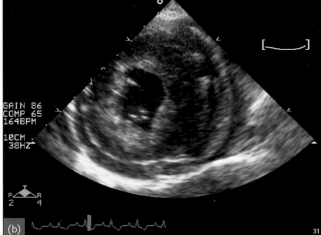

9.149 (continued) (e) A 10-year-old Jack Russell Terrier with severe pulmonary arterial hypertension associated with a form of interstitial lung disease (cause not identified). Continuous wave Doppler, from the right parasternal short-axis view, optimizing with the pulmonic regurgitation jet seen on colour Doppler. Peak velocity (PR Vmax) was 4.03 m/s (reference value <2.2 m/s) corresponding to a diastolic PA–RV pressure gradient (PR maxPG) of 65 mmHg (reference value <20 mmHg). This is severe diastolic pulmonary arterial hypertension. (f) Pulmonary flow (pulsed wave spectral Doppler) from a dog with pulmonary hypertension due to angiostrongylosis (same dog as in Figure 9.147). This shows steep acceleration and delayed deceleration with mid-systolic notching in the pulmonary envelopes. However, this must be interpreted with caution since it can be artefactual if there is suboptimal alignment with pulmonary flow.

Myocardial infiltrative disease

The myocardium can be affected by infiltration, but it is unusual. These infiltrations are normally neoplastic (e.g. lymphoma). Animals are usually presented for investigation of other, non-cardiac signs. Cardiac dysrhythmias, such as ventricular tachycardia, may be clinically important.

Radiography: Thoracic radiographs may or may not indicate any abnormalities in the cardiac silhouette. Radiographs may reflect the presence of the primary lesion.

Doppler echocardiography: Echocardiographic findings include:

- Infiltration into the myocardium is usually generalized and results in the impression of thickened myocardial walls (Figures 9.150 and 9.151)

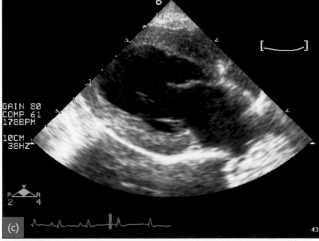

9.150 (a) Right parasternal long-axis four-chamber view and (b) short-axis view from a crossbreed dog. The myocardium appears thickened with a heterogeneous patchy increased echogenicity. There is a small amount of pericardial effusion. This was sampled and cytology confirmed the diagnosis of cardiac lymphoma. (c) After 9 days of staged chemotherapy, the walls had reduced thickness.

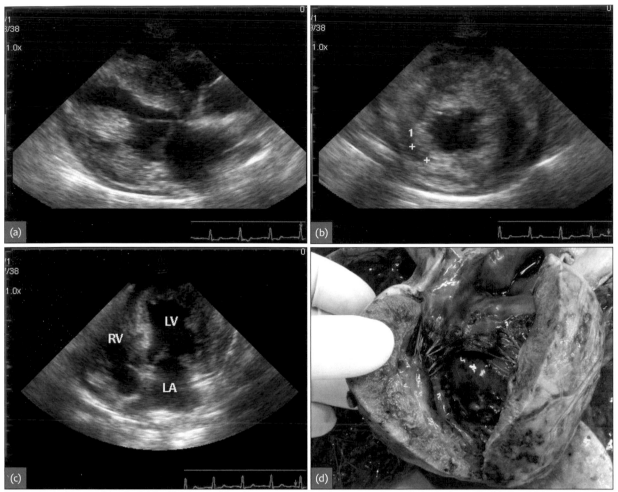

9.151 An 11-year-old male Golden Retriever with collapse, anaemia and paroxysmal ventricular tachycardia. (a) The right parasternal long-axis four-chamber view, (b) short-axis view and (c) left apical four-chamber view all show evidence of thickened myocardial walls, with disrupted architecture and numerous hypoechoic lesions of various sizes. (d) Post-mortem examination showed the entire myocardium was affected by a disseminated haemangiosarcoma.
(Courtesy of R. Irvine)

Acquired valvular heart disease

Myxomatous mitral valve disease

There are a number of synonyms for MMVD, including myxomatous degenerative valvular disease, valvular endocardiosis, chronic valvular disease and mitral valve disease. This is the most common cardiac disease in dogs, and its prevalence approaches 100% in certain small-breed dogs (especially Cavalier King Charles Spaniels). Small-breed dogs are over-represented with premature onset of disease but large-breed dogs may also be affected. The valvular degenerative changes are very common in aged dogs. The pathology does occur in other species, including cats, but not with the same high prevalence or severity noted in dogs. All four heart valves may be affected; the mitral valve is predominantly affected, followed by the tricuspid, aortic and pulmonic valves.

Pathology and pathophysiology

The pathology is characterized by myxomatous degeneration of valve tissue. This is associated with the expansion of the spongiosa layer of the valve with accumulation of glycosaminoglycans and proteoglycans; these changes are more severe at the leaflet tips of the valve, leading to the characteristic myxomatous nodules recognized on pathology and during echocardiography. The resulting redundancy of the leaflet, which is evident in the mitral valve especially, leads to systolic prolapse (i.e. bulging on the atrial side of the mitral valve annulus). The deformity is associated with mitral regurgitation, which eventually results in an audible murmur. With progression of the condition, there can be in-turning of the valve leaflet tips, further expanding the mitral regurgitation orifice.

Mitral regurgitation leads to left atrial and left ventricular volume overload. This eventually results in an increase in the size of these chambers; this can initially be adaptive remodelling (chamber dilatation and eccentric hypertrophy of the LV, leading to preserved relative wall thickness). Maladaptive remodelling is associated with left ventricular dilatation and perturbed left ventricular geometry with rounded shape and reduced relative wall thickness. These changes affect the mitral annulus (it becomes stretched) and further compromise the function of the mitral valve apparatus, leading to further mitral regurgitation (i.e. mitral regurgitation begets mitral regurgitation). Eventually, left atrial pressure increases, leading to increased pulmonary venous and pulmonary capillary pressures, resulting in left-sided CHF in advanced cases. The right heart may also be affected so there may be concurrent right-sided CHF.

Staging

These pathological changes and progression of disease can be documented by imaging (echocardiography, thoracic radiography) and the results of imaging form the basis of the staging of MMVD, as proposed by the ACVIM consensus guidelines (Keene *et al.*, 2019). This gives the different stages of MMVD as shown in Figure 9.152.

Staging for MMVD is important, especially for the identification of advanced preclinical disease prior to the development of CHF. The evaluation of pimobendan in cardiomegaly (EPIC) study showed that dogs with stage B2 MMVD had increased time to end-point of the study (onset of CHF or death) when receiving treatment rather than placebo (Boswood *et al.*, 2016). Prolonging the preclinical phase of the disease has considerable welfare importance and therefore accurate identification of this stage of the disease is vital for the individual dog. Staging to identify stage B2 should precede any treatment, since pimobendan will reduce cardiac size (reverse remodelling), possibly confounding confirmation of Stage B2.

Radiography

Thoracic radiographs are very sensitive at reflecting the volume overload on the left heart resulting from mitral regurgitation. They are considered to be the gold standard for diagnosing actual or imminent left-sided CHF. Radiographs will therefore reflect the stage of the disease:

- Stage A: cardiac silhouette and lungs within normal limits
- Stage B1: no significant left atrial or left ventricular enlargement or generalized cardiomegaly. Unremarkable lung field
- Stage B2: VHS of >10.5 vertebrae (or greater than breed-specific reference values, if known). If echocardiography is unavailable to confirm generalized cardiomegaly, a VHS of >11.5 vertebrae is more specific as a cut-off prior to starting treatment. Evidence of left atrial enlargement and left ventricular enlargement. Pulmonary vasculature and lung field unremarkable in preclinical disease
- Stage C: CHF. Typically, this occurs with slow progression of MMVD and resulting volume overload, so there will be left atrial and left ventricular enlargement and generalized cardiomegaly (the only exception may be with sudden increase in left atrial pressures due to chordal rupture). In decompensated stage C, there will be radiographic evidence of left-sided CHF with pulmonary venous congestion and a predominantly perihilar or caudodorsal pulmonary parenchymal opacification, which may vary in severity from mild interstitial to severe mixed interstitial and alveolar. Concurrent evidence of right-sided CHF or pulmonary hypertension may or may not be present. In compensated stage C (dogs on medication for CHF), the lung field should be clear
- Stage D: Usually refractory or uncontrolled CHF. Radiographic findings depend on presentation and additional problems.

Progression of the disease can be followed from serial radiographs (Figure 9.153). The rate of increase in cardiac silhouette size is exponential about 6 months prior to onset of CHF.

Echocardiography

Echocardiography allows confirmation of the diagnosis and staging of the disease by assessing specific chamber enlargement as well as other markers of severity, such as estimation of left-sided filling pressures, assessment of systolic function and recognition of pulmonary hypertension or other complications of advanced disease.

Assessing the mitral valve: The thick nodular degenerative changes are usually characteristic and can be dramatic in small-breed dogs, which reflects the pathological process of myxomatous degeneration (Figure 9.154). Identification of mitral valve prolapse is also important and may precede development of a heart murmur. Screening Cavalier King Charles Spaniels for presence and severity of premature onset of mitral valve prolapse, even before any significant mitral regurgitation, has been shown to be important in reducing prevalence of MMVD in younger dogs in the Danish Kennel Club scheme (Birkegard *et al.*, 2016) (Figure 9.155).

	Stage A Predisposed	Stage B Preclinical MMVD		Stage C CHF		Stage D End-stage CHF
Murmur grade	None	Progressively louder				
Sub-staging	**N/A**	**Stage B1**	**Stage B2**	**Stage C (decompensated)**	**Stage C (stable)**	**Stage D**
Criteria (echocardiography)	Normal	Evidence of MMVD, MR. Normal LA and LV size; or minimal dilatation of either LA or LV	LA:Ao ≥1.6 **and** LVIDdN >1.7	LA and LV dilatation. Increased left-sided filling pressures (mitral E:IVRT >2.5)	LA and LV dilatation. No overt evidence of increased left-sided filling pressures	Specific problems relating to individual animal
Criteria (radiography)	Normal	Normal – no overt evidence of left atrial enlargement or generalized cardiomegaly	VHS >10.5 v (if no echocardiography, VHS >11.5 v)	Left-sided or generalized cardiomegaly. Pulmonary venous congestion. Signs of pulmonary oedema	Left-sided or generalized cardiomegaly. No evidence of overt pulmonary oedema	Likely to be uncontrolled CHF and severe cardiomegaly

9.152 Staging of MMVD based on the ACVIM consensus guidelines for the diagnosis and treatment of MMVD in dogs (Keene *et al.*, 2019). Ao = aorta; LVIDdN = left ventricular internal diameter in diastole normalized for bodyweight by allometric scaling; MR = mitral regurgitation.

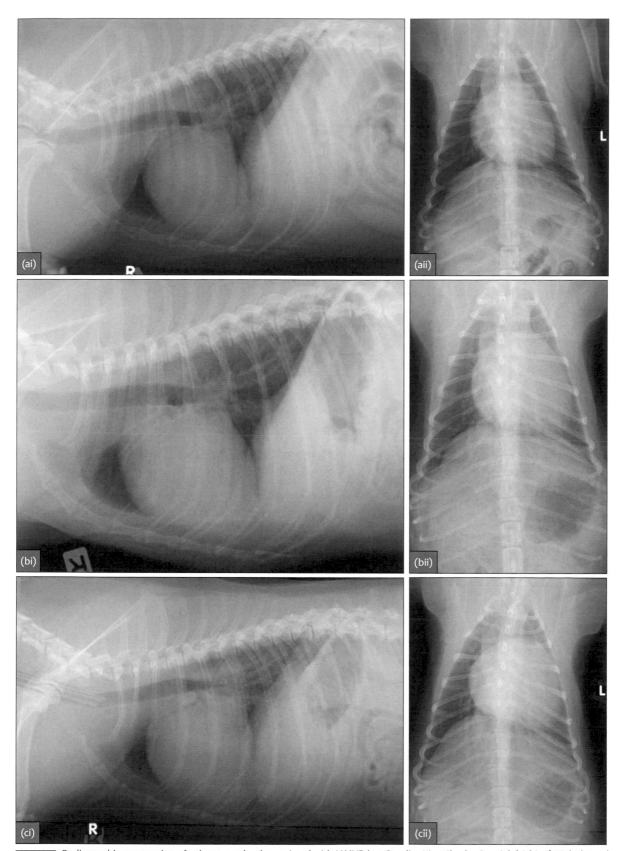

9.153 Radiographic progression of volume overload associated with MMVD in a Cavalier King Charles Spaniel. (ai, bi, ci) Right lateral and (aii, bii, cii) DV views. (a) Initial radiographs (at 7 years and 1 month of age) to investigate an increase in grade of heart murmur, which had been first detected at least 18 months prior to imaging. Mild left-sided cardiomegaly is evident on the lateral view (VHS 11.75 v). Echocardiography did not fully meet stage B2 criteria at this time. (b) Radiographs repeated 9 months later. The cardiomegaly has progressed (VHS 12.25 v). The DV view shows an increase in left atrial size, with greater lateral deviation of the left caudal lobar bronchus. Echocardiography was consistent with advanced stage B2 MMVD. Treatment with furosemide was initiated 3 months later after an increase in resting respiratory rate. (c) Radiographs repeated 16 months after initial radiographs, to further investigate a problematic persistent cough. The cardiomegaly has continued to progress (VHS 13 v). There has been a further increase in left atrial and left ventricular enlargement. The pulmonary veins are mildly congested and there is a perihilar unstructured interstitial pattern which is attributed to the enlarged left atrium and may be cardiogenic pulmonary oedema. These radiographs were obtained under anaesthesia prior to tracheobronchoscopy, which revealed bronchial collapse associated with bronchomalacia and mild tracheal collapse.

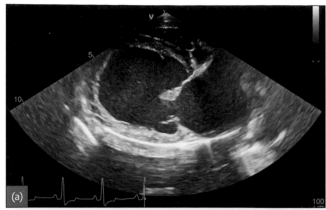

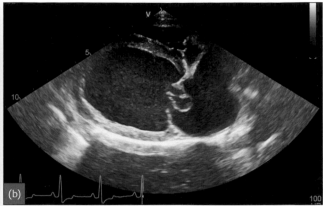

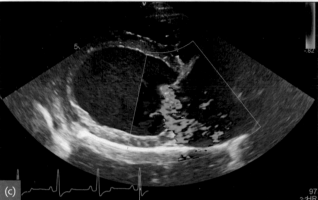

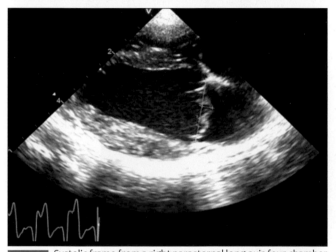

9.154 A Whippet with advanced, stage B2 MMVD. (a) The nodular thickening of the anterior leaflet tip can be seen (diastolic frame). (b) In systole, there is severe prolapse of the anterior leaflet giving the impression of a parachute valve (systolic frame). (c) This is associated with severe mitral regurgitation with an eccentric jet (systolic frame).

9.155 Systolic frame from a right parasternal long-axis four-chamber view of a Cavalier King Charles Spaniel with Stage B1 MMVD, showing mitral valve prolapse. A line is drawn along the mitral annulus. In the Danish system of screening for mitral prolapse (shown here), lines are drawn perpendicular to the annulus line to the atrial side of the valve at three sites: the anterior (cranial or septal) leaflet, the coaptation point and the posterior (caudal or mural) leaflet, and the values in millimetres are summed. In the new UK scheme, the maximum prolapse distance is measured, rather than all three distances (which can sometimes be difficult to optimize on a single systolic frame).

Large-breed dogs can also develop myxomatous valvular degeneration but often do not show the florid valve thickening or severity of prolapse seen in small-breed dogs, even if they have severe mitral regurgitation.

Assessing chamber size and staging of MMVD: The left atrial and left ventricular size reflect the volume overload and therefore the severity of the mitral regurgitation. It is most important to measure the left atrial size, most commonly by the early diastolic LA:aortic diameter ratio (LA:Ao)

and the left ventricular internal diameter at end-diastole normalized for bodyweight by allometric scaling (LVIDdN, usually measured by M-mode). Stage B2 requires both the LA (LA:Ao ≥1.6) and the LV (LVIDdN >1.7) to be dilated. Note that stage B2 can range from barely meeting these criteria to very advanced (Figure 9.156). The LA does not expand in all directions at a similar rate. One of the earliest signs of left atrial dilatation can be flaring of the interatrial septum to the right, seen from a right parasternal long-axis four-chamber view. This maximal left atrial diameter can be measured at end-systole and indexed to the aortic annulus diameter (obtained from the right parasternal five-chamber view, measuring between the open aortic valve leaflets) to produce the LAmax:Ao annulus ratio (Strohm *et al.*, 2018) (Figure 9.157). These may be more repeatable measurements than those for the short-axis LA:Ao.

Assessing severity of mitral regurgitation: Mitral regurgitation colour flow jet area, qualitatively or semi-quantitatively compared with left atrial area, is commonly used to estimate severity of mitral regurgitation. However, this is misleading, since the jet area will be affected by the frequency of the transducer, Nyquist limit, image quality and other factors. If the Nyquist limit is set as high as possible, the colour flow jet width at the narrowest part of the jet (the vena contracta) and the presence of an isovelocity colour flow change on the ventricular side of the valve can reflect more severe mitral regurgitation (Figure 9.158).

Spectral Doppler analysis of transmitral flow including mitral regurgitation is performed from the left apical four-chamber view. Mitral regurgitation causes volume overload of the LA, resulting in increased transmitral flow returning to the LV, which increases the early transmitral E wave velocity (pulsed wave Doppler). In addition, the E wave velocity will be affected by the early diastolic left atrial–left ventricular pressure gradient. A mitral E velocity of >1.2 m/s is associated with more advanced disease and poorer prognosis.

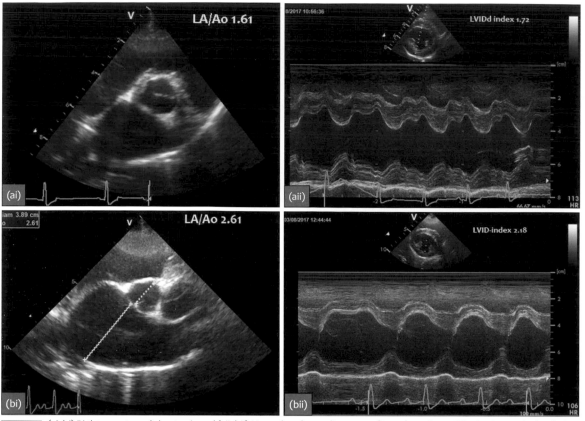

9.156 (ai, bi) Right parasternal short-axis and (aii, bii) M-mode echocardiograms of two dogs. Stage B2 criteria require both the LA:Ao and LVIDdN to be increased (≥1.6 and >1.7, respectively). Therefore, there can be a range in severity for stage B2, from (a) very mild (LA:Ao 1.61; LVIDdN 1.72) to (b) advanced (LA:Ao 2.61; LVIDdN 2.18). Both these dogs would meet inclusion criteria for the EPIC study and may, therefore, benefit from being prescribed pimobendan.

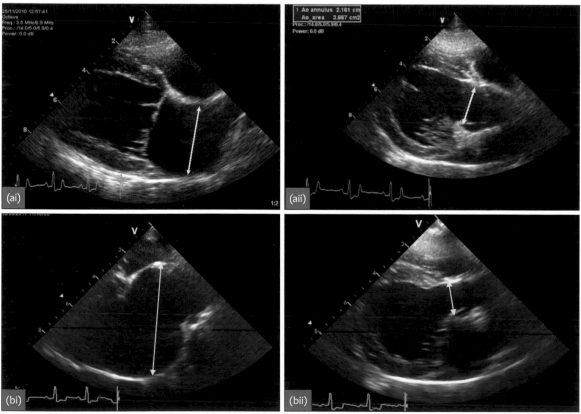

9.157 (a) Normal LA with a square appearance during systole in a dog with MMVD stage B1. (b) Stage C decompensated MMVD, with bowing of the interatrial septum and rounded appearance to the LA, consistent with increased left atrial pressure. (ai, bi) Right parasternal long-axis four-chamber views, showing measurement of left atrial diameter at the end of systole (LA max). (aii, bii) Right parasternal long-axis five-chamber views showing the aortic annulus. The aortic annulus diameter is measured on a systolic frame, between open aortic valve leaflets. The ratio (LA max:Ao annulus) is calculated; normal values are <2.5.

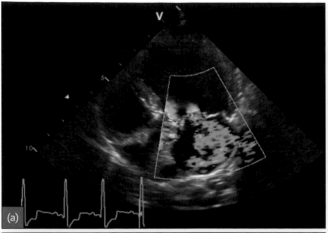

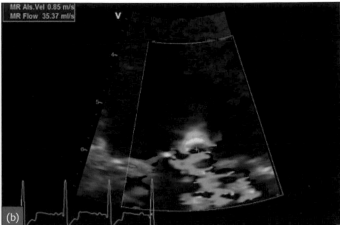

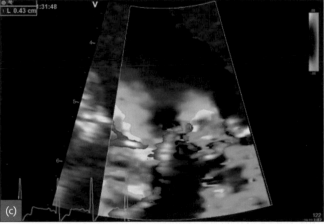

9.158 Use of colour flow Doppler to estimate severity of mitral regurgitation. Left apical four-chamber views with colour interrogation of the mitral valve, during ventricular systole, from a Cavalier King Charles Spaniel with end-stage biventricular CHF. (a) Colour flow showing the mitral regurgitation jet area almost filling the LA. However, it should be noted that jet area is not recommended to assess severity of mitral regurgitation as it is influenced by a range of other factors.
(b) Magnified image. The flow convergence leading to a semicircle of colour aliasing on the ventricular side of the mitral valve, prior to the regurgitant orifice, is consistent with severe mitral regurgitation if the Nyquist limit is high. With a central jet of mitral regurgitation, the proximal isovelocity surface area (PISA) can determine the mitral regurgitant volume, but this is not applicable with eccentric or multiple jets, common in MMVD.
(c) Magnified image. The width of the vena contracta (width of jet as it becomes turbulent through the mitral regurgitant orifice) correlates with severity of mitral regurgitation. It can be indexed to aortic annulus diameter.

Because of the large pressure gradient between the LV and LA and resulting high-velocity mitral regurgitation, continuous wave spectral Doppler is required. The image may need to be altered to optimize parallel alignment with the colour flow mitral regurgitant jet. Peak mitral regurgitation velocity is typically 5–6 m/s. Lower mitral regurgitation velocities may be seen with reduced left ventricular systolic function and/or increased left atrial pressure. Higher velocity mitral regurgitation can be associated with systemic hypertension, which may be situational (i.e. caused by stress during echocardiography) or genuine. A complete, dense continuous wave envelope is consistent with severe mitral regurgitation. Mild mitral regurgitation is often associated with incomplete spectral Doppler envelopes. The continuous wave envelopes are typically tongue-shaped. More pointed envelopes are consistent with increased left-sided filling pressures (Figure 9.159).

Assessing left-sided filling pressures:

- Mitral E wave velocity: the higher the E wave velocity, the more mitral regurgitation and/or increased left atrial pressure.
- The mitral E:A ratio is influenced by diastolic function. Dogs with MMVD tend to be older; in older healthy dogs, the mitral E:A velocity ratio may be <1, which is a sign of impaired relaxation (a normal aging change). If this is seen, left-sided filling pressures are not likely to be increased.
- A pseudo-normal (mitral E:A ratio 1–2) or restrictive (mitral E:A ratio >2) transmitral flow pattern can be consistent with increased left atrial pressure (especially if E velocity >1.2 m/s) and/or reduced left atrial function, secondary to significant dilatation.

- The best echocardiographic estimate of left-sided filling pressures is the E:IVRT. A ratio of >2.5 in MMVD is consistent with significant increased left atrial pressure and left-sided CHF (Schober *et al.*, 2010).

Assessing systolic function: Mitral regurgitation results in low afterload on the LV, and a significant proportion of the total left ventricular stroke volume is regurgitant rather than forward stroke volume into the aorta. Left atrial pressure is significantly less than aortic pressure, even in the presence of CHF. This low afterload results in apparently hyperkinetic left ventricular function – especially apparent in the IVS, recognized in both 2D and LV M-mode. Therefore, measurements such as fractional shortening and ejection fraction will be high, and do not reflect intrinsic left ventricular systolic function (contractility). Since systolic function is inversely proportional to the left ventricular size at end-systole, assessing systolic size better reflects LV systolic function. It is impaired if:

- M-mode LVIDs is greater than the breed-specific reference range
- M-mode LVIDs normalized for bodyweight by allometric scaling (LVIDsN) is >1.26 (reference range 0.71–1.26)
- Simpson's method of discs or length–area monoplane calculation of left ventricular ESV is increased to above breed-specific reference range
- Calculation of ESVI. Values of >30 ml/m^2 are consistent with impaired systolic function, but actual values vary with breed and size of dog
- If fractional shortening or ejection fraction are 'normal' in the presence of severe mitral regurgitation, systolic function is likely to be impaired as a hyperkinetic LV is expected.

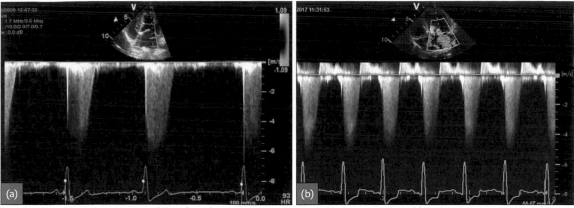

9.159 Continuous wave spectral Doppler echocardiograms showing mitral regurgitation. (a) Cocker Spaniel with stage B2 MMVD. Typical mitral regurgitation spectral Doppler envelopes are tongue shaped, but the full spectral Doppler is not always evident unless mitral regurgitation is severe. The third spectrum is complete and could be used to measure mitral regurgitation velocity (normally 5–6 m/s). (b) Cavalier King Charles Spaniel with stage D MMVD and biventricular CHF. The mitral regurgitation continuous wave spectral Doppler envelopes are more pointed with high left-sided filling pressures.

Impaired systolic function is more likely in large-breed dogs with MMVD, such as German Shepherd Dogs, Border Collies, Airedale Terriers. However, myocardial failure may develop in any case of end-stage MMVD.

Pulmonary hypertension: Dogs with advanced MMVD may develop post-capillary (type 2) hypertension (see 'Pulmonary hypertension (and cor pulmonale)', above). High left atrial pressure (even compensated left-sided CHF in animals receiving medication) results in pulmonary venous, pulmonary capillary and then pulmonary arterial hypertension. As tricuspid regurgitation is common in

dogs with MMVD, its velocity can be measured and used to estimate the pulmonary arterial systolic pressure (having excluded pulmonic stenosis or other causes of increased right ventricular systolic pressure). Clinical signs suggestive of pulmonary hypertension include shortness of breath without overt, decompensated left-sided CHF, exercise intolerance or syncope. Small-breed dogs may have concurrent respiratory disease, so may have pre-capillary or mixed causes of pulmonary hypertension. Severe pulmonary hypertension may lead to right-sided CHF (Figure 9.160).

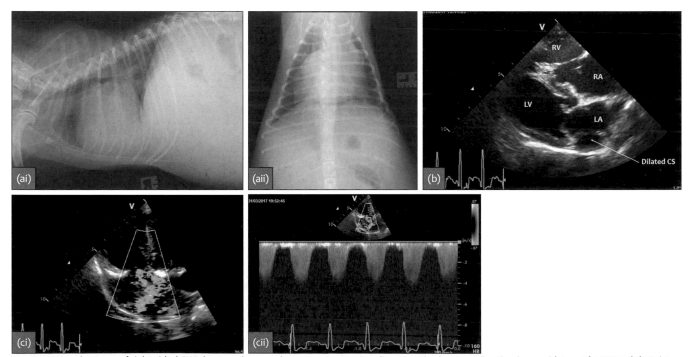

9.160 Development of right-sided CHF due to pulmonary hypertension in a Cavalier King Charles Spaniel with advanced (stage D) MMVD. (ai) Right lateral and (aii) DV thoracic radiographs showing ascites, consistent with right-sided CHF. There is generalized cardiomegaly, with left atrial and left ventricular enlargement, resulting in apex shifting to the right. The lateral view with increased sternal contact suggests concurrent right ventricular enlargement. The DV view shows pulmonary venous congestion; the lobar pulmonary arteries are also increased in size. (b) Right parasternal long-axis four-chamber view showing marked right heart enlargement with flattening of the IVS, consistent with right ventricular pressure overload (pulmonary hypertension). There is a dilated coronary sinus (CS), initially thought to be due to a PLCrVC, but this reduced to normal size after treatment of the CHF and pulmonary hypertension. (ci) Left apical four-chamber view from the time of presentation, showing severe tricuspid regurgitation at increased velocity. (cii) Tricuspid regurgitation velocity was approximately 4 m/s (pulmonic stenosis was excluded). Therefore, from the modified Bernoulli equation, the RV–RA pressure gradient was calculated to be approximately 64 mmHg. The right atrial pressure was increased, as evidenced by the right-sided CHF signs, so pulmonary arterial systolic pressure was over 64 mmHg.

Potential sequelae of end-stage MMVD: The most common consequences of end-stage MMVD are development of systolic dysfunction or pulmonary hypertension. Arrhythmias are also common, especially atrial fibrillation (which reflects atrial stretch), the development of which may lead to further decompensation as cardiac output is further reduced.

Additional sequelae, which can result in acute presentation, include ruptured chordae tendinae and left atrial tear.

Ruptured chordae tendinae: The myxomatous degenerative process can affect the chordae tendinae, and ruptured minor chordae are fairly common. However, rupture of a primary cord can result in a sudden increase in left atrial pressure and acute decompensation into stage C CHF with fulminant pulmonary oedema. Chordae can sometimes be seen flicking into the LA during systole (Figure 9.161), or the tip of a leaflet may flail if a primary cord is ruptured (Figure 9.162).

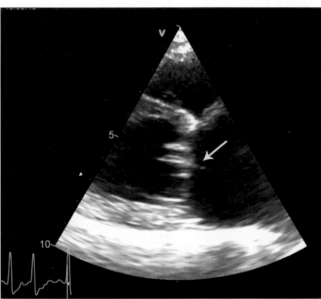

9.161 Right parasternal long-axis four-chamber view from a dog with MMVD and rupture of a chorda tendina; this slender cord can be seen flicking into the LA during ventricular systole (arrowed).

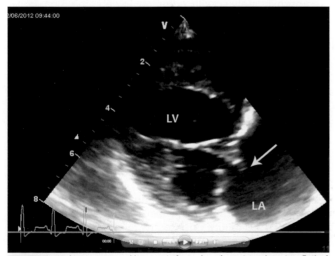

9.162 Right parasternal long-axis four-chamber view showing flail of the tip of the anterior mitral valve leaflet in early systole (arrowed), reflecting rupture of a major chorda tendina.

Left atrial tear: Mitral regurgitation can result in jet lesions of the left atrial endocardium, which can lead to a full thickness left atrial tear and pericardial haemorrhage. This can result in collapse of the dog. It should be suspected in a dog with marked left atrial dilatation with a pericardial effusion with cardiac tamponade (Figure 9.163); sometimes a clot can be seen in the pericardial effusion.

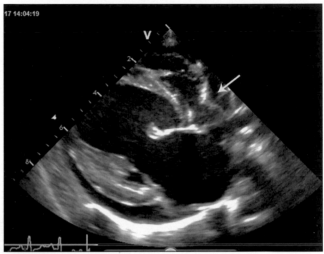

9.163 Right parasternal long-axis four-chamber view from a small crossbreed dog receiving treatment for advanced MMVD with CHF. The dog had suddenly collapsed and was found to have a pericardial effusion with cardiac tamponade (diastolic collapse of the right atrial wall; arrowed). In a dog with a very dilated LA and cardiac tamponade, the possibility of a left atrial tear and pericardial haemorrhage must be considered.

Infectious endocarditis

Endocarditis is inflammation that mainly affects heart valves, although occasionally it can be mural. In dogs and cats, the mitral and aortic valves are most likely to be affected. Dogs with aortic stenosis are predisposed, possibly reflecting endocardial injury due to the shear stresses of high-velocity turbulent flow. However, dogs with MMVD do not appear to show increased risk for endocarditis. Endocarditis follows bacteraemia; common sources of bacteraemia include dental disease and procedures, periodontal disease, urinary tract infections and septic arthritis (immune-mediated polyarthropathy as a consequence of endocarditis is also possible). Affected animals may have fever and shifting lameness. A new heart murmur may or may not be present. Since a murmur is not reliably present, echocardiography is indicated in any case with fever of unknown origin, where endocarditis is a potential differential diagnosis.

Diagnosis is made depending on a combination of major and minor criteria, called the Duke criteria, some of which depend on imaging. The major criteria are:

- Echocardiographic evidence of a vegetative oscillatory lesion or erosive lesion
- New valvular incompetence associated with the lesion
- Positive blood cultures (≥ 2 sites).

Minor criteria (non-imaging) include fever, size of dog (>15 kg), aortic stenosis, thromboembolic disease, immune-mediated disease (polyarthropathy, glomerulonephropathy, positive blood culture) and positive *Bartonella* serology.

Radiography

Radiography is not usually informative, but may show cardiomegaly depending on chronicity and degree of volume overloading. Occasionally, CHF may develop.

Echocardiography

Vegetations are highly consistent with endocarditis, usually associated with thrombus formation. These are oscillatory lesions, which move independently of the valve. This distinguishes them from myxomatous nodules associated with MMVD. They may initially be hypoechoic and poorly defined, but they become more echogenic and organized once long-standing. The very earliest lesions are erosions in the valve associated with new valvular incompetence (mitral regurgitation (possible systolic murmur) or aortic regurgitation (possible diastolic murmur), depending on which heart valve is affected). A very small thrombus associated with this may be appreciated, but this becomes progressively larger and more organized. Eventually, the lesion may contribute to valve stenosis, however it may not be possible to exclude pre-existing aortic stenosis in the case of the aortic valve. Examples are shown in Figures 9.164 and 9.165.

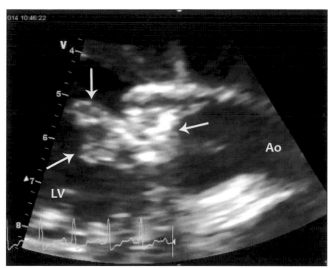

9.165 Right parasternal long-axis five-chamber view of a Boxer with aortic valve vegetative endocarditis. A large, hyperechoic lesion can be seen on the ventricular side of the aortic valve in this diastolic frame (arrowed). Ao = aorta.

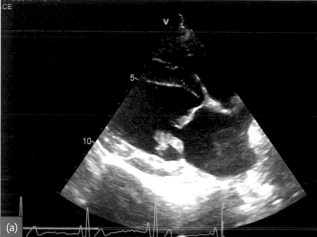

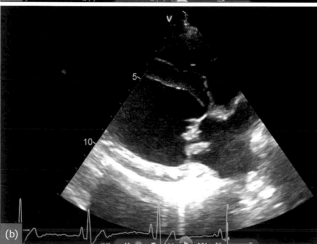

9.164 Right parasternal four-chamber views from a Labrador Retriever with right thoracic limb lameness, fever and subsequent development of neurological signs and a new heart murmur detected during hospitalization. (a) A vegetation can be seen on the ventricular side of the posterior mitral valve leaflet in diastole, which (b) flicked into the LA during systole. A smaller vegetation can be seen on the anterior leaflet during systole.

Pericardial disease

The normal pericardium is not essential to life, but it maintains the heart in its normal position in the mediastinum and thoracic cavity, prevents excessive dilatation of heart chambers in the presence of cardiac disease and preserves normal ventricular interdependence. The small amount of pericardial fluid between the visceral and parietal layers of the serous pericardium provides lubrication, but this fluid is not normally visible on ultrasound examination.

Pericardial effusions and cardiac tamponade

An increase in pericardial effusion is readily identified by ultrasonography as an anechoic space between the heart and parietal layer of pericardium. In dogs, idiopathic pericardial effusions and effusions associated with neoplasia are approximately equally common. In cats, the most common reason for a pericardial effusion is CHF.

If the pericardial pressure exceeds right atrial pressure, venous return to the right heart will be adversely affected, which may result in signs of right-sided CHF in the chronic situation. Diastolic collapse of the right atrial wall (and also sometimes the right ventricular wall) may be observed; this is called cardiac tamponade (Figure 9.166). Any animal with a pericardial effusion should be assessed for presence of cardiac tamponade, as this is an indication for pericardiocentesis. If the fluid accumulates suddenly, a small pericardial effusion may result in tamponade (e.g. left atrial tear with MMVD (see Figure 9.163)). However, if the fluid builds up slowly, the compliant pericardium can slowly expand and a very large effusion may develop. Sudden onset cardiac tamponade can lead to forward failure prior to any evidence of right-sided CHF. Affected animals may be collapsed and may have weak pulses including pulsus paradoxus (weaker pulse during inspiration than expiration) and systemic hypotension (cardiogenic shock).

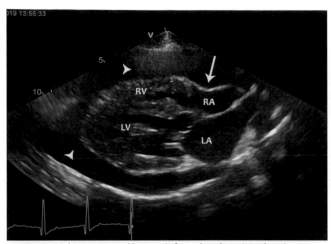

9.166 Right parasternal long-axis four-chamber view showing pericardial effusion (arrowheads) as an anechoic region surrounding the heart. The right atrial wall shows some collapse (arrowed); this is cardiac tamponade and it indicates that pericardial pressure exceeds right atrial pressure.

Important tips

As long as the animal is reasonably haemodynamically stable, the anechoic pericardial effusion makes it easier to appreciate any right atrial or heart base masses. Assess for cardiac neoplasia prior to pericardiocentesis.

Prior to sedation and pericardiocentesis, especially if the animal shows signs of cardiogenic shock and even if there is evidence of right-sided CHF, intravenous fluids are indicated to improve venous return to the right side of the heart to maintain cardiac output. These should be discontinued after the procedure.

Pericardial effusions in dogs

- Idiopathic pericardial effusion or haemorrhage, also known as idiopathic pericarditis.
  - Common in middle-aged to older large or giant breeds of dog, including Labrador Retrievers, Golden Retrievers, St Bernards and Newfoundlands.
  - Unknown aetiology.
  - No masses.
  - The effusion is haemorrhagic and often of large volume prior to causing cardiac tamponade.
  - May recur at some point in the future (prompting pericardiectomy).
- Cardiac neoplasia is commonly associated with pericardial effusions.
- Left atrial tear (see 'Potential sequelae of end-stage MMVD', above).
- Septic pericarditis. Rare, but can be seen in scenting dogs, likely due to migrating foreign organic material.
- Trauma or coagulopathy: pericardial haemorrhage is possible.
- Systemic diseases: small pericardial effusions can be seen with uraemia in dogs and cats, and in systemic inflammatory response syndrome. Conditions associated with hypoalbuminaemia may result in pericardial effusion as well as other body cavity effusions. These conditions do not usually result in cardiac tamponade (see Figure 9.145).

Pericardial effusions in cats

- CHF: normally, this is a small pericardial effusion as a manifestation of biventricular CHF; therefore, it may be seen in association with a pleural effusion. It rarely results in cardiac tamponade and pericardiocentesis is rarely necessary (Figure 9.167).
- Feline infectious peritonitis: the pericardial effusion rarely needs to be drained, although fluid analysis may be rewarding. Other clinical signs usually predominate.
- Lymphoma: usually not of significance haemodynamically. Cytology may be rewarding if pericardiocentesis is carried out.

Radiography

In dogs, and in cats with large pericardial effusions (Figure 9.167a), radiographic findings include a globular cardiac silhouette with no evidence of specific chamber enlargement and a sharp outline (due to loss of systolic–diastolic movement blur of the heart itself). In cats with the more commonly seen mild or moderate pericardial effusion, the cardiac silhouette often appears ovoid rather than globular. The appearance then resembles the normal shape of a canine cardiac silhouette (Figure 9.167c). There may be signs of right-sided CHF with a distended CdVC and ascites.

Echocardiography

Ultrasonography is extremely sensitive for detection of fluid so pericardial effusions are readily documented on echocardiography (Figure 9.167b). A pericardial effusion needs to be distinguished from a pleural effusion, although both may occur together. With sufficient depth of imaging, a pericardial effusion is circular, surrounding the heart, and 'attached' to the atrial walls dorsally. In large pericardial effusions, the heart may be seen to swing within the effusion. Moving cranial or caudal to the cardiac silhouette, observation of mediastinal structures, or fluid dorsal to the atria, indicates the presence of a pleural effusion.

It is important to assess for the presence of cardiac tamponade (see Figure 9.166) and heart base masses.

Cardiac neoplasia: Although echocardiography is the most commonly used imaging modality to detect cardiac masses, CT offers superior imaging for regions surrounded by lung, which precludes an acoustic window. With recent increased access to CT, more pericardial effusions are attributed to a known cause, rather than being idiopathic. Cardiac neoplasia is most commonly diagnosed associated with pericardial effusion. However, it can also result in arrhythmias or be detected during imaging.

- Haemangiosarcoma is the most frequent cardiac neoplasm (most commonly involving the right atrial appendage or right atrioventricular groove) (Figures 9.168 and 9.169). Although German Shepherd Dogs and Golden Retrievers are predisposed, it can be seen in many different breeds and their crosses. Dogs are usually older.
- Heart base neoplasia (e.g. chemodectoma) is most common in brachycephalic breeds. It may occasionally be recognized as an incidental finding during assessment of another cardiac disease not associated with pericardial effusion. It can be the cause of a pericardial effusion in some animals, however. Chemodectomas are typically periaortic, reasonably

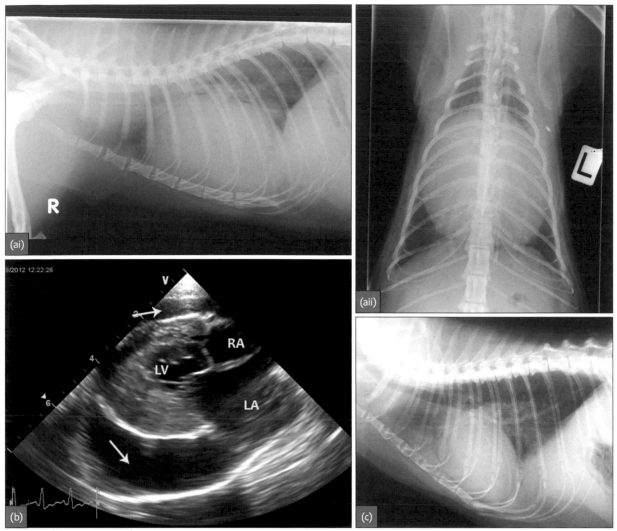

9.167 (ai) Lateral and (aii) DV thoracic radiographs of a 5-year-old cat with HCM and biventricular CHF. Unusually, this was associated with a large, recurrent pericardial effusion contributing to global generalized enlargement of the cardiac silhouette, without radiographic evidence of specific chamber enlargement. (b) Right parasternal four-chamber view of the same cat as in (a), showing a large pericardial effusion (arrowed). Asymmetrical hypertrophy of the LVFW can be seen, with left atrial dilatation. 72 ml of serosanguinous effusion was drained. (c) Lateral thoracic radiograph of an 11-year-old cat with a moderate pericardial effusion; the cardiac silhouette is ovoid and resembles a normal canine cardiac silhouette.

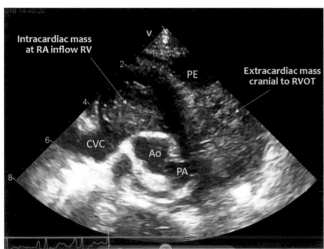

9.168 Right parasternal short-axis view showing right ventricular inflow and outflow from a Border Terrier presenting with cranial caval syndrome. There is a heterogeneous mass in the region of the tricuspid valve, located mainly in the RA. There is a small pericardial effusion (PE) and an extensive extracardiac mass, only part of which is seen, outside the RVOT. This was an extensive haemangiosarcoma. Ao = aorta; CVC = caudal vena cava; PA = pulmonic trunk.

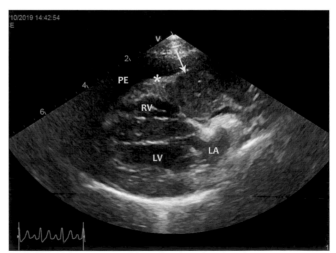

9.169 Right parasternal four-chamber view showing a heterogeneous mass (arrowed) affecting the right atrioventricular groove of a 12-year-old Dachshund. Pericardial effusion (PE) had been drained one day previously, but residual effusion is evident. The myocardium of the RVFW also appears abnormal (*) suggesting infiltration. A presumptive diagnosis of haemangiosarcoma was made.

homogeneous, hyperechoic, well circumscribed masses (Figure 9.170). Neuroendocrine tumours can also occur within the heart itself.

- Myxoma: these are rare intracardiac tumours, usually located in the RA or LA (Figure 9.171).
- Other extracardiac (heart base) masses that may result in pericardial effusion (e.g. ectopic thyroid carcinoma).
- Mesothelioma: this neoplasm is not usually associated with distinct mass lesions. Difficult to diagnose even on cytology or histopathology of pericardium post pericardiectomy.
- Neoplasia may also result in myocardial infiltration (see 'Myocardial infiltrative disease', above, and Figures 9.150 and 9.151).

Computed tomography

CT is not constrained by lung interference and is superior at assessing the full extent of cardiac neoplasia as well as any pulmonary (or other) metastases or other organ involvement (Figures 9.172 and 9.173).

Herniated, incarcerated fat: Occasionally, a very small amount of herniated or incarcerated material may result in a pericardial effusion. With a very small peritoneopericardial diaphragmatic hernia (PPDH), herniated fat or other abdominal contents (pseudo-mass lesions) may be evident on echocardiography (Figure 9.174). See also 'Peritoneopericardial diaphragmatic hernia', below and Chapter 8.

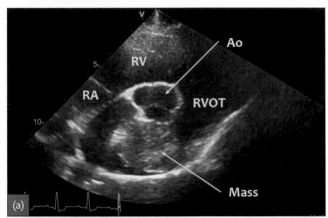

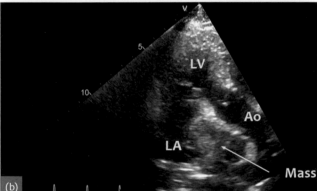

9.170 (a) Right parasternal short-axis view at the level of the aortic valves and (b) left apical three-chamber view of a Staffordshire Bull Terrier with ventricular tachycardia. There was no pericardial effusion, but a periaortic heart base mass (possible chemodectoma) is shown. Ao = aorta.

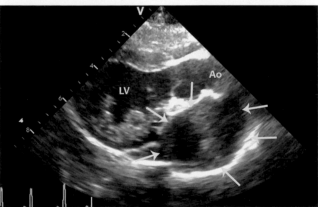

9.171 Right parasternal long-axis five-chamber view, optimizing an isoechoic, homogeneous mass within the LAA (arrowed) of a 10-year-old neutered Cavalier King Charles Spaniel bitch with preclinical MMVD. The appearance is most consistent with a myxoma, but this was not confirmed. LAA masses are rare. Ao = aorta.

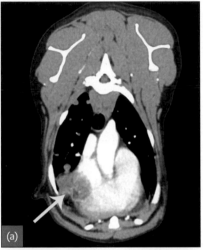

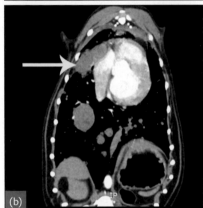

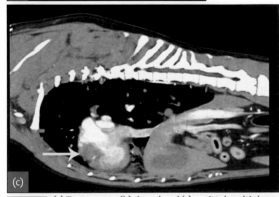

9.172 (a) Transverse, (b) dorsal and (c) sagittal multiplanar reformatted contrast-enhanced thoracic CT images (soft tissue reconstruction) of a large, rounded, heterogeneous soft tissue attenuating, mildly rim enhancing mass (probable haemangiosarcoma) arising from the region of the RA/atrioventricular groove (arrowed) in a dog. Multiple small soft tissue attenuating nodules are also visible within the lungs (disseminated metastasis).

(Courtesy of Will Humphreys, University of Liverpool)

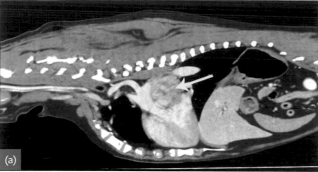

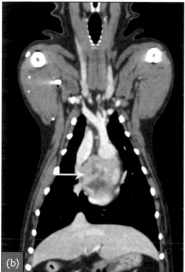

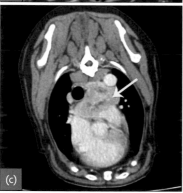

9.173 (a) Sagittal, (b) dorsal and (c) transverse multiplanar reformatted contrast-enhanced CT thoracic images (soft tissue reconstruction) showing a large globoid, sharply marginated but heterogeneously contrast enhancing mass at the heart base (arrowed) displacing the caudal trachea to the right (possible chemodectoma).
(Courtesy of Will Humphreys, University of Liverpool)

Constrictive or constrictive–effusive pericardial disease

Constrictive pericardial disease is rare and may be a late consequence of chronic or recurrent pericardial effusion. If a residual pericardial effusion is also present, the diagnosis is easier to make as this is easily identified using ultrasonography. If the pericardium is severely thickened or fibrotic, it becomes non-compliant and constrains filling of the cardiac chambers. This is a difficult diagnosis to make and it must be distinguished from a type of RCM. Documentation of increased ventricular interdependence by Doppler echocardiography can help diagnose constrictive pericardial disease. The pathophysiology of constrictive pericardial disease can be simplified:

- The heart chambers are all constrained by the non-compliant pericardium
- It normally leads to increased systemic venous return to the right side of the heart during inspiration (this can be identified with increased diastolic transtricuspid velocities during inspiration). This is because of negative thoracic pressure increasing venous return to the thorax from the head, neck and abdomen via the venae cavae
- This increased blood in the right heart during inspiration will reduce the ability of the left heart to fill. Transmitral or PVF velocities are reduced during inspiration and greater during expiration (Figure 9.175). This demonstrates increased ventricular dependence. The increased blood in the right heart can also affect aortic outflow; therefore, pulses may be weaker during inspiration than expiration (pulsus paradoxus). The left heart is not normally affected by respiratory phase, so documentation of >25% variation in transmitral E waves with reduction during inspiration is highly suggestive of pericardial disease. It is important that the dog is breathing normally, and not panting, when this is observed
- The flow propagation velocity of the early ventricular filling in the LV will be high (steep slope on mitral flow colour M-mode). In contrast, this will have reduced velocity (more shallow slope) with an RCM.

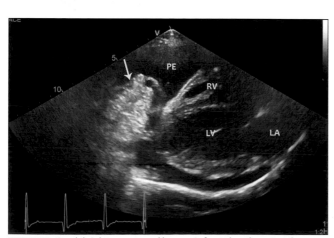

9.174 Caudal right parasternal long-axis four-chamber view from a 1-year-old male German Shepherd Dog with a pericardial effusion (PE) resulting in cardiac tamponade and right-sided CHF. There is a hyperechoic 'mass' in the PE (arrowed), attached not to the heart but to the parietal pericardial wall. This was subsequently confirmed to be herniated fat associated with a very small PPDH.

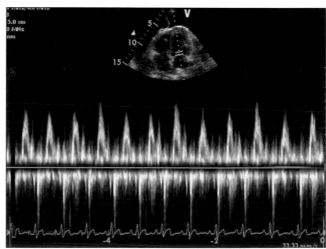

9.175 Continuous wave spectral Doppler showing respiratory variation in transmitral flow velocities in a dog with constrictive–effusive pericardial disease.
(Courtesy of Urszula Bartoszuk)

Peritoneopericardial diaphragmatic hernia

A PPDH is a relatively common congenital developmental defect resulting in an abnormal communication between the peritoneal and pericardial cavities that arises during development of the diaphragm (septum transversum). Depending on the size of defect, it may allow herniation of abdominal contents into the pericardial sac. It must be differentiated from a traumatic diaphragmatic rupture, which usually does not involve the pericardial space. Animals with PPDH may present in different ways:

- Completely asymptomatic: an incidental finding during imaging for another reason; may be of minor or major importance
- It may result in a pericardial effusion (see above)
- It may result in gastrointestinal obstruction if parts of the gastrointestinal tract are herniated
- Auscultation may identify muffled or absent cardiac sounds, or displacement of the heart

- A PPDH may be associated with congenital heart disease or abnormal midline abdominal body wall closure.

Various forms of imaging should successfully identify abdominal contents within the pericardial cavity. Discontinuity of the diaphragm may be evident (Figure 9.176).

More rarely, other congenital peritoneopleural diaphragmatic hernias can be recognized.

Pericardial cyst

Pericardial cysts are rare in dogs and cats. They may represent residual tissue from a closed PPDH, which may accumulate fluid and then exert similar effects on the adjacent heart chambers (typically the right heart) to a pericardial effusion. Some may be associated with pericardial effusions. Mostly, they consist of a fibrous, thick-walled capsule containing haemorrhagic fluid (Figure 9.177). True coelomic (thin-walled) cysts seem to be even more rare.

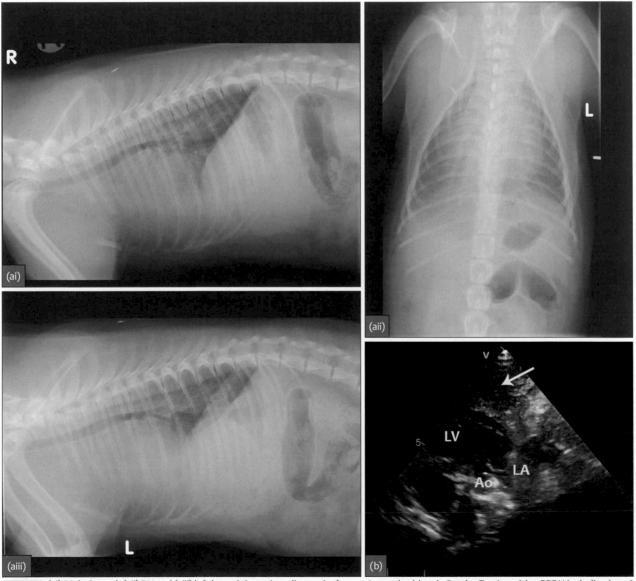

9.176 (ai) Right lateral, (aii) DV and (aiii) left lateral thoracic radiographs from a 4-month-old male Border Terrier with a PPDH including herniated liver in the pericardial sac. The dog also had a sternal cleft and large abdominal hernia. Generalized enlargement of the cardiac silhouette is seen, with a poorly defined diaphragmatic line. (b) Modified left apical five-chamber view from the same dog, showing the liver (arrowed) adjacent to the left ventricular wall. Ao = aorta.

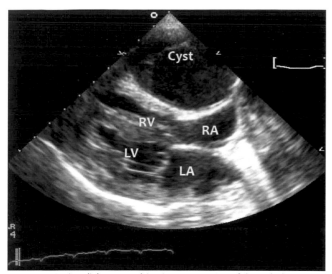

9.177 Pericardial cyst resulting in compression of the right heart in a 4-year-old crossbreed dog that had episodic collapse on severe exertion and, more recently, signs of right-sided CHF. The cyst is relatively thick-walled and filled with haemorrhagic contents.
(Reproduced from Loureiro *et al.* (2009) with permission)

Pericardial defects

Pericardial defects are most likely congenital developmental abnormalities where part of the pericardium is absent. They are most often reported as an incidental finding at post-mortem examination. However, if part of the heart (e.g. an atrial appendage) herniates through the defect and there is subsequently enlargement of the affected heart chamber, this can result in incarceration, necrosis, shock or at least a reduction in that chamber's function, compromising cardiac output. The right atrial appendage is most commonly reported as being affected. It can be difficult to confirm this from imaging modalities as the normal pericardium surrounding the defect or herniated region is very thin. A suspected LAA herniation is shown in Figure 9.178. A post-mortem example of a herniated RV is shown in Figure 9.179.

Surgical pericardial windows may be created as part of the management of pericardial effusions or during other surgical procedures (e.g. epicardial pacemaker lead placement). If these windows are too large (or small), they can also result in herniation of part of the heart. Herniation may be more likely if there is development of chamber enlargement (e.g. with acquired cardiac disease).

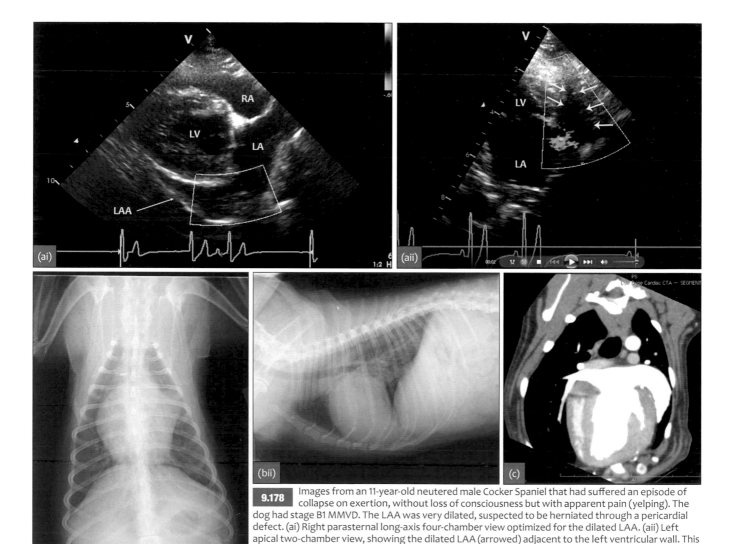

9.178 Images from an 11-year-old neutered male Cocker Spaniel that had suffered an episode of collapse on exertion, without loss of consciousness but with apparent pain (yelping). The dog had stage B1 MMVD. The LAA was very dilated, suspected to be herniated through a pericardial defect. (ai) Right parasternal long-axis four-chamber view optimized for the dilated LAA. (aii) Left apical two-chamber view, showing the dilated LAA (arrowed) adjacent to the left ventricular wall. This was associated with apparent turbulence suggesting some mild obstruction associated with atrial systole (colour flow Doppler). (bi) DV and (bii) right lateral thoracic radiographs from the same dog, showing LAA enlargement on the DV view. (c) Transverse thoracic CT image with intravascular contrast material confirming the enlargement of the LAA. The pericardium could not be directly imaged to confirm LAA herniation outside the pericardium.

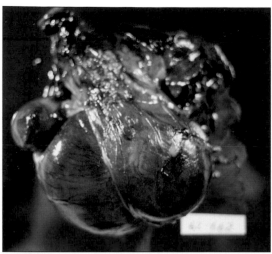

9.179 Canine heart with herniation and incarceration of the RV through a large pericardial defect.
(Courtesy of J. Buchanan)

Acquired vascular disease

Peripheral vascular disease is rare in animals compared with its frequency associated with ageing in humans.

Systemic vascular disease
Systemic hypertension

From the thoracic imaging point of view, one may identify the consequences of systemic hypertension, such as echocardiographic evidence of concentric left ventricular hypertrophy or high-velocity mitral regurgitation (see Figure 9.146). Older cats can sometimes show aortic redundancy.

Arterial thromboembolism

FATE is a well known, devastating consequence of cardiac disease in cats associated with left atrial dilatation. Thrombi within the LA can embolize downstream in the arterial system, commonly to the caudal aorta. In any cat presenting with FATE, investigations of probable underlying cardiac disease are indicated (see 'Feline myocardial disease', above). The pain and stress of the condition may precipitate onset of CHF. Rarely, neoplastic emboli may be associated with pulmonary neoplasia.

In dogs, systemic ATE does not result in such a peracute onset as in cats, nor is it associated with such apparently severe pain. ATE or arterial thrombosis is generally associated with another condition that may result in vascular disease or a hypercoagulable state:

- Endocrine disease (e.g. hypothyroidism, hyperadrenocorticism)
- Protein-losing conditions (e.g. protein-losing nephropathy or enteropathy)
- Inflammatory conditions (e.g. immune-mediated haemolytic anaemia, steroid-responsive meningoarteritis).

The caudal aorta is most commonly affected, which results in ischaemia of the affected limb (if unilateral) or limbs (if bilateral) and consequent pelvic limb weakness or collapse on exercise. Femoral pulses may be absent,

and differential cyanosis may be observable in unpigmented footpads or nailbeds apparent on exertion, even if not at rest.

ATE is not normally associated with cardiac disease, so thoracic imaging is less important in dogs. However, some of the conditions that may result in ATE may also cause PTE (see 'Pulmonary thromboembolism', below).

Pulmonary vascular disease
Parasitic

Dirofilariasis: Heartworm disease, caused by the nematode *Dirofilaria immitis*, is common in certain parts of the world, mainly tropical or subtropical regions, where the mosquito vector is common. However, with pet travel and pet rescue from different countries, it may also be seen in the UK even though it is not endemic in Northern Europe. It can affect both dogs and cats, but dogs are most frequently recognized with clinical disease.

Adult heartworms live in the pulmonary arteries and in severe infestations may also be present in the RV. These are large (approximately 15–25 cm in length) and, therefore, can significantly obstruct the pulmonary arteries especially in smaller animals and those with high worm burdens. Microfilariae produced by the adult female heartworm are released into the circulation. These are then ingested by feeding female mosquitos, in which they undergo several moults to form an infective stage transmitted by the mosquito into another canine or feline host. About 3 months later the parasite reaches an immature adult stage and enters the vascular system. It then migrates to the heart and lungs where it matures into the adult worm. The pulmonary arterial response to heartworms in the cat is more severe than that in the dog, and in general the clinical manifestations of the disease tend to be more severe in this species.

The manifestations of heartworm disease depend on the number of worms, the chronicity of infection and on interactions between the parasite and host. Most dogs with heartworm infestation are asymptomatic. Presenting signs in symptomatic dogs may include lethargy, coughing, poor condition, ascites and syncope. More serious consequences of heartworm disease, such as parasitic eosinophilic pneumonitis, may occur. Rare complications include eosinophilic granulomatosis, thromboembolic disease, pulmonary hypertension, glomerulonephritis, caval syndrome and disseminated intravascular coagulation.

Clinical signs in cats are often chronic and nonspecific. These include anorexia, weight loss, vomiting, dyspnoea and coughing. They usually present with respiratory signs, which must be differentiated from feline asthma. This is called heartworm-associated respiratory disease (Garrity *et al.*, 2019).

More acute signs are usually due to aberrant worm migration (more common in cats than dogs) or worm embolization, and include shock, salivation, haemoptysis, neurological signs, vomiting, syncope and even death.

Radiography: Radiographic findings include:

- Dogs (see Figures 9.148 and 9.180). Changes primarily reflect the pulmonary hypertension that results from physical obstruction to outflow by adult worms living in the RV and pulmonary outflow tract, as well as changes to the walls of the pulmonary arteries:
  - Enlargement of the right side of the heart ('reversed D' appearance on DV or VD view)
  - Enlargement of the pulmonic trunk (Figure 9.181)

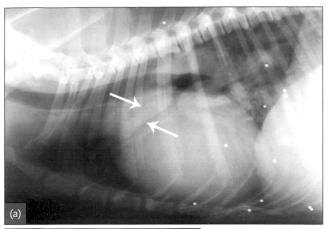

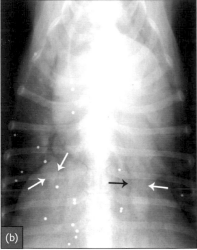

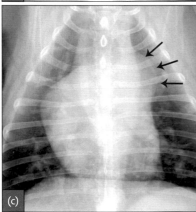

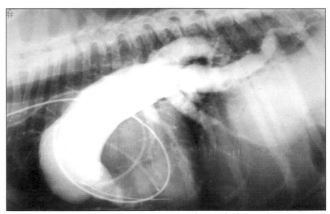

9.181 Selective lateral angiogram in a dog with chronic heartworm disease. Several catheters are present but angiography was performed via a catheter in the pulmonic trunk. The contrast medium fills a markedly dilated pulmonic trunk and its branches. The caudal lobar pulmonary arteries are also tortuous and truncated.

9.180 (a) Lateral and (b) VD thoracic radiographs of a 12-year-old male Golden Retriever with heartworm disease. The pulmonary arteries are extremely enlarged and tortuous (arrowed). The cardiac silhouette is rounded and right-sided cardiomegaly is present. Incidental tiny metallic opacities represent lead shot from a previous injury. (c) DV thoracic radiograph of a 4-year-old Staffordshire Bull Terrier with heartworm disease. This radiograph was acquired 3 months after treatment for caval syndrome and heartworm disease. Severe right-sided cardiac enlargement and pulmonic trunk enlargement (arrowed) are still evident.

- Enlargement and tortuosity of the (particularly caudal) lobar pulmonary arteries (Figures 9.148 and 9.181)
- Right-sided heart failure may be evident in advanced disease
- There may be a diffuse bronchointerstitial pulmonary pattern due to eosinophilic infiltrates associated with an allergic response
- Patchy pulmonary opacification (interstitial to alveolar patterns) may be seen, associated with PTE

- Cats (Figure 9.182):
    - Most commonly enlargement of the caudal lobar pulmonary arteries (>1.6 times the width of the ninth rib on the VD view)
    - Tortuosity of these vessels and enlargement of the right side of the heart is much less common than in dogs
    - Bronchointerstitial or even alveolar pulmonary patterns and pulmonary hyperinflation, mimicking feline bronchial disease, have also been reported
    - Changes may also be seen in cats that ultimately resist heartworm infestation and are eventually negative for the disease.

Echocardiography: Ultrasonography can be a useful adjunctive test in dogs and can provide definitive evidence of infection in cats when other tests are equivocal.

- Adult worms in dogs are usually present in the pulmonary arteries and, therefore, may not be seen on ultrasound examination.

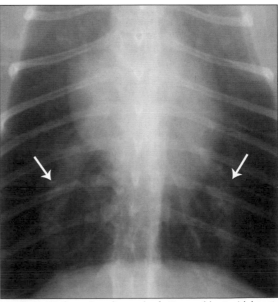

9.182 VD thoracic radiograph of a 7-year-old cat with heartworm disease, showing moderate to severe enlargement and lack of tapering of the caudal lobar pulmonary arteries (arrowed).

- However, they may be found in the pulmonic trunk, the right and left caudal lobar arteries (Figure 9.183a), and occasionally the RA, RV or across the tricuspid valve (Figure 9.183b). The latter has particularly been described in dogs with caval syndrome.
- On 2D echocardiography, adult worms appear as strongly echogenic short parallel lines (Figure 9.183a).

Supportive echocardiographic findings of the diagnosis in the absence of visible adult worms predominantly occur as a consequence of pulmonary hypertension and include (Figure 9.184):

- Right ventricular eccentric hypertrophy
- Right atrial and pulmonic trunk dilatation
- Septal flattening and paradoxical motion
- Tricuspid regurgitation can be identified in dogs with advanced pulmonary hypertension or if adult worms are present across the valves.

Angiostrongylosis: *Angiostrongylus vasorum* is a meta-strongylid nematode that infests domestic dogs. *A. vasorum* has a worldwide distribution and within Europe is endemic in most of England, Wales, France, Ireland and Denmark. Foxes are presumed to act as a wildlife reservoir for the parasite. The adult worms are 1.5–2.0 cm long and located in peripheral pulmonary arteries and are not imaged in the right heart or pulmonary arteries near the heart. The adult worm is oviparous. The eggs are carried to the pulmonary capillaries. The eggs hatch and first-stage (L1) larvae migrate through the alveolar epithelium, are coughed up, swallowed and passed in the faeces. The life cycle is indirect and larvae undergo subsequent moults within a molluscan intermediate host, to become third-stage (L3) larvae. When a dog ingests an intermediate host, infective L3 larvae are liberated into the dog's small intestine. The L3 larvae undergo two further moults in the mesenteric lymph nodes and the L5 larvae migrate via the liver to the right side of the heart, completing the life cycle.

The most common clinical signs associated with angiostrongylosis are coughing and dyspnoea caused by the inflammatory response to the eggs and migrating larvae at the level of the alveolar membrane. The second common manifestation of angiostrongylosis is a coagulopathy. Subcutaneous, mucosal and internal haemorrhages may be seen. Neurological signs associated with cerebral haemorrhage may also occur. Bleeding may

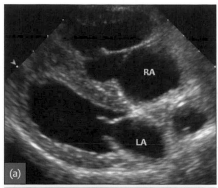

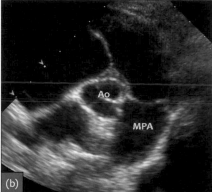

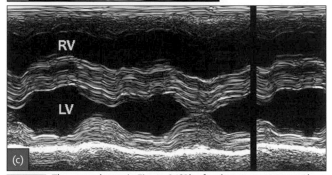

9.184 The same dog as in Figure 9.183b after heartworm removal. (a) Right parasternal long-axis view. Note the enlarged RA and compare its size to that of the LA. (b) Right parasternal short-axis view obtained at the heart base and optimized for the pulmonic trunk (MPA). The MPA is enlarged both before and after the pulmonic valve. Usually, the MPA diameter is close to the diameter of the aorta (Ao) at this level. (c) M-mode obtained at the level of the papillary muscles from a right parasternal location. The RV is markedly dilated. The LV is also labelled for comparison.

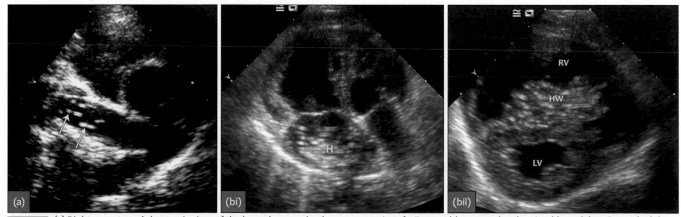

9.183 (a) Right parasternal short-axis view of the heart base and pulmonary arteries of a 7-year-old neutered male mixed-breed dog. Several adult worms can be seen in the right pulmonary artery (arrowed). (b) A 4-year-old Staffordshire Bull Terrier with caval syndrome due to heartworm disease. (bi) Left parasternal long-axis four-chamber view. A large mass of adult heartworms (H) is present in the enlarged RA. They are identified as parallel echogenic lines. (bii) Right parasternal short-axis view obtained at the level of the papillary muscles. During diastole the worms (HW) moved through the tricuspid valve and into the enlarged RV.

occur with or without concurrent respiratory disease and the pathogenesis of the coagulopathy is undetermined. A minority of dogs suffer collapse episodes or sudden death, possibly due to aberrant larval migration into the myocardium. Aberrant parasite migration may also affect the central nervous system or the eye, resulting in neurological or ocular signs. The majority of affected dogs are young and Cavalier King Charles Spaniels appear particularly predisposed to clinical disease.

Angiostrongylosis should be suspected in any young dog presenting with compatible clinical signs and a typical radiographic pattern (see below), especially in endemic areas. The diagnosis is confirmed by demonstrating the presence of L1 larvae in the faeces (rectal mucosal swab or faecal Baermann's test) or airway or lung aspirate cytology samples. The Angio Detect in-clinic test (IDEXX) rapidly confirms presence of antigen. Other diagnostic findings are variable. Eosinophilic inflammation in airway cytology samples is less common than might be expected. The results of coagulation function testing are inconsistent and in some cases may be normal.

Radiography: Significant thoracic radiographic abnormalities are present in almost all clinically affected dogs (see Figure 9.147).

- Most common findings are alveolar pattern and bronchial thickening (seen in approximately 80% and 70% of dogs, respectively). Typically, the alveolar infiltrate has a multifocal or peripheral distribution (see Figure 9.147). Less commonly, a mild generalized interstitial pattern may be seen.
- Note that the same thoracic radiographic changes are also seen in most dogs with *A. vasorum*-associated coagulopathy, even in the absence of clinical signs of respiratory disease.
- Less common findings include a small-volume pleural effusion and right ventricular enlargement (see Figure 9.147).
- Although *A. vasorum* is a pulmonary vascular parasite, significant radiographic changes affecting the pulmonary arteries are not usually seen.
- Radiographic improvement may lag behind clinical resolution.
- Residual alveolar pattern may still be present 1 month after successful treatment and an interstitial pattern may persist for up to 3 months.

Computed tomography: Thoracic CT findings have been reported from dogs with both naturally occurring (Coia *et al.*, 2017) and experimental (Dennler *et al.*, 2011) angiostrongylosis. They reflect the radiographic changes, confirming a more peripheral distribution of lesions from diffuse, multifocal nodules of ground-glass opacity to consolidated lung with air bronchograms (Figure 9.185). Filling defects within pulmonary arteries can sometimes be appreciated on contrast CT images, consistent with thromboembolism.

Ultrasonography and echocardiography: Given the peripheral lung distribution and lung consolidation, lesions adjacent to the thoracic body wall can be imaged by ultrasonography. Fine-needle aspiration yields samples for cytological evaluation and confirmation of the diagnosis of angiostrongylosis. The focal hypoechoic consolidated lesions evident on ultrasound images are not specific for the diagnosis of angiostrongylosis.

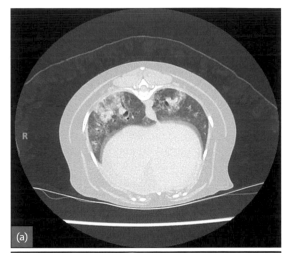

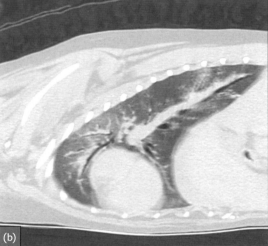

9.185 (a) Transverse (level of diaphragm) and (b) sagittal thoracic CT images of a 2-year-old neutered male mixed-breed dog diagnosed with angiostrongylosis (same dog as in Figure 9.147). There is a diffuse mild ground-glass opacity, multiple irregular regions of parenchymal consolidation and scattered ill-defined heterogeneous hyperattenuating nodular regions. These have a moderately peripheral distribution and are more severe in the caudodorsal parts of both caudal lung lobes.

Angiostrongylus worms cannot be seen on ultrasound examination in the heart or left and right pulmonary arteries. Echocardiographic findings, when present, usually reflect the development of pulmonary hypertension. This does not occur in all cases, but if it does, it might lead to the development of right-sided CHF. Echocardiographic findings include:

- Right atrial and right ventricular enlargement (mainly dilatation) (Figure 9.186)
- Flattening of the IVS with significant increase in right ventricular pressure (severe pulmonary hypertension) (Figure 9.186)
- Dilated pulmonic trunk and lobar pulmonary arteries
- Increased velocity of tricuspid regurgitation and pulmonary regurgitation spectral Doppler envelopes, consistent with increased pulmonic trunk systolic and diastolic pressures respectively (in the absence of RVOT obstruction) (see 'Secondary myocardial disease', above)
- The pulmonary outflow spectral Doppler envelopes can be abnormal in pulmonary hypertension (see Figure 9.149f).

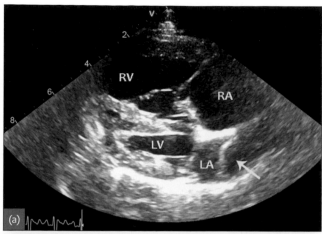

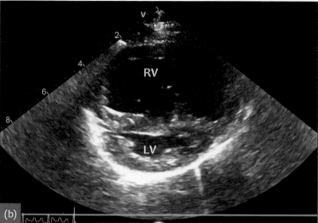

9.186 (a) Right parasternal long-axis four-chamber and (b) short-axis views of a 2-year-old neutered male mixed-breed dog with severe pulmonary hypertension associated with angiostrongylosis (same dog as in Figures 9.185 and 9.147). Marked flattening of the IVS can be seen, leading to left-sided underfilling. Dorsal to the LA, the right pulmonary artery is very dilated (arrowed).

The reason that pulmonary hypertension does not occur in all cases may be due to recruitment of arteriovenous anastomosis shunts in some dogs (Novo Matos et al., 2016). These can be detected by an echocontrast study:

- Saline (possibly mixed with colloid; approximately 0.5 ml/kg) is agitated between two syringes and a three-way valve, then injected into a peripheral vein during echocardiography. Contrast appears in the right side of the heart, but it should not appear in the left side of the heart in a healthy animal, as the bubbles do not traverse the pulmonary capillary bed
- If bubbles appear almost immediately in the left heart, there may be a right-to-left shunt (e.g. patent foramen ovale)
- If bubbles appear in the left heart after three or more cardiac cycles, then there is evidence for pulmonary arteriovenous anastomoses, bypassing the pulmonary capillary bed.

Pulmonary hypertension

See 'Pulmonary hypertension' under 'Secondary myocardial conditions', above, for the classification and description of pulmonary hypertension. Pulmonary hypertension secondary to parasitic infestation such as angiostrongylosis and dirofilariasis has its own classification (type 5) (Reinero et al., 2020), in contrast to the human classification. Rarely, idiopathic pulmonary hypertension

(type 6) is seen where no known cause is evident, but this is less common in animals than in human patients.
Criteria for the diagnosis include:

- Exclusion of pulmonic stenosis or other RVOT obstruction
- Estimation of pulmonary arterial pressure in systole from tricuspid regurgitation velocity (TRv) (if present) and calculation of the pressure gradient (PG) by the modified Bernoulli equation ($PG \approx 4(TRv)^2$). The pressure gradient is approximately equal to the pulmonary arterial systolic pressure. A TRv of >3.4 m/s (or >3.0 m/s in the presence of supporting anatomical features) gives high or intermediate probability of pulmonary hypertension (see Figure 9.149d)
- Presence of one or more anatomical sites supporting presence of pulmonary hypertension:
  - Right ventricular enlargement, flattening of the IVS, underfilling of the LV (see Figures 9.149ab and 9.186) or right ventricular systolic dysfunction
  - Pulmonic trunk dilatation, annulus diameter:aortic annulus diameter ratio of >1, right pulmonary artery:pulmonary vein ratio of >1 (dorsal to LA on right parasternal four-chamber view) (see Figures 9.149c and 9.186) or reduced pulmonary artery distensibility (<30%)
  - Right atrial dilatation or caudal vena caval dilatation.

Other features:

- Estimation of diastolic pulmonary arterial pressure from the pulmonic regurgitation velocity (PRv) and calculation of diastolic pulmonic trunk–right ventricular pressure gradient. Increased if early diastolic PRv is >2.5 m/s (see Figure 9.149e)
- Abnormal systolic notching of the pulmonary outflow spectral Doppler envelope (provided this is not created by artefact or poor alignment) (see Figure 9.149f).

Pulmonary thromboembolism

Any condition that affects pulmonary vascular endothelium, including dirofilariasis, angiostrongylosis and pulmonary hypertension, may result in thrombus formation. Conditions resulting in a hypercoagulable state may also result in pulmonary thrombi or thromboembolism. These include endocrine disease (e.g. hyperadrenocorticism), protein-losing conditions (e.g. glomerular disease), neoplasia and inflammatory diseases such as immune-mediated haemolytic anaemia. PTE may cause pulmonary hypertension or be a consequence of it.

Clinical signs and presentation depend on the size of thrombus or number of thrombi and might include sudden onset dyspnoea with severe ventilation–perfusion mismatch. Diagnosis may be based on increased D-dimer results (confirming presence of cross-linked fibrin), or arterial blood gas analysis that confirms increased alveolar–arterial gradient and the ventilation–perfusion mismatch.

Radiography: Plain radiographs are not usually informative but help to exclude other causes of dyspnoea.

Computed tomography: CT is helpful in the presence of large thrombi in major pulmonary vessels, where contrast material may terminate in the vessels or thrombi may result in filling defects (Figure 9.187).

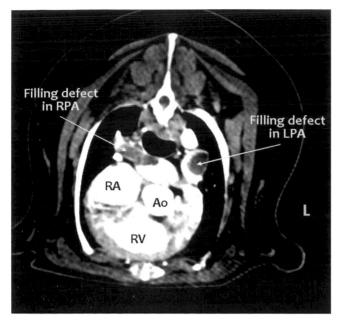

9.187 PTE in a 5-year-old neutered Cavalier King Charles Spaniel bitch; reason for the thromboembolism was not determined in this case. Transverse contrast-enhanced thoracic CT image showing both right and left pulmonary arteries with filling defects, consistent with large thrombi. The right heart is dilated and echocardiography confirmed presence of pulmonary hypertension. Ao = aorta; LPA = left pulmonary artery; RPA = right pulmonary artery.

Echocardiography: Ultrasonography is only able to image the pulmonic trunk and the pulmonary arteries near the heart, so thrombi are not imaged unless they are in this location and very large (Figure 9.188). However, echocardiography may increase the suspicion of PTE if the pulmonic trunk or lobar arteries are dilated or there is evidence of pulmonary hypertension. The RV may be dilated and show septal flattening if pulmonary hypertension or PTE cause increased pressure load on the RV.

Budd–Chiari-like syndrome

In animals, this term describes post-sinusoidal hypertension and the development of a high-protein peritoneal effusion due to the obstruction of hepatic venous return to the heart. The obstruction may involve the:

- Junction of the hepatic veins with the CdVC
- CdVC itself between the entry of the hepatic veins and the heart
- RA.

Causes include thrombosis, caval syndrome associated with heartworm disease, compression or invasion of the CdVC by tumours or other masses, trauma-induced stricture, fibrosis, diaphragmatic hernia and congenital cardiac (e.g. CTD) or caval (e.g. membranous obstruction) anomalies.

Radiography: Other than signs of ascites, radiographic features are not specific. Congenital developmental absence of the CdVC, masses, hernias or other abnormalities in the region of the caudal mediastinum, diaphragm or liver may be seen.

Contrast studies: A caudal vena cavagram (e.g. via lateral saphenous injection) may demonstrate invasion, compression or obstruction of the CdVC.

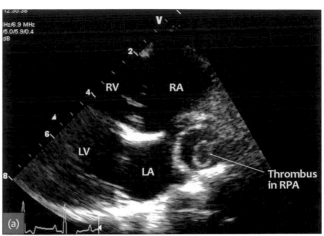

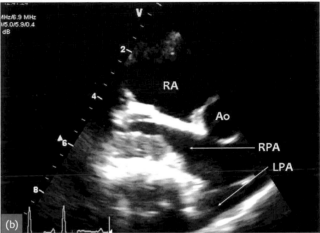

9.188 A 5-year-old neutered Cavalier King Charles Spaniel bitch (same dog as in Figure 9.187) with a large thrombus in the right pulmonary artery (RPA). (a) Right parasternal long-axis four-chamber view showing a very dilated RPA dorsal to the LA, containing a thrombus. (b) Cranial right parasternal short-axis view, optimizing the pulmonic trunk bifurcation into the pulmonary arteries. The same thrombus is visible in the RPA and a poorly defined thrombus is possibly present in the left pulmonary artery (LPA). Ao = aorta.

Ultrasonography: Abdominal ultrasonography may identify abnormalities of the liver or the abdominal portion of the CdVC. Doppler interrogation may identify abnormal or retrograde flow. Colour Doppler evaluation of the hepatic veins and CdVC provides the most information regarding the presence and direction of blood flow within the hepatic veins and CdVC.

Computed tomography: CT may demonstrate structural abnormalities or masses (Figure 9.189). CT angiography may be necessary to demonstrate vascular abnormalities.

Cranial vena cava syndrome

CrVC syndrome results from obstruction of the CrVC with resulting impairment of the venous return from the cranial parts of the body to the heart. Reported causes include great vessel invasion or compression (tumour), granuloma (e.g. blastomycosis) and thromboembolism. Thromboembolism has been described associated with a pacemaker lead. Predisposing factors include conditions that contribute to a hypercoagulable state (immune-mediated disease, sepsis, glomerulonephritis, cardiac disease, neoplasia, corticosteroid administration, central venous catheters in pre-existing conditions).

The clinical signs include symmetrical, simultaneous swelling of the head, neck and thoracic limbs.

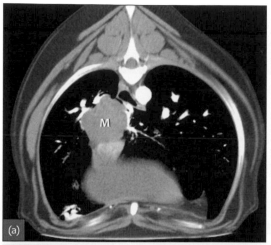

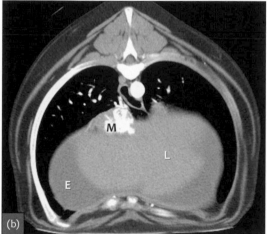

9.189 (a) Post-contrast transverse CT image (soft tissue algorithm and window) of a 6-year-old neutered male Labrador Retriever with a Budd–Chiari-like syndrome due to a CdVC mass. The image was obtained caudal to the heart. The mass (M) is seen as a large soft tissue attenuating structure with a small amount of contrast medium within the CdVC ventral to it. There is also atelectasis of the ventral tip of the right caudal lung lobe. (b) A more caudal image from the same CT series. The caudal part of the mass (M) has large regions of mineralization (these were also hyperdense before contrast administration). The peritoneal effusion (E) is evident on this image, surrounding the liver lobes (L).

Radiography

Radiographs may be normal or may demonstrate the cause of the obstruction (e.g. cranial mediastinal mass). CrVC obstruction near the heart may lead to pleural effusion.

Contrast studies: Angiography may demonstrate intraluminal filling defects, extraluminal compressive masses or other causes of CrVC obstruction. Non-selective angiography via the jugular vein is preferred but may be difficult in the face of swelling of the soft tissues of the neck; cephalic vein administration of contrast medium should also provide excellent opacification (Figure 9.190).

Ultrasonography: In the presence of radiographic abnormalities of the cranial mediastinum, ultrasonography may provide additional information with regard to masses or other abnormalities. If thoracic radiographs are normal, ultrasonography is unlikely to provide additional information and angiography is recommended.

Computed tomography: CT angiography provides an alternative means of evaluating the CrVC for filling defects or compressive lesions.

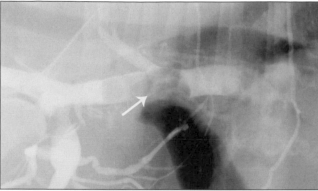

9.190 Lateral angiogram of an 11-year-old neutered Labrador Retriever bitch with recurrence of severe oedema of the head, neck and thoracic limbs 1 week after removal of a thymoma. Non-selective angiography via the cephalic vein demonstrated a large intraluminal filling defect (arrowed) consistent with a thrombus in the CrVC at the level of the costocervical vein. A repeat angiogram 2 weeks later showed the thrombus to be approximately half the size. (Courtesy of D. Davies)

Coronary artery disease

See 'Pulmonic stenosis' under 'Congenital cardiac disease', above, for an outline of congenital developmental abnormalities of the coronary arteries. Congenital coronary artery abnormalities are more common in animals than acquired coronary artery disease.

Coronary arterial and ischaemic heart disease

Ischaemic heart disease is rare in dogs and cats. Myocardial infarction can occur secondary to atherosclerosis or other forms of arteriosclerosis in both the dog and cat. Arteriosclerosis is arterial wall hardening, loss of elasticity and thickening, which leads to luminal narrowing. Specific forms of arteriosclerosis include:

- Lipid deposition and thickening of the intimal cell layers within arteries (atherosclerosis)
- Calcification of the tunica media of muscular arteries
- Thickening of the walls of small arteries or arterioles due to cell proliferation or hyaline deposition (arteriolosclerosis).

Atherosclerosis has been strongly associated with diabetes mellitus and hypothyroidism (but not with hyperadrenocorticism). Mineralization of the walls of the coronary arteries may occur in chronic cases of arteriosclerosis. The gradual occlusion of the coronary arteries leads to myocardial ischaemia, myocardial infarction and fibrosis. The outcome may be sudden death or acute or chronic heart failure.

Ischaemic heart disease has been postulated as a cause of sudden death during anaesthesia or sedation. Myocardial infarction (generally of the LVFW; see 'Imaging findings', below) has also been reported secondary to HCM in the cat. Ischaemic heart disease can also rarely occur as a result of incarceration of the LV in a pericardial defect (congenital) or tear (traumatic) with strangulation of one or both coronary arteries.

Imaging findings: Survey radiographs may reveal coronary artery mineralization in dogs (Figure 9.191). It can be difficult to distinguish coronary mineralization from aortic mineralization radiographically without the use of angiography. Coronary angiography is the diagnostic technique of choice but is seldom used in animals.

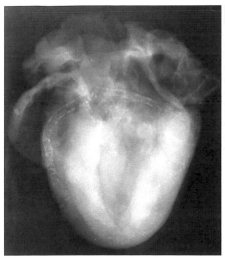

9.191 Post-mortem radiograph of a dog's heart with mineralized coronary arteries due to atherosclerosis. The dog also had hypothyroidism, which has been strongly linked with this condition.

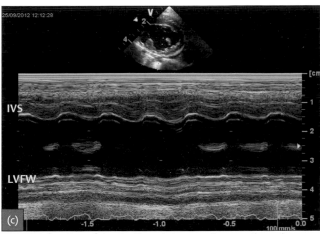

9.192 (continued) A cat with end-stage cardiomyopathy and biventricular CHF including small pericardial and pleural effusions. There is a very thin segment affecting most of the heart's length to the apex, excluding the base of the LVFW. This was believed to represent a region of myocardial infarction with replacement fibrosis. (c) Left ventricular M-mode, which shows the LVFW is thin and relatively akinetic.

With echocardiography, ischaemic myocardium can show thinning, regional hypokinesis or akinesis and reduced or absent contractility. Focal wall thinning can be seen in cats with severe myocardial disease, and this has been pathologically shown to be a consequence of myocardial infarction and replacement fibrosis (Figure 9.192). A focal hyperechoic region within the myocardium may represent a more acute myocardial infarct (Figure 9.193).

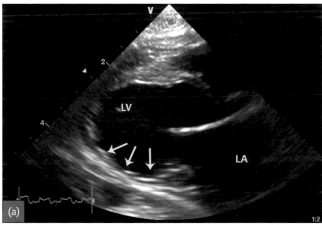

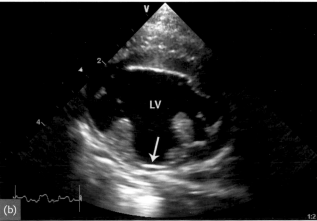

9.192 A cat with end-stage cardiomyopathy and biventricular CHF including small pericardial and pleural effusions. There is a very thin segment affecting most of the heart's length to the apex, excluding the base of the LVFW. This was believed to represent a region of myocardial infarction with replacement fibrosis. (a) Right parasternal four-chamber view, showing the abrupt thinning of the LVFW (arrowed) after the basal segment. (b) Right parasternal short-axis view, showing focal thinning of the LVFW between the papillary muscles (arrowed). (continues)

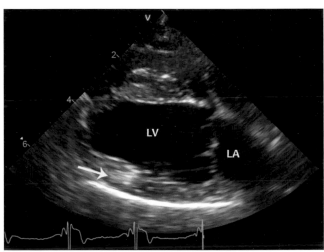

9.193 Right parasternal long-axis four-chamber view of an 11-year-old neutered male Shih Tzu with thromboembolic stroke (confirmed by MRI). There is a focal hyperechoic region within the LVFW (arrowed), possibly representing a myocardial infarct. Cardiac Troponin I level was very high. The dog also had stage B1 MMVD.

Acknowledgement

The author and editors gratefully acknowledge the contributions of the following authors to this chapter in the first edition of this manual: Peter Chapman, Kerstin Hansson, Victoria Johnson, Nola Lester, Wilfried Maï and Federica Morandi.

References and further reading

Arbustini E, Narula N, Dec GW et al. (2013) The MOGE(S) classification for a phenotype-genotype nomenclature of cardiomyopathy: endorsed by the World Heart Federation. *Journal of the American College of Cardiology* **62**, 2046–2072

Bavegems V, Van Caelenberg A, Duchateau L et al. (2005) Vertebral heart size ranges specific for whippets. *Veterinary Radiology & Ultrasound* **46**, 400–403

Beier P, Reese S, Holler PJ et al. (2015) The role of hypothyroidism in the etiology and progression of dilated cardiomyopathy in Doberman Pinschers. *Journal of Veterinary Internal Medicine* **29**, 141–149

Belanger MC, Cote E and Beauchamp G (2014) Association between aortoseptal angle in Golden Retriever puppies and subaortic stenosis in adulthood. *Journal of Veterinary Internal Medicine* **28**, 1498–1503

Biasato I, Zanatta R, Maniscalco L et al. (2018) Left subclavian artery dissection associated with connective tissue abnormalities resembling Marfan-like syndrome in an English Bulldog. Journal of Veterinary Cardiology 20, 136–142

Birkegard AC, Reimann MJ, Martinussen T et al. (2016) Breeding restrictions decrease the prevalence of myxomatous mitral valve disease in Cavalier King Charles Spaniels over an 8- to 10-year period. Journal of Veterinary Internal Medicine 30, 63–68

Boswood A, Häggström J, Gordon SG et al.. (2016) Effect of pimobendan in dogs with preclinical myxomatous mitral valve disease and cardiomegaly: The EPIC study-a randomized clinical trial. Journal of Veterinary Internal Medicine 30, 1765–1779

Brown CS, Johnson LR, Visser LC, Chan JC and Pollard RE (2020) Comparison of fluoroscopic cardiovascular measurements from healthy dogs obtained at end-diastole and end-systole. Journal of Veterinary Cardiology 29, 1–10

Buchanan JW (1990) Pulmonic stenosis caused by single coronary artery in dogs: four cases (1965–1984). Journal of the American Veterinary Medical Association 196, 115–120

Buchanan JW (2001) Patent ductus arteriosus morphology, pathogenesis, types and treatment. Journal of Veterinary Cardiology 3, 7–16

Buchanan JW and Bücheler J (1995) Vertebral scale system to measure canine heart size in radiographs. Journal of the American Veterinary Medical Association 206, 194–199

Burti S, Longhin Osti V, Zotti A and Banzato T (2020) Use of deep learning to detect cardiomegaly on thoracic radiographs in dogs. Veterinary Journal 262, 105505

Bussadori C, Amberger C, Le Bobinnec G and Lombard CW (2000) Guidelines for the echocardiographic studies of suspected subaortic and pulmonic stenosis. Journal of Veterinary Cardiology 2, 15–22

Chetboul V, Charles V, Nicolle A et al. (2006) Retrospective study of 156 atrial septal defects in dogs and cats (2001–2005). Journal of Veterinary Medicine Series A 53, 179–184

Chetboul V, Damoiseaux C, Poissonnier C et al. (2018) Specific features and survival of French Bulldogs with congenital pulmonic stenosis: a prospective cohort study of 66 cases. Journal of Veterinary Cardiology 20, 405–414

Chetboul V, Passavin P, Trehiou-Sechi E et al. (2019) Clinical, epidemiological and echocardiographic features and prognostic factors in cats with restrictive cardiomyopathy: A retrospective study of 92 cases (2001–2015). Journal of Veterinary Internal Medicine 33, 1222–1231

Chetboul V, Poissonnier C, Bomassi E et al. (2020) Epidemiological, clinical, and echocardiographic features, and outcome of dogs with Ebstein's anomaly: 32 cases (2002–2016). Journal of Veterinary Cardiology 29, 11–21

Coia ME, Hammond G, Chan D et al. (2017) Retrospective evaluation of thoracic computed tomography findings in dogs naturally infected by Angiostrongylus vasorum. Veterinary Radiology & Ultrasound 58, 524–534

Cornell CC, Kittleson MD, Della Torre P et al. (2004) Allometric scaling of M-mode cardiac measurements in normal adult dogs. Journal of Veterinary Internal Medicine 18, 311–321

Cuddy LC, Maisenbacher HW, Vigani A and Berry C (2013) Computed tomography angiography of coarctation of the aorta in a dog. Journal of Veterinary Cardiology 15, 277–281

Dennis R, Kirberger RM, Wrigley RH and Barr F (2001) Handbook of Small Animal Radiological Differential Diagnosis. WB Saunders, Philadelphia

Dennler M, Makara M, Kranjc A et al. (2011) Thoracic computed tomography findings in dogs experimentally infected with Angiostrongylus vasorum. Veterinary Radiology & Ultrasound 52, 289–294

Dukes-McEwan J, Borgarelli M, Tidholm A, Vollmar AC and Häggström J (2003) ESVC taskforce for canine dilated cardiomyopathy proposed guidelines for the diagnosis of canine idiopathic dilated cardiomyopathy. Journal of Veterinary Cardiology 5, 7–19

Esser LC, Borkovec M, Bauer A, Häggström J and Wess G (2020) Left ventricular M-mode prediction intervals in 7651 dogs: Population-wide and selected breed-specific values. Journal of Veterinary Internal Medicine 34, 2242–2252

Fox PR (2004) Endomyocardial fibrosis and restrictive cardiomyopathy: pathologic and clinical features. Journal of Veterinary Cardiology 6, 25–31

Fox PR, Basso C, Thiene G and Maron BJ (2014) Spontaneously occurring restrictive nonhypertrophied cardiomyopathy in domestic cats: a new animal model of human disease. Cardiovascular Pathology 23, 28–34

Fox PR, Maron BJ, Basso C, Liu SK and Thiene G (2000) Spontaneously occurring arrhythmogenic right ventricular cardiomyopathy in the domestic cat: A new animal model similar to the human disease. Circulation 102, 1863–1870

Garrity S, Lee-Fowler T and Reinero C (2019) Feline asthma and heartworm disease: Clinical features, diagnostics and therapeutics. Journal of Feline Medicine and Surgery 21, 825–834

Häggström J, Andersson AO, Falk T et al. (2016) Effect of body weight on echocardiographic measurements in 19,866 pure-bred cats with or without heart disease. Journal of Veterinary Internal Medicine 30, 1601–1611

Holler PJ and Wess G (2014) Sphericity index and E-point-to-septal-separation (EPSS) to diagnose dilated cardiomyopathy in Doberman Pinschers. Journal of Veterinary Internal Medicine 28, 123–129

Jepsen-Grant K, Pollard RE and Johnson LR (2013) Vertebral heart scores in eight dog breeds. Veterinary Radiology & Ultrasound 54, 3–8

Keene BW, Atkins CE, Bonagura JD et al. (2019) ACVIM consensus guidelines for the diagnosis and treatment of myxomatous mitral valve disease in dogs. Journal of Veterinary Internal Medicine 33, 1127–1140

Kimura Y, Fukushima R, Hirakawa A, Kobayashi M and Machida N (2016) Epidemiological and clinical features of the endomyocardial form of restrictive cardiomyopathy in cats: a review of 41 cases. Journal of Veterinary Medical Science 78, 781–784

Kraetschmer S, Ludwig K, Meneses F, Nolte I and Simon D (2008) Vertebral heart scale in the beagle dog. Journal of Small Animal Practice 49, 240–243

Laborda-Vidal P, Pedro B, Baker M et al. (2016) Use of ECG-gated computed tomography, echocardiography and selective angiography in five dogs with pulmonic stenosis and one dog with pulmonic stenosis and aberrant coronary arteries. Journal of Veterinary Cardiology 18, 418–426

Lamb CR (2000) Ability to visualise the cardiac silhouette in animals with pleural fluid: the pericardial fat stripe. Veterinary Radiology & Ultrasound 41, 519–520

Lamb CR, Wikeley H, Boswood A and Pfeiffer DU (2001) Use of breed-specific ranges for the vertebral heart scale as an aid to the radiographic diagnosis of cardiac disease in dogs. Veterinary Record 148, 707–711

Lenz JA, Bach JF, Bell CM and Stepien RL (2015) Aortic tear and dissection related to connective tissues abnormalities resembling Marfan syndrome in a Great Dane. Journal of Veterinary Cardiology 17, 134–141

Loureiro J, Burrow R and Dukes-McEwan J (2009) Canine intrapericardial cyst – complicated surgical correction of an unusual cause of right heart failure. Journal of Small Animal Practice 50, 492–497

Luciani MG, Withoeft JA, Pissetti HMC et al. (2019) Vertebral heart size in healthy Australian cattle dog. Anatomia Histologia Embryologia 48, 264–267

Luis Fuentes V, Abbott J, Chetboul V et al. (2020) ACVIM consensus statement guidelines for the classification, diagnosis, and management of cardiomyopathies in cats. Journal of Veterinary Internal Medicine 34, 1062–1077

Malcolm EL, Visser LC, Phillips KL and Johnson LR (2018) Diagnostic value of vertebral left atrial size as determined from thoracic radiographs for assessment of left atrial size in dogs with myxomatous mitral valve disease. Journal of the American Veterinary Medical Association 253, 1038–1045

Marin LM, Brown J, McBrien C et al. (2007) Vertebral heart size in retired racing Greyhounds. Veterinary Radiology & Ultrasound 48, 332–334

McKenna WJ, Maron BJ and Thiene G (2017) Classification, epidemiology, and global burden of cardiomyopathies. Circulation Research 121, 722–730

Minors SL, O'Grady MR, Williams RM and O'Sullivan ML (2006) Clinical and echocardiographic features of primary infundibular stenosis with intact ventricular septum in dogs. Journal of Veterinary Internal Medicine 20, 1344–1350

Novo Matos J, Malbon A, Dennler M and Glaus T (2016) Intrapulmonary arteriovenous anastomoses in dogs with severe Angiostrongylus vasorum infection: clinical, radiographic, and echocardiographic evaluation. Journal of Veterinary Cardiology 18, 110–124

Novo Matos J, Pereira N, Glaus T et al. (2018) Transient myocardial thickening in cats associated with heart failure. Journal of Veterinary Internal Medicine 32, 48–56

Oliveira P, Domenech O, Silva J et al. (2011) Retrospective review of congenital heart disease in 976 dogs. Journal of Veterinary Internal Medicine 25, 477–483

Puccinelli C, Citi S, Vezzosi T, Garibaldi S and Tognetti R (2021) A radiographic study of breed-specific vertebral heart score and vertebral left atrial size in Chihuahuas. Veterinary Radiology & Ultrasound 62, 20–26

Reinero C, Visser LC, Kellihan HB et al. (2020) ACVIM consensus statement guidelines for the diagnosis, classification, treatment, and monitoring of pulmonary hypertension in dogs. Journal of Veterinary Internal Medicine 34, 549–573

Schober KE, Fox PR, Abbott J et al. (2022) Retrospective evaluation of hypertrophic cardiomyopathy in 68 dogs. Journal of Veterinary Internal Medicine 36, 865–876

Schober KE, Hart TM, Stern JA et al. (2010) Detection of congestive heart failure in dogs by Doppler echocardiography. Journal of Veterinary Internal Medicine 24, 1358–1368

Schrope DP (2015) Prevalence of congenital heart disease in 76,301 mixed-breed dogs and 57,025 mixed-breed cats. Journal of Veterinary Cardiology 17, 192–202

Simpson KE, Gunn-Moore DA, Shaw DJ et al. (2009) Pulsed-wave Doppler tissue imaging velocities in normal geriatric cats and geriatric cats with primary or systemic diseases linked to specific cardiomyopathies in humans, and the influence of age and heart rate upon these velocities. Journal of Feline Medicine and Surgery 11, 293–304

Strohm LE, Visser LC, Chapel EH, Drost WT and Bonagura JD (2018) Two-dimensional, long-axis echocardiographic ratios for assessment of left atrial and ventricular size in dogs. Journal of Veterinary Cardiology 20, 330–342

Summerfield NJ, Boswood A, O'Grady MR et al. (2012) Efficacy of pimobendan in the prevention of congestive heart failure or sudden death in Doberman Pinschers with preclinical dilated cardiomyopathy (the PROTECT Study). Journal of Veterinary Internal Medicine 26, 1337–1349

Suter PF (1984) Thoracic Radiography. A Text Atlas of Thoracic Diseases of the Dog and Cat. Peter F. Suter, Wettswill

Taylor CJ, Simon BT, Stanley BJ, Lai GP and Mankin KMT (2020) Norwich terriers possess a greater vertebral heart scale than the canine reference value. Veterinary Radiology & Ultrasound 61, 10–15

Vezzosi T, Puccinelli C, Tognetti R, Pelligra T and Citi S (2020) Radiographic vertebral left atrial size: A reference interval study in healthy adult dogs. Veterinary Radiology & Ultrasound 61, 507–511

Wess G, Domenech O, Dukes-McEwan J, Häggström J and Gordon S (2017) European Society of Veterinary Cardiology screening guidelines for dilated cardiomyopathy in Doberman Pinschers. Journal of Veterinary Cardiology 19, 405–415

Chapter 10

The mediastinum

Elizabeth Baines and Karine Gendron

In general terms, a mediastinum is a membranous partition between two parts of an organ or two body cavities. Specifically, the thoracic mediastinum lies within the thoracic cavity, roughly conforms to the median plane of the body, and divides the thorax into left and right halves. It is a connective tissue septum that lies between the left and right pleural cavities and forms a space for the passage of viscera, nerves and blood vessels. It lies between the vertebral column and sternum, between the thoracic inlet and diaphragm, and is bounded laterally by the mediastinal pleurae (a component of the parietal pleura). It encloses all midline thoracic structures (i.e. all intrathoracic structures except the lungs and pleural cavities) and is continuous with the connective tissue of the neck (cervical fascia) via the thoracic inlet and the retroperitoneal space via the aortic hiatus. Anatomists split the mediastinum into five sections relative to the pericardium, although no physical barrier exists between the different parts (Figure 10.1).

- The cranial mediastinum lies cranial to the pericardium, attaches to the longus colli muscles dorsally, and contains the trachea, oesophagus, thymus, cranial sternal and cranial mediastinal lymph nodes, and many blood vessels and nerves (Figure 10.2).

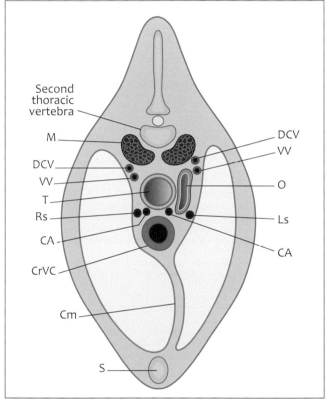

10.2 Transverse aspect of the cranial mediastinum at the level of the second thoracic vertebra. The cranial mediastinum is between the longus colli muscles (M) and sternum (S), between the left and right mediastinal pleurae, and is wider dorsally to accommodate the thoracic viscera. All thoracic viscera except the lungs are in the mediastinum. CA = right and left common carotid arteries; Cm = cranioventral mediastinal reflection; CrVC = cranial vena cava; DCV = right and left deep cranial vertebral veins; Ls = left subclavian artery; O = oesophagus; Rs = right subclavian artery; T = trachea; VV = right and left vertebral veins.
(Redrawn after Suter (1984))

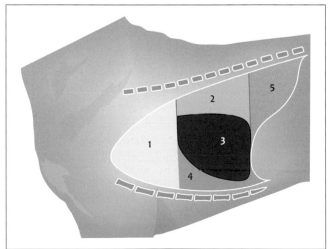

10.1 Lateral aspect of the median plane. The mediastinum divides the thoracic cavity into left and right sides and is partitioned relative to the pericardium. 1 = cranial mediastinum; 2 = dorsal mediastinum; 3 = middle mediastinum; 4 = ventral mediastinum; 5 = caudal mediastinum.

- The dorsal mediastinum is between the vertebrae and pericardium and contains the aorta and its initial branches, azygos vein, thoracic duct, tracheal bifurcation, oesophagus and tracheobronchial lymph nodes. At the tracheal bifurcation, the mediastinal pleura reflects at the lungs and transitions to the pulmonary pleura.
- The middle mediastinum contains the heart and pericardium, which is fused to the mediastinal pleura.

The vagus and phrenic nerves run on the left and right sides of the pericardium and are deep to the mediastinal pleurae.

- The ventral mediastinum is between the sternum and pericardium and contains the thymus cranially and the phrenicopericardial ligament caudally.
- The caudal mediastinum (see Figure 10.19) lies caudal to the pericardium and may be fenestrated in carnivores to allow communication between the two pleural cavities. Dorsally, it contains the descending aorta, thoracic duct and azygos vein: in cats, it is ventral to the cranial aspect of the psoas muscles. Slightly more ventrally, it contains the oesophagus and vagus nerves. Ventrally, it is deflected to the left, contains the left phrenic nerve, and attaches to the diaphragm. A separate fold of the right caudal mediastinal pleura, the plica venae cavae, extends from the pericardium to the diaphragm and contains the caudal vena cava and right phrenic nerve.

Imaging anatomy

The five anatomical divisions may be differentiated on lateral thoracic radiographs and during thoracic computed tomography (CT). However, the dorsal, middle and ventral mediastina summate with each other on dorsoventral (DV) and ventrodorsal (VD) thoracic radiographs. Therefore, it is also customary to divide the mediastinum into cranial, middle and caudal thirds relative to the cardiac silhouette (Figures 10.3).

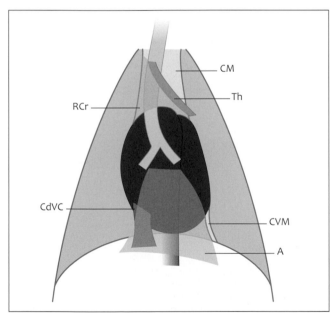

10.3 Ventral aspect of the thorax. On DV and VD views, the dorsal, middle and ventral mediastina summate with each other and therefore the mediastinum is simply divided into thirds relative to the heart. The cranial mediastinum (CM) is cranial to the heart, caudal to the thoracic inlet, and between the left and right cranial lung lobes. The ventral portion of the right cranial lobe (Rcr) crosses to the left, outlining the right side of the cranioventral mediastinal reflection, which is the position of the vestigial thymus (Th). The middle mediastinum is at the level of the heart. The caudal mediastinum is caudal to the heart, cranial to the diaphragm, and the ventral portion is displaced to the left by the accessory lobe of the right lung (A) and called the caudoventral mediastinal reflection (CVM). The accessory lobe is in the mediastinal recess, which lies between the CVM and the plica venae cavae (not depicted). The plica venae cavae surrounds and is ventral to the caudal vena cava (CdVC).
(Redrawn after Suter (1984))

In general, the mediastinum is wider (left-to-right) at the level of the heart and dorsally to accommodate most of the mediastinal structures (e.g. aorta, oesophagus). The ventral portions of the cranial and caudal mediastina have substantially reduced connective tissue and form sheet-like membranes between the right and left lungs. During imaging, these structures appear as thin linear soft tissue opacities when viewed tangentially or in cross-section and represent only four layers of pleurae (pulmonary and visceral pleurae of the right and left lungs) contrasted by gas in the two lungs. These structures are commonly referred to as 'mediastinal reflections' and can be differentiated from the wider dorsal portion of the mediastinum (Figure 10.4).

- The cranial mediastinal reflection (cranioventral mediastinal reflection) crosses the midline and lies obliquely between the right and left cranial lung lobes (Figure 10.5 and 10.6).
- The caudal mediastinal reflection (caudoventral mediastinal reflection) lies between the left caudal and the accessory lung lobes (Figure 10.7).
- The plica venae cavae is a similar appearing structure that is derived from the right mediastinal pleura and lies between the caudal and accessory lobes of the right lung. It is also ventrally located, not extending dorsal to the caudal vena cava except to surround it.

In some normal animals, these three mediastinal structures can appear thick due to physiological fat deposition. The caudal mediastinal reflection and plica venae cavae are lateral to the median plane and the space between them, the mediastinal recess, is an evagination of the right pleural cavity that crosses the median plane and houses the accessory lung lobe (see Figures 10.3 and 10.19).

Most mediastinal structures are covered by adventitia and not by serosa, except for a small portion of the oesophagus that is adjacent to the mediastinal serous cavity (a minor serous cavity discussed below). The major serous cavities of the thorax are the pleural and pericardial cavities. Serous cavities are hollow potential spaces. In contrast, the mediastinum is an actual space that is filled with structures interconnected by connective tissue and is continuous with the connective tissue of the neck and retroperitoneal space. Adventitia is a type of loose fibrous connective tissue, containing collagen and elastin fibres, that forms the outer covering of certain structures (tunica adventitia). This tissue also occupies the space between these structures, joining them, and provides a place for fat deposition. Serosa is another type of loose connective tissue within the thoracic cavity that also forms the outer covering of some structures (tunica serosa) but is structurally and functionally different (see Chapters 7 and 11).

During imaging, it is important to remember that the pathological spread of fluid, gas and inflammatory or neoplastic cells through the mediastinum is not typically free as would be observed in a serous cavity because the mediastinum is not a hollow potential space. Rather, the spread is more akin to that of disease through connective tissue elsewhere in the body (e.g. the spread of subcutaneous emphysema, ventral oedema or suppurative fasciitis/cellulitis through the body wall). Loose connective tissue, however, allows disease to spread and tears more easily than dense connective tissue.

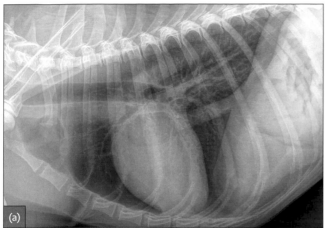

(a)

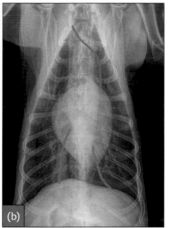

(b)

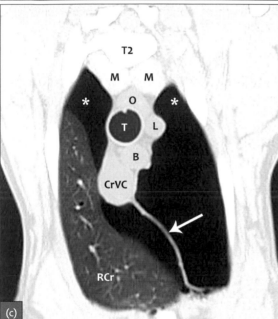

(c)

10.4 (a) Lateral and (b) VD thoracic radiographs of an adult dog showing the location of the mediastinum (green). All thoracic structures except the thoracic boundaries, lungs and pleural cavities are within the mediastinum and adhered by connective tissue. On lateral views, the mediastinum summates with all structures within the thoracic cavity. On DV and VD views, the mediastinum summates with the midline structures, the caudal vena cava, and portions of the lung. The mediastinum is widest where it surrounds the heart and dorsally to accommodate structures like the oesophagus, trachea and aorta. The amount of connective tissue in the ventral portion of the cranial and caudal mediastina is substantially reduced to two apposing serous membranes. However, mediastinal fat accumulation may occur in overweight and obese animals and some dog breeds (e.g. Bulldogs). The thinner ventral portions of the mediastinum and the plica venae cavae are occasionally seen on DV and VD radiographs (darker green lines). The ventral part of the cranial mediastinum contains lymph nodes and internal thoracic blood vessels, and the thymus in juvenile animals. (c) Transverse CT image (lung window) of an adult dog with bilateral pneumothorax. The image was obtained at the level of the second thoracic vertebra (T2). Both pleural cavities are enlarged and filled with gas (∗). The gas contrasts with the normal cranial mediastinum (green), which makes the shape of the mediastinum more obvious. The ventral portion of the cranial mediastinum (arrowed) is narrow and is deflected towards the left. The dorsal portion is roughly in the median plane and wider to accommodate the oesophagus (O), trachea (T), left subclavian artery (L), brachiocephalic trunk (B) and cranial vena cava (CrVC). These mediastinal structures are bound together by loose connective tissue (adventitia), which also joins to the longus colli muscles (M). In the image, the connective tissue is the fat attenuating substance that connects the viscera, blood vessels and muscles. Unlike normal pleural cavities, which are potential spaces, the mediastinum is an actual space that is filled with tissues and organs that are mostly tubular. RCr = right cranial lung lobe.

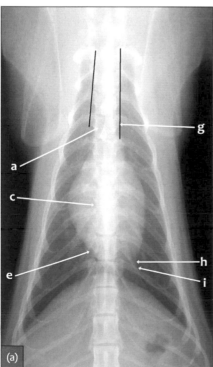

(a)

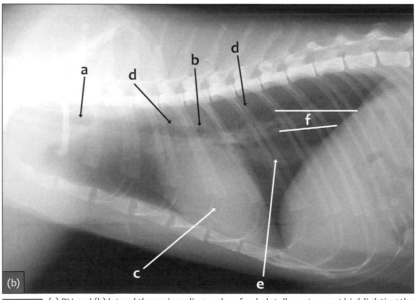

(b)

10.5 (a) DV and (b) lateral thoracic radiographs of a skeletally mature cat highlighting the structures normally visible in the mediastinum. On DV and VD views, the cranial mediastinum of cats is not wider than the summated vertebral column. a = trachea; b = end-on tracheal bifurcation approximating the location of the carina; c = cardiac silhouette; d = aorta; e = caudal vena cava; f = position of oesophagus; g = width of cranial mediastinum; h = cardiac silhouette apex; i = caudoventral mediastinal reflection.

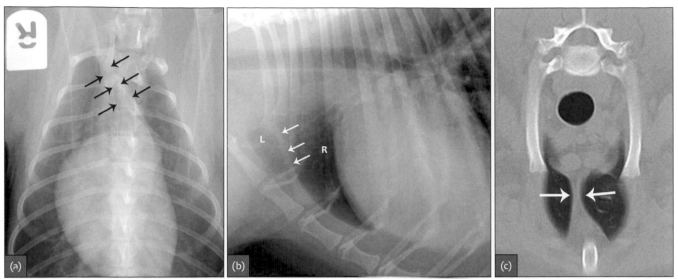

10.6 (a) DV thoracic radiograph of a mature dog showing the ventral part of the cranial mediastinum (arrowed). The dog is slightly rotated and has accumulated fat, which accentuates this structure. (b) Close-up of a right lateral thoracic radiograph of a 2-year-old dog showing a portion of the cranioventral mediastinum (arrowed) as a thin line of soft tissue opacity between the left (L) and right (R) cranial lung lobes. (c) Transverse CT image obtained at the level of the first rib (window width 2000 HU, window level –500 HU). The cranioventral mediastinum is clearly seen between the left and right cranial lung lobes (arrowed).

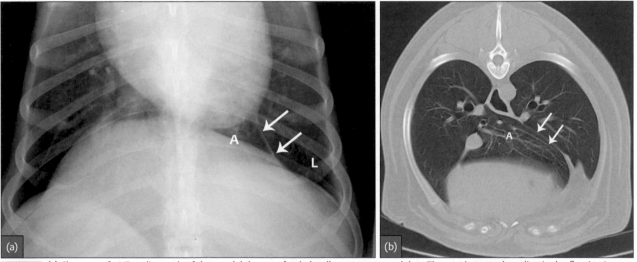

10.7 (a) Close-up of a VD radiograph of the caudal thorax of a skeletally mature normal dog. The caudoventral mediastinal reflection is seen as a narrow band of soft tissue opacity (arrowed) separating the accessory (A) and left caudal (L) lung lobes. (b) Transverse thoracic CT image obtained at the level of the accessory lobe (window width 2000 HU, window level –500 HU). The caudoventral mediastinal reflection is clearly delineated (arrowed). The extension of the accessory lobe (A) across the midline and dorsal to the caudal vena cava can be seen.

Radiographic observation of structures

As the mediastinum is a difficult area to examine clinically, diagnostic imaging plays an important role in the detection and investigation of mediastinal abnormalities. Survey thoracic radiography is the imaging modality of choice for initial study of the mediastinum, which should be assessed on at least two orthogonal views. The lateral view allows examination of many of the normally visible structures but does not allow assessment of width or mediastinal shift (see 'Interpretative principles', below). The DV or VD view allows full assessment of the position of the mediastinum and is more sensitive for diagnosing mediastinal fluid and masses. The VD view allows a more complete assessment of the caudal mediastinum than the DV view, as the heart moves slightly away from the diaphragm in dorsal recumbency. Inflation of the cranial lung lobes is also typically better when the animal is in dorsal recumbency.

Optimal radiographic quality is vital to examine the mediastinum. On lateral radiographs, particular care must be taken to ensure that the thoracic limbs are extended cranially to avoid summation of the triceps muscles with the cranioventral thorax, which would mimic a cranioventral mediastinal mass. On DV and VD radiographs, rotation can lead to a false detection of mediastinal shift and nearly all mediastinal structures summate with the back and sternum making it difficult to distinguish most structures. In addition, summation of the thoracic girdle with the cranial thorax may be problematic. This summation may be eliminated by obtaining a VD view with the animal's thoracic limbs lying lateral to the thoracic wall and the X-ray beam centred slightly more cranially than a standard VD view. This procedure is well tolerated and provides superior visibility of the cranial mediastinal margins. This view is commonly called the 'humanoid VD' view because the position of the animal is similar to the position of a human during posteroanterior chest radiography (Figure 10.8).

The width of the normal cranial mediastinum

- The dorsal part of the cranial mediastinum is wider than the ventral part to accommodate structures like the trachea, oesophagus and cranial vena cava. The ventral part forms the cranial mediastinal reflection.
- In dogs, the maximum width of the cranial mediastinum on a DV or VD radiograph (especially the ventral part) should be less than twice the width of the vertebral column at this level.
- In cats, the width of the cranial mediastinum on a DV or VD radiograph should not be greater than the width of the thoracic vertebral column.

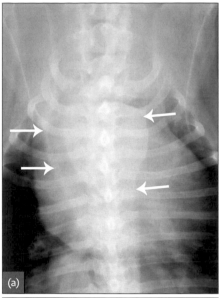

(a)

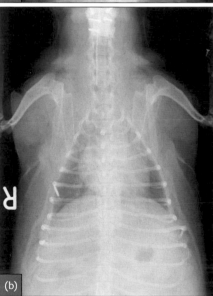

(b)

10.9 (a) DV thoracic radiograph of an 8-year-old Bulldog bitch. The width of the cranial mediastinum (arrowed) and location of the trachea are within normal limits for this breed. (b) DV thoracic radiograph of a 7-year-old male Chihuahua with tracheal collapse. The cranial mediastinum is wide, which could be due to a mass lesion. The presence of large subcutaneous fat deposits, however, supports a conclusion of physiological mediastinal fat deposition.

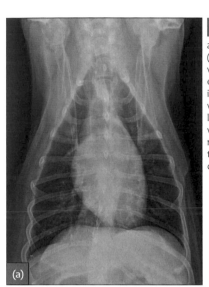

(a)

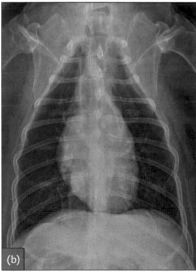

(b)

10.8 VD thoracic radiographs of an adult dog positioned (a) in the usual position with thoracic limbs extended cranially and (b) in a 'humanoid' position with the thoracic limbs lying lateral to the thoracic wall. The latter position reduces summation of the thoracic girdle with the cranial thorax.

The width of the normal mediastinum is greater dorsally *versus* ventrally and may vary with amount of fat, according to body condition and breed conformation. On DV and VD thoracic radiographs of obese or brachycephalic breeds, the mediastinum may be wider due to larger fat deposits, especially in the cranial mediastinum. This normal condition can be difficult to differentiate from a cranial mediastinal mass (Figure 10.9a), but consideration of the animal's body condition and breed may aid interpretation (Figure 10.9b). On lateral radiographs, excess fat will not efface cardiac margins nor reduce contrast as occurs with pleural fluid. Ultrasonography often assists in the differentiation.

Some mediastinal structures are visible on all or only some radiographic views (Figure 10.10). Other mediastinal structures, however, are not normally visible due to insufficient differential absorption of the X-ray beam. This may be because the structures are too small to have a perceptible effect or may be a result of the low-contrast radiographic technique for the thorax not allowing mediastinal fat to sufficiently contrast with other structures. Insufficient differential absorption of the X-ray beam produces border effacement (border obliteration) and the formation of radiographic silhouettes that do not necessarily represent only one structure.

Except for the trachea and oesophagus, which may contain intraluminal gas, mediastinal structures typically have a soft tissue opacity and form a radiographic silhouette with each other. Even large mediastinal fat deposits are usually insufficient to provide enough contrast to outline structures. More mediastinal structures are

Normally visible
• Trachea, including its bifurcation and the origins of the bronchi • Heart within the pericardium • Aorta • Caudal vena cava (usually seen better on the VD than the DV view due to shifting of the heart when the animal is in dorsal recumbency) • Thymus in young animals • Oesophagus (sometimes but not always seen; visible particularly on left lateral views and if it contains air or fluid; rarely seen on DV or VD view in a normal animal)
Not normally visible
• Cranial vena cava (except for the ventral border in the cranial mediastinum on a lateral view) • Brachiocephalic trunk • Left subclavian artery • Azygos vein • Pulmonic trunk • Vagus nerve • Recurrent laryngeal and phrenic nerves • Thoracic duct • Tracheobronchial, mediastinal and cranial sternal lymph nodes

10.10 Mediastinal structures normally visible and not normally visible on survey radiographs.

discernible on lateral views than DV and VD views because the structures are spread farther apart and sufficiently contrasted by mediastinal fat or gas in the lungs, but many still combine to form a silhouette.

On lateral radiographs, the mediastinum can be roughly divided dorsally and ventrally by a dorsal plane through the carina, which is the dorsoventral ridge of soft tissue at the tracheal bifurcation (see Figure 10.69). Most mediastinal structures lie dorsal to this line, the heart being the most obvious exception. In normal animals, the tracheobronchial lymph nodes and the great vessels form a silhouette with the heart base and the azygos vein forms a silhouette with the aorta and the ventral longitudinal ligaments of the vertebrae.

The most ventral margin of the mediastinum is contiguous with the dorsal surface of the sternum. Radiographically, there is often a band of soft tissue opacity dorsal to the sternum, which is a composite shadow (silhouette) of the transverse thoracic muscle, internal thoracic artery and vein, cranial sternal lymph nodes and other structures. There is often a large 'retrosternal' fat deposit in the ventral mediastinum at the level of and extending caudally to the xiphoid process. This often contrasts with the cardiac apex due to differences in opacity. The ventrally located structures within the mediastinum should not be confused with pleural or mediastinal fluid.

Mediastinal reflections and folds

Ventral part of the cranial mediastinum:

- Cranial mediastinal reflection (see Figures 10.2, 10.3 and 10.5):
  - Obliquely oriented (right cranial to left caudal) sheet-like structure that crosses the midline and contains the internal thoracic arteries, veins and lymphatic vessels
  - VD radiograph (dogs): thin curvilinear opacity between the left and right cranial lung lobes
  - Lateral radiograph (dogs): curvilinear soft tissue opacity running caudoventrally from the level of the first rib to the sternum.

Ventral part of the caudal mediastinum (see Figure 10.19):

- Left of midline – caudal mediastinal reflection (see Figures 10.3 and 10.5):
  - Appears as a fine band of soft tissue opacity running between the cardiac apex and the left side of the diaphragm
  - Seen better on VD than DV radiographs but inconsistently visible
  - Not seen on lateral radiographs
  - Sometimes mistaken for the phrenicopericardial ligament (cardiophrenic ligament or sternopericardiac ligament), which is not radiographically visible
- Right of midline – plica venae cavae:
  - Envelops the caudal vena cava and attaches the pericardium to the right side of the diaphragm
  - Radiographically indistinguishable as an individual structure.

Lymph nodes

The thoracic lymph nodes can be divided into a parietal group that drains the body wall and a visceral group that drains the internal organs of the thoracic cavity. Each group comprises two lymph centres.

- The ventral thoracic lymph centre consists of the cranial sternal lymph nodes (previously known as sternal, retrosternal or presternal lymph nodes). These nodes are usually paired, although variation exists, and lie just dorsal to the second sternebra in dogs and slightly more caudal in cats (typically dorsal to the third sternebra).
  - The sternal lymph nodes receive afferent lymphatic vessels from parts of the thoracic boundaries, mammary glands, serous membranes and thymus. They also drain the peritoneal cavity via lymphatic vessels in the diaphragm and can therefore act as sentinels for peritoneal disease.
  - In contrast, much of the abdominal and pelvic viscera drain via the thoracic duct to the cranial vena cava. The thoracic duct also receives drainage from the limbs.
- The dorsal thoracic lymph centre includes the aortic thoracic lymph nodes, which primarily drain the dorsolateral body wall, diaphragm and mediastinum. They are frequently absent and rarely seen during imaging in dogs and cats.
- The mediastinal lymph centre consists of the cranial mediastinal lymph nodes, which vary in number. These nodes lie in the cranial mediastinum adjacent to the cranial vena cava, brachiocephalic trunk, left subclavian artery and trachea.
  - The cranial mediastinal lymph nodes receive lymph from many parts of the body, including the neck and cranial parts of the thoracic boundaries. Within the thoracic cavity, they drain the mediastinal structures, including the other thoracic lymph nodes.
- The bronchial lymph centre comprises pulmonary and tracheobronchial lymph nodes. The pulmonary nodes are often absent. There are three tracheobronchial lymph nodes: middle, right and left.
  - The middle, or bifurcational, tracheobronchial lymph node is the largest of the group and forms a V shape lying between the principal bronchi at the

heart base, caudodorsal to the tracheal bifurcation. The apex of the middle tracheobronchial lymph node fits neatly into the angle formed by the tracheal bifurcation (Figure 10.11a).

- The right and left tracheobronchial lymph nodes lie lateral to their respective bronchus. They sit immediately cranial to the tracheal bifurcation, the right just ventral to, and the left just dorsal to the trachea (Figure 10.11a).
- The tracheobronchial lymph nodes primarily drain the lungs and bronchi, but also the pulmonary lymph nodes (when present), the diaphragm and some mediastinal structures.

Lymph node mineralization may be seen as a sequel to fungal (see Figure 10.11b) or mycobacterial disease, or aspiration of barium suspension. Normal thoracic lymph nodes are not visible on radiographs, but some may be seen during cross-sectional imaging (e.g. thoracic CT). Specific radiographic features are seen when these lymph nodes are enlarged (Figures 10.12 to 10.15).

Juvenile mediastinum

The thymus may be visible due to its relatively large size in puppies and kittens. The thymus lies in the ventral part of the cranial mediastinum and the cranial part of the ventral mediastinum and might contact the left cranioventral aspect of the pericardium. In the cat, this is best seen on the lateral view as a crescent-shaped opacity paralleling the cranial border of the heart in the cranioventral thorax (Figure 10.16). In the dog it can be best seen on the DV view as a triangular opacity, extending from the midline towards the left side, the so-called thymic sail sign (Figure 10.17). It may occasionally be seen cranial to the cardiac silhouette on the lateral view.

The thymus (Figure 10.18) reaches its maximum size at 4 months old, and then progressively undergoes involution until it is no longer visible at about 1 year of age. Occasionally, a persistent thymic remnant may be seen in older animals. On DV and VD thoracic radiographs, this may appear as a linear to triangular soft tissue opacity in the position of the previous thymus.

Mediastinal serous cavity

The mediastinal serous cavity is a hollow potential space (like the pleural cavity) located in the caudal mediastinum ventral to the aorta, to the right of the oesophagus, from the heart base to the diaphragm (Figure 10.19). It derives embryologically from a portion of the omental bursa becoming trapped within the caudal mediastinum as the diaphragm develops. It is also known as the cavum mediastini serosum, infracardiac bursa, Sussdorf's space, and persistent right pneumoenteric recess. It is a potential space for herniation of abdominal organs and a rare site of inflammatory, neoplastic and traumatic diseases (Figure 10.20).

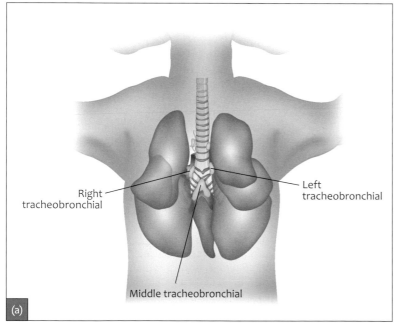

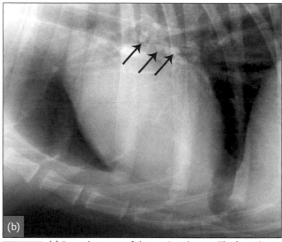

10.11 (a) Dorsal aspect of the canine thorax. The location of the tracheobronchial lymph nodes relative to the tracheal bifurcation is shown. (b) Lateral radiograph of an 8-year-old neutered Labrador Retriever bitch with chronic systemic coccidioidomycosis. Many small pulmonary, tracheobronchial and cranial mediastinal lymph nodes are faintly mineralized (some arrowed).

Lymph nodes	Radiographic features when enlarged
Tracheobronchial (see Figure 10.13)	All slightly increased in size Hazy increase in perihilar opacity There are other differentials for this appearance
Cranial sternal (see Figure 10.14)	Broad-based sessile soft tissue opacity dorsal to the second sternebra, creating an extrapleural sign
Cranial mediastinal (see Figure 10.15)	Wide cranial mediastinum on DV and VD views Difficult to perceive on lateral views

10.12 Radiographic features of enlarged mediastinal lymph nodes.

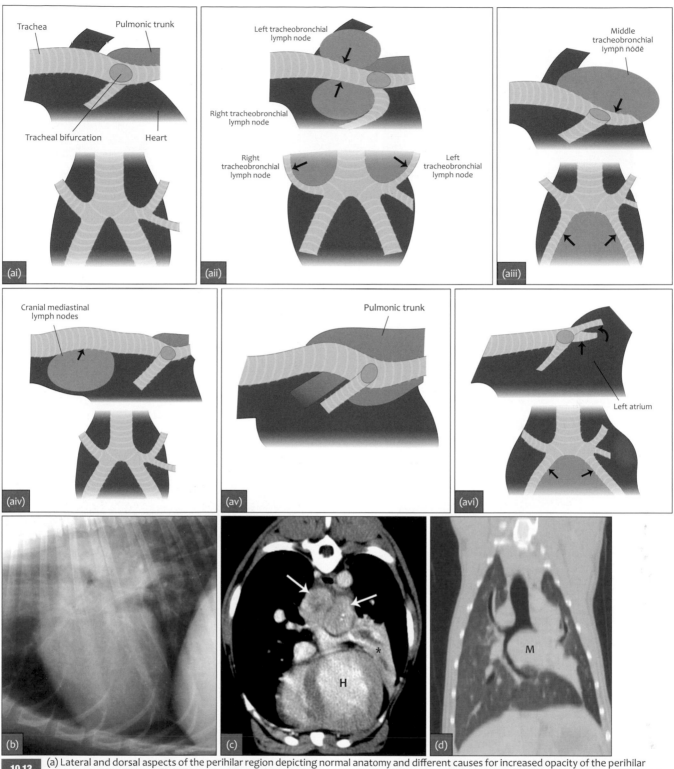

10.13 (a) Lateral and dorsal aspects of the perihilar region depicting normal anatomy and different causes for increased opacity of the perihilar region based on differences in location and mass effects. (ai) Normal perihilar structures. Note that the angle between the principal bronchi can vary with breed and centring of the X-ray beam. (aii) Left and right tracheobronchial lymph node enlargement. Both nodes can accentuate the ventral deflection of the trachea at the carina. The right sits just ventral to, and the left just dorsal to, the trachea. (aiii) Middle tracheobronchial lymph node enlargement. Note that the lymph node lies between the principal bronchi and, when enlarged, displaces the principal bronchi laterally and ventrally. (aiv) Cranial mediastinal lymph node enlargement. If these nodes are large enough, they can displace the trachea dorsally, cranial to the carina. Note that heart base tumours are often located in this region and can produce a similar effect. (av) Pulmonary artery enlargement. Enlarged pulmonary arteries (and sometimes veins) can be mistaken for enlarged lymph nodes. This is a diagram of enlargement of the pulmonic trunk (main pulmonary artery) in dirofilariasis. (avi) Left atrial enlargement. On DV and VD radiographs, both left atrial enlargement and middle tracheobronchial lymphadenomegaly cause lateral displacement of the principal bronchi. However, with lymphadenomegaly, there are usually no other concurrent signs of cardiomegaly. On lateral radiographs, the lymphadenomegaly displaces the bronchi ventrally, whereas left atrial enlargement displaces the carina and principal bronchi (especially the left) dorsally. (b) Close-up of a lateral thoracic radiograph of a 3-year-old male neutered crossbreed dog with enlarged right, left and middle tracheobronchial lymph nodes due to systemic fungal disease. Note the ventral depression of the trachea and principal bronchi. (c) Transverse thoracic CT image (soft tissue window). The enlarged middle tracheobronchial lymph node (arrowed) is dorsal to the heart (H). The adjacent left cranial lung lobe (caudal part) is consolidated (∗). (d) Dorsal thoracic CT reconstruction (lung window). The middle tracheobronchial lymph node (M) displaces the principal bronchi laterally. (continues)

(a, Redrawn after Suter (1984))

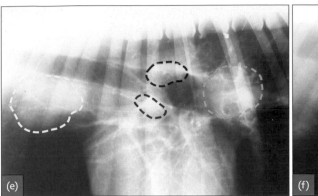

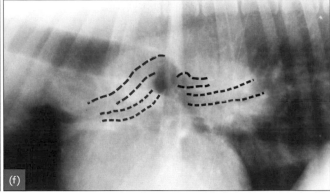

10.13 (continued) (e) Close-up of a lateral thoracic radiograph of a dog with multicentric lymphoma. The middle (light blue), right (red) and left (dark blue) tracheobronchial and cranial mediastinal (yellow) lymph nodes are moderately enlarged. (f) Close-up of a lateral thoracic radiograph of a 5-year-old Cocker Spaniel with multicentric lymphoma. The tracheobronchial lymph nodes are large, causing ventral displacement and separation of the cranial lobar bronchi (red) and caudal lobar bronchi (blue). Ventral displacement of the bronchi is an important feature that distinguishes increased opacity of the hilar region due to lymphadenomegaly from left atrial enlargement, which causes dorsal bronchial displacement.

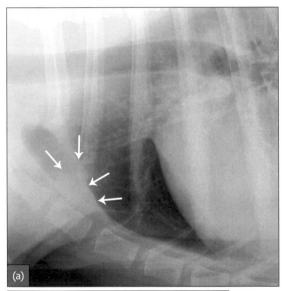

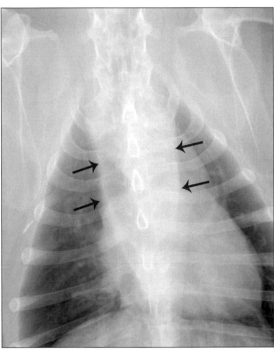

10.15 Close-up of a VD radiograph of the cranial thorax in an 8-year-old Border Collie with lymphadenomegaly of the mediastinal lymph nodes. The cranial mediastinum is wide and mildly convex (arrowed).

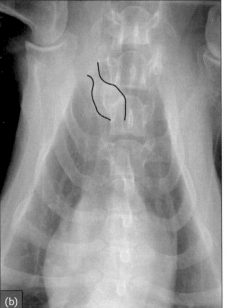

10.14 (a) Lateral and (b) VD thoracic radiographs of a 6-year-old Australian Cattle Dog with mild lymphadenomegaly of the cranial sternal lymph nodes (arrowed in (a), red lines in (b)) secondary to abdominal neoplasia.

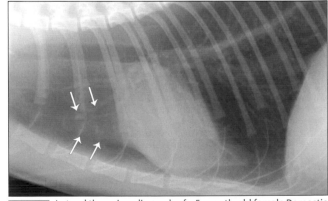

10.16 Lateral thoracic radiograph of a 5-month-old female Domestic Shorthaired cat. The thymus is seen as a faint triangular soft tissue opacity (arrowed) cranial to the heart. It was not visible on the DV view.

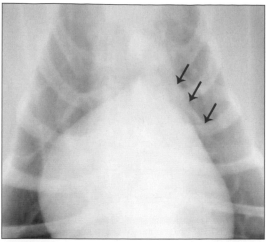

10.17 DV thoracic radiograph of a 1-year-old Boxer bitch, showing a small thymic sail sign (arrowed) just cranial to the heart and to the left of the midline.

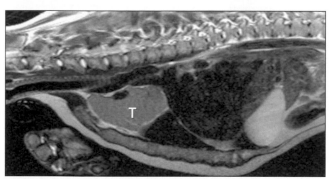

10.18 Sagittal T2-weighted MRI scan of the thorax of a 3-month-old Italian Spinone bitch. The thymus (T) is seen as a hyperintense solid soft tissue structure cranial to the heart.

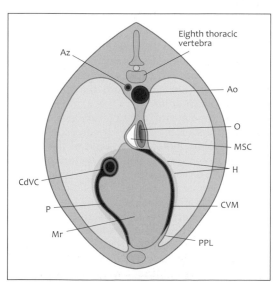

10.19 Transverse aspect of the caudal mediastinum at the level of the eighth thoracic vertebra. The caudal mediastinum is between the vertebral column and sternum, between the pericardium and diaphragm, and between the left and right pleural cavities. The caudal mediastinum is wider dorsally to accommodate the intrathoracic structures like the aorta (Ao), azygos vein (Az), and oesophagus (O). In addition, the dorsal part of the caudal mediastinum contains the mediastinal serous cavity (MSC). The ventral part of the mediastinum (caudoventral mediastinal reflection (CVM)) is thin and displaced to the left by the accessory lung lobe, which lies in the mediastinal recess (Mr). The right boundary of the mediastinal recess is the plica venae cavae (P), which surrounds and is ventral to the caudal vena cava (CdVC). The CVM should not be mistaken for the phrenicopericardial ligament (PPL). H = Outline of position of the heart.
(Redrawn after Suter (1984))

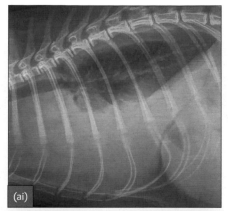

(ai)

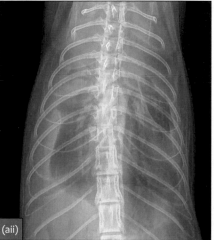

(aii)

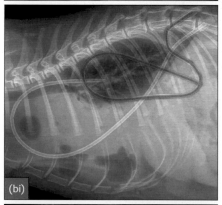

(bi)

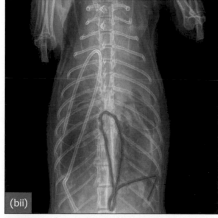

(bii)

10.20 The mediastinal serous cavity is in the dorsal part of the caudal mediastinum to the right of the oesophagus (o) between the heart base and diaphragm. (ai, bi, ci) Lateral and (aii, bii, cii) orthogonal thoracic radiographs in an adult cat with severe bilateral pleural fluid: (a) on presentation, (b) after placement of bilateral chest tubes. The left chest tube (red) pierces the left caudal lung lobe and loops upon itself in the mediastinal serous cavity. (continues) ▶

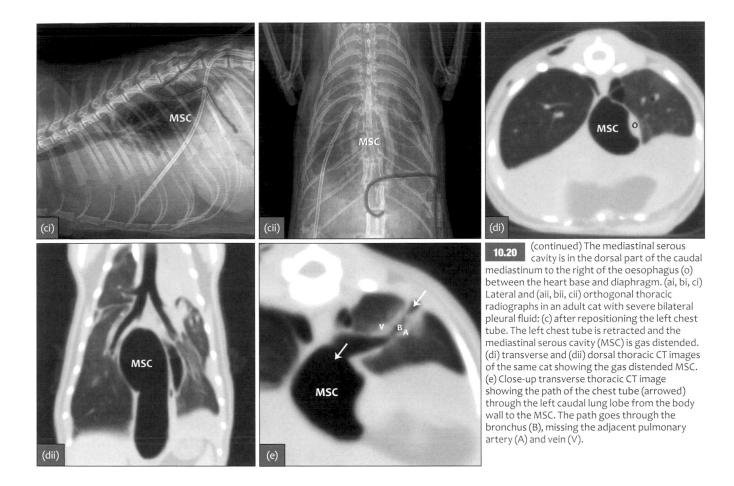

10.20 (continued) The mediastinal serous cavity is in the dorsal part of the caudal mediastinum to the right of the oesophagus (o) between the heart base and diaphragm. (ai, bi, ci) Lateral and (aii, bii, cii) orthogonal thoracic radiographs in an adult cat with severe bilateral pleural fluid: (c) after repositioning the left chest tube. The left chest tube is retracted and the mediastinal serous cavity (MSC) is gas distended. (di) transverse and (dii) dorsal thoracic CT images of the same cat showing the gas distended MSC. (e) Close-up transverse thoracic CT image showing the path of the chest tube (arrowed) through the left caudal lung lobe from the body wall to the MSC. The path goes through the bronchus (B), missing the adjacent pulmonary artery (A) and vein (V).

Interpretative principles

Mediastinal shift

A mediastinal shift is any deviation of the mediastinal structures towards one side of the thorax. This finding does not usually signify mediastinal disease but is a valuable sign of disease on either side of the mediastinum. The mediastinum is mainly a midline structure, so displacement to the left or right is a strong indicator of change in the volume of one side of the thorax. This is an important radiographic sign to recognize as it may indicate disease of the lung, pleural cavity or thoracic boundary. Identification of mediastinal shift can be very important in correct diagnosis and prompt treatment of potentially life-threatening diseases such as diaphragmatic hernia, pneumonia or tension pneumothorax. Mediastinal shift is recognized by a change in the position of the heart, trachea, aortic arch or caudal vena cava, or by asymmetry between the sizes of the two lungs or two pleural cavities. Mediastinal shift may persist after the active disease process has resolved, due to adhesions or lobar collapse.

On DV and VD thoracic radiographs, assessment of the position of the mediastinum depends on the animal being correctly positioned and free from rotation, as rotation of the animal will falsely suggest mediastinal shift (Figure 10.21). If the cardiac apex appears to be displaced in the same direction as the sternum, then any apparent mediastinal shift might be an effect of rotation. If the apex of the heart appears to be displaced away from the sternum, then true mediastinal shift must be present. Where there is doubt, a new radiograph without rotation should be obtained. Mediastinal shift cannot be evaluated on lateral radiographs although secondary changes may be observed. For example, when there is unilateral or asymmetric lung collapse, a mediastinal shift towards the side of greater collapse occurs and causes the cardiac silhouette to appear dorsally displaced from the sternum on lateral radiographs (see Chapter 11).

Although there are several possible causes, mediastinal shift is most commonly due to relative decreased lung volume on one side, increased volume of the pleural cavity or lung on one side, or a combination of these processes. Some causes include:

- Unilateral atelectasis (collapse) due to any reason
- Asymmetrical or unilateral pleural effusion
- Asymmetrical or unilateral pneumothorax
- Pulmonary hyperinflation due to unilateral pulmonary emphysema or compensatory hyperinflation
- Large pulmonary mass or masses
- Diaphragmatic rupture with herniation of abdominal viscera
- Pleural adhesions
- Deformities of the vertebral column or thoracic wall, such as scoliosis or pectus excavatum
- Thoracic wall mass.

The presence or absence of mediastinal shift can help differentiate the underlying cause of some conditions. For example, increased opacity of the right middle lung lobe with a mediastinal shift towards the affected lobe indicates lobar collapse, which may be pathological (e.g. bronchial obstruction) or a technical complication

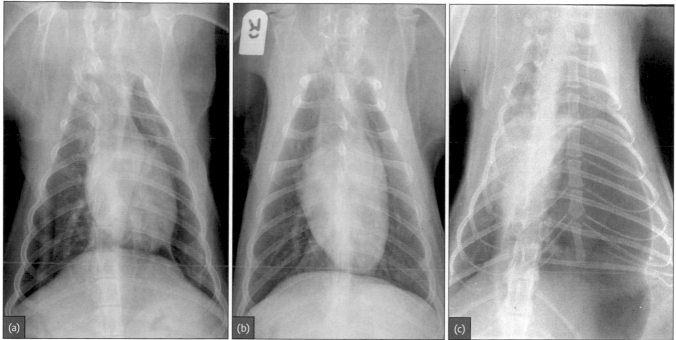

10.21 (a) VD thoracic radiograph of a mature dog with moderate rotation of the thorax. Note that the cardiac silhouette has moved in the same direction as the sternum. A true mediastinal shift is likely absent. (b) VD thoracic radiograph of the same dog. The dog is well positioned and the spinous processes summate with the vertebral bodies and sternebrae. Note that the cardiac silhouette is in a normal position and there is no mediastinal shift. The previous displacement of the cardiac silhouette was simply due to rotation. (c) DV thoracic radiograph of an 8-year-old neutered male Oriental cat with a unilateral tension pneumothorax. The mediastinum is shifted to the right due to severe expansion of the left pleural cavity. Although the cat is poorly positioned with marked rotation, the cardiac apex is rotated in the opposite direction to the sternum, confirming the mediastinal shift.

(e.g. atelectasis associated with recumbency). Increased opacity of the right middle lung lobe with a mediastinal shift away from the lobe indicates lobar expansion due to space-occupying disease such as lung neoplasia or lung lobe torsion. The direction of displacement of the mediastinum (towards or away from the side of disease) depends more on whether the underlying condition produces increased or decreased volume, pressure or both on the more severely affected side of the thorax than on the underlying cause. For example, gas in a pleural cavity can cause either a mediastinal shift towards (normotensive) or away (tension pneumothorax) from the side of pneumothorax. In general:

- Relatively decreased lung volume on one side of the thoracic cavity causes a shift towards that side (ipsilateral shift) (Figure 10.22a)
- Relatively increased lung or pleural space volume on one side of the thoracic cavity causes a shift away from that side (contralateral shift) (Figure 10.22b)
- The presence of a large intrathoracic mass may cause a shift away from that side (contralateral shift) (Figure 10.22c)

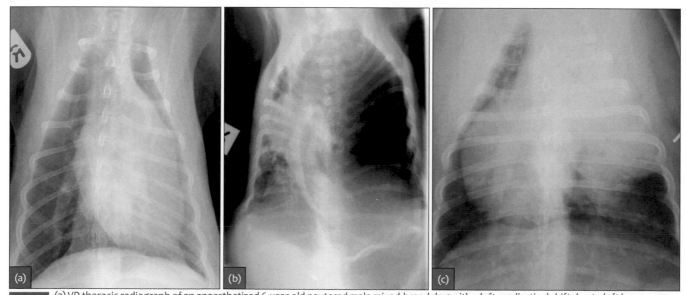

10.22 (a) VD thoracic radiograph of an anaesthetized 6-year-old neutered male mixed-breed dog with a left mediastinal shift due to left lung atelectasis. The cardiac silhouette has moved towards the left due to diminished left lung volume (ipsilateral shift). (b) DV thoracic radiograph of a puppy with a right mediastinal shift due to congenital lobar emphysema. The trachea and cardiac silhouette are markedly shifted into the right side of the thorax due to the presence of the hyperinflated left lung lobe (contralateral shift). (c) DV thoracic radiograph of a dog with a right mediastinal shift due to a left cranial lobar pulmonary mass. The cardiac silhouette is displaced towards the right, away from the mass (contralateral shift).

- Adhesions secondary to chronic inflammatory pleural effusion may cause a more complicated mediastinal shift
- Multiple mechanisms may occur concurrently (e.g. lung lobe collapse on one side and lung hyperinflation on the opposite side).

Abnormal observation of mediastinal structures

It is unusual to see all the mediastinal reflections and structures during radiography; an observable mediastinal reflection, or deformation of a mediastinal reflection, may be a sign of disease. In addition, the ability to differentiate mediastinal structures more clearly indicates the presence of a contrasting substance between them. In extremely obese animals and some deep-chested dogs, it can be normal to have increased visibility of some cranial mediastinal structures on lateral views. In most other instances, the ability to observe more mediastinal structures than typical is due to an abnormal condition. The most common clinical situation in which mediastinal structures become abnormally visible is when gas contrasts with the adventitial or outer surfaces of the structures, indicating pneumomediastinum (see below). A rare but concerning scenario is the presence of an infiltrating metal opacity outlining the adventitial surfaces of mediastinal structures, suggesting extravasation of a previously administered positive contrast agent.

Mediastinal masses

Masses in the mediastinum may be neoplasms, inflammatory lesions (i.e. abscess, granuloma), localized fluid accumulations (e.g. cyst, paraoesophageal empyema), foreign bodies or normal anatomical variation. It is important to distinguish pathological masses from normal anatomical variation. Dogs with a wide shallow thoracic conformation, such as brachycephalic breeds, often have a wide mediastinum that appears mass-like (see Figure 10.9a). Obese dogs will have increased fat deposits in the mediastinum (see Figure 10.9b), again mimicking a mediastinal mass. True masses may be accompanied by clinical signs that further support the diagnosis of a mass, such as dyspnoea and exercise intolerance.

Determining the cause of the mass is also important. As with abnormalities in other body parts, one of the most important steps in determining the cause of a mass is to establish its anatomical location as precisely as possible because this may suggest the organ or tissue of origin. For example, a perihilar mediastinal mass is likely to be due to tracheobronchial lymphadenomegaly or a heart base mass. Mediastinal masses may be located anywhere within the mediastinum, depending on their aetiology and tissue of origin. To simplify the process, mediastinal masses can be divided into five main possible locations (Figure 10.23). It may be impossible to localize a mass to only one location as large masses can involve multiple parts. Furthermore, a mass can be so large that its origin is difficult to determine, even using CT. Occasionally, it is difficult to determine whether a mass near the midline originates from the mediastinum or from the lung adjacent to the mediastinum. Factors that may assist in differentiation are shown in Figure 10.24 (see also 'Masses', below, and Figure 10.32).

Another way to determine the origin of a mediastinal mass is to assess the displacement of other intrathoracic structures. Most masses are of soft tissue opacity, thus not permitting further differentiation based on radiographic appearance, but masses may occasionally be mineralized (e.g. teratoma) or of fat opacity (e.g. mediastinal lipoma). Ultrasonography can be very useful in further assessment of these lesions, either using the heart or liver as an acoustic window or, if the mass is large enough, by a direct transthoracic technique.

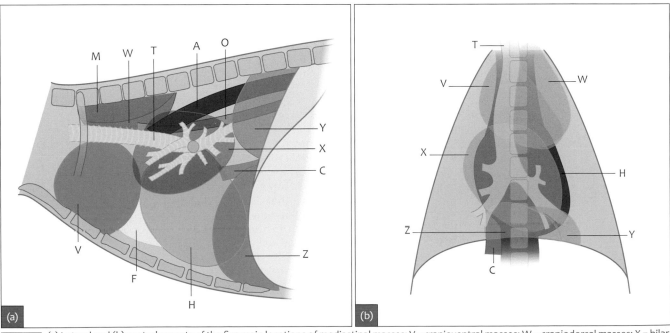

10.23 (a) Lateral and (b) ventral aspects of the five main locations of mediastinal masses: V = cranioventral masses; W = craniodorsal masses; X = hilar and perihilar masses; Y = caudodorsal masses; Z = caudoventral masses. Several structures are labelled for reference: A = thoracic descending aorta; C = caudal vena cava; F = mediastinal fat; H = heart; M = shadow of intrathoracic part of longus colli muscle; O = oesophagus; T = trachea.
(Redrawn after Suter (1984))

- The DV or VD radiograph may reveal whether the mass is in the midline
- Lateral displacement of the medial lung margin may be seen with a mediastinal mass, similar in appearance to an extrapleural sign
- A mediastinal mass will usually be equal in size and similar in appearance on both lateral views, whereas a pulmonary mass may have different appearances on opposite lateral views due to magnification and inflation of the surrounding lung
- Displacement and effacement of mediastinal structures suggest a mediastinal origin but may also occur if a pulmonary mass is large and adjacent to the midline
- If a suitable acoustic window is attainable, then ultrasonography may be useful in differentiating the two anatomical compartments by evaluating the motion of the mass with lung movement (see Chapter 2)

10.24 Factors that may help in distinguishing a mediastinal mass from a lung mass adjacent to the mediastinum.

Mediastinal fluid

Excluding the lumen of hollow structures, mediastinal fluid is not generally freely moveable because the mediastinum is not a hollow space like the pleural cavity. When fluid accumulates within the mediastinum, it does so in the interstitial spaces, the lumens of hollow organs (e.g. oesophagus, trachea, blood vessels, lymphatic vessels), the mediastinal serous cavity, pathologically created cavities caused by disruptions of the loose connective tissue, or in abnormal masses (e.g. cysts, neoplasms, abscesses, haematomas). Abnormal fluid accumulation in the heart chambers and pericardial cavity is discussed separately (see Chapter 9).

Generalized or diffuse mediastinal fluid generally causes further border effacement of the contents of the mediastinum during radiography and widespread increased mediastinal width. The abnormal fluid accumulates within the tissues themselves (e.g. interstitial oedema, inflammation, haemorrhage) or in abnormal cavities caused by disruption or tearing of the connective tissue. Fluid that accumulates within abnormal pockets or cavities is 'loculated fluid' (trapped fluid, encapsulated fluid). When sufficiently large, loculated mediastinal fluid can result in a focal widening of the mediastinum that produces a space-occupying lesion. The location of the loculated fluid may be helpful to determine its cause, but other radiographic signs are usually not specific enough to determine the cause of focal mediastinal widening. During conventional radiography, it might be impossible to differentiate a solid soft tissue mass from loculated fluid. Concurrent pleural fluid is also possible and positional radiography may displace free pleural fluid and aid in the detection of loculated mediastinal fluid or mass (see Chapter 11). Reverse fissures may occasionally be visible on DV and VD radiographs as smooth triangular soft tissue opacity projections, extending caudolaterally from the midline (Figure 10.25).

Alternative imaging of the mediastinum

Due to the limitations of radiographic assessment of the mediastinum it is important to realize the role of alternative imaging techniques in investigation of this region.

Transthoracic ultrasonography of the normal mediastinum is generally unrewarding due to the presence of air-filled lung between the thoracic wall and the mediastinum. However, many structures within the normal mediastinum can be identified using ultrasonography when pleural fluid is present (see Chapter 11). In animals

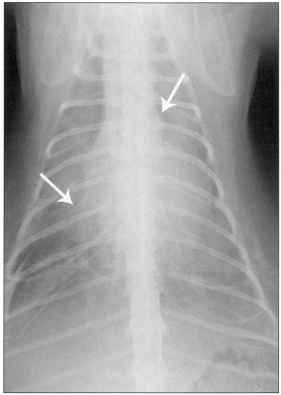

10.25 DV thoracic radiograph of a 10-year-old neutered male Domestic Shorthaired cat with pleural and mediastinal fluid due to congestive heart failure. Triangular 'reverse fissures' that might represent mediastinal fluid can be seen (arrowed).

with mediastinal disease, ultrasonography is very useful in differentiating mediastinal fluid from a mass, determining the cause of a focally wide mediastinum and determining the extent of a mass. Ultrasonography also facilitates guided fine-needle aspiration (FNA) or tissue biopsy. The cranial mediastinum can be accessed via parasternal, intercostal or thoracic inlet windows, the middle mediastinum via the cardiac notch, and the caudal mediastinum either parasternally or via a transhepatic approach. Transoesophageal ultrasonography has been used in dogs to examine the heart base and great vessels, but this technique requires general anaesthesia and specialized equipment and is not widely available (see Chapter 2).

CT and, to a lesser extent, magnetic resonance imaging (MRI) are very useful for examining the mediastinum in both dogs and cats (Figure 10.26). Both allow evaluation of the mediastinum without summation from other structures and have better contrast resolution than standard radiography, allowing distinction between solid, fatty, cystic, calcified and vascular structures. CT images of the mediastinum should usually be viewed using a soft tissue window and acquired before and after intravenous contrast medium administration. CT angiography is particularly helpful in distinguishing mediastinal blood vessels from masses. The speed of CT acquisition results in minimal movement blur and, as advanced multidetector helical CT scanners and respiratory and cardiac gating have become more widely available, this has revolutionized imaging of the mediastinum. However, this does not mean that CT is required for every case.

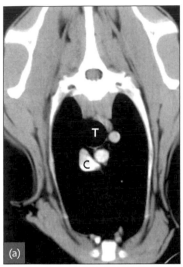
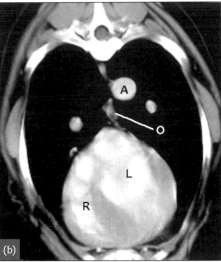
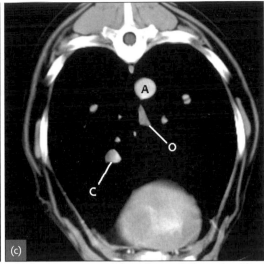
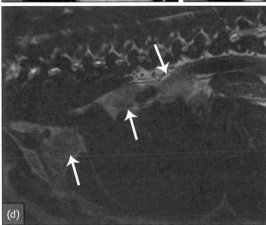

10.26 Transverse CT images obtained from a normal dog using a soft tissue algorithm at the level of the (a) second thoracic vertebra, (b) heart base and (c) ninth thoracic vertebra. All images were acquired after intravenous administration of non-ionic iodinated contrast medium and are displayed with a soft tissue window (window width 300 HU, window level 40 HU). (b) Contrast medium can be seen within the left and right ventricles. The unlabelled hyperattenuating structures within the lungs (seen as small round structures) are the pulmonary arteries and veins beginning to fill with contrast medium. (d) Sagittal thoracic MRI image of a 4-year-old Staffordshire Bull Terrier bitch. Although cardiac movement impedes full interpretation, enlarged cranial mediastinal and tracheobronchial lymph nodes (arrowed) are seen. A = aorta; C = vena cava (cranial in (a), caudal in (c)); L = left ventricle; O = oesophagus; R = right ventricle; T = trachea.

Diseases

Pneumomediastinum

In the mediastinum, gas is normally present in the tracheal lumen and can be present in the normal oesophageal lumen. Gas dissecting through the loose connective tissue, often contrasting with the adventitial margin of organs is abnormal and is called pneumomediastinum. The abnormally located gas is usually air from cervical, tracheal, oesophageal, body wall or pulmonary injury, but bacterial production is possible. Pneumomediastinum always results from another disease process and the key to investigating and treating the condition lies in identifying the underlying cause. Several of the many possible causes are listed in Figure 10.27.

Pneumomediastinum may occur in isolation (spontaneous, idiopathic) or may be accompanied by other abnormalities, including pneumothorax, subcutaneous emphysema, pneumoretroperitoneum or suppurative inflammation of the deep cervical fascia. With chronic cough or mechanical hyperventilation, pulmonary interstitial emphysema can develop with gas trapped in the peribronchovascular interstitium of the lungs. This gas drains into the mediastinum rather than the pleural space, leading to a localized pneumomediastinum. Clinical signs often reflect accompanying conditions, such as dyspnoea or tachypnoea secondary to pneumothorax, discomfort secondary to subcutaneous emphysema, or systemic signs of sepsis. Rarely, a large-volume pneumomediastinum may compress the thin-walled veins of the mediastinum (i.e. cranial vena

Cause	Comments
Thoracic wall, tracheal, oesophageal or cervical injury	Blunt thoracic trauma resulting in bronchial or alveolar rupture Perforating injury to skin or neck (e.g. puncture wounds, pharyngeal stick injuries) Iatrogenic cervical or tracheal injury (e.g. jugular venepuncture, transtracheal washing, tracheostomy) Tracheal rupture (e.g. secondary to overinflation of endotracheal tube cuff) Oesophageal rupture (e.g. foreign body, bite wound, iatrogenic)
Spontaneous	For example following severe cough, respiratory disease (such as paraquat toxicity), pulmonary interstitial emphysema
Lung lobe torsion causing bronchial rupture	Rare
Idiopathic	No cause identified

10.27 Causes of pneumomediastinum.

cava, caudal vena cava and azygos vein) and lead to diminished venous return and circulatory collapse. Treatment of pneumomediastinum is usually by treatment of the underlying cause without the removal of air from the mediastinum.

Pneumomediastinum may be mild to severe, may resolve spontaneously with time, or may progress to pneumothorax. If pneumomediastinum and pneumothorax are present simultaneously, then the pneumomediastinum may have led to the pneumothorax. Pneumothorax does not lead to pneumomediastinum as the mediastinum is collapsed by the pressure of the pleural gas.

Radiography

Radiography is essential in the diagnosis of pneumomediastinum. It allows assessment of the extent of the condition, shows associated lesions and complications, may identify the cause, and allows assessment of the resolution or progression of the condition. Radiographic appearance is similar in all cases (Figure 10.28):

- Decreased opacity of the mediastinum due to the presence of dissecting, infiltrating, linear gas opacities that contrast the external (adventitial) surfaces of mediastinal structures (e.g. aorta, trachea, oesophagus and cranial mediastinal blood vessels) making them easier to outline
- Ventral border of longus colli muscles can be seen inserting on the ventral border of the sixth thoracic vertebra
- Both the luminal and adventitial surfaces of the trachea are contrasted by gas
- Extensive subcutaneous emphysema may also be present, making radiographic interpretation more challenging due to the superimposition of linear and reticulated gas shadows
- Radiographs of the neck or abdomen may demonstrate the causative lesion, such as a penetrating foreign body or fracture, or extension of gas into the retro-peritoneal space (Figure 10.29)
- Pneumoretroperitoneum originating from pneumomediastinum is usually an incidental finding of minor consequence but should be differentiated from spread of suppurative inflammation or rupture of a hollow abdominal viscus, which is a surgical emergency (see Figure 10.28c). Pneumomediastinum usually leads to pneumoretroperitoneum, rather than pneumoperitoneum
- Oesophageal perforation will typically produce concurrent mediastinal fluid accumulation.

Contrast studies: If oesophageal perforation is suspected, then intraluminal administration of 5–10 ml of a non-ionic iodinated contrast medium, such as iohexol, may be used to confirm the diagnosis and identify the site of perforation. Orthogonal radiographs should be obtained immediately and 5–10 minutes after oral administration to allow time for extravasation of the contrast medium. If tracheal perforation is suspected, tracheoscopy is recommended.

Other imaging modalities

Due to the presence of gas, ultrasonography is not useful. Advanced imaging techniques, such as CT or MRI, are rarely needed to make the diagnosis, although they may assist in identifying the cause. CT is of value in the investigation of penetrating pharyngeal or oesophageal injuries (Figures 10.30 and 10.31).

Masses

Masses are produced by several neoplastic, inflammatory, degenerative and developmental causes, and are differentiated from infiltrative tumours by their more-or-less demarcated, space-occupying, roughly spherical shape. Most have a soft tissue opacity, but the opacity varies with different conditions and may be fat, mineral or gas.

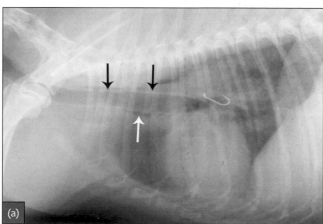

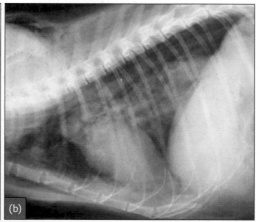

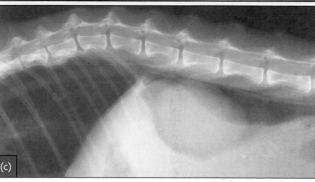

10.28 (a) Lateral thoracic radiograph of a 5-year-old mixed-breed dog with subtle pneumomediastinum secondary to a perforating oesophageal foreign body (a fishhook). The small amounts of gas contrasting with the outer surface of the trachea (arrowed) are an important radiographic finding. (b) Lateral thoracic radiograph of an 8-year-old neutered female Domestic Shorthaired cat with pneumomediastinum, pneumothorax, extensive subcutaneous emphysema, and pulmonary contusions after a road traffic accident. A ruptured trachea was identified on endoscopic examination. (c) Close-up of a lateral trunk radiograph of an emaciated 12-year-old Domestic Shorthaired cat with extension of pneumomediastinum to pneumoretroperitoneum. The thoracic and abdominal aorta and kidneys are contrasted by gas. Minimal trauma to the aortic hiatus allows gas tracking into the retroperitoneal space. This finding is typically of minor consequence but should be differentiated from gas originating from ruptured abdominal organs.

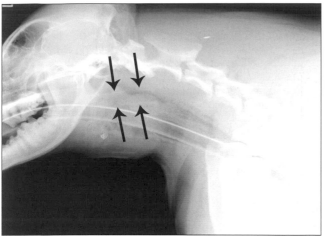

10.29 Left lateral neck radiograph of a 6-year-old neutered crossbreed bitch with a penetrating pharyngeal injury. Summating with the oropharynx and the retropharyngeal soft tissues are two fine parallel linear radiopacities (arrowed) that are consistent with a stick. In addition, there are multiple linear gas opacities tracking along the deep cervical fascia and cranial mediastinum, contrasting with the adventitial surface of the trachea and the brachiocephalic trunk and consistent with deep fascial emphysema and pneumomediastinum.

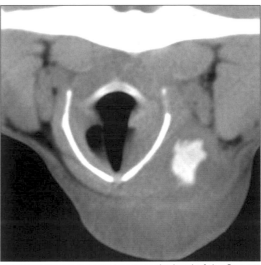

10.31 Transverse CT image at the level of the first cervical vertebra of a 3-year-old male Labrador Retriever with pneumomediastinum due to a penetrating injury (window width 300 HU, window level 50 HU). Left and ventral to the larynx, there is a hyperattenuating structure surrounded by soft tissue swelling. During exploratory surgery, this structure was found to be a stick.

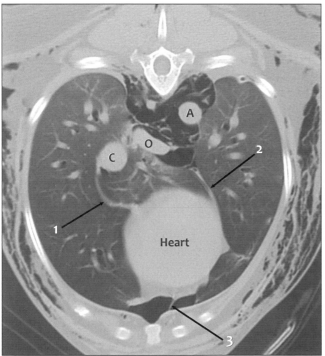

10.30 Transverse CT image (lung window) of a 5-year-old Siberian Husky with severe pneumomediastinum, severe subcutaneous emphysema and mild bilateral pneumothorax. The image was obtained at the level of the eighth thoracic vertebra. The dorsal part of the caudal mediastinum is wide and contains a large volume of gas (pneumomediastinum) that dissects through the connective tissue and contrasts with the adventitia surrounding the aorta (A) and oesophagus (O). The body wall contains a large volume of gas (subcutaneous emphysema) that dissects through the connective tissue (fascia). In the ventral part of the thoracic cavity, the normal plica venae cavae (1), caudoventral mediastinal reflection (2) and phrenicopericardial ligament (3) are seen as thin, soft tissue opacities. The former two are between lung lobes and define the boundaries of the mediastinal recess. The latter is contrasted by gas in both pleural cavities (bilateral pneumothorax). Note how the gas in the mediastinum and body wall is interrupted by numerous internal soft tissue septa, which provide a barrier to flow. The gas-filled spaces in the mediastinum and body wall are pathologically created by the disruption of the connective tissue. The pleural cavities are pre-existing potential spaces that do not have internal septa. C = caudal vena cava.

Masses can occur anywhere within the mediastinum, with the most common sites being the ventral part of the cranial mediastinum (cranioventral) and the dorsal mediastinum (perihilar). Clinical signs usually depend on the size and position of the mass, which determine whether there is any effect on adjacent structures (e.g. tracheal compression). Occasionally, tumours will produce substances that have a distant effect (e.g. hyperthyroidism). Animals with cranial mediastinal masses usually present with signs of dyspnoea, coughing and exercise intolerance. Occasionally gagging, vomiting or regurgitation may be present, secondary to either oesophageal compression or megaoesophagus due to paraneoplastic myasthenia gravis, usually associated with thymoma. Horner's syndrome, vocalization changes and laryngeal paralysis may result from peripheral nerve compression by masses in the cranial mediastinum, especially dorsally. Mediastinal masses may also compress vascular or lymphatic structures. This may lead to head, neck and possibly thoracic limb oedema when the cranial vena cava is involved, or ascites when the caudal vena cava is involved. Causes of mediastinal masses and their main radiographic signs are listed in Figure 10.32.

Radiography

Radiographic appearance depends on the position and size of the mass:

- Masses typically produce a focal abnormal soft tissue opacity that may be circumscribed or indistinctly margined
- Small masses may form silhouettes with other soft tissue structures and only be visible as subtle focal bulging of the mediastinum
- Larger masses may be visible and cause displacement of nearby or associated structures. Commonly, there is border obliteration between a cranial mediastinal mass and the cardiac silhouette, which can make it difficult to assess the heart. Large masses will push the heart caudally and displace the trachea. On lateral radiographs, observing the tracheal bifurcation caudal

Causes	Radiological signs	Additional information	Image
Craniodorsal			
• Oesophageal diseases • Tumours of neural or neuroendocrine origin • Paravertebral or vertebral tumours • Aortic aneurysm • Exceptional location of chemodectoma or thymoma	• Trachea depressed ventrally and to the right • Silhouette sign with aorta • Can be very difficult to see unless mineralized or very large	• Check for oesophageal abnormalities • Check for vertebral abnormalities including ventral new bone formation and a widened intervertebral foramen	 A craniodorsal oesophageal mass in a 10-year-old male Border Collie
Cranioventral			
• Lymphoma • Thymic lesions (thymoma, thymic lymphoma, thymic branchial cyst, thymic haematoma (has been reported secondary to anticoagulant toxicity in juvenile dogs), thymic hyperplasia, thymic amyloidosis) • Cranial sternal lymph node enlargement • Mediastinal cysts (most common location) • Ectopic thyroid and parathyroid tumours • Chemodectoma • Pericardial cyst • Mediastinal haemorrhage	• Trachea elevated ± compressed • Increase in soft tissue opacity in cranioventral thorax with loss of radiolucent space cranial to the heart • Wide cranial mediastinum • Caudal displacement of heart and carina • Caudal displacement ± compression of cranial lung lobes	• Paraneoplastic disease may occur in association with thymoma; megaoesophagus secondary to myasthenia gravis in dogs; exfoliative dermatitis in cats • Obesity can cause similar signs and should be ruled out	 A large thymoma in an 11-year-old neutered male Domestic Short-haired cat

10.32 Sites, causes and main radiographic signs of mediastinal masses. CdVC = caudal vena cava; PPDH = peritoneopericardial diaphragmatic hernia. (continues)

Causes	Radiological signs	Additional information	Image
Perihilar (dorsal)			
• Chemodectoma or other heart base tumour • Perihilar lymphadenopathy (lymphosarcoma, metastatic disease, fungal disease, tuberculosis, nocardiosis, actinomycosis) • Vascular or cardiac enlargement mimicking a mass (pulmonic trunk, aorta, atrial mass) • Bronchogenic cysts • Oesophageal foreign body	• Increased perihilar opacity, often poorly defined • Peripheral displacement of heart base structures • Accentuated ventroflexion of caudal trachea • Impingement and displacement of carina and principal bronchi ± lung lobe collapse if complete • Bronchial obstruction • Often wide caudal lobar bronchi on DV and VD views (see Figure 10.13)	• Enlarged lymph nodes elsewhere may support lymphadenomegaly as the cause of the perihilar mass effect	 Enlarged tracheobronchial lymph nodes in a 5-year-old Domestic Shorthaired cat with mycobacterial disease
Caudodorsal			
• Oesophageal lesions • Neural tumours • Hiatal hernia • PPDH • Migrating foreign bodies • Diaphragmatic lesions (abscess, mass, haematoma)	• Wide caudal mediastinum • Displacement of oesophagus or impingement on lumen • Border obliteration or effacement with diaphragm		 A paravertebral sarcoma in an 8-year-old Rottweiler bitch. The lesion was destructive and entered the vertebral canal

10.32 (continued) Sites, causes and main radiographic signs of mediastinal masses. CdVC = caudal vena cava; PPDH = peritoneopericardial diaphragmatic hernia. (continues)

Causes	Radiological signs	Additional information	Image
Caudoventral			
• Hernias (PPDH, hiatal less common) • Traumatic rupture • Pericardial cyst • Diaphragmatic mass lesions (abscess, mass, haematoma)	• Displacement or impingement of the CdVC • Border obliteration or effacement with caudal border heart ± diaphragm	• Diaphragmatic hernia and rupture – the abdomen and diaphragm should be closely examined	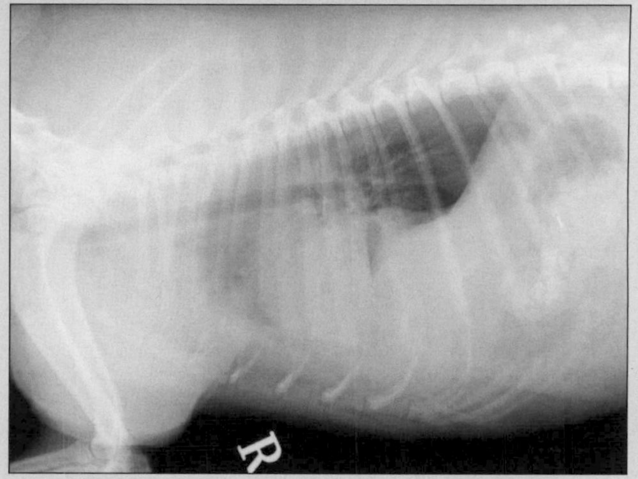 A ventrally located diaphragmatic rupture in a 5-year-old neutered male mixed-breed dog. The liver herniated into a pleural cavity
Any mediastinal location			
• Abscess • Granuloma (including secondary to migrating foreign body) • Haematoma • Primary mediastinal tumours (e.g. haemangiosarcoma, fibrosarcoma, histiocytic sarcoma, lipoma, squamous cell carcinoma) • Pleural tumours • Bronchial tumours	• Displacement of adjacent structures (depending on location)		

10.32 (continued) Sites, causes and main radiographic signs of mediastinal masses. CdVC = caudal vena cava; PPDH = peritoneopericardial diaphragmatic hernia.

- to the sixth intercostal space is a sign of cardiac displacement by a cranial mediastinal mass, rather than cardiac enlargement (Figure 10.33a)
- DV and VD views are the most useful views to differentiate a mediastinal mass from a mass in the cranial lung lobes (see Figures 10.24 and 10.33a)
- Small lesions with a fat or soft tissue opacity and eggshell-like mineralization are occasionally seen in the mediastinum in cats. These are foci of nodular fat necrosis and are of no clinical significance (Figure 10.33b)
- Mediastinal fluid, pleural fluid or both commonly occur with mediastinal masses, resulting in further border effacement of mediastinal structures. With large cranial mediastinal masses combined with pleural effusion, the mass and the cardiac margins are often completely obliterated by pleural fluid
- Additional radiographic views using a horizontal beam may be useful to differentiate a mass from free pleural fluid (see also Chapter 11)
- The accessory lung lobe sits in the mediastinal recess, which can become filled with pleural fluid, making it difficult to differentiate caudal mediastinal masses from loculated pleural fluid or accessory lobe or diaphragmatic consolidation
- Caudal mediastinal masses may also appear as relatively well defined ovoid masses of homogeneous soft tissue opacity, extending from the tracheal bifurcation to the diaphragm (Figure 10.33c) and summated with the oesophagus

- Mediastinal haemorrhage can lead to haematoma formation with mass effect. The margins of the haematoma can be somewhat moulded to the mediastinal border, which helps to distinguish it from other types of mediastinal mass (Figure 10.33d)
- Additional concurrent abnormalities (e.g. megaoesophagus, abdominal lymphadenopathy and hepatosplenomegaly) may help prioritize the differential diagnosis.

Further imaging techniques, such as contrast studies, ultrasonography and CT, may be required to further identify the site of the lesion.

Contrast studies:

- Oesophagography may identify involvement or displacement of the oesophagus.
- Angiography may be useful to delineate masses or identify vascular invasion, malformation or involvement.
- Positive contrast peritoneography may be performed to investigate cases of suspected congenital peritoneopericardial diaphragmatic hernia, congenital or acquired pleuroperitoneal diaphragmatic hernia, or diaphragmatic rupture.

These radiographic procedures are rarely necessary and have been largely superseded by ultrasonography and CT.

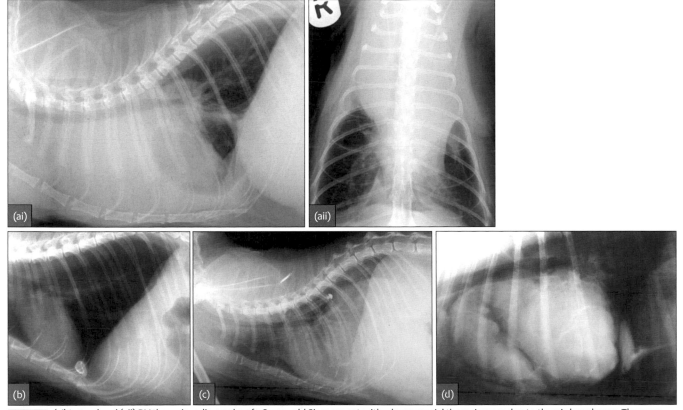

10.33 (ai) Lateral and (aii) DV thoracic radiographs of a 3-year-old Siamese cat with a large cranial thoracic mass due to thymic lymphoma. The mass has a homogeneous soft tissue opacity with indistinct margins. On the lateral view, the tumour displaces the carina to the seventh intercostal space, suggesting that the mass is cranial to the heart. On the DV view, the origin of the mass is clearly mediastinal as the tumour is in the midline and displaces both cranial lung lobes caudolaterally. The tracheobronchial lymph nodes are also enlarged and a small volume of pleural fluid is present. (b) Lateral thoracic radiograph of a Himalayan cat with nodular fat necrosis in the caudoventral aspect of the mediastinum. Nodular fat necrosis is usually an incidental finding of minor consequence and more commonly seen in the abdomen. The eggshell-like mineralization is a typical feature. (c) Lateral thoracic radiograph of a 13-year-old neutered male Domestic Shorthaired cat with a caudal mediastinal abscess. The abscess forms a relatively well defined rounded soft tissue mass between the cardiac silhouette and the diaphragm, summated with the caudal vena cava. An oesophagostomy feeding tube is in place. (d) Lateral thoracic radiograph of a dog with a mediastinal haematoma and pneumothorax following a road traffic accident. The haematoma forms a large mass in the cranial and ventral mediastina with dorsal tracheal displacement, an irregular margin and slightly heterogeneous soft tissue opacity.

Ultrasonography

Ultrasonography is invaluable for assessing mediastinal masses, particularly those located in a cranioventral position where a suitable transthoracic acoustic window can be accessed. The caudal mediastinum is harder to image with ultrasonography, but a subcostal or parasternal approach may be successful. Assessment can be made of the echogenicity and margination of the mass and any involvement of the other mediastinal structures. Mediastinal origin of a mass may be confirmed by identifying movement of the right and left lungs over the static mass. The use of contrast-enhanced ultrasonography may allow differentiation between types of mediastinal masses.

Ultrasonography allows guided FNA or biopsy for cytological or histological diagnosis, and hence appropriate treatment to be instigated. It is essential to obtain a coagulation profile before performing a biopsy as the mass may represent a large mediastinal blood clot in a coagulopathic animal.

Ultrasonography is also particularly helpful in distinguishing cranial mediastinal fat or fluid from a solid soft tissue mass:

- Fat has a characteristic hyperechoic and hyperattenuating appearance and usually surrounds but does not displace vessels (Figure 10.34)

- Fluid will usually be anechoic (see below)
- Masses vary in appearance but are often hypoechoic to fat, displace mediastinal blood vessels, may have central blood flow identified with colour Doppler and may be accompanied by effusion (Figure 10.35).

It is impossible to confirm the cause or origin of a mediastinal mass using ultrasonography alone (Figure 10.36); masses caused by many different conditions often appear identical on ultrasonograms. Biopsy is the gold standard for definitive diagnosis; however, certain ultrasonographic features such as location may be useful in narrowing the differential list:

- Mediastinal lymph node enlargement and lymphoma:
  - Lymphoma may be represented by several enlarged nodes or a focal mass, often in the cranial mediastinum, in the region of the thymus
  - Cranial mediastinal and cranial sternal lymph nodes are usually easily identified as hypoechoic nodular masses surrounding the mediastinal blood vessels (Figure 10.37). They occasionally may be cystic or heterogeneous
  - Multicentric lymphoma may cause caudal mediastinal space-occupying lesions. This region is more challenging to interrogate ultrasonographically

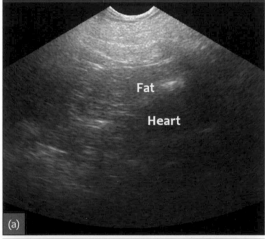

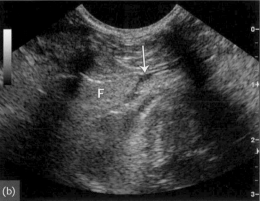

10.34 The appearance of mediastinal fat on ultrasonography. (a) Dorsal plane image of the cranial mediastinum of an obese 6-year-old Cocker Spaniel. Cranial to the heart and internal to the thick hyperechoic thoracic wall, the mediastinal fat appears as a large amount of homogeneous tissue with a coarse echotexture. (b) Dorsal plane image of the cranial thorax of a 9-year-old neutered male Maltese. A triangular region of hyperechoic tissue (F) is seen cranial to the heart: a very small amount of pleural fluid surrounds the tip (arrowed). The tissue was presumed to be mediastinal fat and confirmed by FNA.
(Courtesy of G. Seiler)

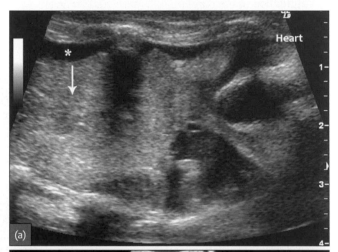

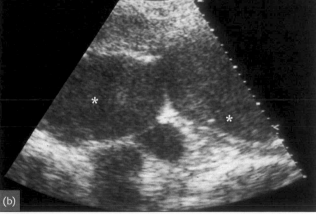

10.35 (a) Dorsal plane image of the cranial thorax of a 10-year-old neutered female Domestic Shorthaired cat with biopsy-confirmed carcinoma and haemorrhage. In the cranial mediastinum, the tumour is seen as a large heterogenous mass (arrowed) that is cranial to the heart and surrounded by fluid in both pleural cavities (*). (b) The cranial mediastinum of a 5-year-old neutered Flat-Coated Retriever bitch with a lobulated mass (*) attributed to a round cell sarcoma. Enlarged mediastinal lymph nodes are also present.
(a, Courtesy of G. Seiler)

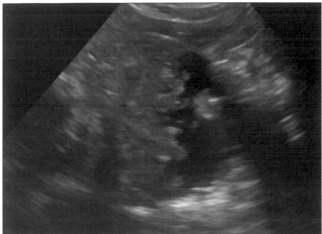

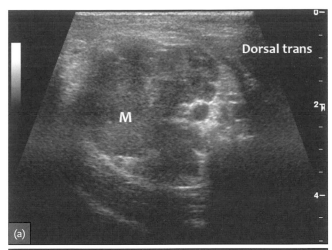

Dorsal trans

M

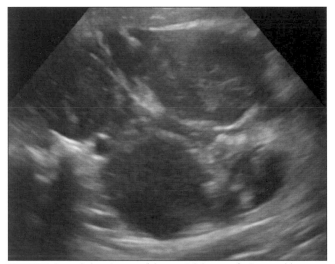

10.36 Dorsal plane image of the cranial thorax of a 10-year-old neutered crossbreed bitch with metastatic melanoma. There are large, relatively homogeneous masses with anechoic crescentic caudal borders in the cranial mediastinum. Definitive histopathological diagnosis was not made.

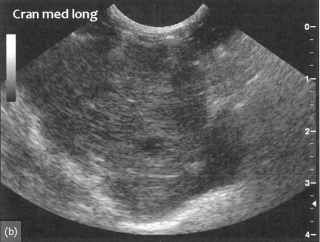

Cran med long

(a)

(b)

10.37 Dorsal plane image of the cranial thorax of a 3-year-old neutered male British Shorthaired cat. Adjacent to the cranial vena cava, there are three well defined, relatively hypoechoic, rounded structures (consistent with enlarged lymph nodes) and a scant amount of pleural fluid.

10.38 (a) Transverse plane left intercostal image of a biopsy-confirmed thymoma; dorsal is to the right. In the cranial mediastinum, the tumour is seen as a large, hypoechoic, lobulated mass (M) that partially surrounds mediastinal blood vessels. The blood vessels are seen as round hypoechoic structures dorsal to the mass. (b) Dorsal plane image of a thymoma. The cranial mediastinum is filled by a hypoechoic lobulated mass.
(Courtesy of G. Seiler)

- Certain ultrasonographic features may be more suggestive of malignant neoplasia rather than reactive inflammatory nodal change. These require further investigation and include abnormal size and shape, abnormal (non-hilar) angioarchitecture, altered echogenicity of the hilus and evidence of nodal necrosis. Contrast harmonic ultrasonography has potential for the evaluation of malignant nodes
- FNA often provides cytological confirmation of the diagnosis without the need for tissue biopsy
- Thymoma:
  - Ultrasonographic appearance may vary and may be identical to that of thymic lymphoma (Figure 10.38)
  - Large thymomas are often echogenic with small to large cystic regions
  - Small thymomas may mimic abnormal lymph nodes
  - On occasion, thymomas may invade the cranial vena cava
- Oesophageal abnormalities: rarely, it is possible to identify an oesophageal mass using transthoracic ultrasonography (see 'Oesophagus', below). This

detection is facilitated by the presence of pleural fluid and a transhepatic route usually provides the best acoustic window
- Mediastinal cyst (see 'Cysts', below)
- Mediastinal haematoma:
  - Varies greatly in appearance with time since haemorrhage occurred
  - A simple haematoma is avascular and usually shows ultrasonographic resolution with time
  - The presence of central vasculature within the mass suggests the presence of an underlying haemorrhagic lesion (i.e. the mass is not purely a large haematoma)
  - Coexisting effusion is often present
- Paraoesophageal abscess, empyema or neoplasia:
  - With involvement of the mediastinal serous cavity, soft tissue masses in the dorsal part of the caudal mediastinum will appear relatively well circumscribed and will be situated caudal to the cardiac silhouette and parallel to the right side of the oesophagus. Suppurative processes are referred to as empyema. Neoplastic and haemorrhagic conditions have been described in this space and can appear similar to empyema

- Empyema of the mediastinal serous cavity is often found in association with lobar pneumonia. Pleural fluid may also be present
- Abscesses adjacent to the oesophagus may occur secondary to perforating material. Their location is less predictable and they have less well defined margins
- The wall may be irregular with complex or echogenic fluid content in the lumen (Figure 10.39).

Computed tomography

CT has revolutionized the diagnosis and evaluation of mediastinal masses (Figure 10.40). It provides further information on radiographically identified masses and can also identify masses not seen or only suspected on standard radiographs (Figure 10.41). CT potentially allows distinction between different types of tumours, as well as differentiating abscesses/empyema, cysts and haematomas. Thymomas tend to be more heterogeneous than

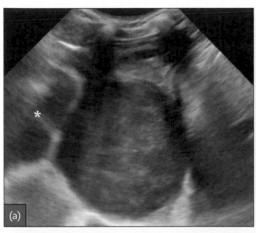
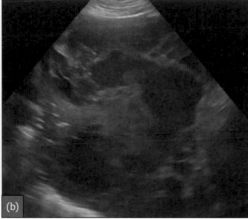

10.39 (a) Dorsal plane image of the caudal thorax of a 13-year-old neutered male Domestic Shorthaired cat with a caudal mediastinal abscess. Between the heart (*) and the diaphragm, the abscess forms a large space-occupying lesion that is round, relatively well defined and homogeneous. (b) Transverse plane image of the caudal thorax of a 2-year-old neutered crossbreed bitch. There is a large, complex, loculated mass with a slightly irregular but relatively well defined wall.

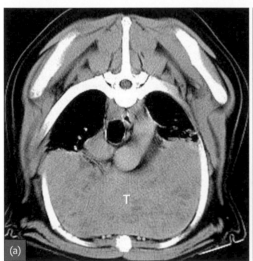
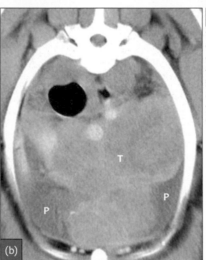

10.40 (a) Transverse CT image at the level of the fifth intercostal space of a 7-year-old neutered Labrador Retriever bitch with a thymoma (T) (window width 300 HU, window level 50 HU). (b) Post-contrast transverse CT image at the level of the fifth intercostal space of a 5-year-old neutered male crossbreed dog with a thymoma (T) (window width 300 HU, window level 50 HU). Pleural effusion (P) is also present.

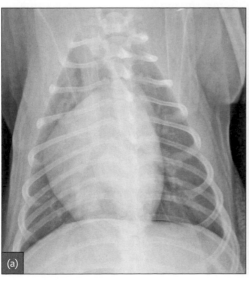
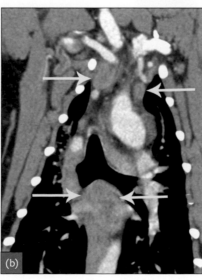

10.41 (a) DV thoracic radiograph of a 4-year-old Staffordshire Bull Terrier bitch with subtle increased mediastinal width. (b) Reformatted dorsal oblique contrast CT image at the level of the heart base allowing observation of enlarged cranial mediastinal and middle tracheobronchial lymph nodes (arrowed) (window width 400 HU, window level 40 HU).

lymphomas, particularly in larger masses, with a cystic component, and may demonstrate increased vascular invasion.

Biopsy is the gold standard for diagnosis and CT-guided biopsy (Figure 10.42) may be performed for masses that are not amenable to ultrasound-guided biopsy. CT is also extremely useful to guide surgical intervention or radiation therapy.

Intravenous contrast medium should be administered unless there is a clinical contraindication. Pre- and post-contrast techniques allow assessment of the margins and vascularity of the lesion and the association between the mass and the blood vessels within the mediastinum, allowing possible differentiation between masses that are locally invasive and those that are not. CT angiography with a rapid injection pump will allow assessment of both arterial supply and venous drainage and facilitate surgical planning. Tumour staging may also be carried out, with assessment of local lymphadenopathy and distant metastatic spread, including of occult skeletal lesions (Figure 10.43).

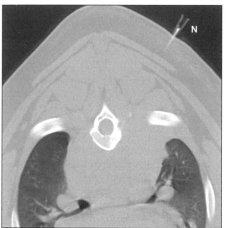

10.42 Transverse CT image at the level of the seventh intercostal space of a 2-year-old neutered Dogue de Bordeaux bitch with lymphoma undergoing CT-guided biopsy (window width 2000 HU, window level –500 HU). The lymphoma is seen as a large, soft tissue attenuating tumour in the dorsal mediastinum between the vertebrae, heart and both lungs. The needle (N) is shown within the skin and from this position is advanced further into the mass (see Chapter 3).

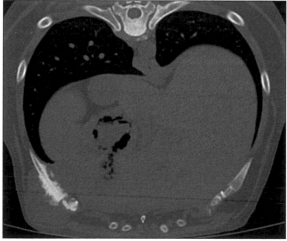

10.43 Transverse CT image at the level of the seventh rib of a 10-year-old neutered crossbreed bitch with metastatic melanoma (window width 1500 HU, window level 300 HU). CT was performed to determine the extent of disease. Just dorsal to the right seventh costochondral junction, there is an irregularly marginated osteolytic lesion with a spiculated periosteal reaction and an associated soft tissue mass. Assessment of the acquired CT images using all appropriate windows will maximize the available information (see also Chapter 3).

Scintigraphy

Scintigraphy using sodium ^{99m}Tc-pertechnetate or iodine-123 can be used to identify neoplastic ectopic thyroid tissue. Radionuclide uptake in a mass is indicative of thyroidal origin of the tissue (Figure 10.44).

Larger, more heterogeneous and irregularly marginated masses are more likely to be malignant (ectopic thyroid carcinoma or metastatic thyroid carcinoma infiltrating cranial mediastinal lymph nodes), although scintigraphic appearance is not definitive. Smaller and less intense masses may also represent hyperfunctioning ectopic thyroid tissue (especially in hyperthyroid animals or animals that have previously undergone thyroidectomy). Evaluation of the scintigram considering the animal's history and hormonal status is mandatory; a biopsy sample is needed for definitive characterization of benign *versus* malignant disease.

Scintigraphy performed with indium-111-labelled white blood cells may be used to identify occult abscesses.

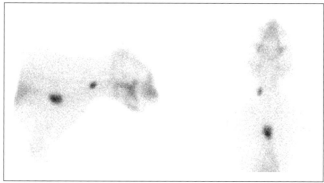

10.44 Right lateral and ventral scintigrams of the head, neck and cranial thorax of a 12-year-old hyperthyroid Domestic Shorthaired cat, obtained 20 minutes after intravenous injection of sodium ^{99m}Tc-pertechnetate. Thoracic radiographs obtained prior to the study revealed a poorly defined cranial mediastinal mass. There is a focus of uptake associated with the right thyroid lobe, much higher in intensity than the salivary glands. The left thyroid lobe is not visible. A second intense focus of uptake is seen in the thorax, corresponding to the lesion seen on radiographs. Final diagnosis was hyperthyroidism with ectopic hyperfunctioning thyroidal tissue in the cranial mediastinum.
(Courtesy of F. Morandi)

Cysts

In imaging, a cyst is a focal accumulation of fluid that is contained by a thin membrane. In pathology, true or primary cysts are lined by epithelium. Therefore, a cyst detected during imaging may be a true cyst or may be a secondary cyst or other type of fluid accumulation. A variety of mediastinal cysts may be observed during thoracic imaging of cats and, less frequently, dogs. These include cysts of pleural, branchial, thymic, lymphatic, bronchogenic and neoplastic origin. Mediastinal cysts are often benign incidental findings, though compressive effects may be present. It should also be noted that cyst rupture may occasionally lead to chronic mediastinitis.

Idiopathic cranial mediastinal cysts are commonly seen in older cats. These are usually solitary lesions, benign, and asymptomatic unless very large. The contents are usually of low cellularity and FNA is usually unnecessary.

In dogs, large fluid-filled structures are occasionally identified in the dorsal part of the caudal mediastinum. The exact cause of these cyst-like abnormalities cannot always be determined, but paraoesophageal empyema, cystic lung neoplasms or parasitic cysts are possible.

Radiography

Findings are as for other mediastinal masses.

- A cranioventral location is most common.
- Small idiopathic mediastinal cysts in cats may appear as faint, barely visible soft tissue opacities cranial to the heart on a lateral view (Figure 10.45a).

Ultrasonography

Findings are diagnostic for cystic lesions (Figure 10.45b):

- Thin-walled anechoic structure(s)
- Complex cysts may have a more echogenic fluid content
- Cysts may be associated with neoplasia (such as cystic thymoma).

Computed tomography

Findings are diagnostic for cystic lesions (Figure 10.45c):

- Thin-walled fluid-filled structure
- Possible contrast-enhancing rim
- CT-guided aspiration can be performed, if required.

Effusion

Mediastinal fluid alone, without concurrent pleural fluid, is uncommon. Fluid accumulation in the medial part of the pleural cavity (adjacent to the mediastinum) may spuriously make the mediastinum appear wide on radiographs as the mediastinum cannot be distinguished from pleural fluid. Effusions include pus, lymph, blood, chyle, transudate and modified transudate.

In chylomediastinum, effusion from the thoracic duct will initially be limited to the mediastinum, but the fluid has usually entered the pleural space by the time the animal shows clinical signs.

Haemomediastinum may result from trauma. This may occur due to bleeding from one of the great vessels (usually rapidly fatal) or the haemorrhage may extend into the mediastinum from trauma to the neck. Other causes of mediastinal haemorrhage include coagulopathy, neoplastic erosion of vessels and, rarely, rapid involution of the thymus (usually fatal).

Oesophageal perforation results in mediastinitis, and initially small volumes of fluid may distribute evenly throughout the mediastinum.

Some neoplastic masses may produce a modified transudate.

Radiography

A DV view (Figure 10.46a) is usually the most useful, but changes can be subtle:

- Reverse fissures are visible at the heart base
- Increased width of both the cranial mediastinum and the caudoventral mediastinal reflection may be seen.

On lateral views (Figure 10.46b), the cranial border and apex of the heart and the cranioventral mediastinal reflection may be obscured.

Ultrasonography

Ultrasonography has limited use in the presence of small volumes of fluid due to the difficulty in locating a suitable

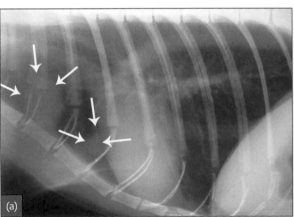

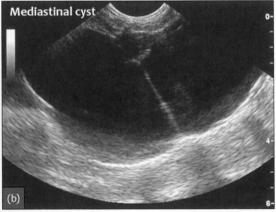

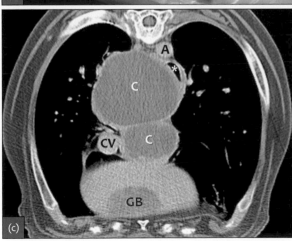

10.45 (a) Left lateral thoracic radiograph of a 12-year-old Siamese cat with two small cranial mediastinal cysts (arrowed). (b) Dorsal plane image of the cranial thorax of a 12-year-old spayed female Domestic Shorthaired cat with an ultrasonographically confirmed mediastinal cyst. On radiographs (not shown), the cyst appeared as a round soft tissue opacity cranial to the heart. Ultrasonographically, the cyst appears as an anechoic fluid-filled structure separated into two cavities by a thin septum. (c) Transverse CT image of the caudal mediastinum of an 11-year-old St. Bernard with confirmed cystic adenocarcinoma arising from the accessory lung lobe. The neoplasm produces two large fluid-filled cystic structures (C) in the dorsal part of the caudal mediastinum, adjacent to the left and right caudal lung lobes, caudal vena cava (CV), oesophagus (∗) and aorta (A). The appearance of the larger cyst is similar to that of empyema of the mediastinal serous cavity. GB = gallbladder.
(b, Courtesy of G. Seiler)

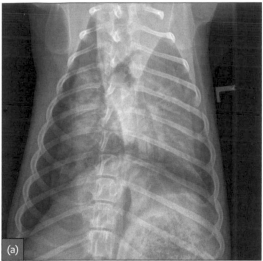

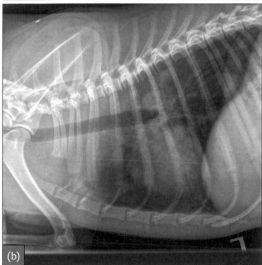

10.46 (a) DV and (b) left lateral thoracic radiographs of a 2-year-old Cocker Spaniel bitch following a road traffic accident. The cranial mediastinum is wide with caudal retraction of the lungs from the thoracic inlet and has a homogeneous soft tissue opacity that effaces the borders of the cardiac silhouette. In addition, the lungs are slightly retracted from the body wall and surrounded by gas, consistent with pneumothorax.

acoustic window but may be useful to guide sampling techniques. It can be difficult to differentiate pleural and mediastinal fluid based on ultrasonography alone. However, this distinction is easier in the cranial thorax where more typical appearances are identified:

- In the cranial thorax, fluid in the two pleural cavities is seen as two discrete pockets separated by the narrow ventral part of the cranial mediastinum (Figure 10.47)
- Cranial mediastinal fluid causes a wide mediastinum, and the mediastinal blood vessels are separated from fat by irregularly shaped fluid pockets.

Computed tomography

CT is much more sensitive for small volumes of mediastinal fluid and allows identification of pocketed fluid. Attenuation can be measured (CT number), which may provide useful additional information about the nature of the fluid, particularly if a sample is unobtainable. Altering the position of the animal (e.g. ventral *versus* dorsal recumbency) and repeating a CT sequence will assist in displacing pleural fluid, allowing better evaluation of coexisting lesions.

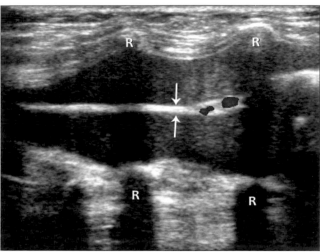

10.47 Dorsal plane image of the ventral aspect of the cranial mediastinum of a 3-year-old cat with a moderate bilateral pleural effusion. The entire width of the cat is included in the image. Note the left and right ribs (R). The cranial mediastinum is seen as a narrow echogenic band (between arrows) between the left and right pleural spaces, which are expanded and filled with anechoic fluid. Note the small blood vessels identified within the mediastinum with colour Doppler.

Mediastinitis

Mediastinitis implies infection or inflammation in the mediastinum. Acute mediastinitis is characterized by a thick irregularly marginated mediastinum and exudate production due to the infiltration of inflammatory cells and fluid. Fat stranding may be observed as an increased attenuation that is usually ill defined but may have linear components. With chronic mediastinitis, abscess or granuloma formation is also possible. Mediastinitis can develop from a primary disease process, such as fungal (*Histoplasma* or *Cryptococcus* species) or bacterial (including *Actinomyces* and *Nocardia* species) infection. Spirocercosis and pythiosis have also been associated with mediastinitis (Figure 10.48).

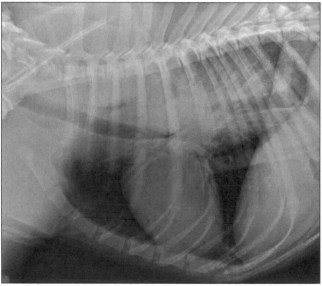

10.48 Lateral thoracic radiograph of an adult dog with pythiosis (infection by *Pythium insidiosum*, a fungus-like organism). The dorsal part of the mediastinum has a generalized increased opacity that is worst near the lung hilus and extends caudodorsally towards the diaphragm. No loss of definition of the cardiac silhouette is detected.

Mediastinitis may occur secondary to perforation of the trachea or oesophagus, or as an extension of an infectious or inflammatory process from the cervical soft tissue, pericardium, pulmonary parenchyma or pleural cavity. The most common cause is oesophageal perforation. Migrating foreign body is another cause. It is unusual for mediastinitis to occur alone; it more frequently occurs in association with pleuritis.

Clinical features may include tachypnoea, dyspnoea, pain, cough, regurgitation, vocal changes (secondary to recurrent laryngeal nerve involvement) and head and neck swelling.

Radiography

Radiographic changes are often subtle.

- Increased width and possible increased opacity of the mediastinum may be seen, particularly on DV and VD views.
- If the inflammation is focal then discrete masses may be seen, which must then be differentiated from neoplastic causes.
- Pneumomediastinum may be present, especially when the mediastinitis is secondary to tracheal, pharyngeal, or oesophageal perforation.

Contrast studies: If oesophageal perforation is suspected, then oral administration of a small volume (5–10 ml) of non-ionic water-soluble iodine-containing contrast medium, such as iohexol, may identify the site. Orthogonal views should be obtained to look for evidence of extravasation of the contrast medium. If no extravasation is seen on initial films, then repeat films should be taken 5–10 minutes later to look for slow leakage.

In cases of chronic oesophageal perforation, the original perforation may have closed, in which case no contrast leakage will be evident.

Ultrasonography

The usefulness of ultrasonography depends on the site and extent of the mediastinitis and whether any fluid or increased mediastinal thickness is loculated or focal. Ultrasonography allows guided sampling of the abnormal tissue. This is particularly useful for culture and sensitivity. Appearance of mediastinitis includes:

- Gross increased thickness and echogenicity of the mediastinal pleurae
- Small to moderate amounts of echogenic fluid
- Enlarged lymph nodes and gas may also be identified.

Computed tomography

As with mediastinal fluid, CT is very sensitive to small volumes of exudate or subtle increases in the thickness of the mediastinum. Fat stranding may be seen. Small volumes of mediastinal gas are easily seen when present. Contrast-enhanced CT images should show areas of inflammation or necrotic areas and allow the extent of the disease to be assessed (Figure 10.49).

Mediastinal oedema

Abnormal interstitial fluid accumulation in the mediastinum (i.e. mediastinal oedema) may accompany any condition that alters Starling forces and produces oedema elsewhere. It is often overlooked due to the concurrent presence of other mediastinal disease but may be more readily

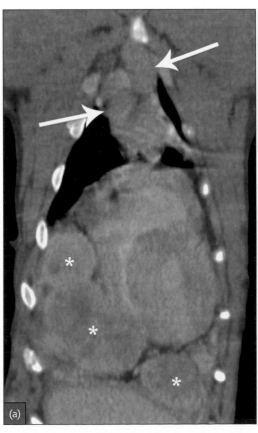
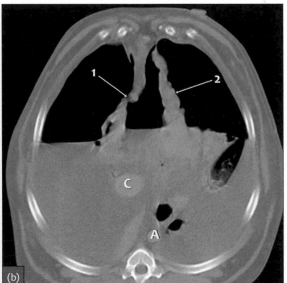

10.49 (a) Reformatted dorsal oblique contrast CT image of the ventral thorax of a 4-year-old neutered German Shorthaired Pointer bitch with *Actinomyces* infection showing irregular, peripherally enhancing masses in the caudal thorax (*) and enlargement of the cranial sternal lymph nodes (arrowed). (b) Transverse contrast CT image (soft tissue window) obtained at the level of the tenth thoracic vertebra of an 8-year-old Boxer with spread of suppurative inflammation throughout the thoracic cavity. The dog has bilateral pneumothorax. The dog was positioned in dorsal recumbency; note the gravity-dependent distribution of the pleural fluid and gas. The fluid was consistent with pyothorax (pleural empyema). The gas contrasts with the plica venae cavae (1) and caudoventral mediastinal reflection (2). Both are severely thickened and irregularly margined due to the infiltration of inflammatory cells and fluid, consistent with mediastinitis. A = aorta; C = caudal vena cava.

recognized now that CT and MRI are more commonly used to evaluate the mediastinum. During CT, mediastinal oedema may appear as regions of fat stranding and thick mediastinal pleurae. Fat stranding due to inflammation (mediastinitis) looks similar.

Oesophagus

Imaging anatomy

The oesophagus is located in the neck, thorax and cranial abdomen. It is the muscular tube that connects the pharynx to the stomach and is bounded at each end by functional sphincters (rather than true annular muscular sphincters). Cranially, the cricopharyngeal sphincter is composed of the pharyngeal constrictors including the cricopharyngeal and thyropharyngeal muscles, which are paired and largely fused. Caudally, the anatomy of the sphincter mechanism is complex due to contributions from focally thick oesophageal musculature, gastric rugal folds, muscular support from the diaphragm and stomach, the acute angle of the gastro-oesophageal junction, and positive intra-abdominal pressure.

The oesophageal wall is composed of four layers or tunics: mucosa, submucosa, muscularis and adventitia. In the caudal mediastinum, however, a portion of the oesophagus is covered by serosa and not adhered to adjacent structures (see 'Mediastinal serous cavity', above). In the dog, the mucosa forms longitudinal linear striations and the muscularis layer is striated muscle. In the cat, the caudal third of the muscularis layer is smooth muscle with the overlying mucosa having characteristic herringbone-like folds. During dynamic imaging, normal oesophageal motility may be observed as a coordinated series of constrictions and dilatations that propel lumen contents towards the stomach (peristalsis). A bolus entering the cranial part of the oesophagus initiates a primary peristaltic wave that conveys the bolus to the stomach. Any remaining lumen content is cleared by secondary peristaltic waves originating from anywhere along the path of the oesophagus. The bolus is typically caudally convex and cranially tapered.

In all animals suspected of having oesophageal disease, thoracic (including the stomach area) and cervical (including the pharyngeal area) radiographs should be obtained to examine the entire course of the oesophagus. The oesophagus is rarely visible on survey radiographs, although occasionally a portion of it may be visible on lateral views as a poorly defined, tubular, faint soft tissue opacity between the heart base and the diaphragm (Figure 10.50). Its visibility may be accentuated in emaciated animals and on left lateral views. In the neck, caudal to the pharynx, the oesophagus is dorsal to the trachea. In the mid-cervical and cranial thoracic regions, the oesophagus is more mobile but typically continues along the left dorsolateral aspect of the trachea. In the mid-to-caudal thorax, the oesophagus continues its course dorsal to the tracheal bifurcation to the stomach.

Small amounts of oesophageal air may be observed in four typical sites in normal dogs:

- In the most cranial aspect of the cervical oesophagus as a triangular gas opacity
- Cranial to the first rib
- Craniodorsal to the heart base
- Caudal to the cardiac silhouette, between the aorta and caudal vena cava.

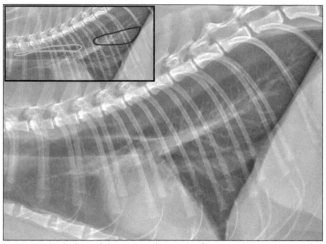

10.50 Right lateral thoracic radiograph of a normal oesophagus of an 8-year-old cat under general anaesthesia. The oesophageal lumen contains a small amount of gas dorsal to the heart (blue on inset) and a small amount of fluid cranial to the diaphragm (red on inset) that redistributed on other views.

Aerophagia, dyspnoea, excitement and sedation are all commonly associated with larger quantities of gas. General anaesthesia may cause marked generalized dilation of the normal oesophagus, mimicking megaoesophagus. Further studies may be warranted in animals with clinical signs of oesophageal disease and oesophageal air visible on survey radiographs.

Oesophageal disease may be present despite a normal radiographic appearance. Other signs of oesophageal disease may include:

- Aspiration pneumonia
- Pneumomediastinum
- Ventral displacement of the trachea
- Mediastinitis
- Pleural fluid
- Hypertrophic osteopathy.

Interpretative principles

Tracheal stripe sign

The tracheal stripe sign (Figure 10.51) is most prominent on left lateral radiographs but may be seen on right lateral radiographs and is known as the dorsal tracheal band or tracheo-oesophageal stripe sign. It is commonly seen as a thin band of soft tissue opacity with uniform height that is contrasted by gas on both sides. The soft tissue silhouette is formed by the combination of the ventral oesophageal wall draping over the dorsal tracheal wall. The gas opacities are in the lumens of the trachea (ventrally) and oesophagus (dorsally). Detection of the tracheal stripe sign indicates oesophageal luminal air, which may be of minor consequence (aerophagia) or a sign of oesophageal disease (especially when the length of the stripe is the same as the length of the thoracic part of the trachea). Due to the high variability in conformation of veterinary species, no ranges have been established for its normal thickness. Care should be taken not to confuse a tracheal stripe sign with a pneumomediastinum, where mediastinal gas may surround the external surface of the trachea and oesophagus.

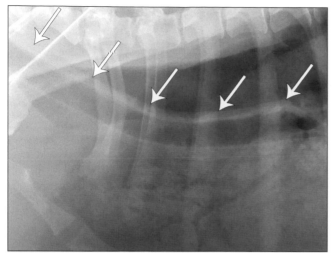

10.51 Close-up of a lateral thoracic radiograph of a dog with a diffusely enlarged, gas-filled oesophagus and cranioventral lung consolidation (aspiration pneumonia). The soft tissue stripe (arrowed) is a silhouette of the tracheal and oesophageal walls, contrasted dorsally and ventrally by gas.

Redundant oesophagus

A redundant oesophagus is one that is longer than expected and therefore may have a tortuous course. This is an occasional finding that is usually of minor consequence. Differentiating this condition from oesophageal disease is important. A redundant oesophagus is usually identified in the thoracic inlet as a ventral, but occasionally lateral, deviation of the oesophagus, mainly in young dogs of brachycephalic breeds (Figure 10.52) and the Shar Pei. It has also been described in the cat.

Diseases

Oesophageal enlargement is one of the most common imaging signs associated oesophageal disease. Overall diameter enlargement due to lumen enlargement is the most common form, but increased mural thickness can occur. Like most hollow organs, the enlarged oesophagus may be distended or flaccid depending on lumen

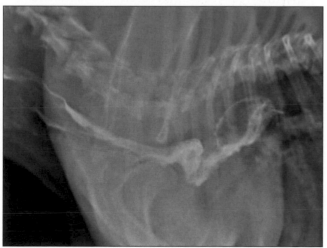

10.52 Fluoroscopic oesophagram with orally administered liquid barium suspension in a 1.5-year-old French Bulldog with severe laryngeal collapse and possible regurgitation. At the level of the second rib pair, the oesophagus has a sinuous course, which completely resolved with neck position and oesophageal peristalsis, consistent with a redundant oesophagus.

content and pressure. The enlargement may affect parts of (focal or segmental enlargement) or the entire (generalized enlargement) oesophagus. Recognizing the different types of oesophageal enlargement is important for prioritizing the differential diagnosis. Focal enlargement is usually due to a mass (e.g. neoplasm, abscess, granuloma) or foreign body. Segmental enlargement is usually due to lumen obstruction with secondary dilatation cranial to the obstruction (e.g. vascular ring anomaly, oesophageal stricture, foreign body). Generalized enlargement may be due to a caudal oesophageal obstruction (e.g. foreign body, neoplasm), oesophagitis, anaesthesia or neuromuscular dysfunction.

Megaoesophagus

Megaoesophagus is generalized or diffuse oesophageal enlargement with neuromuscular dysfunction and commonly produces decreased oesophageal peristalsis and regurgitation. However, some people use the term generically to indicate any type of oesophageal enlargement. This is most commonly an acquired condition, although congenital disease is occasionally encountered. German Shepherd Dogs, Golden Retrievers and Irish Setters have an increased risk for developing acquired megaoesophagus. The underlying cause often remains undetermined (idiopathic), although it may be secondary to one of many possible aetiologies (Figure 10.53).

A familial predisposition for congenital megaoesophagus has been suggested in the Irish Setter, Great Dane and German Shepherd Dog as well as several other breeds, presenting as either delayed oesophageal maturation or congenital myasthenia gravis. Congenital segmental oesophageal dysfunction has been reported in Shar Pei and Newfoundland dogs. Congenital megaoesophagus in cats is rare, but Siamese cats may be predisposed. Animals with megaoesophagus usually present with regurgitation or may occasionally be asymptomatic. In congenital cases, signs are usually first noticed after weaning.

Neuromuscular disease
• Idiopathic
• Myasthenia gravis
• Systemic lupus erythematosus
• Polymyositis/polymyopathy
• Glycogen storage disease
• Dermatomyositis
• Dysautonomia
• Distemper
• Tetanus
Caudal oesophageal obstruction
• Neoplasia
• Stricture
• Foreign body
Toxicity
• Lead
• Organophosphate
Miscellaneous
• Hypoadrenocorticism
• Oesophagitis
• Thymoma (paraneoplastic myasthenia gravis)
• Gastric dilatation–volvulus
• Hypothyroidism

10.53 Causes of generalized or diffuse oesophageal enlargement.

Key points

It is important to note that many animals without oesophageal disease will show incidental oesophageal dilation with a gas-filled lumen due to:

- Excitement
- Aerophagia
- General anaesthesia and sedation
  - If the history is suggestive of oesophageal disease, then consider repeating radiography in the conscious animal.

Radiography: Findings include:

- Generalized or focal oesophageal dilatation (Figure 10.54)
- Tracheal stripe sign
- Stark interface between oesophagus and longus colli muscles
- Rightward and ventral displacement of trachea
- May depress the heart (giving the impression of a small cardiac silhouette)
- Thin, soft tissue stripes representing oesophageal walls converging towards the diaphragm may be the only visible sign of a gas-distended oesophagus. Scrutiny is required as this sign may be easily overlooked (Figure 10.55)
- Increased amount of gas in the stomach or persistent gaseous gastric distension in the absence of torsion or pyloric obstruction
- Aspiration pneumonia is a common complication.

Contrast studies: In cases where survey radiographs are not definitive, then positive contrast oesophagrams may provide useful information about the presence and degree of oesophageal dilatation and previously undetected mural or lumen structural abnormalities, and oesophageal function (particularly when acquired with fluoroscopy). Risks of the procedure should be carefully weighed against potential diagnostic gains as these animals are at risk of aspiration pneumonia or asphyxiation. To lessen the risk of aspiration, consider horizontal views with the animal standing or in ventral recumbency.

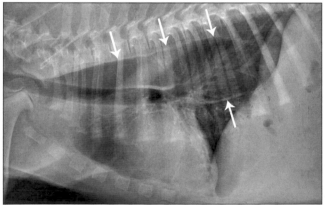

10.54 Right lateral thoracic radiograph of a 2-month-old Siberian Husky with regurgitation due to congenital megaoesophagus. The oesophagus is severely enlarged and distended, primarily with gas. Thin lines of soft tissue opacity represent the stretched oesophageal walls (arrowed), and the trachea and cardiac silhouette are mildly ventrally depressed. Note a tracheal stripe sign is less apparent in right lateral recumbency due to the redistribution of gas and fluid within the oesophageal lumen. Ventral to the fifth thoracic vertebra, the dorsal oesophageal wall is focally indented by the bronchoesophageal artery. Summating with the heart, the ventral tip of the left cranial lung lobe (caudal part) has mildly increased pulmonary opacity, consistent with aspiration pneumonia.

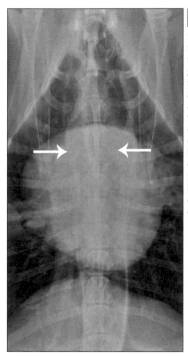

10.55 VD thoracic radiograph of a 5-year-old hound with acquired megaoesophagus due to myasthenia gravis. Note the gas-filled oesophagus, indented on the left by the aorta and on the right by the azygos vein (arrowed). The soft tissue stripes, representing the oesophageal wall, converge caudally at the oesophageal hiatus of the diaphragm. The dog also has aspiration pneumonia, seen here causing border effacement of portions of the left and right sides of the cardiac silhouette.

Oesophagitis

Oesophageal inflammation can be caused by chemical injuries from ingested substances (corrosives, pill or capsule retention), gastro-oesophageal reflux (secondary to general anaesthesia, hiatal defects, persistent vomiting, mispositioned feeding tubes), foreign bodies or structural abnormalities (e.g. neoplasm). It has been demonstrated to be a risk factor for the development of megaoesophagus in dogs. Oral dry administration of tablets (particularly tetracycline or doxycycline) has been associated with development of oesophagitis in cats.

Once oesophagitis has developed, a vicious cycle can ensue whereby inflammation decreases the tone of the caudal oesophageal sphincter, which leads to more reflux and inflammation. The prognosis for uncomplicated oesophagitis tends to be good.

Radiography: Radiographs are usually normal. Acute inflammation can cause increased wall thickness and functional disturbances such as reluctance to swallow and gastro-oesophageal reflux. Chronic inflammation can lead to fibrosis and stricture formation (see 'Oesophageal strictures', below). All these findings are difficult or impossible to detect during plain radiography. Observable findings that might be present include generalized or focal oesophageal dilatation (the lumen may be filled with air, ingesta or fluid) and the underlying cause (e.g. hernias, neoplasms or foreign bodies).

Contrast studies: Oesophagitis is an endoscopic diagnosis. Barium oesophagography is infrequently performed but may confirm:

- Motility disturbances
- Oesophageal dilatation
- Irregular mucosal surface, prominent mucosal folds
- Prolonged retention of contrast medium
- Signs of ulceration or perforation (Figure 10.56)
- Stricture formation.

When present, radiographic changes are often most evident in the caudal oesophagus.

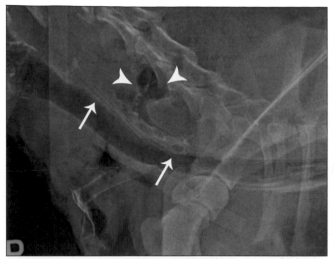

10.56 Lateral fluoroscopic oesophagram of a 2-year-old mixed-breed dog a week after a dog fight. A low-osmolar, non-ionic contrast medium was orally administered to examine for suspected oesophageal perforation. The oesophageal lumen is opacified by the contrast medium and has normal linear striations (arrowed). In the mid to caudal neck, contrast medium has leaked out of the oesophagus and into a large gas-filled pocket (arrowheads) between the oesophagus and vertebral column. In the caudoventral neck, deep wounds and a Penrose drain are visible.

Fluoroscopy with contrast medium: Dynamic swallowing studies (e.g. fluoroscopy) are more accurate than static contrast studies for the diagnosis of gastro-oesophageal reflux and the abnormalities that predispose to it, and oesophageal spasticity.

Oesophageal strictures

An oesophageal stricture is a circular band of scar tissue that forms secondary to severe oesophagitis. Typically 1–3 weeks following injury, progressive healing of the deeper oesophageal wall layers by fibrosis results in wall constriction and obstruction to food passage. The most common causes of stricture are gastro-oesophageal reflux (secondary to general anaesthesia) and trauma from oesophageal foreign bodies. Rarely, strictures are secondary to congenital or extraluminal disease (e.g. perioesophageal fibrosis due to mediastinitis or external compression due to perioesophageal mass).

Radiography: Plain radiographic findings are usually normal. Oesophageal dilatation with gas, fluid or ingesta within the lumen may be seen cranial to the stricture.

Contrast studies: Positive contrast studies (orally administered) are often needed to confirm stricture and assess location, length and degree of narrowing. Strictures are characterized by persistent luminal narrowing on sequential radiographs. Oesophageal dilatation cranial to the stenosis may be evident. Normal longitudinal striations tend to converge and/or become irregular at the site of injury to the mucosa. Subtle strictures may go unnoticed using only liquid contrast material and, therefore, mixing contrast material with semi-solid food or kibble can be helpful.

Fluoroscopy with oral contrast medium: This enables optimal evaluation of the length of strictures and maximal diameter of the narrowed segment and assessment of motility (Figure 10.57).

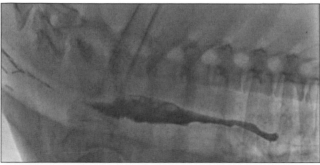

10.57 Lateral fluoroscopic oesophagram (inverted grayscale) with orally administered liquid barium suspension in a 2-year-old Labrador Retriever, 2 weeks after surgical repair of an oesophageal rupture that occurred during balloon dilation of strictures secondary to general anaesthesia. The oesophageal luminal surface is highly irregular due to scar tissue formation and inflammation (oesophagitis). At the cranial edge of the image, haemoclips partially summate with a trace of barium coating the lumen.

Ultrasonography: This modality is useful in diagnosing compressive strictures caused by an extramural mass. Ultrasound-guided FNA may be performed.

Oesophageal diverticulum

A diverticulum is an outpouching of a hollow viscus that is typically lined by epithelium (mucosa). True diverticula contain all wall layers and false diverticula involve herniation of the mucosa through a defect in the muscular and adventitial or serosal layers. Oesophageal diverticula are rare and may be congenital or acquired. The accumulation of food particles within diverticula leads to oesophagitis, mechanical obstruction and altered motility. Congenital diverticula are herniations of the mucosa through the muscularis, and most commonly occur in medium- to small-breed dogs. Acquired diverticula may be further classified by different mechanisms of formation:

- Pulsion diverticulum, from increased intraluminal pressure secondary to obstruction such as a stricture or foreign body
- Traction diverticulum, from perioesophageal inflammation and fibrosis. These are often small and insignificant.

When severe, diverticula may eventually perforate, resulting in mediastinitis. Diverticula should not be confused with normal redundancy of the oesophagus. Extending the animal's neck should smooth out any equivocal undulations. Diverticula also should not be confused with segmental oesophageal enlargement, which produces a circumferential enlargement (*versus* a focal outpouching).

Radiography: This is usually normal. When present, findings include:

- Pouch-like sacculation of the oesophagus (gas/ingesta)
- Ingesta more commonly collects in pulsion than traction diverticula.

Contrast studies: Findings include:
- Contrast medium within a pouch-like sacculation of the oesophagus
- Large multiloculated diverticula may only partially fill with contrast medium

- Pulsion diverticula usually have rounded or multilobed borders, a thin wall, and a neck similar in size to the diverticulum itself
- Traction diverticula usually have a triangular shape with a wide base at the oesophagus, a thick wall and a tip pointing to the area of adhesion.

Oesophageal neoplasia

Oesophageal neoplasms are rare and constitute less than 0.5% of all neoplasms in dogs and cats. In endemic areas, fibrosarcoma and osteosarcoma developing from malignant transformation of *Spirocerca lupi* granulomas (see 'Spirocercosis', below) are the most common malignant oesophageal neoplasms in dogs. Neoplasms may be primary oesophageal, perioesophageal (thyroid, thymus, heart base or lymph nodes) or metastatic (thyroid, pulmonary and gastric carcinomas). In dogs, primary neoplasms include leiomyoma, leiomyosarcoma, carcinoma and chondrosarcoma, while in cats, squamous cell carcinoma is the most diagnosed primary tumour. Leiomyomas have a slow growth rate and often have an indolent clinical course.

Radiography: Findings include:

- Oesophageal dilatation cranial to the lesion
- Formation of a mass or thick wall
- Displacement of the oesophagus by a perioesophageal tumour
- Mineralization of the oesophageal mass (rare)
  - Differential diagnoses for this finding include foreign body with mineral, accumulation of ingesta with mineral particles, coating of abnormal mucosa by oral medication of mineral opacity (e.g. bismuth).

Contrast studies: Positive or negative (pneumo-oesophagram) contrast medium may be used. A mural mass or filling defect and/or obstruction with pooling of contrast medium cranially to the abnormality may be demonstrated.

Ultrasonography: In most cases, this modality will be limited to examining the oesophagus in the cervical region, thoracic inlet, and caudal thoracic and cranial abdominal regions. Consider ultrasound-guided FNA of accessible lesions.

Computed tomography: This is particularly recommended when surgery is contemplated. It is the most sensitive diagnostic imaging tool for pulmonary metastasis (Figure 10.58) and allows evaluation of regional lymph nodes. Oral positive contrast material is not recommended due to beam hardening artefacts and risk of aspiration; however, insertion of an oesophageal tube confirms the position of the lumen in larger masses.

Oesophageal foreign body

Oesophageal foreign bodies are common in dogs (particularly young dogs and terriers) and unusual in cats. Most oesophageal foreign bodies occur due to ingestion but foreign bodies that perforate the pharynx or body wall may also affect the oesophagus. Retained intraluminal oesophageal foreign bodies may cause partial or complete mechanical obstruction to the caudal movement of ingesta, accentuated by muscle spasms and tissue oedema. Oesophageal foreign bodies commonly lodge at the level of the thoracic inlet, heart base or oesophageal hiatus. Radiographs should be obtained of the neck and thorax, from the pharynx to the stomach.

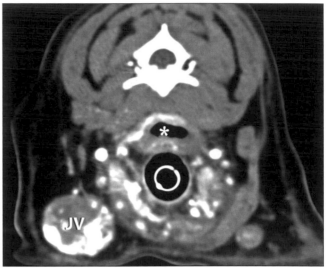

10.58 Transverse CT angiogram (arterial phase, soft tissue window) of the cranial neck of an adult mixed-breed dog with extensive regional and distant metastasis of a thyroid carcinoma, including large tumour thrombi in the jugular vein (JV). Associated with the neoplasm, there is a collection of anomalous blood vessels with arteriovenous shunting ventral to the oesophagus (*) and surrounding the trachea (note the tracheal tube). Arising from this, a vessel enters the cranial oesophageal wall, which is moderately irregularly thick and abnormally enhancing.

Complications, such as aspiration pneumonia or oesophageal perforation (with secondary pneumomediastinum, mediastinitis, pleural fluid, pleuritis, tracheo-oesophageal fistula) and underlying abnormalities that may have caused the foreign body to become stuck should be ruled out. The longer the foreign body has been lodged, and the sharper it is, the greater the chance of perforation and the greater the risk of rupture during retrieval (Figure 10.59). Radiographs are recommended after retrieval to assess for rupture and complete removal of the foreign body.

Radiography: Findings include:

- Focal structure localized to the oesophagus
  - Opacity may range from lucent to soft tissue (e.g. rawhide), mineral (e.g. bone) or metal (e.g. sewing needle, fishhook) depending on the composition. A foreign body with soft tissue opacity can resemble other masses such as neoplasms, granulomas, abscesses and paraoesophageal empyema (Figure 10.60)
- Variable oesophageal dilatation (gas/ingesta) cranial to the obstruction
- Small areas of gas accumulation within or around the foreign body
- Mass effect, most often with ventral and rightward displacement of the trachea
- Occasionally, no abnormality is detected
- Signs of complications (e.g. aspiration pneumonia, perforation and secondary mediastinitis, pleuritis and fistula)
- The dorsal portion of the cricoid cartilage is frequently mineralized enough to be visible on radiographs. This normal finding should not be mistaken for an oesophageal foreign body.

Contrast studies: Some foreign bodies are undetectable on plain radiographs and may require oral administration of contrast medium for diagnosis. If oesophageal perforation is suspected, it is important to use non-ionic, low-osmolar

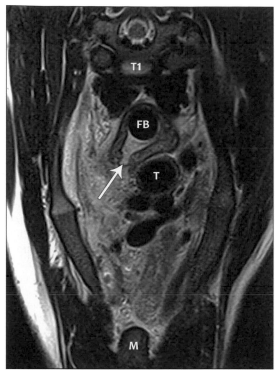

10.59 Transverse T2-weighted MRI image at the thoracic inlet of a 6-month-old Boxer with mediastinitis and brachial plexitis secondary to a perforating oesophageal foreign body (stick). The stick (FB) is located within the oesophageal lumen and has caused a focal wall rupture (arrowed). Surrounding the oesophagus and trachea (T), the mediastinum is severely swollen and hyperintense. The first thoracic vertebra (T1), manubrium (M) and first rib pair can be seen.

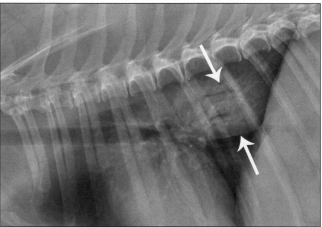

10.60 Right lateral thoracic radiograph of a 12-year-old terrier with a rawhide toy lodged in the caudal oesophagus (arrowed). The thoracic oesophagus is enlarged, and the lumen contains gas and a focal soft tissue opacity with linear gas striations attributed to the rawhide toy. An oesophageal foreign body with soft tissue opacity may resemble a focal mass, but the parallel gas lines facilitated the diagnosis in this case.

iodinated agents such as iohexol. Contrast studies will help differentiate between partial and complete obstruction. Findings include:

* Partial or completely obstructed caudal flow of contrast material
* Luminal filling defect (*versus* mural filling defect)
* Oesophageal dilatation cranial to the obstruction
* Contrast coating of the foreign body (persistent contrast material in the oesophageal lumen)
* Altered oesophageal motility (peristalsis) on dynamic studies.

Fluoroscopy: This may be used to guide the retrieval of the foreign body when performed with forceps but is unnecessary with endoscopy.

Vascular ring anomaly

Vascular ring anomalies are congenital malformations formed when arteries (or their atretic portions) partially or completely encircle the trachea and oesophagus, potentially constricting these structures (see also Chapter 9). Various vascular ring anomalies have been described but the most common approximately 90% of cases) involve persistence of the right fourth aortic arch (PRAA). Structures need to be present on both sides of the trachea and oesophagus to produce a 'ring' around these structures. With PRAA, the second part of the ring is usually the left ligamentum arteriosum. Other less common vascular anomalies include anomalous right or left subclavian arteries, double aortic arch, persistent right aorta, left aortic arch, right ligamentum arteriosum and aberrant intercostal arteries. Frequently, additional cardiovascular anomalies (such as a persistent left cranial vena cava) are present but may not be of clinical significance. The condition is likely heritable in German Shepherd Dogs, Labrador Retrievers and Greyhounds. Vascular ring anomalies are less common in the cat.

Certain clinical signs are common to all vascular ring anomalies. In carnivores, oesophageal obstruction is typically more problematic than airway obstruction; only double aortic arch anomalies produce significant tracheal stenosis and dyspnoea. Most cases present as thin and stunted with a history of regurgitation of solid food at the time of weaning. Rarely, the ductus arteriosus may remain patent, in which case clinical signs of a machinery or continuous heart murmur and radiographic signs of patent ductus arteriosus (PDA) are likely to be present (see Chapter 7).

Prognosis after surgical correction is guarded. Prognostic indicators are not established. No consistent relationship has been identified between age at surgery and prognosis, and oesophageal dilatation persisting following surgery does not appear to carry a poor prognosis. Affected animals should be expected to have an increased lifetime risk of regurgitation and aspiration.

Radiography: Findings include:

* Segmental oesophageal dilatation cranial to the stricture with abrupt caudal tapering at the heart base, around the level of the fourth–sixth intercostal space (Figure 10.61)
  * The enlarged lumen of the oesophagus has a variable appearance reflecting the nature of the contents (gas, fluid, ingesta)
* Ventral deviation of the thoracic trachea
* On DV and VD views, in dogs with a PRAA, moderate focal leftward curvature of the trachea may be observed near the cranial border of the heart because the aortic arch is abnormally positioned on the right side of the trachea (Figure 10.62). Oesophagography is not necessary to confirm diagnosis
  * The descending aorta (caudal to the aortic arch) is usually in the midline, although this may be difficult to assess radiographically
* If a well defined and normal left aortic arch is visible on a DV or VD view, then one of the less common vascular ring anomalies should be considered
* Moderate focal narrowing of the trachea

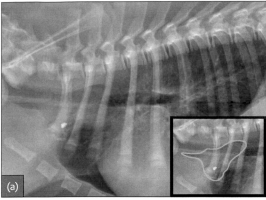

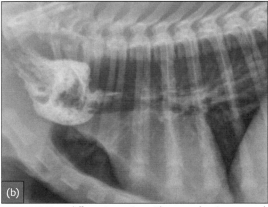

10.61 Two different puppies with a vascular ring anomaly comprising PRAA and segmental oesophageal dilatation cranial to the heart base. In both puppies, the cranial thoracic oesophagus is moderately distended. (a) Lateral thoracic radiograph. The oesophageal lumen is gas filled to the level of the third rib (outlined blue in inset) and contains a few mineral particles ventrally (gravel sign). (b) Lateral oesophagram. The oesophageal lumen is filled with barium and has a filling defect that is highly suggestive of indentation by the right aortic arch.

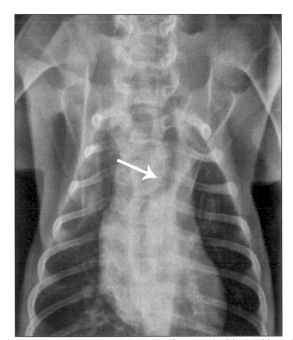

10.62 VD thoracic radiograph of a 12-week-old mixed-breed dog with PRAA that contributes to a vascular ring anomaly. At the level of the fourth thoracic vertebra, the abnormal right aortic arch causes severe leftward deviation of the trachea (arrowed). Also note that the cranial mediastinum is wide due to the segmental enlargement of the oesophagus.

- Focal tracheal stenosis and malformation of tracheal rings are suggestive of double aortic arch anomaly, although causes other than a vascular ring anomaly are possible
- Aspiration pneumonia is a common complication of a vascular ring anomaly
- Fibrous bands within the oesophagus may mimic vascular ring anomalies but angiography or oesophagoscopy will confirm the diagnosis.

Contrast studies: Orally administered contrast medium during radiography or fluoroscopy may assist diagnosis by confirming segmental oesophageal enlargement, location of the oesophageal obstruction and the severity of oesophageal distention. Contrast studies do not provide information about vascular anatomy, which may be needed for surgery. Altered oesophageal motility observed during fluoroscopy might offer additional prognostic information. During radiography, the right lateral view best demonstrates a curved filling defect associated with PRAA (see Figure 10.61).

Selective angiography: Selective angiography has been mostly supplanted by CT angiography. Angiography may reduce diagnostic uncertainty by confirming the type and location of the vascular anomaly.

Ultrasonography: Echocardiography is advised in cases of PDA and is useful to exclude other congenital cardiac abnormalities.

Computed tomography: CT angiography is recommended when there is suspicion of an atypical vascular ring anomaly or concurrent PDA and PRAA. CT angiography (arterial phase) is most useful for the characterization of these arterial malformations. A classification scheme for vascular ring anomalies has been proposed:

- In types 1–3 (Figure 10.63), the aortic arch is to the right of the trachea and oesophagus (dextropositioned)
  - Type 1 is the most common and results from a left ligamentum arteriosum connecting the aorta and pulmonic trunk dorsally, constricting the oesophagus ventrally against the trachea
  - Type 2 and 3 anomalies involve an aberrant left subclavian artery that crosses the oesophagus dorsally and laterally
  - In type 2, the ligamentum arteriosum is right-sided and does not constrict the oesophagus
  - In type 3, the normal left ligamentum arteriosum is present (as in type 1) and there are two sites of compression
- Type 4 anomalies represent double aortic arches that join caudal to the heart base to form a single descending aorta
- Other vascular malformations such as anomalous subclavian arteries may also result in entrapment of the oesophagus
- Except when a PDA is present, the thin ligamentum is not distinctly seen because of its size and lack of opacification (it is isoattenuating to the oesophagus so there is no contrast between the structures).

Spirocercosis

The nematode *Spirocerca lupi* may lead to the development of oesophageal granulomas and neoplasms. The condition is common in endemic areas (most tropical and

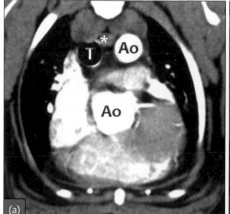
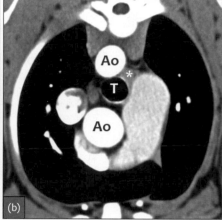
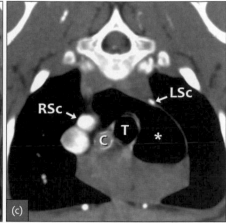

10.63 Transverse CT angiograms at the cranial aspect of the heart in three different dogs. Diagnosis of a vascular ring anomaly hinges on identifying the spatial arrangement of the blood vessels, trachea and oesophagus. However, the ligamentum arteriosum is not usually identifiable except in cases with PDA. Diagnosis also depends on identifying the result of a vascular ring (e.g. segmental oesophageal enlargement). (a) Normal arrangement. The oesophagus (*) and aortic arch (Ao) are to the left of the trachea (T). (b) Type 1 PRAA. The aortic arch circles to the right of the trachea and oesophagus. The oesophagus is compressed between the aorta, the pulmonic trunk on the left and the ligamentum arteriosum dorsally. (c) Type 3 PRAA with an aberrant left subclavian artery (LSc). Cranial to its origin on the descending aorta, the left subclavian artery runs dorsally and laterally to the oesophagus and contributes to the compression. Not shown on this slice, the right subclavian artery (RSc) has a separate origin from the trunk (C) that gives rise to both common carotid arteries.

subtropical countries) but otherwise very rare. Although any breed can be affected, the condition is seen more commonly in large-breed dogs. Infections in cats are reported. Eggs containing first-stage infective larvae are eaten by coprophagous dung beetles. Dogs then ingest the beetle or a paratenic host and the larvae penetrate the gastric wall, migrate through arteries and reach the thoracic aorta in about 3 weeks. After 10–12 weeks in the aorta, the larvae migrate to the oesophagus, and it is here that the adult develops within nodules in the oesophageal wall. With time, a granuloma forms and is typically situated in the caudal oesophageal wall. In atypical cases, it may be at the level of the lung hilus and be smaller. Granulomas may undergo neoplastic transformation to fibrosarcomas or osteosarcomas (26–41% of cases). Animals typically present with regurgitation (or, less commonly, vomiting) or an oesophageal mass may be identified as an incidental finding of major importance. Complications can occur due to perforation of the oesophagus (mediastinitis, pleuritis, mediastinal haematoma, aberrant migration with abscess formation) or rupture of the aortic aneurysm (acute haemothorax). Parotid salivary gland hypertrophy with hypersalivation may occur.

Radiography: Findings include:

- In clinically affected animals, a typical oesophageal mass will usually be seen on radiographs
  - On DV and VD views, a midline bulge with soft tissue opacity may be seen in the caudal thorax (Figure 10.64)
  - On the lateral view, an ill-defined soft tissue opacity may summate with the caudal oesophagus
  - Rarely, the mass may be in an atypical location such as the cranial or mid-thoracic oesophagus
- Ventral displacement of the caudal vena cava
- Oesophageal dilatation (gas/ingesta) cranial to the granuloma
- Signs of spondylitis of the caudal thoracic vertebrae (pathognomonic)
- 'Pseudospondylosis' (more lamellar spondylosis extending to midventral vertebral bodies)
- Mineralized foci within the granuloma (trapped mineralized ingesta or metaplasia into osteosarcoma)

- Metastasis to lungs
- Aortic aneurysm
- Hypertrophic osteopathy
- Periosteal reaction on ribs
- Signs of complications.

Contrast studies: A positive contrast oesophagram using barium mixed with canned food (barium burger) or a pneumo-oesophagram may show abnormalities: the former is preferred. A mass or mural filling defect may be seen (often dorsally) (Figure 10.65).

Ultrasonography: Oesophageal masses adjacent to the diaphragm can be seen via a transhepatic window. Ultrasonography may be useful to investigate mediastinal complications, guide sampling when indicated and characterize a hypertrophic parotid salivary gland.

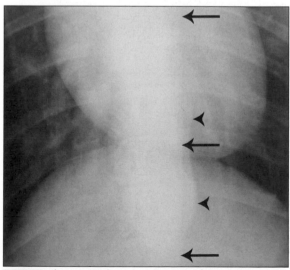

10.64 Close-up DV thoracic radiograph of the caudal oesophagus in a mature dog. In cases of suspected *S. lupi* infection, it is essential to follow the left outline of the aorta (arrowed). A second bulge in this area (arrowheads) is consistent with an oesophageal *S. lupi* granuloma, aortic aneurysm secondary to *S. lupi* infection or both.

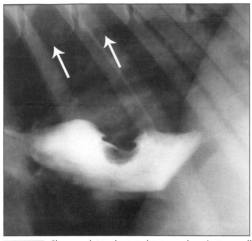

10.65 Close-up lateral oesophagram showing a small dorsal oesophageal wall filling defect consistent with *S. lupi* granuloma. Thoracic spondylitis (arrowed) is considered to be pathognomonic for *S. lupi* infection, especially in endemic areas. Spondylosis deformans is also present caudally and is an incidental finding of minor consequence unrelated to the infection.

Computed tomography: CT is recommended when considering surgical mass resection. Adding air to the oesophagus prior to scanning improves delineation of oesophageal masses (Figure 10.66). CT is excellent for early detection of thoracic metastases, focal aortic mineralization and signs of early spondylitis, and is best performed with the animal in ventral recumbency.

Pythiosis

Pythium insidiosum is an aquatic oomycete more closely related to algae than to fungi with a worldwide tropical and subtropical distribution. Pythiosis typically affects young, immunocompetent large-breed dogs and most commonly affects the small intestine, and with lesser frequency the stomach and colon, in its gastrointestinal form. Strict oesophageal involvement is infrequent. The disease is sporadically reported in cats. Zoospores exhibit chemotaxis towards wounds and damaged

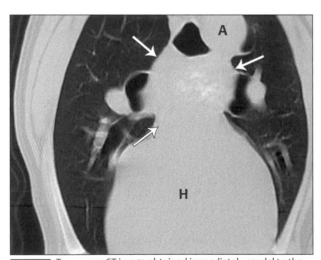

10.66 Transverse CT image obtained immediately caudal to the carina of an 8-year-old neutered male Dalmatian (window level -215 HU, window width 1996 HU (lung window)). An *S. lupi* granuloma is visible in the oesophagus (arrowed). The mineralization within is indicative of malignant transformation (osteosarcoma or fibrosarcoma). Dorsal to the mass, the oesophageal lumen contains a small amount of gas and the wall of the aorta (A) is partially mineralized. H = heart.

mucosal surfaces. Following entry, the infection provokes severe granulomatous inflammation of the alimentary tract and associated tissues.

Radiography: Findings include:

- Variably defined oesophageal mass with soft tissue opacity (Figure 10.67)
- Mediastinal infiltrations may blur the margins of the mass
- Cranial and caudal to the lesion, the oesophagus may contain gas
- Thick tracheal stripe
- Ventral deviation of the trachea and cardiac silhouette.

Contrast studies: Positive contrast oesophagrams may facilitate the recognition of the process as circumferential to the oesophagus and compressive. An irregular mucosal surface is expected.

Ultrasonography: If an acoustic window can be found, then the lesion will present as a circumferential hypoechoic oesophageal mass. Ultrasonography may be useful in assessing the degree of mediastinal involvement.

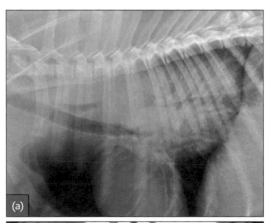
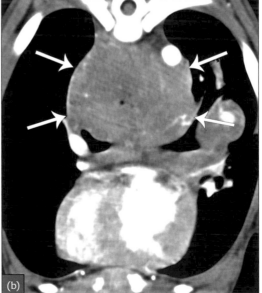

10.67 A 2-year-old Boxer with a history of hyporexia and regurgitation due to oesophageal pythiosis. (a) Lateral thoracic radiograph. An ill-defined dorsal mediastinal mass is present. Moderate oesophageal gas is dorsally displaced and interrupted at the level of the heart base. (b) Transverse CT image. The oesophagus (arrowed) is severely circumferentially thick, and this infiltrative process extends into the mediastinum and along the pulmonary vasculature.

Computed tomography: CT findings include:

- Circumferentially thick oesophageal wall (Figure 10.67)
- Strongly vascular lesion
- Moderate to severe lymphadenomegaly
- Mediastinal and peribronchial/perivascular extension
- Oesophageal extension to the stomach or cervical region.

Gastro-oesophageal intussusception

Gastro-oesophageal intussusception is a rare condition and results from the invagination of the stomach, with or without other abdominal viscera (spleen, duodenum, pancreas and omentum), into the caudal oesophageal lumen. Predisposing factors include megaoesophagus, congenital oesophageal abnormalities, incompetency of the caudal oesophageal sphincter mechanism and chronic vomiting. It has been reported to be more common in younger dogs (<3 months). The highest prevalence has been reported in large-breed dogs, particularly German Shepherd Dogs.

The clinical signs include regurgitation, vomiting and distress. Rapid deterioration occurs if a large portion of the stomach prolapses into the oesophagus. While the condition constitutes a surgical emergency, new studies show better survival rates (88% in one series (Grimes *et al.*, 2020)) than suggested in the earlier literature. Occasionally, gastro-oesophageal intussusception may be an intermittent problem or include only parts of the stomach.

Radiography: The radiographic signs are usually sensitive and specific enough for accurate and timely diagnosis. Lateral views tend to be the most helpful, but the orthogonal view may be helpful to confirm the mediastinal location of the displaced stomach. Findings include:

- Well demarcated soft tissue opacity or heterogeneous mass within the caudal oesophagus (Figure 10.68)
  - The cranial margin of the soft tissue opacity is usually cranially convex and contrasted by gas in the oesophageal lumen
- Gastric rugae extending into the mass
- Oesophageal dilatation (gas) cranial to the displaced stomach
- The gastric silhouette may be absent from the cranial abdomen or, when gas-distended, its lumen may reveal a defined communication with the mass
- Aspiration pneumonia is common.

Contrast studies: Rarely necessary and contraindicated if surgery is contemplated due to increased risk of aspiration and prolonged time to intervention. Findings include:

- Abrupt cessation of the passage of barium in the oesophagus
- Oesophageal dilatation at and cranial to the displaced stomach
- Gastric rugae are present within the oesophagus
- Contrast medium may outline transverse folds between the dilated oesophageal lumen and the displaced stomach.

Fluoroscopy with or without contrast medium: This may be useful to demonstrate intermittent disease. A false-negative result is possible with intermittent gastro-oesophageal intussusception.

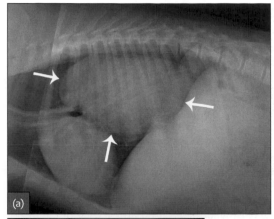
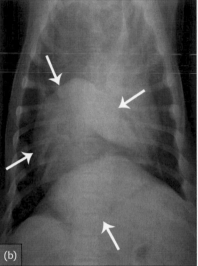

10.68 (a, b) Orthogonal thoracic radiographs in a dog with gastro-oesophageal intussusception. The stomach (arrowed) is displaced cranially into the caudal oesophagus. The displaced stomach appears as a large, circumscribed mass with homogeneous soft tissue opacity. Note the characteristic cranially convex margin of the stomach that is contrasted by gas within the oesophageal lumen. The oesophagus is severely enlarged and displaces the cardiac silhouette and trachea ventrally.

Ultrasonography: Abdominal ultrasonography helps document in real time the oesophageal location of the stomach, its vascularity and whether changes are dynamic.

Computed tomography: CT is usually unnecessary for diagnosis; however, if performed, findings may include:

- Stomach displaced into the lumen of the caudal oesophagus
- Concentric rings of oesophageal and gastric wall
- Gastric rugal folds are seen on the outer surface of the intussusceptum
- The gastric mucosa is expected to enhance in the early vascular phase. Absent or weak enhancement indicates vascular compromise
- Gastric and oesophageal wall oedema may be variable, depending on vascular compromise and duration, and present as thick hypoattenuating layers
- Gastric vasculature being drawn into the oesophagus
- Cranial displacement of abdominal organs (spleen, duodenum, pancreas, omentum).

Hiatal hernia

For information on hiatal hernias, see Chapter 8.

Trachea

Imaging anatomy

The trachea is a relatively non-collapsible tube that connects the larynx to the bronchial tree. Caudally, the trachea divides into two principal bronchi (left and right). At this level, called the tracheal bifurcation, the airway becomes focally wide. It is common to see a circular air opacity on lateral radiographs, which is an end-on air-filled bronchial lumen, summating with the tracheal bifurcation. This lucency is used to surmise the location of the tracheal carina, which is a dorsoventrally oriented ridge of soft tissue at the caudal aspect of the trachea between the principal bronchi (Figure 10.69). In normal dogs and cats, the tracheal bifurcation is located at the level of the fourth or fifth intercostal space (Figure 10.70).

Unlike most other hollow organs, the trachea is relatively non-collapsible because the wall is reinforced by C-shaped cartilages (often called tracheal rings). This emphasizes that one of the most important aspects of assessing the trachea for disease is maintenance of its lumen size. In addition to the tracheal cartilages, the trachea also comprises interconnecting tracheal ligaments, respiratory mucosa and a gas-filled lumen. Dorsally, the open-ringed cartilages are connected by the trachealis muscle and connective tissue; this membranous portion of the tracheal wall is called the paries membranaceus or, more commonly, the dorsal tracheal membrane.

- In carnivores, the normal adventitial surface of the tracheal wall is distinguishable from neighbouring cervical and mediastinal soft tissue. Therefore, it is often impossible to assess wall thickness. This margin may be seen with pneumomediastinum when gas contrasts with the external surface of the trachea. The cartilaginous rings within the wall may be seen and provide an estimate of wall thickness, especially ventrally.
- In cross-section, the canine and feline trachea is slightly wider (left-to-right) than it is tall (dorsoventrally).
- The tracheal diameter is larger in the cranial cervical region and narrows at the thoracic inlet.
- Radiographs should be obtained with the head and neck in neutral position to avoid artefacts associated with positioning.
- The cervical and thoracic trachea should be radiographed separately as exposure and positioning requirements differ.
- Mild dorsal deviation of the trachea at the level of the first intercostal space (Figure 10.71) is a normal anatomical variant mostly seen in terriers. It results from the passage of the right subclavian artery ventral to the trachea.
- Contrast radiographic studies are no longer recommended for the evaluation of tracheal disease, as aspiration of contrast media may result in pulmonary oedema or asphyxiation. Tracheobronchoscopy and CT have superseded these techniques.

Interpretative principles

Tracheal size, shape and opacity

The normal tracheal diameter is variable among breeds and species. The tracheal diameter is usually assessed subjectively, but the ratio of tracheal diameter to thoracic inlet diameter (TD:TI) on lateral thoracic radiographs has been used as an objective way to quantify lumen size (Figures 10.72 and 10.73). In dogs, the TD:TI significantly

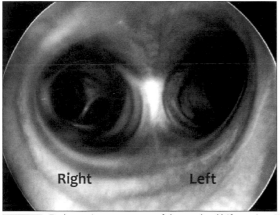

10.69 Endoscopic appearance of the tracheal bifurcation. The left and right principal bronchi are clearly visible, with the carina in the middle.
(Reproduced from the BSAVA Manual of Canine and Feline Endoscopy and Endosurgery; courtesy of T McCarthy)

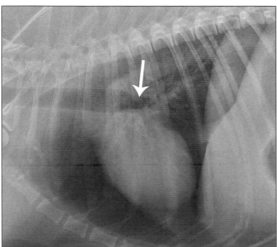

10.70 Left lateral thoracic radiograph of a 9-year-old crossbreed dog. In animals with a deep thorax conformation, such as this dog, the trachea diverges from the vertebral column with a more pronounced angle. The tracheal bifurcation (arrowed) is located at the fifth intercostal space.

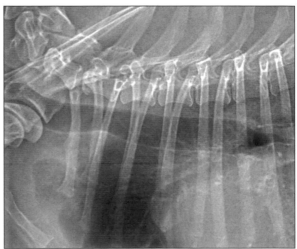

10.71 Lateral thoracic radiograph of a dog with mild dorsal elevation of the ventral tracheal wall at the first intercostal space. This appearance is a normal variant usually observed in shallow-chested dogs, such as terriers, and results from the right subclavian artery coursing ventral to the trachea at this level.

Skull shape	Normal tracheal diameter:thoracic inlet ratio
Meso- and dolichocephalic	0.21 ± 0.03
Brachycephalic (Bulldogs)	0.11 ± 0.03
Brachycephalic (other)	0.16 ± 0.03

10.72 Normal TD:TI for different canine skull shapes. These values do not apply to young dogs until about 9 months of age.

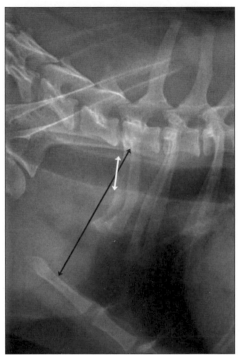

10.73 Close-up lateral thoracic radiograph of a normal Dachshund depicting calculation of the TD:TI. The thoracic inlet distance (black arrow) is measured from the ventral aspect of the vertebral column at the midpoint of the most cranial rib to the dorsal surface of the manubrium at its point of minimal thickness. The tracheal diameter (white arrow) is measured between the internal surfaces of the tracheal wall oriented perpendicularly to the tracheal long axis at the point where the thoracic inlet line crosses the midpoint of the tracheal lumen. In this dog, the TD:TI is 0.2.

changes during early growth and should not be applied before the age of 9 months.

- The tracheal lumen should be smoothly outlined. In the Dachshund and other chondrodystrophic breeds, the tracheal lumen can be irregularly outlined.
- Mild to moderate cartilage mineralization is a normal feature in skeletally mature dogs and cats. Marked cartilage mineralization can frequently be seen in giant-breed and chondrodystrophic dogs at all ages and is of no clinical importance.
- Conditions that promote metastatic calcification (e.g. hyperadrenocorticism) can diffusely affect the tracheal cartilages along with other soft tissues.
- In the normal dog and cat, the tracheal luminal diameter does not significantly change between inspiration and expiration.

Tracheal location

The trachea is mobile and therefore its position within the neck and thorax will vary with positioning or displacement by some space-occupying abnormalities. Differentiating normal anatomical and physiological variations from disease is important. The location of a displacement can indicate the underlying cause.

On lateral radiographs:

- In the cervical region, the trachea courses ventral and roughly parallel to the cervical vertebral column
- In the thorax, the trachea diverges from the vertebral canal, forming an angle that varies with body type (approximately 10–20 degrees)
  - The most caudal part of the trachea is further away from the vertebral column. This may not be the case in shallow-chested breeds
- Ventral neck flexion typically results in dorsal bowing (dorsal convexity) of the trachea, not to be mistaken for a sign of a cranial mediastinal mass.

On DV and VD radiographs:

- The trachea mostly summates with the vertebral column and sternum and leans slightly right of midline, especially in small barrel-chested breeds and obese animals. Displacement of the trachea from the midline is usually a sign of inappropriate positioning or mass effect.

Apparent tracheal narrowing of minor consequence

On lateral radiographs of dogs, the tracheal lumen near the thoracic inlet may appear narrow due to the presence of a broad-based band of soft tissue opacity that summates with the dorsal aspect of the tracheal lumen. This normal variation in the appearance of the trachea may be seen in animals with and without respiratory signs, is likely due to several different causes (e.g. altered cross-sectional shape of trachea, position of trachea, summation of soft tissue structures like the trachealis muscle, oesophagus and cervical musculature), and should not be mistaken for tracheal collapse without other evidence of tracheal collapse. This phenomenon has also been referred to as a 'pseudocollapse' (Figure 10.74), which is a misnomer because:

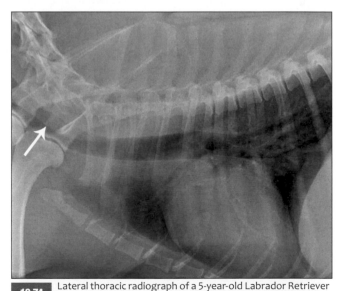

10.74 Lateral thoracic radiograph of a 5-year-old Labrador Retriever bitch without respiratory signs depicting pseudocollapse of the trachea. Note the band of soft tissue opacity summating with the dorsal portion of the cervical tracheal lumen (arrowed). The dorsal tracheal wall is visible in a normal position. This normal finding should not be mistaken for tracheal collapse.

- A true narrowing of the tracheal lumen is always present, but probably not permanent or marked enough to cause clinical signs
- The dorsally located trachealis muscle allows partial invagination of itself or extratracheal structures into the tracheal lumen (sometimes referred to as 'redundant tracheal membrane', although there is no redundant tissue)
- Extension of the head and neck promotes compression and narrowing of the tracheal lumen.

Although not commonly observed during imaging, contraction of the trachealis muscle normally narrows the tracheal lumen to increase intraluminal pressure (e.g. during coughing).

Dynamic height changes with respiration

The tracheal luminal diameter should not change markedly between inspiration and expiration. Dynamic variation in the tracheal luminal diameter is increased by:

- Softening of the tracheal rings
- Flaring of the tracheal rings
- Obstruction to air flow
- Respiratory effort.

Pharyngeal, laryngeal and intrathoracic conditions can influence tracheal dynamics and therefore these areas should also be assessed radiographically. The phase of respiration is important in the diagnosis of tracheal collapse and thus radiographs should be taken during both inhalation and exhalation, including both the cervical and thoracic parts of the trachea.

Echotracheography

The cervical trachea can be evaluated ultrasonographically; however, anatomical factors and luminal air may limit visibility of the dorsal wall. Identification of tracheal collapse is possible with this modality in the cervical region only, seen as a crescentic trachea during collapse. Intrathoracic portions of the trachea are practically inaccessible with ultrasonography wherever intervening aerated lung is present.

Computed tomography

Indications and limitations: Tracheal CT is a useful technique to investigate:

- Rupture
- Collapse
- Mass
- Obstruction or stenosis
- Stent placement.

Tracheoscopy remains the gold standard for the evaluation of rupture or collapse. Advantages of tracheal CT compared with other modalities include:

- Cross-sectional evaluation of the entire length of the trachea
- Real-time evaluation during the respiratory cycle (dynamic cine-CT or shuttle acquisitions)
- Images acquired during apnoea and positive-pressure ventilation can be compared to show dynamic differences in the trachea associated with intraluminal pressure changes.

The technique is limited by anaesthetic requirements:

- Intubation may be necessary to keep airways open but often masks the pathology
- Compliant, stable animals may do well with sedation only
- Dynamic studies are preferentially performed in conscious animals, which is only rarely possible.

When tracheoscopy is unavailable, tracheal CT is very useful for the follow-up examination of dogs with intraluminal stent placement for tracheal collapse. CT allows differentiation of intraluminal fluid accumulation from excessive granulation tissue, which is otherwise a difficult task.

Diseases

Tracheal diseases can be categorized according to morphological and dynamic nature, or by origin (intraluminal, mural or extramural) (Figure 10.75).

Tracheal hypoplasia

Tracheal hypoplasia is a congenital developmental anomaly characterized by abnormal narrowing of the tracheal lumen by at least 50% of the cross-sectional area, affecting the entire length of the trachea. The tracheal rings are almost complete with negligible dorsal muscle.

- Bulldogs and Mastiffs are more commonly affected than other breeds.
- The smallest TD:TI in Bulldogs without clinical signs of respiratory disease is 0.09.
- Has been described in the Labrador Retriever, German Shepherd Dog, Weimaraner and Basset Hound.
- Rare in cats.
- Tracheal hypoplasia is one component of canine brachycephalic obstructive airway syndrome, which can include stenotic nares and elongated soft palate along with other nasal and oropharyngeal anatomical abnormalities.

Morphological – intraluminal and mural disorders

• Tracheitis
• Tracheal oedema, inhalational injury
• Tracheal stricture:
  • Generalized – hypoplastic trachea
  • Localized – segmental stricture, scarring
• Tracheal foreign body
• Tracheal neoplasm
• Endotracheal granuloma – parasites, infection
• Tracheal trauma – bite wounds, laceration

Dynamic disorders – tracheal collapse syndrome
• Caudal cervical – inspiratory • Intrathoracic – expiratory • Generalized – inspiratory/expiratory
Extramural disorders
• Cervical mass – thyroid gland, abscess • Cranial mediastinal mass – lymphoma, thymoma, abscess • Cardiomegaly • Craniodorsal mediastinal mass (rare) – soft tissue sarcoma, vertebral body tumour • Megaoesophagus and oesophageal foreign body • Perihilar mass – lymphoma, granuloma, heart base tumour

10.75 Classification of tracheal diseases.

- Concurrent congenital abnormalities (e.g. megaoesophagus, pulmonic stenosis, aortic stenosis) have also been identified.
- Caution should be exercised before diagnosing this condition in puppies before the age of 6 months. The TD:TI is significantly smaller in dogs <9 months of age (Figure 10.76).
- Affected animals may present with stridor, dyspnoea, reduced exercise tolerance and coughing.

Imaging findings:

- Radiographically, the trachea appears uniformly narrow compared with the variation of luminal size along the length of the trachea seen with tracheal collapse.
- Increased wall thickness (Figure 10.77) may be identified and can be a result of chronic inflammation or genetic factors.

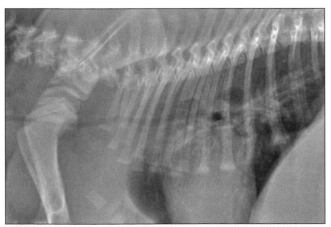

10.76 Lateral thoracic radiograph of a 2-month-old Bulldog puppy with dyspnoea of 3 weeks' duration. The tracheal diameter is diffusely very small and consistent with tracheal hypoplasia (a congenital developmental anomaly). However, although tracheal hypoplasia may have contributed to the severity of the clinical signs, the clinical signs fully resolved following treatment for severe concurrent laryngitis and suspected bronchitis.

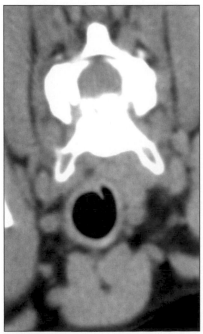

10.77 Transverse CT image of the trachea at the level of the sixth cervical vertebra of a Beagle cross with mucopolysaccharidosis VII. The tracheal cartilages are thick for the breed and overlap, resulting in a reduced tracheal lumen.

Focal tracheal stricture

Focal tracheal stricture is a rare condition resulting in abnormal focal narrowing of the trachea, usually affecting all wall layers, and may involve:

- Strictures secondary to trauma such as bite wounds, prolonged intubation or tracheal surgery
- Congenital segmental tracheal stenosis, for which different configurations have been described (e.g. laterolateral)
- In some instances, severe tracheal collapse (see below) may be mistaken for a focal tracheal stricture, mostly in Yorkshire Terriers. In the caudal cervical region, the tracheal cartilages are abnormally shaped such that the ventral aspect of the cartilage is statically dorsally convex and projects into the tracheal lumen, mimicking tumours, foreign bodies or strictures (Figure 10.78).

Focal tracheal stricture may occur without clinical signs despite a reduction of up to 80% in the size of the tracheal lumen in cross-section. In severe cases, the stricture may result in exertional dyspnoea, wheezing and coughing, with the potential for cyanosis, syncope or asphyxiation.

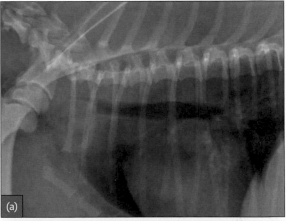

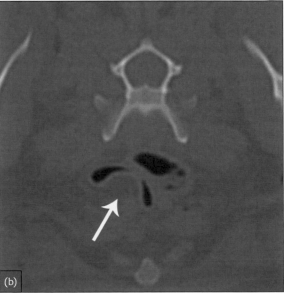

10.78 Caudal cervical tracheal malformation in a small-breed dog. (a) Lateral thoracic radiograph. At the level of the thoracic inlet, the tracheal lumen is severely narrowed by a smooth, broad-based mass effacing the ventral tracheal wall. (b) Transverse CT image of the neck. The apparent mass is due to buckling and rigid inward bowing of the tracheal rings. Note the trachea has a 'W' shape typical of this condition (arrowed).

Imaging findings:

- Focal narrowing of the trachea.
- Length may be variable.
- Irregular margin of the stricture attributed to soft tissue proliferation due to loss of cartilage support.
- CT can be very helpful for determining the exact location and extent of stricture.
- In some instances of tracheal collapse: dorsally convex with a smooth bulge and unchanged appearance in dynamic imaging. Easily differentiated from other conditions with CT or tracheoscopy.

Interventional radiology procedures: Balloon dilation or intraluminal tracheal stent placement can alleviate airway obstruction.

Tracheal collapse

Tracheal collapse is narrowing of the tracheal lumen due to loss of wall support. The narrowing may be static or dynamic during inhalation and exhalation. In most instances, tracheal collapse is a progressive, degenerative disease that causes gradual weakening of the tracheal cartilages, predominantly affecting middle-aged to older small- and toy-breed dogs.

- Cartilage rigidity is decreased due to hypocellularity and reduced glycosaminoglycan and calcium content.
- Soft tracheal cartilages result in dynamic tracheal collapse during respiration.
- Elongation of the dorsal tracheal membrane, and lateral flaring of the tracheal cartilages, results in a flattening of the trachea into a crescent shape.
- Tracheal collapse may be:
  - Inspiratory, involving the cervical region
  - Expiratory, involving the thoracic region
  - Mixed, involving the entire trachea.
- The location and degree of collapse are variable, and a mild degree of tracheal collapse is commonly seen in older small and toy breeds, often without clinical signs. Collapse often extends to the bronchi.

Clinical signs range from a mild, intermittent 'honking' cough to severe respiratory distress and cyanosis.

- Coughing can be elicited by tracheal compression and may be exacerbated by excitement, such as pulling against a collar or drinking cold water.
- Tracheal collapse may be associated with tracheobronchitis, laryngeal oedema, emphysema, hepatomegaly, left heart failure or cor pulmonale.
- Tracheobronchoscopy is very useful for the diagnosis of tracheal collapse and a scoring system has been developed, which serves as the gold standard (Figure 10.79).

Cervical tracheal collapse can occur during inhalation due to laryngeal or nasopharyngeal airway obstruction (e.g. laryngeal paralysis, masses, laryngitis, nasopharyngeal polyps) causing a sufficient negative intratracheal pressure to exceed the strength of the cartilaginous rings and collapse the tracheal lumen.

- In cats, tracheal collapse is nearly pathognomonic of upper respiratory tract obstruction. In this species, cartilage ring degeneration has only been described in mucopolysaccharidosis.

Imaging findings: Radiography, fluoroscopy and CT are all used in the diagnosis of clinically significant tracheal collapse.

- The lateral radiographic view is most useful in demonstrating the tracheal lumen.
- DV radiographs may demonstrate a fusiform widening of the trachea in areas that are narrowed on the lateral view.
- Historically, the craniocaudal tangential view of the thoracic inlet was used to demonstrate tracheal collapse. This technique was supplanted by endoscopy, fluoroscopy and CT as it is difficult to perform, results in personnel exposure and shows a limited portion of the trachea.
- Fluoroscopy is particularly useful to demonstrate dynamic changes in phase with respiration.
- Inspiratory and expiratory lateral radiographs should be acquired to assess for cervical (extrathoracic) and intrathoracic collapse. Timing of exposure can be challenging as affected animals often suffer from shallow breathing. Figure 10.80 demonstrates the effect of respiration phase on the radiographic appearance of the collapsing trachea.
- At inspiration, an abnormal cervical segment collapses and the thoracic segment dilates (Figure 10.81a).

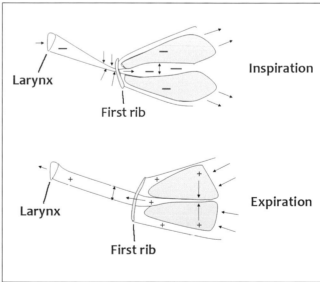

Grade	Degree of tracheal collapse
1 – mild	25%
2 – moderate	50%
3 – severe	75%
4 – total	100%

10.79 Tracheobronchoscopic grading of tracheal collapse.

10.80 The dependence of tracheal collapse on phase of respiration. During inspiration, there is a slightly negative pressure within the lumen of the cervical trachea when air moves towards the thorax. This pressure difference collapses the cervical trachea when the tracheal wall lacks sufficient stability. In the thoracic area, the pressure within the trachea is higher than the pressure within the thoracic cavity, which results in tracheal distention. During expiration, the cervical trachea is distended due to the luminal pressure exceeding the outside pressure when air flows towards the larynx. However, the thoracic pressure exceeds the intratracheal pressure, which collapses the thoracic trachea when the tracheal wall lacks sufficient stability.
(Redrawn after Suter (1984))

- At expiration, an abnormal thoracic segment collapses and the cervical segment is normal (Figure 10.81b).
- Radiography underestimates the degree of tracheal collapse compared with fluoroscopy, correctly identifying the disease in only 59% of cases, but is useful in identifying concurrent pulmonary or cardiac disease.
- The ventral wall of the trachea usually retains a normal shape, while the dorsal border is blurred or irregular due to many factors, including uneven flaring of the tracheal rings, rotation of the trachea, superimposition of structures and inflammatory mucosal changes (Figure 10.82).
- Imaging of the larynx, pharynx and nasal cavities can be helpful to rule out upper airway obstruction as a cause of cervical tracheal collapse, particularly in cats (Figure 10.83).

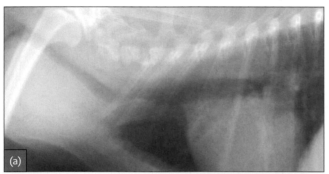

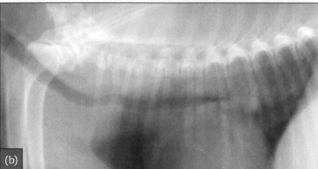

10.81 (a) Lateral radiograph centred on the thoracic inlet of a 15-year-old Miniature Poodle showing partial collapse of the extrathoracic (cervical) portion and a distended intrathoracic portion of the trachea during inspiration. Also notice the well expanded and aerated lungs and height of the principal bronchi. (b) Lateral radiograph demonstrating partial collapse of the intrathoracic portion and normal diameter of the cervical portion of the trachea during expiration. Notice the smaller lung volume, pulmonary opacification and collapsed principal bronchi.

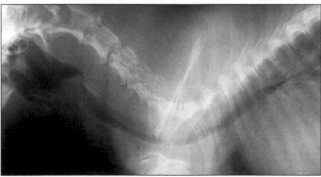

10.82 Lateral cervicothoracic radiograph of a 16-year-old Chihuahua with extensive cervical and thoracic tracheal collapse. Notice the curvilinear ventral and undulating dorsal aspect of the collapsing tracheal wall.

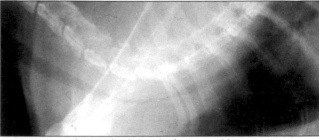

10.83 Lateral cervical radiograph of a 6-year-old Domestic Shorthaired cat with chronic inspiratory stridor. Notice the marked collapse of the caudal cervical trachea. A congenital deformation in the cranial end of the trachea with significant luminal obstruction was found on post-mortem examination.
(Reproduced from Hendricks and O'Brien (1985) with permission

Interventional radiological procedures: Intraluminal tracheal stent placement is a valid technique to treat tracheal collapse in selected cases.

Tracheal laceration and avulsion

Tracheal lacerations or avulsions are rare but serious conditions typically associated with trauma, such as road traffic accidents, bite injuries and overzealous intubation (mostly in cats). Wound dehiscence following tracheal surgery (e.g. for removal of a tracheal neoplasm) and rapid neck hyperextension injury ('whiplash') are rare causes.

- Clinical signs include dyspnoea of variable severity depending on the size of the lesion, subcutaneous emphysema, pneumomediastinum and possible pneumothorax.
- Clinical signs are often delayed and related to subsequent tracheal strictures presenting 10–14 days after the event.

Imaging findings:

- The tracheal wall abnormality itself may not be directly visible, with secondary features being more readily identifiable (Figure 10.84).
- The shape of the trachea may be altered with irregularity of the walls, lumen or both.

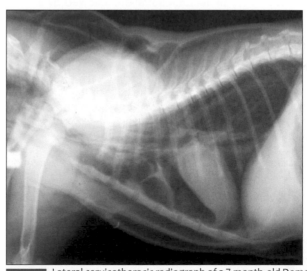

10.84 Lateral cervicothoracic radiograph of a 7-month-old Domestic Shorthaired cat suffering from a tracheal intubation injury sustained during a routine spay procedure. The laceration site is not directly visible but the secondary subcutaneous emphysema and pneumomediastinum are. The tracheal wall is contrasted by gas on both sides.

- Pneumomediastinum is commonly identified and may be localized or generalized. This may occasionally progress to a pneumothorax, pneumoretroperitoneum or pneumoperitoneum.
- Discontinuous tracheal margins may be seen with a complete tracheal rupture. In addition, a 'pseudotrachea' may be identified radiographically, seen as a ballooned focal area of the trachea where a complete rupture has occurred. These may be better seen in the subacute phase. Tracheal rings are absent in this section. Local mediastinal tissues focally distend with air only, giving the impression of an intact tracheal wall (Figure 10.85).

Tracheal masses

Endotracheal masses cause tracheal stenosis and include neoplasms, abscesses, granulomas, polyps and haematomas. Local haematomas may also occur with rodenticide toxicity, although diffuse narrowing of the trachea is more common in this condition due to bleeding into the tracheal wall or mediastinum.

- Tracheal masses are rare and often not identifiable if small or surrounded by fluid. They may be focal and polypoid, sessile or plaque-like.
- Tracheal granulomas can occur due to infection (parasitic, fungal or bacterial) or following tracheotomy or stent placement. Inflammatory masses include lymphoplasmacytic infiltration and lymphoid hyperplasia.
- Tracheal neoplasms are rare in dogs and cats but include lymphoma, epithelial neoplasms (e.g. carcinomas), and mesenchymal neoplasms (e.g. osteochondroma, chondrosarcoma (Figure 10.86)). Tumours that arise external to the trachea may compress or invade the tracheal wall (e.g. thyroid carcinoma, lung neoplasm, aortic body neoplasm, oesophageal tumour) although this is not a common finding.

Clinical signs depend on the degree of stenosis. Up to half the airway may be compromised without the appearance of clinical signs, meaning the condition can go unnoticed until it is advanced. Close examination may reveal a slow inspiratory phase of respiration, followed by a more rapid expiratory phase. Progressively, stridor and rattles, paroxysmal coughing, gagging, dyspnoea and dysphonia may occur.

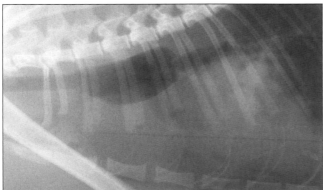

10.85 Lateral thoracic radiograph of a 4-year-old Domestic Shorthaired cat with complete tracheal rupture due to a road traffic accident. Notice the absence of tracheal rings within the ballooned radiolucent area extending from the second to fourth intercostal spaces. This gas bubble contained in local mediastinal tissues is sometimes referred to as a pseudotrachea.
(Courtesy of E. Friend)

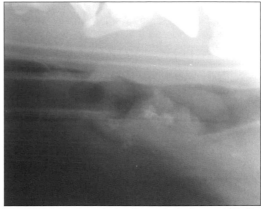

10.86 Lateral cervical radiograph of a 7-year-old Rottweiler with chronic upper respiratory distress. There is a mass of soft tissue and mineral opacity arising from the ventral aspect of the tracheal wall, inhibiting further passage of the endotracheal tube. An oesophageal tube can be seen dorsally. Final diagnosis was a tracheal chondrosarcoma.

Imaging findings: Radiography is relatively sensitive but not specific for the diagnosis of tracheal masses.

- The main radiographic finding is a mass, usually of a soft tissue opacity, that is associated with the tracheal wall and projects into the lumen where it is contrasted by gas.
- Diffuse pulmonary underinflation may be seen with cervical tracheal obstruction.
- Air trapping in the lungs may occur with intrathoracic tracheal obstruction.

Contrast-enhanced CT allows assessment of the exact location and extent of tracheal masses (Figure 10.87).

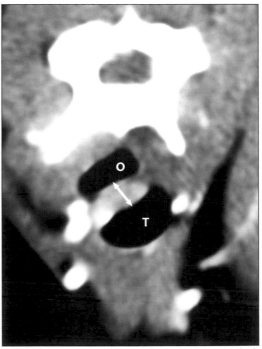

10.87 Transverse contrast-enhanced CT image at the level of the sixth cervical vertebra of a 10-year-old Domestic Shorthaired cat with chronic inspiratory dyspnoea. There is a contrast-enhancing soft tissue mass (arrowed) arising from the dorsal wall of the trachea (T) adjacent to the gas-distended oesophagus (O). Final diagnosis was a tracheal lymphoma. Tracheal resection and chemotherapy maintained this cat in remission for almost 2 years.

Interventional tracheal radiology: Intraluminal stent placement can alleviate airway obstruction caused by tracheal masses that are not readily accessible via surgery, or when surgery is declined or not indicated.

Foreign material in the trachea

The ease with which foreign bodies in the trachea can be seen depends upon the opacity, location and size of the foreign body, and the radiographic view used.

- Tracheobronchial secretions and superimposition of skeletal structures may impair detection of foreign bodies.
- Inhaled foreign bodies are most often found in young animals, with larger types, such as teeth and small stones, lodging at the tracheal bifurcation and smaller foreign bodies, such as grass awns, passing into the bronchi.
- The left caudal lobar bronchus is the most common site for bronchial foreign bodies as it continues in a straight line from the trachea.
- Small foreign bodies may be coughed out, unless they are barbed or pointed, or are surrounded by mucus, which may adhere them to the tracheal wall.

Clinically, animals with tracheal foreign bodies are more likely to present with dyspnoea and respiratory noise, while animals with bronchial foreign bodies more commonly produce a cough of sudden onset. The latter are more commonly working dogs. Haemoptysis may be seen. Chronic cases of plant awn inhalation may progress to abscessation with perforation of the bronchus and the development of pneumonia, pyothorax and infection of distant sites. In cats, the prominent ossified clavicles can summate with the tracheal lumen and should not be confused with a tracheal foreign body.

Imaging findings:
- The foreign body may cause focal reduced size of the gas-filled tracheal lumen without loss of overall tracheal diameter.
- Intraluminal mineral and bone opaque foreign bodies such as stones, bones, teeth and marbles are easily seen (Figure 10.88).
- Intraluminal plastic or organic foreign bodies are less visible, although their non-anatomical shape may help in identification.

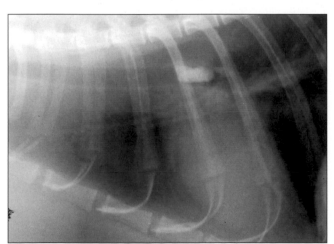

10.88 Lateral thoracic radiograph of a 5-year-old Domestic Shorthaired cat with a mineral opaque foreign body in the caudal trachea.
(Courtesy of E. Friend)

- An endotracheal tube that has been bitten through and dislodged during anaesthetic recovery can be seen radiographically and removed endoscopically.
- Intraluminal mucus surrounding the foreign body may be seen as a focal increase in soft tissue opacity.
- Fluid in the tracheal lumen is not radiographically visible since it does not create clear margins, unless using a horizontal X-ray beam. However, aspirated barium liquid will be easily recognized due to its mineral opacity. Small amounts are of no clinical consequence.
- Bronchial foreign bodies may cause obstructive atelectasis, especially when chronic, or obstructive air trapping, especially when an acute foreign body acts like a valve (see Chapter 7).

Interventional radiological procedures: Interventional radiological techniques are useful for retrieval of foreign bodies in the trachea and principal bronchi. Interventional radiology is particularly valuable in small animals where surgical or endoscopic intervention could severely compromise airway patency.

Tracheitis

Inflammation of the trachea may occur due to viral, bacterial or parasitic infection, or may have a non-infectious cause such as prolonged barking, collapsing trachea, chronic cardiac disease or inhaled irritants (e.g. smoke).

- Irritation by gas, dust or allergy may result in tracheitis, and severe cases may be associated with bronchitis or bronchopneumonia.
- Exudate, necrosis and mucosal proliferation, as well as contraction of the trachealis muscle, may result in narrowing of the tracheal lumen.
- Clinically, a dry, sometimes paroxysmal cough is seen and may be associated with discomfort or rarely dyspnoea. The animal is otherwise healthy in uncomplicated cases of tracheobronchitis.

Imaging findings: Tracheitis is often radiographically unremarkable unless it is severe or complicated by tracheal collapse, cardiac disease or pulmonary disease. Acute severe tracheobronchitis may result in diffuse luminal narrowing due to increased wall thickness and may mimic tracheal hypoplasia. Severe airway collapse (e.g. bronchospasm) is possible and may be life-threatening.

Oslerus osleri *infection:* This parasitic infection, previously called *Filaroides osleri*, is now relatively rare and is usually identified in dogs less than 2 years old and in kennelled dogs, such as racing Greyhounds.

- Direct transmission from dog to dog is possible, including from dam to puppy through faeces and saliva.
- Clinical signs may be absent or, in more advanced cases, wheezing, dyspnoea and weight loss may be observed.
- Clinical signs include a mild to paroxysmal hacking and often unproductive cough, which may end in retching and is unresponsive to antibiotics.
- The trachea is sensitive to palpation and, unless a secondary infection is present, body temperature is normal.
- Bronchoscopy is the method of choice for diagnosis and may identify granulomas, papules or nodules.
- Radiographically, the trachea may be normal or diffusely thick with an irregular surface or soft tissue nodules (Figure 10.89).

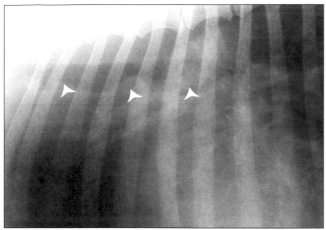

10.89 Lateral thoracic radiograph of a 5-year-old Lurcher with several nodules (arrowheads) in the caudal thoracic trachea representing *Oslerus osleri* granulomas.
(Courtesy of A. Holloway)

Tracheal haemorrhage

Tracheal haemorrhage can occur locally secondary to injury from external or internal trauma, particularly during intubation accidents, or more commonly diffusely secondary to generalized bleeding disorders in dogs and cats. Diffuse, regular increased thickness of the tracheal lining should alert the clinician to the possibility of rodenticide poisoning with submucosal haemorrhagic infiltrate. This finding is often associated with other sites of haemorrhage, particularly in the mediastinum and lungs.

Imaging findings:

- Marked widespread increased thickness of all aspects of the tracheal wall with a reduction in luminal diameter (Figure 10.90).
- Often associated with a wide mediastinum.
- Often associated with patchy pulmonary opacification in multiple lung lobes.

Extrinsic conditions affecting tracheal position and opacity

A variety of conditions of neighbouring organs can affect the radiographic position and opacity of the trachea. In most cases these do not result in clinical signs of tracheal disease. Severe extramural tracheal compression may become clinically apparent.

Enlarged cardiac silhouette: Cardiac enlargement involving the heart base and marked pericardial effusion can cause dorsal deviation of the thoracic trachea.

- Cardiomegaly typically deviates the carina, and therefore the entire trachea is displaced dorsally, becoming more parallel to the vertebral column.
- Bending of the trachea tends to be associated with focal enlargements, such as may occur with heart base tumours. These abnormalities tend to be cranial to the carina.

Imaging findings:

- Dorsal deviation of the thoracic trachea with a straight course parallel to the vertebral column (Figure 10.91).
- Heart base masses can cause focal dorsal and lateral deviation (Figure 10.92).

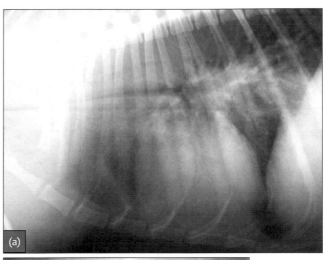

(a)

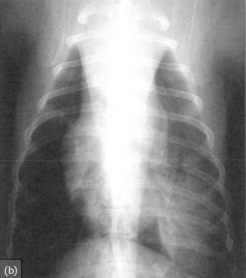

(b)

10.90 A 3-year-old Labrador Retriever with rodenticide toxicity (warfarin) causing submucosal tracheal and pulmonary haemorrhage. (a) Lateral thoracic radiograph. The cranial mediastinum shows increased soft tissue opacity with caudal displacement of the lungs from the first rib pair. At this level, the tracheal lumen is severely narrowed. In addition, there is patchy pulmonary opacification. (b) DV thoracic radiograph. The cranial mediastinum is severely widened, the cranial lung lobes are caudally displaced and there is increased opacity in the left caudal lung lobe.

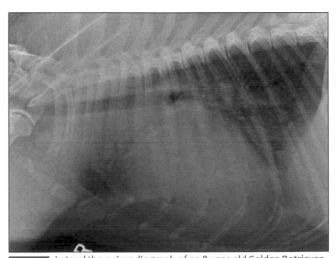

10.91 Lateral thoracic radiograph of an 8-year-old Golden Retriever with dilated cardiomyopathy. Note the general dorsal displacement of the trachea secondary to cardiac enlargement.

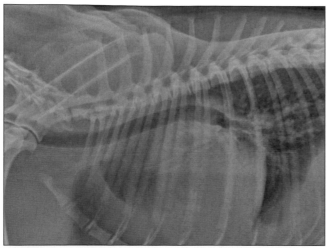

10.92 Lateral thoracic radiograph of an 8-year-old Boxer with recent lethargy. At the level of the heart base, the trachea is focally displaced dorsally by a soft tissue opacity. Moderate pleural effusion is also present. On echocardiography, a heart base mass was seen encircling and compressing vessels and the heart was otherwise structurally normal. The location of the mass is consistent with an aortic body tumour.

- Enlargement of the pulmonic trunk, as seen with post-stenotic dilatation in pulmonic stenosis or dirofilariasis, can protrude dorsally from the cranial heart base and summate with the ventral aspect of the caudal thoracic tracheal lumen. This characteristic feature has been referred to as the 'hat sign' (Figure 10.93). Most dogs with pulmonic stenosis do not demonstrate a hat sign.

Persistence of the fourth right aortic arch: See 'Vascular ring anomaly', above.

Mediastinal masses and pleural fluid: Most observable mediastinal masses in dogs and cats arise from lymphatic, thymic, thyroid or neuroendocrine tissue.

- If large enough, cranial mediastinal masses can cause local dorsal tracheal deviation.
- Vertebral and paravertebral tumours that extend into the cranial mediastinum (e.g. neuroendocrine tumour, nerve sheath neoplasm) can deviate the trachea ventrally.

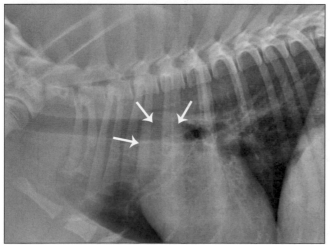

10.93 Lateral thoracic radiograph of a 6-month-old mixed-breed dog with moderate to severe pulmonic stenosis ('hat sign'). The large post-stenotic dilatation of the pulmonic trunk (arrowed) summates with the trachea.

- Tracheobronchial lymphadenopathy may create focal deviation of the caudal trachea, as do heart base masses, and may surround the tracheal bifurcation.
- A gas-filled oesophagus can highlight the tracheal walls but otherwise usually does not affect tracheal appearance unless very large (ventral tracheal displacement is possible).
- Pleural fluid secondary to a cranial mediastinal mass can induce dorsal deviation of the trachea.

Imaging findings:
- Local dorsal tracheal deviation with pivotal point at the carina or cranial mediastinum.
  - With tracheobronchial lymphadenopathy, the caudal trachea can be dorsally or ventrally deviated, depending on the specific lymph node involved (Figure 10.94; see also Figure 10.13).
- Displacement of the tracheal bifurcation caudal to the sixth intercostal space (Figure 10.95).
- Ventral tracheal deviation with masses in the dorsal part of the cranial mediastinum (Figure 10.96).
- With pleural fluid, the tracheal deviation is absent on lateral radiographs (Figure 10.97).

Retropharyngeal and thyroid masses:
- The thyroid gland comprises paired lobes that are lateral or dorsolateral to the first five to eight tracheal rings.
- Thyroid gland enlargement can cause ventral or lateral tracheal deviation.

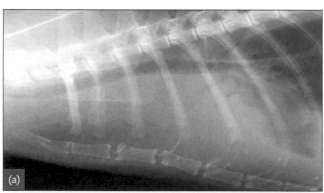

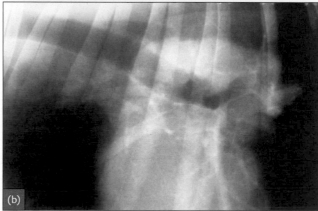

10.94 (a) Lateral thoracic radiograph of a 15-year-old Domestic Shorthaired cat with a mediastinal carcinoma 2 years after successful radiation treatment of a thymoma. Notice the dorsal tracheal deviation pivoting at the level of the fourth rib. There is also visible cranial lung lobe atelectasis (air bronchograms) and pleural effusion. (b) Lateral thoracic radiograph of a dog with tracheobronchial lymphadenopathy causing ventral deviation and compression of the caudal thoracic trachea.

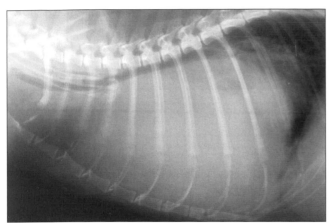

10.95 Lateral thoracic radiograph of an 11-year-old Domestic Shorthaired cat with a large thymoma causing dorsal tracheal deviation and caudal displacement of the carina (eighth intercostal space). The heart is located at the caudodorsal aspect of the mass. The caudal displacement of the carina is pathognomonic for a cranial mediastinal mass.

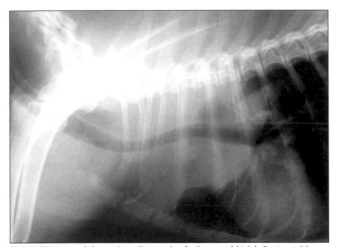

10.96 Lateral thoracic radiograph of a 2-year-old Irish Setter with a neuroendocrine tumour in the dorsal part of the cranial mediastinum causing ventral deviation of the cranial thoracic trachea.

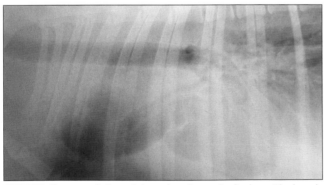

10.97 Close-up of a lateral thoracic radiograph of a dog with pleural effusion. The trachea is straight but parallel to the thoracic vertebral column, a common feature in pleural effusion.

- Retropharyngeal masses (lymphadenopathy, foreign body abscessation) usually cause laryngeal displacement but, if extensive, can also affect the cranial trachea.
- In dogs, thyroid neoplasia is usually a space-occupying lesion that frequently deviates the trachea and may involve the basihyoid bone.
- In cats, thyroid neoplasia typically remains small and rarely causes a mass effect on the trachea.

Imaging findings:
- Marked ventral and lateral deviation of the cranial cervical trachea (Figure 10.98).
- Less commonly, dorsal tracheal deviation.
- Occasionally, mineralization of the mass (Figure 10.99).
- Malignant thyroid neoplasms can be highly vascular and have extensive vascular invasion, which can be observed during angiography, ultrasonography and CT.

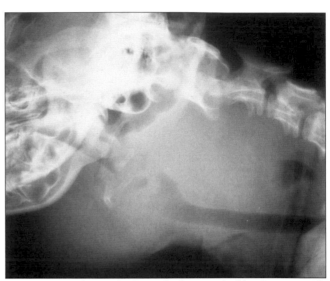

10.98 Lateral cervical radiograph of a 2-month-old Weimaraner with canine strangles. There is severe mandibular and retropharyngeal lymphadenopathy, the latter causing ventral deviation of the larynx and cranial trachea.

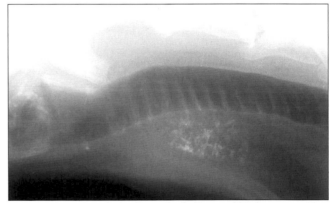

10.99 Lateral cervical radiograph of a 10-year-old Dobermann with a mineralized thyroid tumour causing dorsal deviation of the cranial trachea.

References and further reading

Berryessa NA, Marks SL, Pesavento PA *et al.* (2008) Gastrointestinal pythiosis in 10 dogs from California. *Journal of Veterinary Internal Medicine* **22**, 1065–1069

Bertolini G, Stefanello C and Caldin M (2009) Imaging diagnosis – pulmonary interstitial emphysema in a dog. *Veterinary Radiology & Ultrasound* **50**, 80–82

Grimes JA, Fleming JT, Singh A *et al.* (2020) Characteristics and long-term outcomes of dogs with gastroesophageal intussusception. *Journal of the American Veterinary Medical Association* **256**, 914–920

Hendricks JC and O'Brien JA (1985) Tracheal collapse in two cats. *Journal of the American Veterinary Medical Association* **187**, 418–419

Henninger W and Gutmannsbauer B (1999) CT-anatomy of the canine mediastinum. Abstracts from papers presented at the annual meeting of the EAVDI, Bälsta, Sweden, August 26–29, 1998. *Veterinary Radiology & Ultrasound* **40**, 191

Lhermette P, Sobel D and Robertson E (2020) *BSAVA Manual of Canine and Feline Endoscopy and Endosurgery, 2nd edn*. BSAVA Publications, Gloucester

Morgan KRS and Bray JP (2019) Current diagnostic tests, surgical treatments, and prognostic indicators for vascular ring anomalies in dogs. *Journal of the American Veterinary Medical Association* **254**, 728–730

Petite A and Kirberger K (2011) Mediastinum. In: *Veterinary Computed Tomography*, ed. T Schwarz and J Saunders, pp. 249–260. Wiley-Blackwell, Oxford

Prather AB, Berry CA and Thrall DE (2005) Use of radiography in combination with computed tomography for the assessment of non-cardiac thoracic disease in the dog and cat. *Veterinary Radiology & Ultrasound* **46**, 114–122

Reichle JK and Wisner ER (2000) Non-cardiac thoracic ultrasound in 75 feline and canine patients. *Veterinary Radiology & Ultrasound* **41**, 154–162

Samii VF, Biller DS and Koblik PD (1998) Normal cross-sectional anatomy of the feline thorax and abdomen: comparison of computed tomography and cadaver anatomy. *Veterinary Radiology & Ultrasound* **39**, 504–511

Smallwood JE and George TF (1993) Anatomical atlas for computed tomography in the mesaticephalic dog: thorax and cranial abdomen. *Veterinary Radiology & Ultrasound* **34**, 65–84

Suter PF (1984) *Thoracic Radiography: A Text Atlas of Thoracic Diseases of the Dog and Cat*. Peter F. Suter, Wettswil

Thrall DE (2002) The mediastinum. In: *Textbook of Veterinary Diagnostic Radiology, 4th edn*, ed. DE Thrall, pp. 376–389. WB Saunders, Philadelphia

Wisner ER and Zwingenberger AL (2015) Mediastinum and esophagus. In: *Atlas of Small Animal CT and MRI*, ed. ER Wisner and AL Zwingenberger, pp. 408–422. Wiley-Blackwell, Ames

Yoon J, Feeney DA, Cronk DE, Anderson KL and Ziegler LE (2004) Computed tomographic evaluation of canine and feline mediastinal masses in 14 patients. *Veterinary Radiology & Ultrasound* **45**, 542–546

Zekas LJ and Adams WM (2002) Cranial mediastinal cysts in nine cats. *Veterinary Radiology & Ultrasound* **43**, 413–418

Chapter 11

The pleural space

Mairi Frame and Alison King

Imaging anatomy

A serous membrane (serosa) is a type of epithelium that covers the walls and contents of a body cavity and is attached to underlying tissue by connective tissue. It forms a thin smooth tissue membrane that comprises epithelial (mesothelium) and connective tissue layers (see Chapter 7). Serosa may fold upon itself to create a serous cavity and allow movement between structures. In the thorax, the serosae that cover the lungs, thoracic body walls and diaphragm are called pleurae and they allow movement between these structures. These pleural membranes also divide the thoracic cavity into the left pleural cavity, right pleural cavity and mediastinum (Figure 11.1). The pleurae are further characterized by proximity to other structures.

- Pulmonary pleurae (visceral pleurae) cover the lungs, each of which is a 'viscus' or internal organ.
- Parietal pleurae cover somatic structures and comprise three sections:
  - The diaphragmatic pleura covers the cranial surface of the diaphragm
  - The costal pleura covers the medial surface of the thoracic body wall. It tends to curve slightly medially as it passes over each rib and laterally as it crosses the intercostal spaces
  - The mediastinal pleura forms the medial boundary of each pleural cavity and the lateral boundaries of the mediastinum, which contains the heart, trachea, oesophagus and great vessels.

The visceral and parietal pleurae merge at the lung hilus. The visceral pleurae adhere tightly to the surface of the lungs and are in apposition between adjacent lung lobes (see 'interlobar fissures', below). The mediastinal pleurae attach to the mediastinal structures via loose connective tissue (see Chapter 10). The diaphragmatic and costal pleurae attach to the body wall and diaphragm via the endothoracic fascia, which is the outermost layer of the thoracic cavity that blends with the neck fasciae. A small portion of the parietal pleura is cranially convex, forming a blind end to the pleural cavity that extends cranial to the thoracic inlet; the cranial extension is greater on the left side. This portion of the pleura that is in the neck is called the pleural cupula.

Imaging studies may need to include a portion of the neck to examine the entirety of the pleural cavities. Double layers of the same pleura form connecting pleura such as the left and right pulmonary ligaments, which attach the two lungs to the mediastinum from the lung hilus to the diaphragm. Pulmonary ligaments are not seen during radiography but may be seen during computed tomography (CT) when contrasted by gas in the pleural cavity (pneumothorax).

Each pleural cavity is a serous cavity located between the parietal and visceral pleurae that surrounds nearly the entire ipsilateral lung (except at the lung hilus). It is alternatively called a pleural space; however, the cavity is only a 'potential space' unless it becomes pathologically filled and expanded by fluid, gas or herniated abdominal viscera. Normally, each pleural cavity is less than 1 mm thick and contains only a small volume of serous fluid (usually less than 10 ml) that acts as a lubricant to minimize friction and permit lung movement within the thoracic cavity during inhalation and exhalation. The surface tension of the pleural fluid holds the lungs against the thoracic wall and maintains them inflated against their natural tendency to collapse through elastic recoil, allowing the lungs to remain partially expanded even after complete exhalation. During inhalation, this process also helps maintain expansion of the small airways, which are not supported by cartilage.

Serous fluid is derived from serum, governed by Starling forces, and continuously turned over at a high rate (5–10 litres per 24 hours in humans). Vascular supply to the parietal pleurae is through the systemic circulation via the intercostal and regional arteries. The visceral pleurae are supplied and drained by the pulmonary circulation. This results in an overall movement of pleural fluid from the capillaries of the parietal pleura into the pleural cavity. From there, the serous fluid is absorbed by the capillaries of the visceral pleura and by the lymphatic vessels of the visceral and diaphragmatic pleurae. These lymphatic vessels provide the only means for proteins, red blood cells and particulate matter to return to the cardiovascular system from the pleural cavity. The pleural lymphatic vessels drain to the cranial sternal and cranial mediastinal lymph nodes. Anatomical variation in the route of serous fluid drainage by the visceral pleura may account for the tendency of some cats to develop pleural effusion secondary to left heart failure. However, this pathogenesis is incompletely understood and the literature contains conflicting information.

The pleural cavity also extends into and between lung lobes to form pleural fissures. The fissures between lung lobes are constant and called interlobar fissures. Inconstant (accessory) pleural fissures arising from variable locations on the lung surface are common. The two pleural

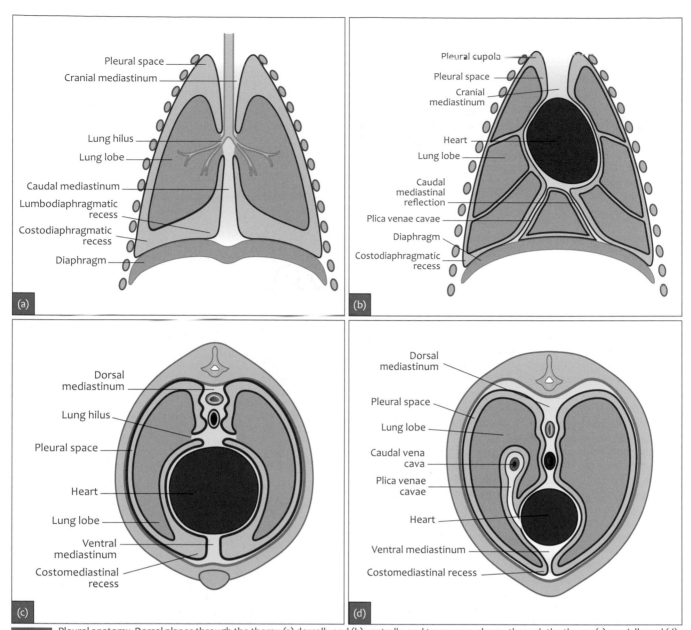

11.1 Pleural anatomy. Dorsal planes through the thorax (a) dorsally and (b) ventrally, and transverse planes through the thorax (c) cranially and (d) caudally. Red lines denote pleurae. The pulmonary and parietal pleurae are joined at the lung hilus. The parietal pleura is divided into continuous costal, mediastinal and diaphragmatic pleurae and folds back upon itself establishing the lines of pleural reflection and forming the pleural recesses. The parietal pleurae extend cranially through the thoracic inlet to form the pleural cupolas. In carnivores, the left and right pleural cavities may communicate with each other via fenestrations in the caudal mediastinum but the pleural cavities do not communicate with the mediastinum.

cavities are distinct from each other and disease may be confined to one cavity. Communication between the two sides is also possible because the caudal mediastinum is fenestrated in carnivores and can be torn during disease. The pleural cavities extend further within the thoracic cavity than the lungs, which means that different portions of the parietal pleurae may reflect upon themselves and be in apposition. This arrangement gives rise to three paired pleural recesses (the costomediastinal, lumbodiaphragmatic and costodiaphragmatic/costophrenic recesses), which are potential spaces that the lungs can fill when expanded. The costomediastinal and costodiaphragmatic recesses are larger than the lumbodiaphragmatic recess, which is the portion of the pleural cavity caudal to the ribs, dorsal to the diaphragmatic crura and cranioventral to the vertebral attachment of the diaphragm. The right pleural cavity also forms the mediastinal recess by extending into the space between the ventral part of the caudal mediastinum (caudal mediastinal reflection) and plica venae

cavae, covering the accessory lung lobe. The mediastinal recess also has an extension between the mediastinum and diaphragm, the left mediastinodiaphragmatic recess, that is rarely observed during imaging.

During thoracic radiography, the size of the costomediastinal and lumbodiaphragmatic recesses are best estimated on lateral views. The costomediastinal recess lies between the ventral border of the lung and the sternum. The lumbodiaphragmatic recess lies within the angle formed by the lumbar vertebral column and diaphragm. The size of the costodiaphragmatic recess is best estimated on dorsoventral (DV) or ventrodorsal (VD) views as the angle formed by the rib cage and diaphragm. The ability to estimate the locations of the lines of pleural reflection (where the parietal pleurae abruptly change direction, e.g. to accommodate the heart) is important because penetration of the thorax (e.g. biopsy) within the delineated area could lead to pneumothorax, haemothorax or the spread of disease into the pleural cavity.

Interpretative principles

Appearance of intrathoracic structures

Pleural membranes

On radiographs, normal pleurae are generally too thin to be visible as distinct structures. However, if the pleurae are oriented parallel to the X-ray beam during radiography, then sufficient X-ray absorption may occur to create visible linear opacities in animals without thoracic disease. These lines are indistinguishable from mildly thick pleurae, small-volume pleural fluid and pleural calcification that may be present in older animals as a degenerative change of minor consequence. Pathological increased pleural thick-ness (e.g. pleuritis, fibrosis, neoplasia) is more likely to produce wider pleural lines (pleural fissures) alongside additional signs of pleural disease. During radiography, normal pleurae do not enhance following intravenous con-trast medium administration.

The parietal pleurae form three mediastinal structures that resemble pleural fissures. In the ventral part of the thorax, the right and left mediastinal pleurae contact each other and form two mediastinal reflections. The cranial or cranioventral mediastinal reflection obliquely crosses the midline cranial to the heart while the caudal or caudoventral mediastinal reflection is located on the left, caudal to the heart. These structures are not pleural fissures as they are not created by the apposition of two layers of visceral pleura (i.e. these mediastinal structures lie between the right and left lungs and not between lobes of the same lung). The plica venae cavae is a struc-ture with similar appearance located caudoventrally between the caudal and accessory lobes of the right lung. This mediastinal structure is also not formed by visceral pleurae, but rather it is a fold of the right media-stinal pleura that surrounds the caudal vena cava between the heart and the right side of the diaphragm (See Chapter 10). Normal fat deposition within the folds may increase the thickness of these structures and be mistaken for pleural or mediastinal disease.

The ventral portion of the cranial mediastinum is fre-quently visible on DV and VD radiographs as an obliquely oriented line between the left cranial and right cranial lung lobes. The ventral portion of the caudal mediastinum is frequently visible on DV and VD radiographs as a soft tissue line running from the cardiac apex to the diaphragm, between the accessory and left caudal lung lobes (Figure 11.2). During imaging, this structure has been mistaken for the phrenicopericardial ligament (also called the cardio-phrenic or sternopericardiac ligament), which is in the ventral mediastinum between the fibrous pericardium and diaphragm. The plica venae cavae is seen mostly during CT as a linear structure.

Pulmonary osseous metaplasia is a potentially mis-leading finding associated with the pleurae that occurs commonly in older dogs and should be differentiated from pulmonary soft tissue nodules. During imaging, this heter-otopic bone formation is often an incidental finding of minor consequence characterized by calcified bodies that either summate with the air-filled lungs or are seen at the periphery of the lungs. These abnormalities appear as multiple tiny, angled and circumscribed opacities that have a generalized random distribution. The angled shape, peripheral location and high opacity of these abnormal-ities, despite their small size, allows these structures to be distinguished from soft tissue pulmonary nodules (Figure 11.3). During radiography, these degenerative

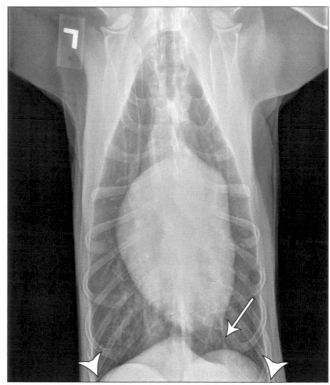

11.2 VD thoracic radiograph of a normal dog demonstrating the caudal mediastinal reflection (arrowed), which is the thin ventral part of the caudal mediastinum. When taking thoracic radiographs, it is important to remember that the pleural space extends beyond the lungs and into the costodiaphragmatic recesses to avoid the caudal margins being missed, as has happened in this case (arrowheads).

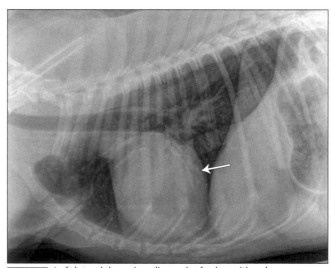

11.3 Left lateral thoracic radiograph of a dog with pulmonary heterotopic osseous metaplasia. These incidental findings are commonly observed in older dogs, are of minor consequence and should not be mistaken for pulmonary nodules. A pleural line is also visible (arrowed).

changes may also resemble end-on pulmonary blood vessels but are frequently seen between blood vessels.

On CT images, the normal pleura is not typically seen unless folded upon itself (e.g. plica venae cavae). However, an opaque line may be seen around the periphery of the thoracic cavity that represents the combination of the parietal and visceral pleurae, the pleural space, some extrapleural fat, the endothoracic fascia and the internal intercostal muscle (Figure 11.4). The visceral pleura between lung lobes may also be visible in places as a faint

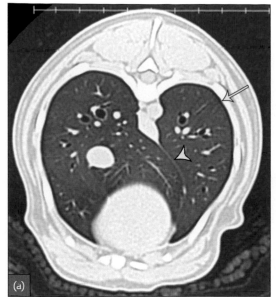

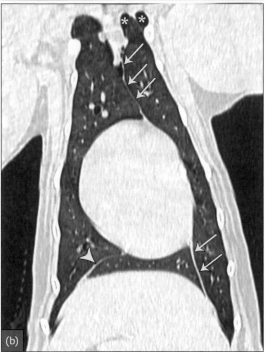

11.4 (a) Transverse, post-contrast thoracic CT image of a dog, displayed in a lung window. The visceral and parietal pleurae cannot be distinguished from each other but are visible as a hyperdense line medial to the intercostal muscles (arrowed). The caudal mediastinal reflection can be seen as a faint hyperdense line running between the left caudal and accessory lung lobes (arrowhead). (b) Dorsal plane thoracic CT image of a dog with mild pneumothorax, displayed in a lung window. The cranial and caudal mediastinal reflections are the ventral portions of the cranial mediastinum and caudal mediastinum, respectively. They are visible as hyperdense lines (arrowed) between the left and right cranial lung lobes and accessory and left caudal lung lobes, respectively. The plica venae cavae appears similarly but is between the right caudal and accessory lobes (arrowhead). A small volume of pleural gas is visible (∗).

hyperdense line but it is usually difficult to define the exact lung lobe margins. The pleurae will be enhanced on CT following intravenous contrast medium administration.

On ultrasound images of normal animals, the visceral pleura is indistinguishable from gas in the underlying lung and the parietal pleura may be observed adjacent to the thoracic body wall. The costal pleura is represented by a smooth, fine, hyperechoic line tracing the internal surface of the intercostal muscles. This lung–wall interface is commonly called the pleural line. The diaphragmatic and mediastinal pleurae are typically undetectable due to air in the lung preventing deeper transmission of the ultrasound beam. However, these serous membranes can sometimes be seen using acoustic windows that do not have lung in the path of the beam (e.g. thoracic inlet, transabdominal). When imaging through intercostal windows, the appearance of the pleural line is described as the 'gator' or 'bat' sign because the pleural line follows the curved contours of the ribs (Figure 11.5a). To-and-fro movement of the pleural line occurs with respiration and may be seen during real-time ultrasonography. This normal appearance is called the 'glide' sign and is usually easiest to identify caudodorsally where thoracic wall and lung movement is greatest. At this level, the most caudal location where the glide sign is observed denotes the most caudal location of aerated lung and approximates with the caudal line of pleural reflection during full lung inflation. A mismatch might indicate lung consolidation, lung collapse, a diaphragmatic mass or displacement, body wall malformation, or expansion of the pleural space. M-mode ultrasonography, directed perpendicularly through the intercostal space, will produce a comparable sign called the 'seashore' sign (Figure 11.5b).

Pleural space

As a potential space, the pleural cavity typically only becomes visible when it is expanded by abnormal content such as gas, excessive fluid or herniated abdominal viscera. Therefore, one of the most characteristic traits of the normal pleural cavity is that the lungs extend all the way to the body wall and diaphragm; there should be no gap between these structures. When the pleural space expands, there is typically a reciprocal change in the adjacent lung. Therefore, pleural disease typically simultaneously produces changes in both the pleural cavity and lung, which can make it difficult to determine whether only pleural disease, or concurrent pleural and pulmonary diseases are present. Typically, secondarily affected lungs become smaller and may have altered opacity due to reduced gas volume uncompensated by hypoxic vasoconstriction and summation with pleural contents (e.g. fluid).

Hemithorax

- Hemithorax is a useful clinical phrase that is an alternate way to describe the left or right side of the thorax.
- Use of this term can be especially meaningful when it is important to convey that the disease cannot be precisely located to a specific anatomical compartment. For example, disease in the left hemithorax might be in the left lung, left pleural cavity, left body wall or some combination of anatomical compartments.
- To reduce confusion due to ambiguity, the term should be avoided when the specific anatomical compartment can be identified. In these situations, the exact anatomical compartment or compartments should be stated (e.g. the left pleural cavity).

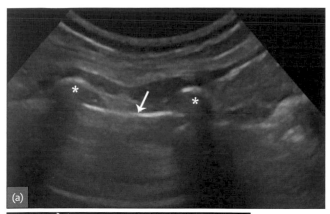

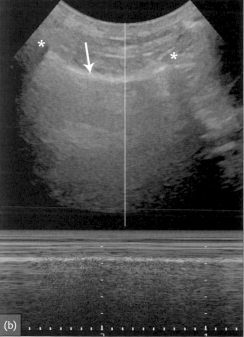

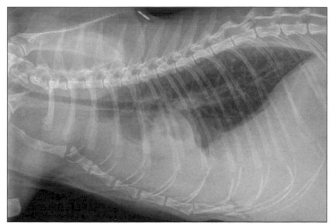

11.6 Right lateral thoracic radiograph of a cat with a large volume of pleural effusion due to lymphoma. In the cranioventral thorax, the pleural cavities are expanded and have a homogeneous fluid opacity that effaces most of the cranial mediastinal structures, cardiac silhouette and cranial border of the diaphragmatic cupula. The cranial lung lobes are severely reduced in size, retracted from the body walls and increased in opacity, and have rounded or scalloped margins. Abdominal effusion (peritoneal fluid) is also present and partially effaces the caudal border of the diaphragmatic cupula.

11.5 (a) Thoracic ultrasound image obtained using an intercostal window in a normal dog. The appearance of the curved pleurae (arrowed) between adjacent ribs (*) has been likened to the eyes of an alligator above the water (gator sign) or the outspread wings of a bat (bat sign). Horizontal reverberation artefacts can be seen (A-lines; see Chapter 2). In real-time imaging, the pleural line can be seen moving against the body wall producing the 'glide' sign – this motion cannot be inferred from the appearance of a static image. The appearance of pneumothorax on a static image is indistinguishable from the presence of normal air-filled lung. (b) B-mode ultrasonogram and resulting M-mode trace. These images were obtained in a normal patient during breathing by directing the sound beam (white line) down through the intercostal space between two ribs (*) and show the 'seashore' sign. In the far field, below the pleural line (arrowed), the normal air-filled lung moves, producing a granular pattern over time (the 'sand'). In the near field, above the pleural line, the static body wall produces horizontal lines (the 'sea').

Pleural fluid: When fluid or gas is introduced into the pleural space, the normal negative pressure is lost, causing the lung to retract from the body wall. The size of the pleural recesses varies with the degree of lung inflation, which is influenced by many physiological and pathological conditions. When abnormally expanded by fluid, the pleural space will have a fluid (soft tissue) opacity and must lie parallel to the X-ray beam to be seen. The appearance of the pleural space will vary with the volume of fluid, and it is impossible to differentiate between types of fluid, fibrin or cellular material simply by radiographic appearance (Figure 11.6). A horizontally oriented X-ray beam generally

does not produce an air–fluid interface unless there is concurrent pneumothorax.

On CT images, expansion of the pleural cavity is easily detected and the density, or attenuation, of the material in the pleural space (measured in Hounsfield units (HU)) will reflect its composition. Fluids have a CT number between 0 and 40 HU, with lower numbers produced by watery and fatty fluid and higher numbers by cellular fluid. Fluid with a CT number below 12 HU is most likely transudate or chylous effusion. A cut off value of 35 HU can be applied to differentiate exudative (<35 HU) from haemorrhagic effusions. Soft tissue structures typically have a CT number from 40 to 80 HU and show contrast enhancement. Visualization of soft tissue attenuating structures is aided by using a soft tissue window when displaying images (Figure 11.7).

On ultrasound images, pleural fluid typically appears anechoic, although increasing cellularity may produce increased echogenicity (Figure 11.8). Soft tissue or fibrinous structures appear echogenic and can be distinguished from the surrounding fluid. On magnetic resonance imaging (MRI), pleural fluid typically appears T1 hypointense and T2 hyperintense.

Pleural gas: On radiographs, pleural gas appears as a gas opacity within the thoracic cavity that is external to the lungs and mediastinum (Figure 11.9). It is differentiated from air-filled lung by its lack of vascular or bronchial markings.

On CT images, pleural gas is non-attenuating (CT number of roughly -1000 HU) and contains no inner architecture. In comparison, air-filled lung has a higher attenuation that varies with the degree of lung inflation and aeration (roughly −850 HU after inhalation and −700 HU after exhalation) (Figure 11.10).

On ultrasound images, pleural gas results in an absent glide sign because, unlike lung tissue, pleural gas does not move with respiration. The static pleural gas appears as a hyperechoic interface just deep to the body wall, with associated acoustic shadowing and reverberation artefact that prevents observation of deeper structures. Pleural gas cannot be differentiated from pulmonary gas based only on static images because it is necessary to observe

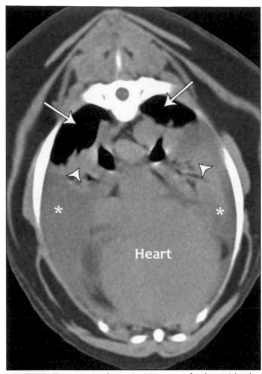

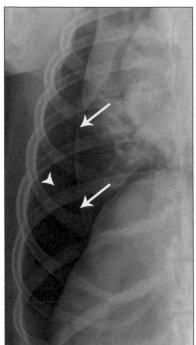

11.9 Close-up of a DV thoracic radiograph of a dog with pneumothorax following lung lobectomy. The right lung is reduced in size and retracted from the body wall (arrowed). The space between the body wall and right lung (the right pleural cavity) is expanded and has a gas opacity that is devoid of vascular markings (arrowhead).

11.7 Transverse thoracic CT image of a dog with a large volume of pleural effusion. The image was obtained with the dog in ventral recumbency and is displayed in a soft tissue window. Both pleural cavities are expanded and filled with fluid-attenuating material that collects ventrally (*). Both lungs are partially collapsed and float on the pleural fluid. The ventral portions of the lungs (arrowheads) are void of air and have a soft tissue opacity. In this image, it is possible to differentiate fluid from soft tissue because of the contrast resolution provided by the soft tissue window display. However, the air-filled portions of the lungs (arrowed) resemble pneumothorax because pulmonary blood vessels and bronchi are not seen extending to the body wall. A lung window would reveal that the pulmonary structures are present and extend to the body wall.

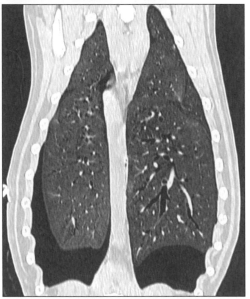

11.10 Dorsal thoracic CT image of a dog in ventral recumbency with bilateral pneumothorax, displayed in a lung window. Both lungs have reduced size and are retracted from the diaphragm. The right lung is also partially retracted from the body wall and mediastinum. Both pleural cavities are non-attenuating and lack internal architecture, indicating the presence of gas.

respiratory movement (the glide sign) to distinguish between gas in the two locations. M-Mode directed through the intercostal space will produce a 'stratosphere' or 'barcode' sign (Figure 11.11). On MRI, gas appears as a signal void on all sequences.

Interlobar fissures

Interlobar fissure lines become visible on radiographs and CT images when there is increased pleural thickness or increased volume of pleural fluid that contrasts with the adjacent air-filled lung. Since only fissures that are parallel with the X-ray beam will be visible on radiographs, knowledge of their normal location is helpful in identifying these findings (Figure 11.12).

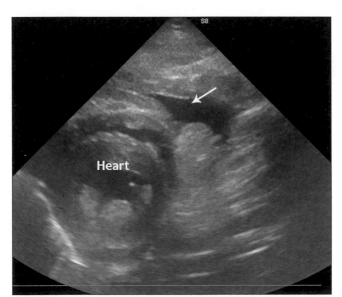

11.8 Thoracic ultrasound image obtained using an acoustic window on the gravity-dependent thoracic wall in a cat with bicavitary effusions (pleural and peritoneal). Small volumes of anechoic fluid are seen in the dependent pleural cavity (arrowed) and in the heart chambers (blood). Pleural fluid is differentiated from pericardial fluid by its angular shape. Pleural fluid is differentiated from mediastinal fluid by its location between the heart and the body wall. Free fluid moves with gravity so small volumes can be more easily identified by scanning from the gravity-dependent surface. Pericardial, mediastinal and peritoneal fluids are not seen in this image.

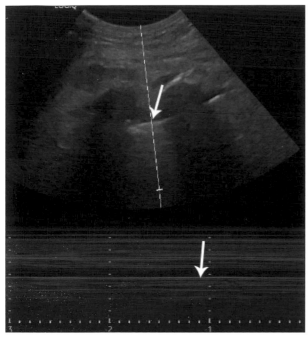

11.11 B-mode ultrasonogram and resulting M-mode trace of a dog with pneumothorax following lung lobectomy and obtained during breathing. On the M-mode trace, the 'barcode/stratosphere' sign results from pleural gas obscuring the lung. The lung is in the far field deep to the pleural line (arrowed). This produces a series of static horizontal lines in the far field deep to the pleural line and replaces the normal granular pattern (sand) produced by lung slide. The appearance of these parallel lines is similar to those produced in the near field by the static body wall. On static B-mode images, it is impossible to distinguish between normal air-filled lung and pneumothorax.

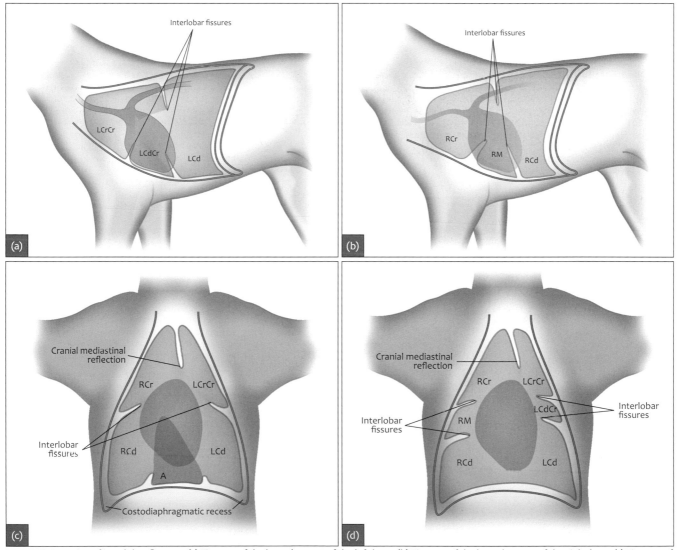

11.12 Location of interlobar fissures. (a) Fissures of the lateral aspect of the left lung. (b) Fissures of the lateral aspect of the right lung. (c) Fissures of the dorsal aspect of the lungs. (d) Fissures of the ventral aspect of the lungs. A = accessory lobe; LCd = left caudal lung lobe; LCdCr = caudal part of the left cranial lung lobe; LCrCr = cranial part of the left cranial lung lobe; RCd = right caudal lung lobe; RCr = right cranial lung lobe; RM = right middle lung lobe.

Thin interlobar fissures produce fine lines of soft tissue opacity that curve towards the heart from the thoracic wall or radiate from the lung hilus and are distinguished from other linear opacities by their location, orientation and the absence of branching. Thick interlobar fissures, as may occur with a large volume of pleural fluid, separate the aerated lung lobes further and produce elongated wedge-shaped or triangular opacities that taper towards the lung hilus from the thoracic wall (Figure 11.13).

Radiographic features:

- Interlobar fissures are thin lines of soft tissue opacity between adjacent aerated lung lobes and typically indicate pleural disease.
- When pleural and pulmonary disease occur together, the distinction between consolidated lung and pleural fluid may be obscured due to border effacement.
- Lung consolidation may create a sharply demarcated border when adjacent to normally aerated lung. This interface, known as a lobar sign, should not be mistaken for a pleural fissure as it indicates lung disease *versus* pleural disease.
- In contrast to pleural fluid, small and moderate volumes of gas do not typically dissect between lung lobes. Therefore, interlobar fissures are not usually visible in patients with mild to moderate pneumothorax.

Lung lobes

In cases with pleural disease, the lungs may have a normal or increased opacity. The appearance of lung parenchymal opacification may be due to summation with pleural fluid, lung collapse, increased blood volume or a combination of factors. When air or fluid is introduced into the pleural space, the normal negative pressure is lost, causing the lungs to lose volume (lung collapse or atelectasis) and therefore retract from the body wall. The degree of retraction in any lung lobe depends on the volume of pleural fluid or gas, the redistribution of pleural fluid or gas according to gravity and any underlying pulmonary disease. The appearance of the collapsed lung can occasionally provide information about the nature of the pleural disease. The most salient features are the size, opacity and shape of the affected lung lobes.

Uniform lung lobe collapse and atelectasis: Normal lung lobes have an inherent elasticity that causes them to collapse uniformly, retaining their normal angled shape. This often occurs when the lung is healthy and pleural disease is acute. On radiographs, the retracted lung lobes may also produce a slightly 'scalloped' border as the lung lobes usually become separated. The opacity of collapsed lung varies with the degree of collapse, presence of underlying lung disease and effectiveness of hypoxic vasoconstriction.

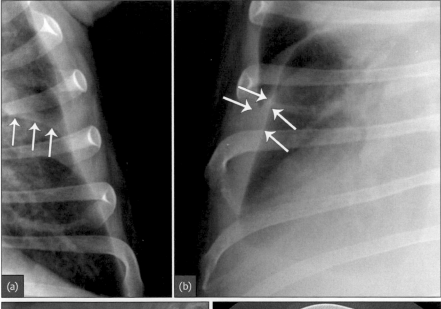

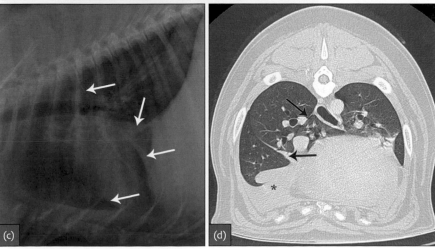

11.13 (a) Close-up of a DV thoracic radiograph of a dog with a moderate volume of pleural effusion demonstrating a thin interlobar fissure (arrowed). (b) Close-up of a DV thoracic radiograph of a dog with a moderate volume of pleural effusion demonstrating a wedge-shaped interlobar fissure (arrowed). (c) Left lateral thoracic radiograph of a dog with a moderate volume of pleural effusion demonstrating multiple interlobar fissures (arrowed). (d) Transverse post-contrast thoracic CT image of a dog with a small volume of pleural effusion, displayed in a lung window. Pleural fluid accumulates in the ventral aspect of the right pleural space (*) and between lung lobes forming interlobar fissures with variably increased thickness (arrowed). The ventral tip of the right lung is deviated in a medial direction due to it 'floating' in the fluid. This displacement demonstrates how mobile lung tissue is in the presence of fluid and therefore how lung lobe torsion can occur in the presence of pleural effusion.

Severe lung collapse can result in pulmonary opacification such that it is impossible to differentiate collapsed lung from pleural fluid on radiographs (see Figure 11.6). On CT images, collapsed areas of lung are primarily reduced in volume and may have normal or increased attenuation. In unenhanced CT images, completely atelectatic lung has a CT number of 50 to 60 HU, which means that it can be difficult to differentiate collapsed lung from pleural fluid. However, following intravascular contrast medium administration, atelectatic lung enhances on CT images and pleural fluid does not (Figure 11.14).

On ultrasound examination, it is easy to differentiate pleural fluid from collapsed lung. Collapsed lung tips are echogenic and triangular with smooth pleural margins and

an internal architecture like liver. Fluid-filled airways appear as anechoic tubular structures and pulmonary blood vessels may be visible. Any remaining air will result in hyperechoic foci with acoustic shadowing and reverberation. The demarcation between the collapsed atelectatic tips and the normally aerated hilar regions is usually also clear (Figure 11.15).

Uneven or asymmetrical lung lobe collapse: In some instances, pleural disease causes non-uniform lung lobe collapse, and the affected lobe does not retain its normal shape. This situation usually occurs when there is underlying pulmonary disease (e.g. a contused or pneumonic lung lobe may collapse more readily than normal lung) or pleural fluid that has been present for some time causing structural changes to the pleura, lung or both. If the pleura becomes substantially thick or the lung loses its elasticity, then the normal angled shape may be lost giving a rounded, more pronounced scalloped appearance to the lobar margins. This can occur in the presence of chronic reactive (e.g. chyle or pus) or neoplastic effusions (Figure 11.16). In the absence of an effusion, this appearance suggests the presence of pleural scarring or fibrosis secondary to severe chronic inflammatory lung disease. This can be a difficult distinction to make as an effusion may develop secondarily around a diseased lung lobe.

Mediastinum and heart

Pleural disease may alter the position of the mediastinum and heart. During imaging, displacement of the mediastinum (or heart) to the left or right side is called a mediastinal shift (or cardiac shift). The normal position of the mediastinum and heart is dependent on both lungs being uniformly inflated and both pleural cavities being of equal size. Unilateral lung collapse, as may occur with unilateral pneumothorax, will cause a mediastinal shift towards the side of lung collapse. In contrast, a unilateral tension pneumothorax will cause over-expansion of one pleural cavity such that the mediastinal shift is away from the side of lung collapse. During thoracic radiography, a

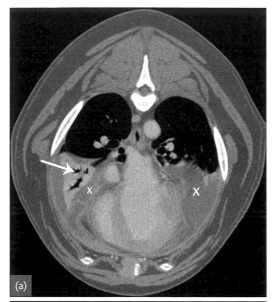

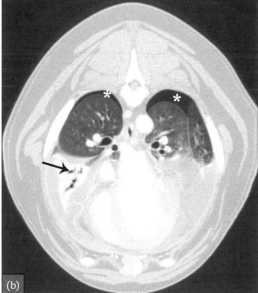

11.14 Transverse post-contrast thoracic CT images of a dog with hydropneumothorax displayed in (a) soft tissue and (b) lung windows. Contrast material was administered intravenously. Both lungs have reduced size and are retracted from the body wall. The expanded pleural cavities contain both fluid (X) and gas (*). In the right lung, the parenchyma of the ventral tip is void of air and is contrast enhancing (arrowed). The pleural fluid does not contrast enhance. The soft tissue window shows greater contrast between the lung tip and adjacent pleural fluid, making it easier to differentiate them. The lung window, however, provides better contrast between lung and gas in the pleural cavity. This demonstrates the importance of maximizing the available contrast resolution by using multiple windows to examine CT images.

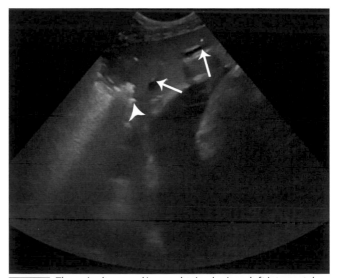

11.15 Thoracic ultrasound image obtained using a left intercostal window in a dog with pleural effusion. The left pleural cavity contains a medium volume of anechoic fluid and the left lung is partially collapsed (reduced size). The ventral portion of the lung is echogenic and triangular with fluid-filled bronchi (arrowed). The dorsal portion of the lung is aerated, and the boundary between the aerated and consolidated portions is clearly seen (arrowhead).

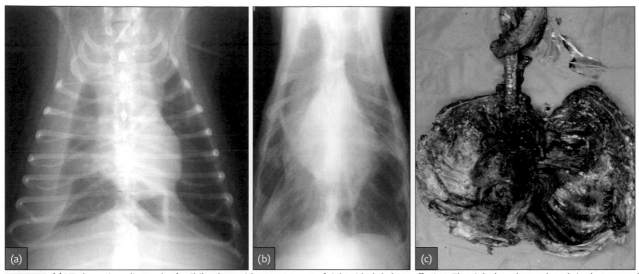

11.16 (a) VD thoracic radiograph of a Chihuahua with recent onset of right sided chylous effusion. The right lung has reduced size but normal shape, forming sharp (acute) angles at the tips. The lung is retracted from the body wall and the moderately expanded pleural space has a fluid opacity. (b) VD thoracic radiograph of an Afghan hound with chronic bilateral chylothorax, which was drained prior to radiography. Both lungs have reduced size with rounded margins and thick interlobar fissures indicating chronicity and scarring of the visceral pleura. The lungs are retracted from the body wall and the mildly expanded pleural spaces have a fluid opacity. The cardiac silhouette is irregularly margined due to prior pericardiectomy. (c) Ventral aspect post-mortem photograph of the opened thorax of the same dog as in (b). Both lungs are collapsed around the heart and covered in multiple layers of fibrinous adhesions. The parietal pleurae also have marked fibrinous changes. These findings are consistent with chronic fibrinous pleuritis.

mediastinal shift is best observed on the DV and VD views. On lateral radiographs, however, the cardiac silhouette may appear dorsally displaced from the sternum. This finding is a common radiographic feature of pneumothorax in dogs and cats, but also may be seen with pleural fluid (particularly in the cat), moderate hypovolaemia, unilateral atelectasis, a large fat accumulation in the ventral mediastinum or pulmonary hyperinflation, or as a normal anatomical variation in deep-chested dogs.

This appearance on lateral radiographs has also been described as 'elevation' of the cardiac silhouette, which may be misleading because elevation is not a recommended term of anatomical direction or orientation, and the heart is not actually elevated. For example, when the patient is in left lateral recumbency, the heart is not displaced to the right, which would be elevated in that position. Rather, the heart slides left and dorsally because of partial or complete collapse of the gravity-dependent lung (i.e. the left lung when the patient is in left lateral recumbency). Unilateral lung collapse cannot maintain the heart in the centre of the thorax, causing an increased distance between the cardiac apex and the sternum (Figure 11.17). If an animal with unilateral pneumothorax or pleural effusion is positioned with the affected side uppermost, then this phenomenon may not be evident.

In patients with pneumothorax, the gap between the heart and the sternum has a gas opacity and generally lacks lung markings due to retraction of the lobes away from the sternum (Figure 11.18). In patients with pleural effusion, the resultant fluid opacity causes varying degrees of border effacement of the cardiac silhouette and may give a false impression of cardiomegaly due to dorsal deviation of the cardiac silhouette and trachea secondary to the effusion. Border effacement of the cardiac silhouette by pleural fluid is dependent on patient positioning and is most pronounced in ventral recumbency (see 'Effect of patient position', below).

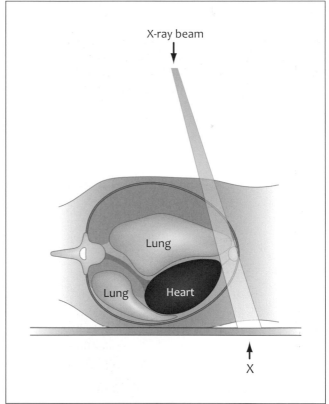

11.17 Altered cardiac position in lateral thoracic radiographs with pneumothorax. The dorsal displacement ('elevation') of the cardiac silhouette seen on lateral radiographs can be explained by loss of the air-filled lung supporting the heart in its normal anatomical position. Note that, in lateral recumbency, the lung closer to the detector collapses more than the uppermost lung due to gravity. Also, less gas is present in the gravity-dependent pleural cavity. These factors cause the heart to shift laterally and the cardiac apex to rotate away from the sternum. (Note the heart sinks laterally and is not elevated dorsally.) The space created between the cardiac apex and the sternum is highlighted by the X-ray beam. The increased distance between the heart and sternum that would be seen on the radiograph is indicated by X.

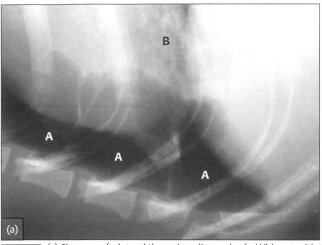

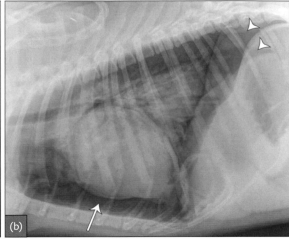

11.18 (a) Close-up of a lateral thoracic radiograph of a Whippet with traumatic pneumothorax showing increased distance between the cardiac silhouette and sternum. The space between the cardiac apex and sternum has a gas opacity with absent lung markings (A). Patchy lung consolidation summating with the heart (B) is likely due to pulmonary contusion. (b) Left lateral thoracic radiograph of a dog with pneumothorax. There is increased distance between the cardiac silhouette and the sternum (arrowed). Both lungs are small but have maintained their triangular shape. They have increased opacity and have retracted from the body walls and diaphragm. The pleural spaces are expanded and have a gas opacity without lung markings. This is especially noticeable in the lumbodiaphragmatic recesses (arrowheads) and costomediastinal recess ventral to the heart (arrowed).

Thoracic boundaries

In the presence of massive pleural effusion or tension pneumothorax, pleural expansion can alter the appearance of the thoracic boundaries by noticeably increasing the thoracic volume, creating a barrel-chested shape. The rib cage is expanded so that the ribs form right angles with the vertebral column (versus their normal caudal angulation). In addition, the intercostal spaces are wider than normal. The diaphragm may be flattened or even show a reversed curvature: its costal attachments may then become visible, a phenomenon known as 'tenting' (Figure 11.19). The extent of these changes is often best understood when pre- and post-drainage radiographs or CT images are compared.

Characteristics of pleural fluid

Free *versus* trapped fluid

Pleural fluid may be free (able to redistribute within the pleural cavity) or trapped (unable to redistribute; also known as encapsulated fluid). Recognizing the difference can be important for diagnosis and for planning thoracocentesis because it is important to know where the fluid is located relative to patient positioning. Pleural fluid is denser than lung, so free fluid always moves towards the gravity-dependent part of the thoracic cavity and the lung floats on top. On CT images, freely movable pleural fluid produces a crescent shape in the dependent part of the thoracic cavity. In contrast, encapsulated, trapped, or loculated fluid – often caused by an inflammatory process – usually appears

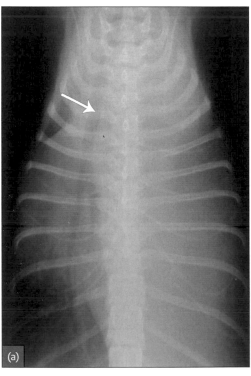

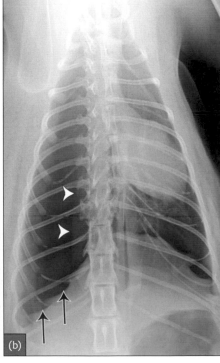

11.19 (a) DV thoracic radiograph of a cat with increased thoracic volume and a unilateral (left) pleural effusion due to pyothorax. Due to thoracic expansion, the ribs are at right angles to the vertebral column and there is an increased distance between ribs. The left pleural space is severely expanded with a homogeneous fluid opacity that effaces the adjacent borders of the mediastinum, body wall and diaphragm. The expanded space severely compresses the left lung and displaces the trachea (arrowed), principal bronchi and heart to the right, compressing the right lung. (b) DV radiograph of a cat with increased thoracic volume due to unilateral (right) tension pneumothorax. As in (a), the ribs are at right angles to the vertebral column and there is an increased distance between them. The diaphragm is flat with 'tenting' of its costal attachments (arrowed). The severely enlarged right pleural cavity has a gas opacity without lung markings. In addition to increased thoracic volume, the pressure within the right pleural space has caused complete collapse and medial displacement of the right lung (arrowheads) and a left cardiac shift.

lenticular or elliptical and its location is unaffected by gravity. On radiographs, differentiating encapsulated fluid from an extrapleural mass can be difficult. Ultrasonography can be helpful in such circumstances, especially once the area in question has been located. Otherwise a systematic examination of the entire thorax is required to identify the sonographic location of pockets of trapped fluid.

Effect of patient position

The distribution of free pleural fluid changes with patient position according to the effects of gravity (Figure 11.20). With the animal in lateral recumbency, fluid moves towards the laterally recumbent side and tends to accumulate in the dorsal and ventral parts of the affected pleural cavities (mostly ventral) as the lungs retract and float towards the highest position. On radiographs, this frequently results in border effacement of the heart and diaphragm, retraction of the ventral lung margins and interlobar fissures in the non-gravity-dependent lung. With the animal in dorsal recumbency, fluid accumulates dorsally in the pleural cavities, including the lumbodiaphragmatic recesses. This pattern of fluid distribution usually allows the heart to remain visible on VD radiographs, because of the differential absorption of the X-ray beam between the heart and pleural fluid. However, in ventral recumbency, pleural fluid will accumulate ventrally and efface the cardiac silhouette on DV radiographs. The heart is in the ventral part of the thorax, which is narrower than the dorsal part and, therefore, the fluid level is relatively higher in ventral than dorsal recumbency so there is a smaller difference in the absorption of the X-ray beam between the heart and pleural fluid on DV views.

In patients with respiratory disease, respiration may be further compromised when the patient is positioned in dorsal recumbency, so this technique should be used only when it is safe for the patient. In addition, small volumes of pleural fluid might not be detected radiographically when the patient is in dorsal recumbency.

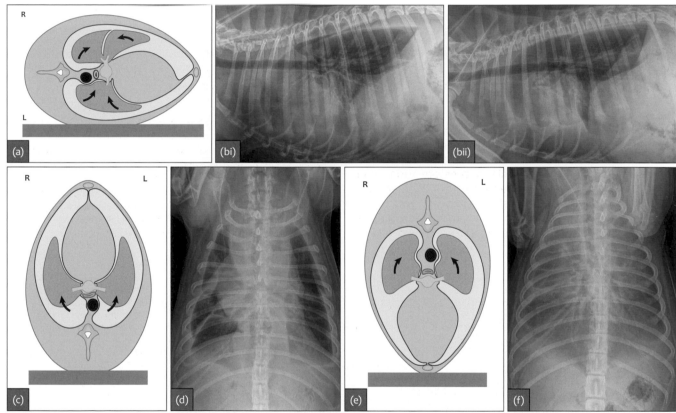

11.20 (a) Pleural fluid distribution in left lateral recumbency. The lungs are small and retracted away from the body wall and mediastinum in the direction of the arrows. There is greater collapse of the left lung due to gravity and the heart shifts to the left side as a consequence. Fluid in the left and right pleural cavities will contribute to diffuse increased opacity of the thoracic cavity relating to the volume of fluid present and create wide interlobar fissures. Fluid in the costomediastinal recesses will efface the ventral border of the cardiac silhouette. (bi) Right and (bii) left lateral thoracic radiographs of a dog with pleural fluid secondary to tricuspid valve dysplasia and Ebstein's anomaly. The lungs are small, retracted from the thoracic boundaries and have scalloped and angled margins. The pleural spaces are expanded and have a fluid opacity that effaces the borders of the heart and diaphragm. Multiple interlobar fissures are visible. (c) Pleural fluid distribution in dorsal recumbency. The lungs are small and retracted away from the body wall and mediastinum in the direction of the arrows. Fluid collects in the dorsal aspect of the left and right pleural cavities and displaces the lungs ventrally. The lungs and fluid are distributed over a wider area than when the animal is in ventral recumbency because the thoracic cavity is wider dorsally and the heart is located ventrally. This allows for greater differential absorption of the X-ray beam between the heart and lungs. (d) VD thoracic radiograph of a dog with pleural fluid secondary to tricuspid valve dysplasia and Ebstein's anomaly. The lungs are small, retracted from the thoracic boundaries, and have scalloped margins. The pleural spaces are expanded and have a fluid opacity that partially effaces the borders of the heart and diaphragm and makes the mediastinum appear wide. Multiple interlobar fissures are visible. (e) Pleural fluid distribution in ventral recumbency. The lungs are small and retracted away from the body wall and mediastinum in the direction of the arrows. Fluid collects in the ventral aspect of the left and right pleural cavities and displaces the lungs dorsally. The lungs and fluid are distributed over a narrower area than when the animal is in dorsal recumbency because the thoracic cavity is narrower ventrally and the heart is located ventrally. This results in similar absorption of the X-ray beam between the heart and lungs. (f) DV thoracic radiograph of a dog with pleural fluid secondary to tricuspid valve dysplasia and Ebstein's anomaly. The lungs are small and retracted from the thoracic boundaries, especially in the cranial thorax and both costodiaphragmatic recesses. The pleural spaces are expanded and have a fluid opacity that completely effaces the borders of the heart and diaphragm. Multiple interlobar fissures are visible. L= left; R = right.
(a, c, e, Redrawn after Suter (1984))

CT is commonly performed with the patient in ventral recumbency so free pleural fluid is usually observed in the ventral aspect of the thoracic cavity with the lungs floating on top (dorsally). The lungs are less mobile near the lung hilus and are more mobile at the periphery. Therefore, it is more common to see the periphery of the lung float laterally or become displaced (see Figure 11.13d). If the patient is scanned in dorsal recumbency, then the fluid redistributes dorsally, and the lung will be located more ventrally than normal. Because the lungs are anchored at the hilus, they retain their normal orientation with the lung tips directed ventrally.

Thoracic ultrasonography is typically performed with the patient in lateral or ventral recumbency or standing. Scanning from the gravity-dependent surface of the thoracic wall will ensure that the fluid is located as close to the transducer as possible and therefore increase the likelihood of it being identified (see Figure 11.8). Note that trapped or encapsulated fluid will be unaffected by changes in patient position on all imaging modalities.

Effect of fluid volume

Imaging signs are greatly influenced by the volume of pleural fluid (Figure 11.21).

On lateral views, pleural fluid is usually first detected dorsal to the sternum where the thin ventral edges of the lung retract easily (Figure 11.22). Depending on the volume of fluid, it may be difficult to detect an increased opacity in this location because the fluid that coats the most ventral part of the lung causes only a slight increased opacity. The lung lobes in this area are more likely to retract because of their ventral location (free pleural fluid tends to accumulate here) and the elasticity of the lung tissue is such that the smaller lobes (right middle and left cranial) and the thinner parts of the lung lobes (periphery) are more likely to collapse under the pressure from the pleural fluid.

As the volume of pleural fluid increases, retraction and separation of the lung lobes from the body wall and each other becomes progressively more pronounced on all radiographic views (see Figure 11.20). With mild to moderate pleural effusions, the degree of retraction of the lung

Volume of effusion	General comments	Lateral view	Ventrodorsal view	Dorsoventral view
Small	Lateral view is preferable to DV and VD views to identify small volumes of effusion. Expiratory views are preferable as lung volume is reduced, so the fluid volume is relatively greater and distributed over a smaller area	Fluid opacity dorsal to sternum causing mild retraction of lung. Ventral margins of the cardiac shadow and diaphragm obscured. Interlobar fissures visible as linear opacities	Very small volumes concealed by mediastinum. Fluid opacity between the lung and lateral thoracic walls, causing mild retraction of the lung. Rounded lung margins at costophrenic angles. Interlobar fissures visible even with small volume of fluid	Mediastinum conceals small volumes or may appear slightly wide. Cardiac silhouette and dome of diaphragm become hazy and partially obscured. Fissure adjacent to the accessory lobe may be visible but others are less likely to be seen
Moderate	Interlobar fissures appear as wedge-shaped opacities extending towards the hilus. As the volume increases they become easier to identify and a larger number become visible, even on DV views. The effusion begins to compress the lungs more and produces an increased opacity throughout the lungs	Overall increased opacity throughout thorax (fluid in costomediastinal recess). Moderate retraction of the lung margins from the sternum. Ventral two-thirds of the cardiac silhouette and diaphragmatic line obscured. Prominent interlobar fissures	Moderate retraction of the lung margins from the lateral thoracic walls but lobes retain their normal shape. Increased area of fluid opacity between the lung margins and the lateral thoracic walls. Prominent interlobar fissures. Wide and rounded costophrenic recesses. Left border of descending aorta obscured. Cardiac silhouette and diaphragmatic line less well visualized. Cranial mediastinum remains visible	Wide mediastinum. Cardiac silhouette and dome of the diaphragm completely obscured. Moderate retraction of the lung margins from the lateral thoracic walls. Narrow area of fluid opacity between the lung margins and the lateral thoracic walls. Peripheral areas of interlobar fissures become visible
Large	Thoracic cavity may appear expanded or barrel-shaped, especially in cats. Diaphragm may be flattened on all views causing caudal displacement of the liver (must be differentiated from hepatomegaly). Interlobar fissures extend to the hilus and separate lobes, producing a leaf-like arrangement. Progressive compression of the lung eventually results in collapse. Smaller lobes (right middle then left and right cranial, then accessory) and peripheral areas of larger lobes are the most compliant, so collapse first. Caudal lobes usually remain inflated. Air bronchograms may be associated with complete collapse. Cardiac silhouette and diaphragm remain visible at greater volumes on VD views than DV and lateral views	Marked retraction of the lung towards the hilus. Lungs float in the fluid causing dorsal displacement of the trachea and lung hilus. Cranial lobes may be completely collapsed and caudally displaced	Wide mediastinum. Lung lobes separated but retain normal shape. Cardiac silhouette and diaphragm obscured. Descending aorta obscured	Marked retraction of the lung margins from the lateral thoracic walls. Lung lobes separated. Cardiac silhouette and thoracic side of the diaphragmatic line obscured

11.21 Radiographic features of different volumes of pleural effusion.

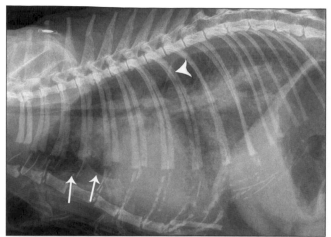

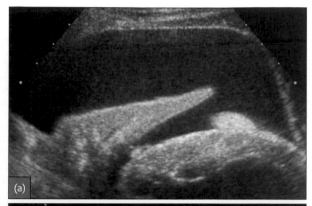

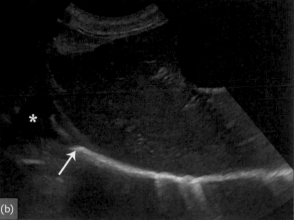

11.22 Right lateral thoracic radiograph of a cat with congestive heart failure. The cardiac silhouette and pulmonary blood vessels are enlarged and there is pulmonary opacification that is most marked caudodorsally. In addition, the lungs have reduced size and are retracted away from the body wall due to fluid in the pleural cavities. Note the fluid opacity dorsal to the sternum and ventral to the lung (arrowed) and an interlobar fissure (arrowhead). The pulmonary opacification is likely a combination of pulmonary oedema, reduced lung inflation and summation with the pleural fluid.

11.23 (a) Thoracic ultrasound image obtained using an intercostal window in a dog with pleural effusion. Deep to the body wall, the pleural space is enlarged and filled with a large volume of anechoic fluid, which was a transudate. The fluid surrounds echogenic collapsed lung. (b) Ultrasound image obtained using an abdominal window in a dog with ulcerative haemorrhagic gastroenteritis. The body wall and liver are in the near field. In the far field, a small volume of anechoic fluid (*) is seen cranial to the diaphragm and adjacent to the ventral tip of a lung lobe (arrowed), which is aerated and not collapsed. The location of the fluid is consistent with pleural effusion, and its irregular and triangular shape distinguishes it from pericardial effusion. This pleural effusion was occult, demonstrating the importance of checking cranial to the diaphragm when performing abdominal ultrasonography as this may be the first indication of pleural disease.

lobes seen on the DV or VD view does not reflect the true extent of the effusion. This is because the fluid accumulates with gravity beneath the lungs and only the fluid lying between the lung and the thoracic wall is struck tangentially by the X-ray beam. With very large volumes of pleural fluid, the lung lobes are even more markedly retracted towards the hilus.

On CT images obtained with the animal in ventral recumbency, fluid accumulates in the ventral aspect of the thorax. Small volumes only mildly dorsally displace the adjacent aerated lung. As the volume of fluid increases, then the area of the thoracic cavity that it occupies will also increase so the displacement is greater and lung compression (secondary collapse or atelectasis) is likely (see Figures 11.7, 11.13d and 11.14).

On ultrasound examination, large volumes of free pleural fluid are likely to be identified from most areas of the thoracic wall where there is no intervening air-filled lung (Figure 11.23). Small volumes of fluid are more likely to be detected when the transducer is placed against the most gravity-dependent area of the thoracic wall (see Figure 11.8). Knowledge of the underlying anatomy is useful to identify acoustic windows through which small volumes of fluid can be located without intervening lung or ribs. The confirmation of small volumes of pleural fluid may be possible via a transdiaphragmatic approach and occult pleural effusions are often first identified during abdominal ultrasonography (Figure 11.23b). In general, the larger the volume of the pleural fluid the larger the distance between the lung surface and body wall or diaphragm, although this is dependent on patient positioning and location of the transducer.

Unilateral *versus* bilateral fluid

Pleural fluid may accumulate in one or both pleural cavities. Because the caudal mediastinum is fenestrated or tears easily in dogs and cats, fluid usually accumulates in both pleural cavities in these species, even when the inciting cause is localized to one side of the thorax. Unilateral or uneven bilateral effusions can result from:

- Closed mediastinal fenestrations, which can be normal anatomical variation or an acquired abnormality in association with chylothorax, haemothorax, or a neoplastic or reactive inflammatory effusion (see Figure 11.16)
- The presence of trapped or encapsulated fluid
- Preferential fluid accumulation adjacent to a collapsed lung lobe. The lung lobe may be collapsed either due to lung disease or secondary to the pleural fluid.

On radiographs, unilateral pleural fluid is easiest to identify on DV and VD views. In general, the typical signs of pleural fluid are only seen on one side of the thorax. A mediastinal shift may also be present, but the direction of the shift depends upon the volume of pleural fluid and the degree of lung collapse. For example, large volumes of fluid may collapse the ipsilateral lung and displace the mediastinum towards the contralateral side (Figure 11.24).

Unilateral effusion is more difficult to identify on lateral views due to summation of the two sides. When the fluid is in the gravity-dependent pleural cavity, it summates with the inflated upper lung and may mimic parenchymal opacification. When the animal is positioned with the fluid in the non-dependent pleural cavity, then more specific signs like

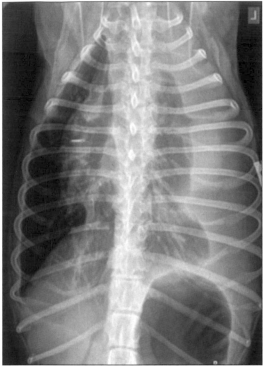

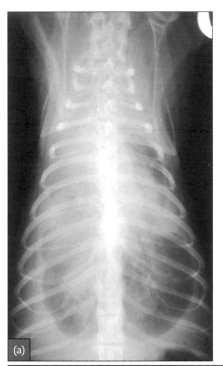

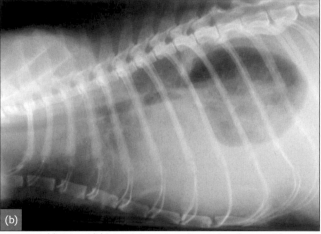

11.24 DV thoracic radiograph of a dog with a large-volume unilateral pleural effusion. The left lung is moderately reduced in size and retracted towards the lung hilus, away from the left body wall and diaphragm. The left pleural cavity is expanded with a homogeneous fluid opacity that effaces the adjacent borders of the cardiac silhouette and diaphragm, and there is also a right mediastinal shift.

11.25 (a) DV and (b) lateral thoracic radiographs of a cat with an uneven bilateral pleural effusion due to pyothorax. Both lungs have reduced size and are unevenly retracted from the body wall and diaphragm. The lung margins are noticeably rounded and scalloped, consistent with a reactive or chronic effusion. Restrictive pleuritis is possible. In addition, there is patchy lung consolidation due to concurrent pneumonia.

fluid opacity dorsal to the sternum and retracted lung margins may also be observed.

Uneven bilateral effusion will also produce asymmetrical changes on DV or VD radiographs, reflecting the volume of fluid present on each side (Figure 11.25). On lateral views, freely movable bilateral effusion typically results in greater collapse of the gravity-dependent lung compared with the non-dependent lung, as fluid moves across the mediastinum with repositioning. Exceptions are possible in cases with concurrent lung disease.

The cross-sectional nature of CT images means that unilateral or uneven bilateral pleural effusions are easy to identify, with the appearance of each pleural cavity reflecting the volume of fluid present. Confirming unilateral pleural effusion using ultrasonography is challenging and requires careful examination to demonstrate the presence of fluid on one side of the mediastinum but not on the other. Likewise, identifying uneven bilateral effusions using ultrasonography is currently impossible as there is no method to accurately determine pleural fluid volume.

Differentiating pleural effusion from other conditions on radiographs

Pseudoeffusions

Some normal anatomical features can produce signs that mimic pleural effusion:

- Mediastinal fat can displace the cardiac silhouette away from the sternum and outline the ventral margins of the lung lobes, causing them to appear rounded on the lateral view, simulating the presence of pleural fluid. This normal feature can be differentiated from an effusion because the cardiac silhouette is not effaced by fat, which has lower opacity than fluid
- Thoracic conformation in certain breeds, notably the Dachshund, may mimic the presence of a small-volume pleural effusion on DV or VD views due to the curvature of the osseous ribs and costal cartilages (Figure 11.26). In dogs with deep narrow chests, the ventral lung margins may be retracted from the sternum, imitating the presence of a small-volume effusion
- In cats, the caudal lung lobes do not extend to fill the angle between the vertebral column and the diaphragm (the lumbodiaphragmatic recess) on lateral radiographs as in dogs. The psoas minor muscle in this region gives rise to a narrow triangle of soft tissue opacity between the caudal margin of the lung and the vertebral column, which should not be misinterpreted as pleural fluid (Figure 11.27).

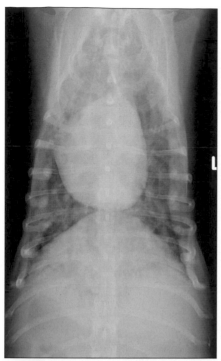

11.26 DV thoracic radiograph of a Dachshund. The shape of the rib cage is typical of what might be seen in some chondrodystrophic dogs. Note the internal deviation of the costochondral junctions creating linear soft tissue opacities that summate with the lateral margins of both lungs. This appearance of the thoracic body wall should not be mistaken for pleural effusion.

Cranial mediastinal mass *versus* pleural effusion

Pleural fluid may mimic or obscure mediastinal masses. Therefore, it can be difficult to diagnose and characterize mediastinal masses when pleural fluid is present. Mediastinal masses tend to be in the midline and will displace other mediastinal structures when large enough.

- In the presence of fluid alone, the heart or trachea should move according to the effects of gravity. Movement that is independent of gravity suggests displacement by a mass (Figure 11.28).
- Moderate to marked volumes of pleural fluid can cause the trachea to become more parallel to the vertebral column, even in the absence of cardiac disease. Dorsal tracheal displacement alone is therefore not an accurate sign of cardiomegaly.
- Compression or distortion of the trachea, and caudal displacement of the carina, usually indicates a cranial mediastinal mass. In the absence of a mass, small volumes of pleural fluid are unable to deviate the trachea dorsally and even large volumes do not compress or distort the trachea nor displace the carina caudally.

Horizontal beam radiography may be useful to observe areas of the thorax concealed by fluid on standard views. CT and ultrasonography are both able to differentiate between cranial mediastinal masses and pleural effusion, and ultrasonography can be useful to help obtain diagnostic samples.

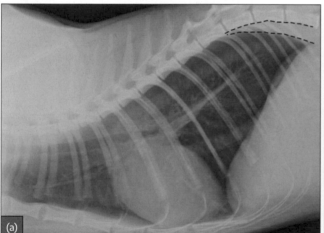

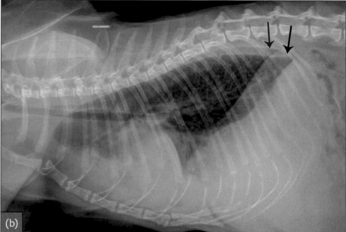

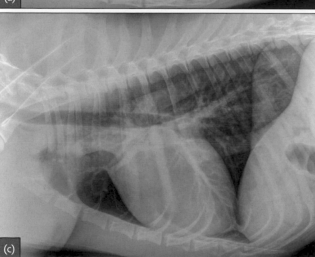

11.27 (a) Lateral thoracic radiograph of a normal cat. In cats, the lumbodiaphragmatic recess is located more ventral to the vertebral column than in dogs due to the morphology of the psoas muscle (dashed line) attachments. The resultant soft tissue opacity between the lung margin and vertebral column represents the muscles and not the lumbodiaphragmatic recess, which is part of the pleural cavity. This soft tissue opacity should not be mistaken for a small volume of pleural effusion in cats. (b) Lateral thoracic radiograph of a cat with pleural effusion. Compared to the normal cat (a), the lungs are rounder and more retracted, and the fluid-filled lumbodiaphragmatic recess (arrowed) is larger, creating a fluid opacity that effaces the adjacent border of the psoas muscles. (c) Lateral thoracic radiograph of a normal dog. In contrast to cats, canine lungs extend further dorsally and often summate with the vertebral column due to the morphology of the ribs and their attachment to the vertebral column.

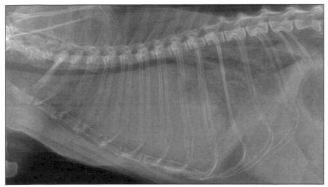

11.28 Lateral thoracic radiograph of a cat with a cranial mediastinal mass and pleural effusion. It can be difficult to localize an abnormal, widespread soft tissue opacity to the pleural cavity, mediastinum, cardiac silhouette or some combination. In this cat, the presence of pleural fluid is confirmed based on retraction and rounding of the caudal lung lobes and a fluid opacity external to the lungs that effaces the cranial margin of the diaphragm. Ventrally, falciform fat contrasts with the caudal border of the diaphragm. Radiographic signs of a concurrent mediastinal mass include severe dorsal displacement of the trachea, caudal displacement of the lungs and caudal displacement of the carina to the seventh intercostal space. The radiograph is well positioned without rotation, which supports that these changes are real and not artefactual.

Lung mass *versus* pleural effusion

Many lung masses are accompanied by pleural fluid so they can be difficult to diagnose and characterize on radiographs. Positional radiography can be helpful to separate masses from small volumes of free pleural fluid. CT can differentiate between lung masses and pleural effusion, although this is more difficult when large volumes of fluid have caused substantial lung atelectasis surrounding the mass. Ultrasonography can be used to identify the pleural effusion and visualize any lung mass located at the periphery of the lung as well as to guide diagnostic sampling.

Thoracic boundary mass *versus* pleural effusion

Body wall and diaphragmatic masses can also be difficult to diagnose and characterize radiographically when accompanied by pleural fluid that obscures details like the presence of an extrapleural sign. Occasionally, tell-tale signs like osteolysis or periosteal reactions may be detected. Positional radiography can be helpful to separate masses from small volumes of free pleural fluid using fluid redistribution but CT and ultrasonography generally provide more useful information.

Characteristics of pleural gas
Effect of patient position and pleural volume

In contrast to pleural fluid detection, pneumothorax is best identified on lateral rather than DV or VD views. Patient positioning is important because free pleural gas rises to the highest point of the thoracic cavity. Consequently, pleural gas frequently contrasts with the caudal lung lobes on lateral and DV radiographs (Figure 11.29). Pneumothorax may be unilateral or bilateral. On lateral views, separation of the cardiac silhouette from the sternum is commonly observed (see Figure 11.18). The greatest separation between cardiac apex and sternum is seen when the affected side is nearer to the cassette (see Figure 11.17).

The degree of retraction of the lung margins is predominantly related to the volume of pleural gas present.

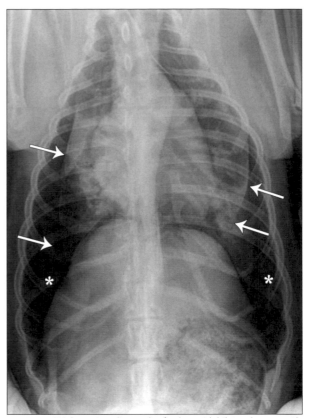

11.29 DV thoracic radiograph of a dog with bilateral pneumothorax. Both lungs are small and retracted from the body wall (arrowed). Both pleural spaces are expanded and have a gas opacity (*). Pulmonary blood vessels do not extend to the periphery of the thoracic cavity.

Small- to medium-volume pneumothorax is often not visible on VD radiographs because the air accumulates in the midline, where it is obscured by summation with the mediastinal and skeletal structures. However, larger volumes are visible. Small-volume pneumothorax will be accompanied by limited retraction of the lung margins. One of the first indications of free pleural gas is the presence of small gas opacities summating with the cardiac apex, because air becomes trapped against the mediastinum in the gravity-dependent pleural cavity.

Most CT images are obtained with the patient in ventral recumbency and, therefore, free gas will accumulate in the dorsal aspect of the thorax (Figure 11.30). CT is very sensitive for the identification of free pleural gas, so even tiny volumes are visible. Small volumes will be located between the pulmonary and costal pleurae and may be visible in several locations. Larger volumes will coalesce dorsally, accompanied by retraction of the lung margins from the body wall. If CT images are obtained with the patient in dorsal recumbency, then the gas will be located ventrally.

Pleural gas is identified using ultrasonography by placing the transducer on the uppermost aspect of the thoracic wall, which varies with patient positioning. A systematic examination is required as small volumes or pockets of gas are more easily missed than large ones. The approximate volume of gas present can be estimated with the patient in ventral recumbency by determining how far ventrally in the intercostal space the gas extends before the retracted lung contacts the costal pleura again, as determined by movement of the pleura with respiration. This is known as the lung point (Figure 11.31).

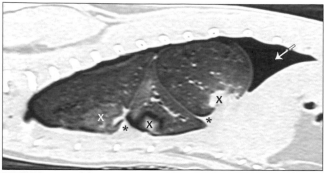

11.30 Sagittal thoracic CT image of a cat in ventral recumbency with pneumothorax and focal inflammatory lung abnormalities (X), displayed in a lung window. The lung lobes are small and retracted from the body wall and diaphragm. The pleural space is expanded and non-attenuating (arrowed). The gas preferentially accumulates in the caudodorsally located lumbodiaphragmatic recess due to gravity. The pleural space also contains a small volume of fluid, which is located ventrally due to gravity (*). The lung margins are rounded, suggesting chronic disease. Free pleural gas can be distinguished from lung gas by the lack of internal architecture when viewed using a lung window.

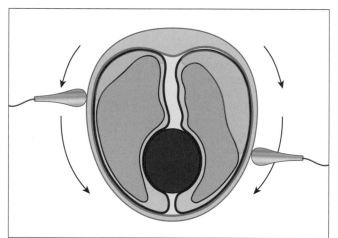

11.31 A transverse section through the thorax showing ultrasound probe placement and movement to estimate the extent of a pneumothorax (blue area) by identifying the lung point, which is where the lung (purple area) regains contact with the costal pleura. Beginning dorsally, move the ultrasound transducer ventrally in the intercostal spaces until a lung point is identified. More severe pneumothorax (right side of the image) will have more ventrally located lung points.

Pleural pressure

Pneumothorax may be due to an injury of the body wall (open pneumothorax) or lung (closed pneumothorax). When the pressure in the pleural cavity is lower than or equivalent to atmospheric pressure, then the pneumothorax may be classified as simple or normotensive. When the pleural pressure exceeds atmospheric pressure, then the pneumothorax is classified as a tension pneumothorax. Tension pneumothorax develops when the injury creates a valve effect that allows more gas into the pleural cavity than is released from it. This increased pleural pressure can rapidly lead to maximal lung collapse and severe medial displacement of the lung and can become life-threatening.

- Bilateral tension pneumothorax can produce a barrel-chested conformation and severe caudal displacement of the diaphragm with 'tenting'.
- Unilateral tension pneumothorax can produce asymmetry of the thorax and a mediastinal shift towards the contralateral side (see Figure 11.19b).

Pseudopneumothorax

A number of conditions can mimic pneumothorax on radiography. Folds of skin running parallel with the long axis of the patient may create a linear air–tissue interface on DV and VD radiographs that summates with the lung periphery (Figure 11.32). These folds can be distinguished from a true pneumothorax as they can be traced beyond the thoracic margins, they contain pulmonary blood vessels and bronchial markings that extend to the body wall, and the direction of the curvature of the lines is different from true interlobar fissures.

Conditions causing pulmonary hyperlucency must also be differentiated from pneumothorax. These conditions include emaciation, lung overinflation associated with asthma or emphysema, and pulmonary hypovascularity due to hypovolaemia (e.g. shock), thromboembolism or reduced cardiac output (e.g. tetralogy of Fallot). Faint vascular markings will usually be seen extending to the thoracic wall in these conditions, and there will be no thin line to mark the edge of a collapsed lung lobe.

Other conditions that can mimic pneumothorax include:

- Overpenetration (overexposure) of thoracic radiographs
- Compensatory hyperinflation of lungs in animals under stress or positive pressure ventilation
- Pulmonary bullae
- Pneumomediastinum
- Subcutaneous emphysema
- Incarceration and gaseous dilatation of herniated stomach or intestine.

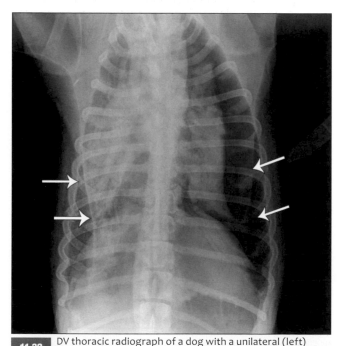

11.32 DV thoracic radiograph of a dog with a unilateral (left) pneumothorax following lung lobectomy. The left lung is small, opaque, and severely retracted from the body wall and diaphragm. The left pleural space is severely expanded and has a gas opacity. On both sides of the dog, there are also prominent skin folds that summate with the lateral aspects of the thorax (arrowed). These linear opacities are differentiated from lung margins because they extend beyond the thoracic boundaries and curve in a different direction than interlobar fissures. Skin folds should not be mistaken for signs of pneumothorax. The ribs on the left side are further apart from each other, indicating increased volume on this side of the thoracic cavity.

Special radiographic views for pleural disease

Radiography is commonly performed in animals with known or suspected pleural disease. Typically, some combination of orthogonal radiographic views is obtained, but a single view may be helpful in severely dyspnoeic patients. Good quality radiographs may be difficult to obtain in dyspnoeic animals and consideration should be given when positioning these animals to avoid precipitating a crisis. It is important to consider oxygen supplementation, creating a calm environment, relieving patient stress or pain and working efficiently. Dorsal recumbency may exacerbate respiratory difficulty in some patients. Drainage of an effusion or pneumothorax prior to radiography may be advisable.

There are many techniques that can be employed to assess pleural disease more effectively. These include altering patient position, beam angulation and making use of different respiratory phases (Figure 11.33). Radiation safety must always be considered and there can be increased risk of exposure when obtaining horizontal beam views or manually restraining a patient (see Chapter 1). Radiographic technique will often require adjustment when pleural disease is suspected. Exposure values based simply on measurements of patient thickness may result in underexposure in the presence of pleural effusion and overexposure in patients with pneumothorax.

Role of cross-sectional imaging of the pleural space

Computed tomography

CT is currently the technique of choice for advanced cross-sectional imaging of the pleural space. Its use depends on availability and usually requires a clinically

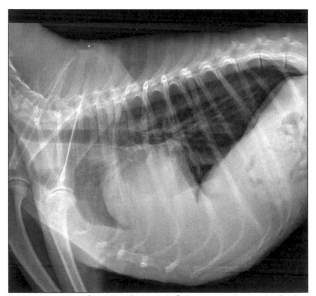

11.33 Lateral (standing/horizontal) thoracic radiograph of a dog with chronic chylothorax. The pleural fluid has accumulated in the ventral aspect of the thoracic cavity according to the effect of gravity, effacing the ventral borders of the cardiac silhouette and diaphragm. This redistribution of fluid demonstrates that the fluid is freely mobile and not compartmentalized, thus allowing the dorsal thoracic structures to be assessed. In the cranioventral thorax, the margin between the lung and pleural fluid should not be mistaken for a horizontal air–fluid interface that may be seen with pneumohydrothorax.

stable patient because sedation or general anaesthesia is often necessary to optimize patient positioning and restraint, and to minimize motion. CT is therefore usually performed as a secondary investigation after initial patient triage and stabilization. However, CT may be performed early in patients with polytrauma. Pre- and post contrast thoracic images are usually obtained in the transverse plane with the patient in ventral recumbency or, in patients without respiratory compromise, dorsal recumbency. In animals with pleural effusion, post-contrast CT images allow differentiation of contrast-enhancing pleura and collapsed lung tissue from non-enhancing pleural fluid. CT images of the thorax are usually obtained during a brief period of induced apnoea after manual inflation of the lungs. This technique should be carried out with care and is contraindicated in patients with suspected pneumothorax, radiographic evidence of bullous lung disease or pulmonary overinflation. A kernel frequency in the medium range should be used without additional edge enhancement to avoid rebound artefacts that may mimic increased pleural thickness or pneumothorax. Images should be viewed using lung and soft tissue windows to evaluate the pleural space (see Figure 11.14).

Ultrasonography

Point-of-care ultrasonography is increasingly used in the investigation of patients with pleural disease, particularly in emergency settings as part of their initial assessment and management. These patients are often clinically compromised and the use of ultrasonography in this way offers several advantages:

- The equipment is portable so examinations can be performed without the need to move the patient
- Sedation is not required, which is beneficial for clinically compromised patients
- The examination can be performed with the patient in ventral recumbency, which is beneficial in patients with respiratory compromise
- The results are obtained immediately, allowing rapid adjustment of patient management.

However, emergency ultrasonographic assessment of the pleural space presents several challenges:

- Accurate assessment of thoracic structures is operator dependent and requires practice
- These patients are often difficult to examine due to clinical signs of respiratory distress
- Global assessment of the pleural cavity requires a thorough and systematic examination of the thorax, particularly if focal lesions are present
- The clinical environment may be bright, noisy and physically cramped, placing additional demands on the operator.

The benefits of thoracic ultrasonography in patients with pleural disease include:

- Rapid differentiation between the presence of fluid, soft tissue and gas within the pleural space
- Rapid differentiation of pleural effusions from pericardial and mediastinal effusions
- Guidance of sampling techniques
- The identification of occult pleural space lesions when performing a cardiac or abdominal examination – the latter via a transdiaphragmatic approach.

Magnetic resonance imaging

MRI has the potential for investigating pleural disease in small animals but there is currently limited evidence supporting its use over other effective modalities. The current role of MRI in patients with pleural disease is:

- The identification of occult pleural space lesions when MRI is performed for other reasons, usually examination of the vertebral column for neurological or musculoskeletal abnormalities
- To further investigate pleural lesions identified using other modalities
- Assessment of thoracic structures if advanced cross-sectional imaging is indicated and CT is unavailable or the use of iodinated contrast medium is contraindicated.

The main limitation of MRI for examining the pleural cavity is image degradation due to respiratory and cardiac motion. Motion artefact can be reduced by:

- Placement of the region of interest closest to the table to reduce movement if this does not significantly impair respiratory function
- Use of a surface coil rather than a birdcage radiofrequency coil when a specific superficial region is under investigation
- Orienting the phase-encoding direction so that any motion artefact avoids areas of importance
- Hyperventilation of patients under general anaesthesia to induce a period of apnoea during which an ultrafast sequence is performed
- Electrocardiogram and/or respiratory gating
- The use of techniques to actively suppress the signal from tissues likely to cause motion artefacts including spatial or spectral saturation, phase reordering and gradient nulling.

Image quality may be improved by increasing the signal:noise ratio by increasing the number of signal averages/excitations, but this does not reduce respiratory blurring and increases scan time. There is no set of pulse sequence protocols for MRI of the pleural structures. Each case is unique and the sequences used should be tailored according to the patient and the pathology.

Diseases

There are many different types of pleural disease, but the most common pathogenic mechanisms are inflammation, trauma and unregulated growth (neoplasia). Pleural disease may affect the pleural cavities, pleurae or both. Most pleural diseases cause expansion of the serous cavity due to the influx of fluid (pleural effusion), gas (pneumothorax) or abdominal content (diaphragmatic hernia). Some pleural diseases alter the morphology and function of the serous membranes making them thick, nodular or fibrotic (stiff). Altered pleura is frequently due to acute or chronic inflammation (pleuritis) or neoplasia (e.g. mesothelioma, carcinomatosis).

Pleural effusion

Pleural effusion is the accumulation of any type of fluid in the pleural space. Small volumes may be tolerated without primary clinical signs, as may larger volumes if they have accumulated slowly. Ongoing fluid accumulation eventually results in pulmonary atelectasis and hypoventilation. It has been suggested that 30 ml/kg of pleural fluid causes subtle dyspnoea and 60 ml/kg results in obvious dyspnoea. Cats may not demonstrate clinical signs unless stressed or near death. Clinical examination may reveal tachypnoea and dyspnoea. Large-volume effusions may result in a barrel-shaped thorax, muffled or absent heart sounds, loss of a palpable apical beat, reduced respiratory sounds (especially ventrally) and dull sounds on percussion. Additional clinical findings may be seen depending on the cause of the effusion. Indications for imaging in animals with pleural effusion include:

- Confirmation of the presence of effusion and determination of the severity
- Identification of small-volume effusions not revealed on clinical examination
- Identification of the primary cause of the effusion
- Identification of fluid pocketing
- Guidance for fluid sampling or drainage.

It may be necessary to stabilize the patient prior to imaging; thoracocentesis may be necessary.

Causes of effusion

Fluid can accumulate in the pleural space due to increased formation, reduced resorption or both. Any process that disrupts capillary or interstitial hydrostatic or oncotic pressures, including lymphatic drainage or vessel integrity, can result in net fluid accumulation. In addition, extension of pathological fluid accumulation from adjacent structures (e.g. parapneumonic spread of infection) can lead to pleural fluid accumulation. Pleural effusions can therefore result from pleural, pulmonary or systemic diseases. In cats, common causes of pleural effusions include feline infectious peritonitis (FIP), congestive heart failure, pyothorax, neoplasia and idiopathic chylothorax.

Hydrothorax: This is the accumulation of aqueous fluid due to an imbalance between oncotic and hydrostatic forces and can be either a transudate or modified transudate.

- A true transudate is a result of hypoproteinaemia (serum albumin below 15 g/l), which is caused by protein-losing enteropathies or nephropathies, chronic hepatic disease, or severe malnutrition. Even a true transudate causes pleural irritation and so will become modified with time.
- A modified transudate is altered by the presence of non-inflammatory cells. This may result from:
  - Systemic hypertension, secondary to right-sided heart failure. Note: Left-sided failure in dogs does not usually result in pleural effusion unless there is concurrent right-sided failure, when it will be accompanied by hepatic congestion and peritoneal effusion (ascites). In cats, pleural effusion is less common with right-sided heart failure, but can occur with left-sided heart failure due to variations in the visceral pleural drainage (see 'Imaging anatomy', above)
  - Reduced pleural lymphatic or venous drainage (e.g. due to cranial mediastinal mass)
  - Protein leakage due to chronic diaphragmatic hernias, especially with liver strangulation
  - Increased pleural hydrostatic pressure due to conditions causing lung lobe collapse or preventing reinflation.

Sterile exudates: Exudates are inflammatory effusions resulting from increased capillary permeability, which are often associated with disease of the pleural surfaces. Exudates may be sterile or septic. Sterile exudates may result from:

* Pneumonia
* Pulmonary or pleural neoplasia
* Exudative pleuritis (e.g. FIP)
* Autoimmune disorders (e.g. systemic lupus erythematosus, rheumatoid arthritis, immune-mediated haemolytic anaemia)
* Pulmonary granulomatous disorders.

Septic exudates: Pyothorax (pleural empyema or purulent pleuritis) may result from contamination by a large range of infectious agents. The most common are *Pasteurella multocida*, *Bacteroides* and *Fusobacterium* in cats, and *Nocardia* and *Actinomyces* in dogs. Contamination may be caused by:

* Direct trauma (e.g. cat bites, penetrating injuries)
* Foreign material (e.g. sticks, grass awns) migrating from the skin surface, oesophagus or respiratory tract (often encountered in hunting dogs)
* Haematogenous or lymphatic spread from a distant septic focus
* Rupture of mediastinal structures (e.g. oesophagus)
* Direct extension from a lung lesion (e.g. ruptured abscess, pneumonia)
* Iatrogenic introduction (e.g. surgery, thoracocentesis).

Haemothorax: This is the accumulation of blood in the pleural space and can result from:

* Erosion or rupture of thoracic blood vessels due to trauma, neoplasia, inflammation, aneurysm (e.g. *Spirocerca lupi*) or iatrogenic causes (e.g. surgery, thoracocentesis)
* Rupture of an intrathoracic mass (e.g. haemangiosarcoma)
* Clotting abnormalities: congenital (e.g. von Willebrand's disease) or acquired (e.g. anticoagulant rodenticides)
* Pulmonary infarcts
* Lung lobe torsion
* Thymic haemorrhage in young dogs.

Chylothorax: This is the accumulation of chyle in the pleural space and can result from:

* Idiopathic chylothorax (common and often a diagnosis of exclusion)
* Cardiac disease (e.g. cardiomyopathy, pericardial effusion, tricuspid dysplasia)
* Heartworm disease
* Cranial mediastinal mass
* Cranial vena caval thrombosis/obstruction
* Fungal granulomas
* Congenital or traumatic lesions of the thoracic duct (rare).

Pseudochyle: This fluid contains lipid breakdown products from malignant or exfoliated pleural cells. Accumulation in the pleural cavity may result from:

* Any longstanding effusion
* Feline cardiomyopathies
* Low-grade pleural infections
* Intrathoracic neoplasia.

Abdominal conditions: Pleural effusion may also occur secondary to abdominal conditions:

* Abdominal fluid may be transported across the diaphragm via the lymphatic drainage, resulting in a concurrent pleural effusion of the same type
* Transport of pancreatic enzymes in animals with pancreatitis may result in a pleural exudate
* Bile in the pleural cavity may occur from transdiaphragmatic transport of bile in animals with extrahepatic biliary tract rupture and bile peritonitis. Alternatively, it may result from a penetrating injury creating a direct tract between the biliary system and thoracic cavity through the diaphragm
* Urothorax may occur where there is trauma to the urinary tract concurrent with diaphragmatic rupture.

Radiography

See 'Interpretative principles', above, for an overview of the features of pleural effusion. Note:

* The decubitus (lateral) radiograph is the most reliable view for identifying small volumes of pleural fluid (5–50 ml in the dog) and assessing changes in volume over time
* Radiographs usually lead to an underestimate of the volume of pleural fluid because the fluid is incompletely seen on each view
* Fluid type cannot be determined based only on radiographic appearance
* Pleural fluid can be indistinguishable from other conditions, for example, adjacent soft tissue masses, lung consolidation and pleural adhesions
* The caudal border of the diaphragm can usually be located by the presence of fat on the abdominal side unless peritoneal effusion is also present.

Radiographic features pointing to the primary cause of the effusion (e.g. cardiac enlargement, mediastinal mass) should be sought. Secondary or concurrent changes (e.g. lung collapse, lung lobe torsion) may provide diagnostic clues or help establish severity.

Chronic or reactive pleural effusion: Chronic pleural effusions of any type will cause the pleura to become thick, forming a rind. This tends to occur more rapidly with reactive effusions (pyothorax, chylothorax, haemothorax) than non-reactive effusions and may also be seen with neoplastic effusions. Reactive effusions may also lead to the formation of fibrous adhesions and trapping or encapsulation of the fluid.
Radiographic findings include:

* Expansion of the pleural space(s) with a fluid opacity and concurrent reduced lung size
* Uneven retraction and collapse of the lung lobes
* Lung margins becoming irregular, undulating and unusually rounded (see Figures 11.16 and 11.25)
* Trapped fluid that is partially restricted by fibrous adhesions and unequally distributed throughout the pleural cavities, but can reposition with gravity
* Encapsulated fluid that is completely confined by fibrous material and has a constant position and shape that are not altered by patient positioning and gravity.

Thoracocentesis: Thoracocentesis can be performed to remove fluid or air from one or both pleural cavities to:

- Relieve respiratory compromise
- Obtain a fluid sample to determine the type of fluid and for possible further analysis (e.g. culture)
- Allow radiographic assessment of intrathoracic structures previously obscured by fluid.

Radiography during drainage or lavage is indicated to assess drain placement. Drainage should be avoided or undertaken with care in animals with bleeding disorders or herniated abdominal contents. Post-drainage radiography is useful to:

- Identify a primary cause of pleural fluid or secondary changes
- Identify incomplete drainage or fluid pocketing
- Identify recurrence of effusion
- Identify restricted lung re-expansion, indicating the presence of adhesions, pleural fibrosis or underlying lung disease
  - Although lung collapse resulting from the effusion may be identified immediately after drainage, this should resolve quickly.

Other radiographic techniques:

- Altering patient position will change the fluid distribution in the pleural cavities and may allow observation of areas concealed by the fluid on standard views.
- Moderately tilting the table in conjunction with conventional views may be sufficient to move free pleural fluid away from specific locations (Figure 11.34).
- VD views often provide a better assessment of the cardiac silhouette, cranioventral lung field and cranial mediastinum in patients with pleural fluid. Cardiac size may be magnified, especially in deep-chested dogs. DV views, however, are generally safer in dyspnoeic patients and better for assessing the pulmonary blood vessels in the non-gravity-dependent caudodorsal lung field.
- Using a horizontally oriented X-ray beam can be helpful to observe air–fluid interfaces or to identify abnormalities obscured by pleural fluid on conventional radiographic views. For example, placing the animal in a vertical (standing) position moves fluid away from the thoracic inlet and towards the diaphragm, allowing cranial mediastinal lesions to be identified on a ventrodorsal (standing/horizontal) radiograph.

Computed tomography

General features of pleural effusion:

- Pleural fluid is easily recognized on CT images using a soft tissue window.
- Free fluid is gravity dependent and is often crescent shaped. Repositioning of the patient can demonstrate that the fluid is not compartmentalized within the pleural space.
- Small fluid volumes may produce wide interlobar fissures.
- Large fluid volumes will occupy more of the pleural space, causing a greater degree of lung retraction.
- Large fluid volumes will cause the lung to float resulting in distortion of lung contours, altered courses of airways and, in some cases, lung lobe torsion.
- Loculated or trapped fluid is more likely elliptical or lenticular and its location is unaffected by gravity.
- Images may reveal an underlying cause of the pleural fluid.

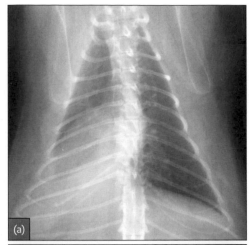

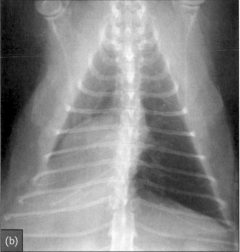

11.34 (a) VD thoracic radiograph of an 8-year-old Siamese cat with lobar resorption atelectasis (obstructive atelectasis) secondary to a bronchial carcinoma. Most pulmonary neoplasms produce a space-occupying tumour, but the most salient feature in this case is the loss of lung volume because the tumour obstructs airflow to the lobe. Note that the right caudal lung lobe is collapsed with an ipsilateral cardiac shift and an increased opacity that effaces the pulmonary blood vessels and adjacent borders of the heart, diaphragm and body wall. In addition, the left lung may have compensatory hyperinflation. A discrete lung tumour contrasted by gas is not seen because of the border effacement. The increased opacity in the right caudal thorax is unlikely encapsulated or trapped pleural fluid because the cardiac shift is towards the abnormality. (b) VD thoracic radiograph of the same cat in the same position with the table and X-ray tube tilted 25 degrees towards the cat's head, allowing free fluid to move cranially within the thorax. In the caudal thorax, the size of the abnormality is slightly reduced. There is a mild overall increased opacity in the cranial thorax. This simple and well tolerated manoeuvre helped identify that there was only a small volume of free pleural fluid.

Fluid type:

- The CT number (in HU) can give an indication of fluid type in dogs, however overlap exists between fluid types and between high-density fluid and low-density soft tissue (Figure 11.35).
- CT number is not as closely associated with fluid type in cats.
- Chronic or reactive effusions may produce uneven or overly rounded lung margins.
- Concurrent thick pleura suggests an exudate or neoplasia rather than a transudate, especially when the thick pleura forms nodular or mass-like lesions.
- Pyothorax is often sedimentary, unilateral or asymmetrically distributed and the fluid may be loculated or trapped. If a large fluid volume is trapped

Suggested cut-off (HU)	Fluid type	Sensitivity	Specificity
<12.5	Transudate/chyle	94%	78%
<34.68	Exudate	96%	95%
>34.68	Haemorrhage	96%	95%
>14	Modified transudate, exudate and haemorrhage	100%	69%

11.35 Suggested cut-off values for determining fluid type in dogs based on CT number.
(Data from Woods et al., 2018; Briola et al., 2019)

and has mass effect, then it may result in a mediastinal shift towards the contralateral side. Pyothorax is commonly accompanied by thick parietal pleura and less commonly by thick pulmonary pleura: this is especially noticeable following intravenous contrast medium administration. The 'split-pleura' sign occurs when thick contrast-enhancing pleurae are separated by non-contrast-enhancing fluid. This can occur between the parietal and visceral pleurae or between parietal pleurae in the costodiaphragmatic recess.

- Haemorrhage may appear heterogeneous due to separation of the cellular and fluid blood components. Over time, settling of the cellular component with gravity may produce linear interfaces within the fluid.
- In patients with chylothorax, thoracic CT or CT angiography, with or without contrast enhancement, can be used to identify cranial mediastinal masses or obstructions in the cranial vena cava (e.g. thrombus). CT lymphangiography can be used to examine the thoracic duct for abnormalities; iodinated contrast

medium may be injected into mesenteric structures, the cisterna chyli or popliteal lymph nodes using ultrasound guidance, or into the metatarsal pads. This procedure has mostly replaced radiographic lymphangiography.

Ultrasonography

Pleural fluid causes separation of the lung from the thoracic wall and produces an acoustic window allowing ultrasonographic detection of intrathoracic structures that are usually obscured by the air-filled lungs. This aids identification of underlying disease processes (e.g. cranial mediastinal mass, lung lobe torsion) and the presence of secondary changes (e.g. pulmonary atelectasis, fibrin tags) (Figure 11.36). Echocardiography may be performed to identify cardiogenic causes of pleural fluid. Ultrasonography may be used to guide thoracic drain placement or fluid sampling.

Pleural fluid can be differentiated from:

- Cranial mediastinal fluid by its location on either side of the thin hyperechoic line formed by the ventral part of the cranial mediastinum (Figure 11.37). In addition, mediastinal fluid tends to increase the width of the mediastinum and accumulates in irregularly shaped pockets within the mediastinal connective tissue. Unlike the pleural cavities, the mediastinum contains blood vessels
- Pericardial effusion by the separation of the lungs from the parietal pleura, the distribution of fluid throughout the thorax, and the angular outline created between fluid and adjacent lung tips. Pericardial effusion is confined by the pericardial sac, forming a roughly circular space around the heart.

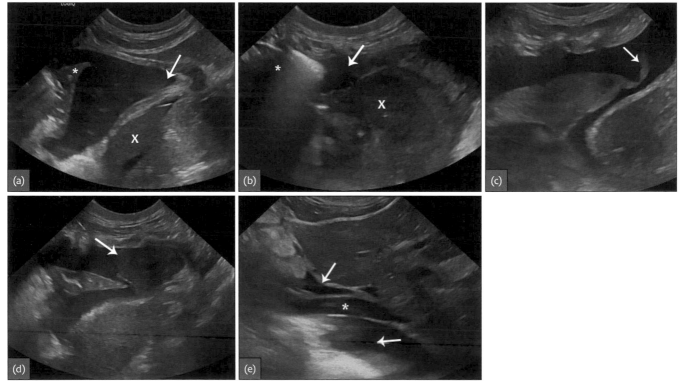

11.36 Thoracic ultrasound images of a cat with a cranial thoracic mass and pleural fluid obtained using multiple acoustic windows with the cat in ventral recumbency. The results of fine-needle aspiration (FNA) analysis were highly suggestive of lymphoma. (a) The pleural space is expanded and contains a large volume of echogenic fluid that fills the costodiaphragmatic recess (arrowed). The echogenicity of the fluid is supportive of an exudate. Collapsed lung (∗) and liver (X) are marked for reference. (b) The cranial thorax contains a space-occupying lesion (X) that is heterogeneously echogenic and surrounded by a small volume of the pleural fluid (arrowed). The fluid has displaced aerated lung (∗), providing an acoustic window for FNA. (c) Extending from the thoracic mass, the presence of a fibrin tag (arrowed) supports the reactive nature of the fluid and the possible presence of pleuritis. (d) Material in the pleural fluid has settled out in the ventral aspect of the thorax due to gravity, creating an interface within the fluid (arrowed). (e) The caudal vena cava (∗) is seen at the level of the caval foramen. Cranial to the diaphragm, the caudal vena cava is surrounded by pleural fluid (arrowed).

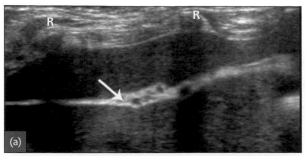

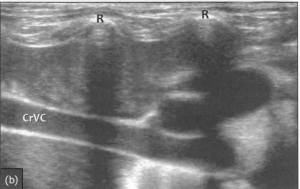

11.37 (a) Thoracic ultrasound image of a 3-year-old Siamese cat with pleural effusion. The image depicts the cranial thorax and was obtained at the level of the costochondral junctions using a linear transducer oriented in a dorsal plane. The near field contains the thoracic wall and two ribs (R). There are acoustic shadows associated with the ribs. In the far field, the left (nearer) and right (further) pleural spaces are markedly expanded and contain slightly echogenic fluid. Between the two pleural cavities, the ventral part of the cranial mediastinum is seen as a narrow hyperechoic band (arrowed). (b) Long-axis ultrasound image of the cranial thorax of a 1-year-old cat with feline infectious peritonitis. The near field contains the thoracic wall and two ribs (R). In the far field, the left and right pleural spaces are markedly expanded and contain echogenic fluid on either side of the cranial vena cava (CrVC).

When pericardial and pleural effusion occur concurrently in cats, the effusions are likely a consequence of the same underlying disease process (e.g. congestive heart failure, FIP, neoplasia) rather than a cause of it.

The echogenicity of pleural fluid typically reflects the cell count. Relatively acellular fluids (transudates, modified transudates and chylous effusions) are usually anechoic. In contrast, cellular fluids (exudates, malignant effusions and haemorrhage) tend to be echogenic (Figure 11.37b). However, echogenicity is an unreliable indicator of the nature of the fluid, as transudates and exudates can be anechoic. Chronic or reactive effusions may lead to fibrin formation, seen as linear echogenic strands that result in septation over time.

There are several ways to perform point-of-care ultrasonography. In emergency settings, thoracic focused assessment with sonography for trauma (tFAST) is one protocol that may be used (Figure 11.38). Pleural fluid is best identified using paracostal or transdiaphragmatic (subxiphoid) windows. The impact of patient position on pleural fluid distribution should be considered when locating small volumes. Ultrasonography has been used to estimate pleural fluid volume by measuring the distance between the ventral lung margins and the sternum in the standing patient. While unable to determine actual volumes, this technique can identify changes over time in individuals and therefore may be useful to monitor patients with pleural effusion.

Trapped, loculated or encapsulated fluid may be unaffected by gravity and easily missed, necessitating a systematic examination via the intercostal spaces. Guidance from other imaging modalities may be useful.

Magnetic resonance imaging

- Pleural fluid is typically homogeneous, T1 hypointense, T2 hyperintense and non-enhancing.
- Motion and flow-related artefacts may be present due to cardiac or respiratory movement, especially if gating is not used.
- Pleural fluid will pool in the gravity-dependent part of the thorax.
- Lung lobes will be displaced, and their margins will retract according to the location and volume of the fluid.
- Fluid due to pyothorax tends to have higher T1 and lower T2W signal intensities than other fluid types.
- Encapsulated fluid or abscessation may produce fluid-filled cavities with contrast-enhancing margins.

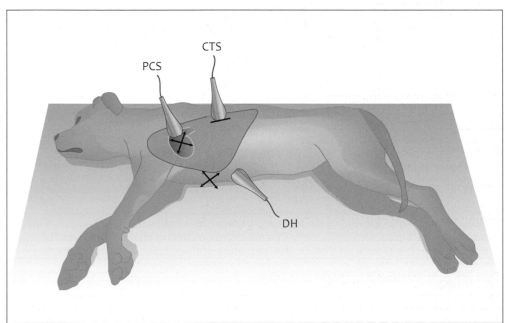

11.38 tFAST is performed on both sides of the thorax with the patient in either ventral or lateral recumbency. The locations for probe placement are indicated: CTS = chest tube sites, dorsal seventh–ninth intercostal spaces; PCS = pericardial sites (same location as parasternal cardiac windows); DH = diaphragmaticohepatic site (abdominal approach through the diaphragm). The CTS are best for detecting pneumothorax and the PCS and DH are best for detecting pleural fluid.

Thick pleura

Increased pleural thickness is usually due to inflammatory or neoplastic causes, but focal pleural haemorrhage associated with trauma may also cause the pleura to become thick. Increased pleural thickness may be uniform (sheet-like) or consist of one or more nodular or mass-like lesions. Pleural nodules typically indicate neoplastic disease or chronic inflammatory disease that has organized into granulomas or abscesses. The distribution may be diffuse, locally extensive, focal or multifocal. Increased pleural thickness may persist in animals after causative factors have been removed.

Pleuritis

Pleuritis is inflammation of the pleura. If pleuritis leads to the production of an exudate, then pleural effusion will result. In cats, the most common cause is FIP, which is often associated with pleural fluid (effusive form). There is also a non-effusive form that causes a focal pyogranulomatous pleuritis. Some other causes of pleuritis in dogs and cats include:

- Local disease extension into the pleural cavity: suppurative lung disease (fibrinous bronchopneumonia, pleuropneumonia), fat herniation through the body wall (trauma), lung or body wall neoplasm, or penetrating body wall trauma
- Irritation from material in the pleural space (e.g. bile, pancreatic enzymes, migrating foreign body)
- Systemic conditions such as septicaemia
- Chronic pleural effusion of any type.

Fibrosing pleuritis (restrictive pleuritis) is usually a result of chronic inflammatory disease and refers to fibrous strand or adhesion formation between pleural surfaces. Chronic inflammation leading to this condition may occur in pyothorax, chylothorax, haemothorax, FIP and mycobacterial disease. This condition is generally more severe as it can restrict lung movement due to the formation of a 'pleural peel', which is a thick fibrous layer produced by the organization of fibrin deposits in the pleural space. Fibrin can adhere to the pleura and extend into the lung parenchyma, reducing lung volume and restricting lung movement. It can even cause adherence of the affected area to the thoracic wall. Progression results in lung lobes becoming enshrouded in fibrin, leading to chronic underinflation (see Figure 11.16bc). Fluid associated with fibrosing pleuritis may be small in volume and may become trapped or encapsulated (Figure 11.39), although the resultant effusion can become severe and bilateral.

Pleural masses

Many conditions can cause pleural masses, including herniated abdominal viscera, granulomas, abscesses, haematomas, pleural adhesions with loculated fluid, pleural peel and neoplasms. Mesothelioma is the only primary neoplasm of the pleura and can be difficult to differentiate from metastatic adenocarcinoma. Mesothelioma does not usually present as a discrete mass lesion but rather as disseminated abnormalities and a large-volume pleural effusion. Diagnosis can be extremely challenging. Metastatic lung neoplasia (carcinoma) may also involve the pleura. Effusion is more commonly associated with pleural masses than pulmonary or extrapleural masses that do not extend into the pleural cavity. Neoplasms that extend into the pleural cavity can also produce imaging signs consistent with fibrosing pleuritis.

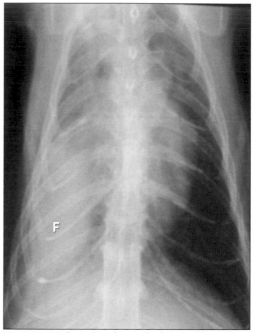

11.39 DV thoracic radiograph of a cat with pyothorax and a large pleural abscess. In the right caudal aspect of the thorax, the abscess can be seen as a large mass with a homogeneous fluid opacity that effaces the adjacent body wall and diaphragmatic borders and displaces the right lung medially. These findings are consistent with an area of encapsulated pleural fluid (F), but a capsule is not apparent on this image.

Radiography

Pleuritis: Thick and irregular pleurae produce linear opacities where they lie tangential to the X-ray beam. Nodular opacities (e.g. abscesses, granulomas) may be seen with chronic organized inflammation.

- These signs are best seen at interlobar fissures but may be observed around the entire lung when severe.
- The signs must also be distinguished from the thick pleurae and calcification that may be seen as an incidental finding of minor consequence in older animals.
- Thick pleura can appear similar to small-volume pleural effusion but moderate-volume effusions result in wedge-shaped rather than linear opacities.
- Tent- or U-shaped opacities may suggest adhesions.

Signs of fibrosing pleuritis:

- Affected lung lobes are reduced in size, have variable opacity, and will not inflate further despite repositioning of the animal
- The difference in lung volume between inspiratory and expiratory views may be minimal
- Following drainage of pleural fluid:
  - Affected areas of lung fail to re-expand normally and retain a rounded outline with an opaque margin, known as cortication
  - Pneumothorax ex vacuo may be observed
  - Re-formation of the effusion may occur due to reduced intrapleural pressure
- Areas of cortication can appear similar to hilar masses and should be differentiated from pulmonary neoplasms (primary or secondary), lung lobe torsion and tracheobronchial lymphadenopathy.

Pleural masses: These are usually associated with pleural effusion, so fluid drainage may be necessary for detection of a mass. A mass is suspected when there is:

- Displacement of the cardiac silhouette or other thoracic structures not associated with gravity or atelectasis
- Uneven lung compression
- A soft tissue opacity not conforming to the linear or triangular shape of the pleural space (often spindle-shaped)
- A soft tissue opacity that maintains its shape and position despite moving the patient. This appearance must be differentiated from trapped or encapsulated fluid.

Computed tomography

Pleuritis:

- Post-contrast enhancement of the pleura can help distinguish it from adjacent fluid, fibrin tags and haemorrhage.
- Diffusely thick, contrast-enhancing pleura is associated with pleuritis and pyothorax (Figure 11.40).
- Increased pleural thickness in the absence of other signs may represent scarring from a previous episode of pleuritis.
- Cranial sternal and cranial mediastinal lymph node enlargement may be observed with pleural disease.
- Localization and characterization of lesions associated with migrating foreign material is possible, including the identification of contrast-enhancing tracts or foreign material.

Pleural masses: There is a considerable overlap in the CT findings between patients with malignant pleural effusion and those with pleuritis. In humans, circumferential or nodular increases in pleural thickness, severe (parietal pleura >1 cm thick) increases in thickness and involvement of the mediastinal pleura are helpful features for differentiating malignant from benign pleural disease.

- Pleural masses can be:
  - Circumscribed or ill defined
  - Nodular or space-occupying lesions (i.e. variable size)
  - Solitary or multiple (usually regionally or asymmetrically distributed)
  - Broad based with the pleura and plaque like.
- Features that are more suggestive of neoplasia include:
  - Severe increased thickness affecting only the parietal pleura
  - Formation of nodules or mass-like tumours
  - Costal pleural masses
  - Signs of thoracic wall invasion.

In dogs, mesothelioma may present as discrete pleural masses. However, the lesions more typically involve widespread pleural changes that may be difficult to detect during imaging. Iatrogenic pneumothorax induced during diagnostic or therapeutic thoracocentesis can provide valuable contrast and reveal abnormalities associated with mesothelioma (Figure 11.41). These lesions enhance with intravenous contrast medium.

Pleural masses with focal mineralization are more likely to be associated with carcinomas than mesotheliomas and must be differentiated from pulmonary osseous metaplasia.

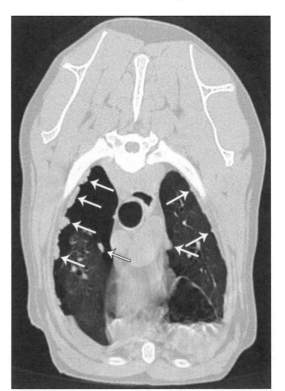

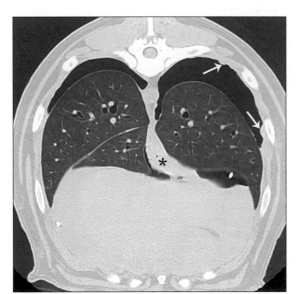

11.40 Transverse thoracic CT image of a 2-year-old German Shepherd Dog with suppurative pleuritis, obtained at the level of the tenth thoracic vertebra and displayed in a lung window. An inciting cause for the inflammation was not determined. The dog had purulent fluid in both pleural cavities consistent with pyothorax (pleural empyema) and gas in both cavities consistent with pneumothorax. The pleural gas contrasts with the pulmonary (visceral) and parietal pleurae. The pulmonary pleura is diffusely mildly thick, which is consistent with pleuritis. The left parietal pleura contains multiple small nodules (arrowed) consistent with marked focal pleuritis or abscesses. The caudoventral mediastinal reflection is also thick and irregularly margined, consistent with mediastinitis (*).

11.41 Transverse post-contrast thoracic CT image of a dog with pleural mesothelioma, displayed in a lung window. The right cranial lung lobe is small and retracted from the body wall. The right pleural cavity is expanded dorsally and has a gas attenuation. The left pleural cavity has a small volume of trapped gas and fluid ventrally, creating a horizontal gas–fluid interface. The neoplasm forms multiple irregular wide-based contrast-enhancing nodular tumours along the parietal and pulmonary pleurae of both pleural cavities (arrowed). The tumours are contrasted by pleural gas, pulmonary gas or both. The pneumothorax may have occurred during drainage of severe bilateral pleural effusion or may have been pre-existing due to intrathoracic disease (pleural masses).

Ultrasonography

Pleural abnormalities are often accompanied by effusion. Ultrasonography can help to identify these underlying abnormalities and the presence of pleural effusion often facilitates ultrasound assessment of the pleurae. Ultrasound-guided aspiration of pleural masses or fluid may contribute to a diagnosis.

- Mild pleural fibrosis appears as mild uniform increased thickness of the pleura.
- Irregularly thick, hyperechoic pleura is more typical of an inflammatory or neoplastic process (Figure 11.42).
- Chronic or reactive effusions are associated with linear echogenic strands of fibrin forming septa in the fluid (see Figure 11.36).
- In patients with pleural peel, the shape of the underlying lung margins may be abnormal.
- The presence of adhesions between the visceral and parietal pleurae can result in loss of the glide sign that is produced by the lung moving normally against the parietal pleura. This should be differentiated from pneumothorax.
- Pleural masses have a variable appearance depending on the underlying cause (Figure 11.43).
- In patients with a diaphragmatic defect, abdominal viscera may be herniated into the pleural cavity.
- Visceral pleural or pulmonary lesions move with respiration while parietal pleural lesions remain still as the lung moves past them. In clinically stable dogs, the nostrils and mouth can be temporarily closed to encourage the dog to take a deep breath to assess for this movement.
- Visceral pleural masses cannot be distinguished from pulmonary masses using ultrasonography.

Magnetic resonance imaging

Pleuritis:

- Normal pleurae and pleural fissures are too thin to be visible on MRI. As with radiography, they only become visible when thick or when pleural fluid is present.
- Pleuritis may cause rounding of the lung margins.
- In humans, septa in pleural effusions may be visible on T2-weighted non-contrast images as areas of low signal intensity, compared with the high signal intensity of the surrounding fluid.
- Foreign objects are usually geometrical and hypointense to signal void on T2* gradient echo images.
- Associated fibrosis, chronic haemorrhage and gas bubbles may produce small areas of hypointensity and therefore must be interpreted with caution.

Pleural masses:

- MRI may be useful to show the origin of a pleural mass or differentiate it from masses arising from intrathoracic structures or the thoracic wall.
- Pleural nodules may appear on T2-weighted images as areas of low signal intensity between the adjacent high signal intensities of the intercostal fat and the accompanying pleural effusion.
- Heterogeneous areas including necrosis or haemorrhage have high intensity on STIR or T2-weighted images.
- In humans, when compared with intercostal muscle, malignant tissue has a higher signal intensity than benign lesions on T2-weighted, proton-density-weighted, pre- and post-contrast T1-weighted and contrast-enhanced fat-saturated T1-weighted sequences.

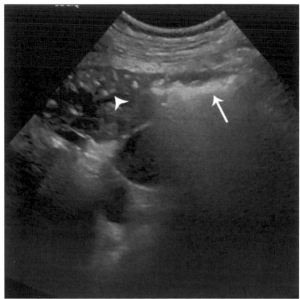

11.42 Thoracic ultrasound image of a dog. The body wall is seen in the near field and consolidated lung with some gas (arrowed) and anechoic fluid (arrowhead) is seen in the mid field. Between the body wall and lung, the pleural surface is irregular, indicating the presence of pleuritis or neoplasia. The results of fine-needle aspiration analysis confirmed the presence of carcinoma.

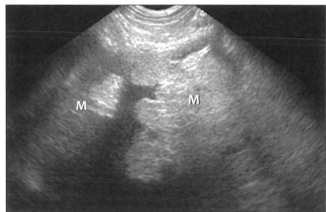

11.43 Thoracic ultrasound image of a 2-year-old Labrador Retriever with a rare neoplasm, telangiectatic osteosarcoma. The neoplasm formed multiple irregular pleural masses (M) and a large volume of haemorrhagic pleural fluid. The masses are cauliflower-like, homogeneously echogenic and surrounded by the fluid.

- On diffusion-weighted imaging, malignant tissue tends to be more compact and structured, producing a hyperintense speckled appearance referred to as 'pointillism'.
- Other features associated with malignant lesions in humans include nodularity, margin irregularity and circumferential involvement or invasion of the diaphragm, thoracic wall or mediastinum.

Pneumothorax

Pneumothorax is the accumulation of gas within one or both pleural cavities, which may develop in a variety of ways (Figure 11.44). Clinical signs of pneumothorax range from subtle to dramatic with progression from rapid shallow breathing to open-mouthed panting or death. The clinical signs usually reflect the volume and rate of gas accumulation. Large volumes of pleural gas are more likely

Traumatic
Open: • Gunshot • Bite • Stab wound • Injury secondary to road accident Closed: • Blunt external trauma • Subpleural bleb, secondary to trauma (goes on to rupture) • Iatrogenic due to thoracocentesis, transthoracic aspiration or biopsy, pericardiocentesis or barotrauma • Extension from pneumomediastinum • Peritoneal gas if a diaphragmatic hernia is present

Spontaneous
Primary: • Lungs are normal • Occurs in northern and deep-chested large breeds of dog, usually middle-aged Secondary: • Lungs are diseased • Examples include emphysema, neoplasia, pneumonia, pulmonary abscessation, parasites (*Oslerus osleri*, *Dirofilaria immitis*, paragonimiasis), migrating foreign bodies, asthma

11.44 Causes of pneumothorax.

to cause substantial compression of the lungs and mediastinal structures, especially when the pressure in the pleural cavity is higher than atmospheric pressure. If the air accumulates slowly, the early signs of respiratory difficulty may only be present on inspiration. Small-volume pneumothorax is often difficult to detect clinically. Pneumothorax can occur as a complication of pneumomediastinum, but the converse is not true. In theory, air may enter the pleural space from the abdomen if a diaphragmatic rupture and free peritoneal gas (pneumoperitoneum) are present.

Causes

Traumatic pneumothorax: Traumatic pneumothorax typically arises from blunt (e.g. vehicular trauma) or penetrating (e.g. gunshot, bite wound, stabbing) injury and is primarily classified according to the route by which gas enters the pleural cavity (i.e. open versus closed).

- Open traumatic pneumothorax is rare and occurs when the thoracic body wall has been breached and gas enters the pleural space directly from the external environment. Typically, air rapidly enters the pleural space through the body wall wound during inspiration until pleural and atmospheric pressures equilibrate.
- Closed traumatic pneumothorax is more common. The thoracic wall is not compromised and gas enters the pleural space from within the animal. This type of injury usually occurs secondary to blunt external trauma causing rupture of a bronchus or area of lung tissue due to a sudden increase in intrathoracic pressure against a closed glottis (diving reflex). Another possibility is that internal shearing forces may create a subpleural bleb that subsequently ruptures. A displaced rib fracture also may penetrate or lacerate the lung without creating a communication with the external environment.
- Iatrogenic traumatic pneumothorax refers to the traumatic introduction of gas into the pleural space during a medical procedure (e.g. introducing air during thoracocentesis or pericardiocentesis, lacerating the lung during these procedures or barotrauma during positive pressure ventilation).

Spontaneous pneumothorax: Spontaneous pneumothorax is typically closed, occurs when no traumatic cause is identified, and is primarily classified by whether the lungs are normal or abnormal (i.e. primary versus secondary).

- Primary spontaneous pneumothorax occurs in association with normal lungs and an underlying cause is not usually identified (i.e. it is idiopathic). The pneumothorax is thought to result from the rupture of blebs or bullae. This condition occurs most commonly in large deep-chested dogs: northern breeds (e.g. Siberian Husky) and hounds are over-represented. There is no sex predilection and middle-aged dogs are more commonly affected.
- Secondary spontaneous pneumothorax is more common and occurs when there is concurrent lung disease, such as emphysema, neoplasia, pneumonia, pulmonary abscess, parasites (including *Dirofilaria* and *Paragonimus*), migrating plant foreign bodies or feline asthma. Pleural adhesions arising from chronic inflammation may also tear, resulting in pneumothorax.

Tension pneumothorax: A simple pneumothorax is one where the pressure in the pleural cavity is lower than or equal to atmospheric pressure (normotensive pneumothorax). When the pleural gas pressure exceeds atmospheric pressure, a tension pneumothorax is present. This occurs when a one-way valve effect exists between the source of the air and the pleural space. Air enters the pleural space with inspiration but cannot exit with expiration, and positive pressure rapidly develops within the pleural space. The pressure rises with each breath, so the condition rapidly becomes life-threatening. The lungs and pulmonary vessels collapse and a fatal decrease in ventilation and cardiac output result. The animal's thorax may be clinically observed to expand as the condition progresses.

Pneumohydrothorax: Pneumohydrothorax refers to the presence of both gas and fluid within one or both pleural cavities and can be called hydropneumothorax if the fluid component has precedence. This condition can arise secondary to trauma (where the fluid is typically blood) or as a complication of pulmonary abscessation, oesophageal perforation, rupture of a cavitary lung neoplasm or migrating foreign material (where the fluid is pus). In addition to gas leakage from the lung, the gas may also result from bacterial production or as a complication of thoracocentesis. Pneumohydrothorax can create bizarre radiographic patterns due to the simultaneous presence of border effacement due to fluid, increased border contrast due to gas and oddly shaped gas opacities.

Radiography

If a body wall defect is detected and shows communication between the pleural cavity and external environment, then it is possible to identify an open pneumothorax. However, not detecting a body wall defect does not definitively identify a closed pneumothorax as small defects may be missed. The determination between open versus closed is usually made during physical examination.

Simple (normotensive) pneumothorax: Radiographic findings vary depending on the volume of pleural gas and severity of lung collapse, and include:

- Expansion of one or both pleural spaces
- Lung margins retracted from the thoracic wall and diaphragm

- Gas opacity surrounding the lung surfaces, medial aspect of the body wall and cranial aspect of the diaphragm
- Collapsed lung lobes that retain their shape
- Normal to increased opacity of collapsed lobe(s) – this may be best observed during exhalation
- No lung markings (e.g. blood vessels) visible external to the collapsed lung lobe(s)
- Separation of the cardiac silhouette from the sternum by gas opacity on lateral views
- Focal air collection between the cardiac silhouette and the sternum on lateral views may be the only indication in a small-volume pneumothorax
- Pneumothorax is commonly bilateral, either due to movement of gas across the mediastinum or bilateral entrance of gas.

Although the underlying causes should be sought, a causal bleb or bulla is often not identified by radiography. Uneven collapse of the lung lobes might point towards concurrent pulmonary disease, for example, contused lung may collapse while normal lung remains inflated. There may be additional findings of thoracic disease.

Tension pneumothorax: In general, the same signs are present as for a simple pneumothorax but they are more severe. Additional radiographic findings include:

- Progression (worsening) of radiographic changes over a short period of time
- The thoracic cavity is markedly hyperlucent due to the large volume of gas in the pleural space
- Severe lung lobe collapse and compression (smaller and opaque lungs that might have a distorted shape)
- Flattened diaphragm with or without 'tenting'
- Overdistension of the thorax with wide intercostal spaces
- Ribs and costal cartilages perpendicular to the vertebral column
- Mediastinal shift away from a unilateral tension pneumothorax.

Pneumohydrothorax: Radiographic features of both pleural effusion and pneumothorax are present, with the appearance depending on the volume of each.

- The pleural space is expanded and has a mix of gas and fluid opacities.
- The distribution of gas and fluid will vary with patient position. In ventral recumbency, free fluid will tend to accumulate ventrally and free gas dorsally.
- Trapped or focal fluid or gas may produce a confusing appearance.
- Reduced lung size with lung margins retracted from the thoracic wall or diaphragm; pulmonary blood vessels do not extend to the periphery of the thoracic cavity.
- Pleural fluid may cause border effacement of the cardiac silhouette or portions of the diaphragm; pleural gas may increase contrast with these structures.
- Radiographs acquired using a horizontally oriented X-ray beam will show a fluid–gas interface.

Other radiographic techniques: Small-volume pneumothorax can be difficult to detect on conventional radiographs. Using a vertically oriented X-ray beam, lateral views are best for detecting pneumothorax, followed by the DV view. The VD view is least useful. End-expiratory radiographs are also useful as the lungs contrast more with the pleural gas because they are more opaque, the costodiaphragmatic angles are blunted and the relative volume of pleural gas is greater compared with the reduced lung volume. Using a horizontally oriented X-ray beam, the ventrodorsal (decubitus/horizontal) view increases the likelihood of detecting a small volume of pleural gas (Figure 11.45). Pneumothorax detection has been shown to be best on either the conventional left lateral view or the ventrodorsal (right decubitus/horizontal) view, while quantity of gas is best evaluated on the conventional right lateral view.

Computed tomography

CT is not usually required to diagnose pneumothorax but may be performed for other reasons in patients with concurrent pneumothorax (e.g. polytrauma evaluation) and can be used to determine the underlying cause in some patients with spontaneous pneumothorax (e.g. rule out ruptured cavitary pulmonic lesions). Identification of the gas-leaking area of the lung is usually not possible. Performing CT following thoracocentesis and under mild positive pressure ventilation may improve evaluation of the lungs and increase patient stability due to reduced atelectasis.

- Bilateral and unilateral pneumothorax are easily recognized on CT images using a lung window.
- A non-attenuating area (-1000 HU) will be present at the highest point of the pleural space between the parietal and visceral pleurae. The size of the area will reflect the volume of gas present.
- As the volume of pleural gas increases, lung lobe volume is progressively reduced, and pulmonary attenuation may increase.
- Tension pneumothorax produces increased thoracic volume, severe lung collapse, and a mediastinal shift.
- Concurrent pleural disease can be easily identified in areas adjacent to the gas and images may also reveal an underlying cause (e.g. ruptured pulmonary bleb, migrating foreign body).
- In patients with pneumohydrothorax, gravity-dependent gas–fluid interfaces will be seen.

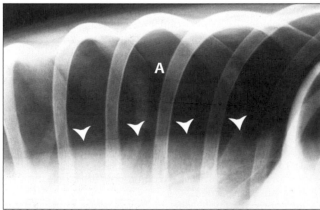

11.45 Ventrodorsal (left decubitus/horizontal) thoracic radiograph of a 2-year-old mixed-breed dog with pneumothorax. Gas redistributes according to gravity. This radiographic view is used to improve detection of pneumothorax. The right lung is small and retracted from the body wall (arrowheads) and the right pleural cavity contains free pleural gas (A).

Ultrasonography

Pneumothorax: Point-of-care ultrasonography is increasingly used in emergency care situations in patients with respiratory distress following trauma or interventional procedures. The examination may be performed using the intercostal spaces as acoustic windows, with the patient standing or in ventral or lateral recumbency. The search for pneumothorax is started at the highest point of the thorax (usually around where a chest drain may be inserted, i.e. the dorsal part of the seventh–ninth intercostal space) and extended caudodorsally (see Figure 11.38).

Pneumothorax cannot be diagnosed from a still image because normal air-filled lung and free pleural gas both produce the same horizontal reverberation artefact (A-lines). Real-time imaging is required to confirm that all structures beyond the parietal pleura are obscured by the gas and that the glide sign, associated with lung movement against the parietal pleura, is no longer visible. M-mode in patients with pneumothorax will produce the barcode or stratosphere sign (see Figure 11.11) rather than the normal seashore sign (see Figure 11.5b).

The extent of the pneumothorax can be estimated by determining how many intercostal spaces are affected and, with the patient in ventral recumbency, by moving the transducer vertically down each intercostal space to determine the lung point (see Figure 11.31). Ventral to this, there will either be a glide sign indicating normal lung or multiple B-lines if the underlying lung is abnormal (Figure 11.46).

- The glide sign is only observed where lung movement can be seen and so may be absent in certain circumstances (e.g. opioid-induced apnoea, large-volume subcutaneous gas accumulation).
- Spurious detection of the glide sign can occur due to patient or probe movement.
- Assessing hyperpnoeic or dyspnoeic animals is challenging due to increased thoracic wall movement. This reduces the positive predictive value of absent lung gliding as a test for pneumothorax.

Pneumohydrothorax: When the patient is in ventral recumbency, pleural fluid will be identified ventrally as an anechoic area, and pleural gas dorsally as an area of reverberation with no visible lung movement. In transverse images obtained through the intercostal space, respiration causes a repetitive ventrodorsal movement of the fluid–gas interface producing the curtain sign. This occurs whenever gas temporarily moves across an area, obscuring the pleural fluid and then revealing it again (likened to the raising and lowering of a curtain). This sign is also associated with peripheral areas of normal lung in the costomediastinal and costodiaphragmatic recesses where they obscure and reveal the underlying regional anatomy during respiration.

Magnetic resonance imaging

Pneumothorax:

- Free pleural gas will appear as a signal void on all MRI sequences.
- Free pleural gas will accumulate in the non-dependent part of the thorax and therefore its location will depend on the position of the patient.
- Lung lobes will retract according to the volume of the gas.
- In patients with pneumohydrothorax, gravity-dependent gas–fluid interfaces will be seen.

References and further reading

Boysen SR and Lisciandro GR (2013) The use of ultrasound for dogs and cats in the emergency room: AFAST and TFAST. *Veterinary Clinics of North America: Small Animal Practice* **43**, 773–797

Briola C, Zoia A, Rocchi P, Caldin M and Bertolini G (2019) Computed tomography attenuation value for the characterization of pleural effusions in dogs: a cross-sectional study in 58 dogs. *Research in Veterinary Science* **124**, 357–365

d'Anjou M-A, Tidwell AS and Hecht S (2005) Radiographic diagnosis of lung lobe torsion. *Veterinary Radiology & Ultrasound* **46**, 478–484

Dennis R (2018) MRI of non-cardiac thoracic conditions. In: *Diagnostic MRI in Dogs and Cats*, ed. W Mai, pp. 710–722. CRC Press, Boca Raton

Lisciandro GR (2008) Evaluation of a thoracic focused assessment with sonography for trauma (TFAST) protocol to detect pneumothorax and concurrent thoracic injury in 145 traumatized dogs. *Journal of Veterinary Emergency and Critical Care* **18**, 258–269

Mai W (2011) Pleura. In: *Veterinary Computed Tomography*, ed. T Schwarz and J Saunders, pp. 279–284. Wiley-Blackwell, Hoboken

Seiler G, Schwarz T, Vignoli M and Rodriguez D (2008) Computed tomographic features of lung lobe torsion. *Veterinary Radiology & Ultrasound* **49**, 504–508

Wisner E and Zwingenberger A (2015) Pleural space. In: *Atlas of Small Animal CT and MRI*, ed. E Wisner and A Zwingenberger, pp. 398–407. Wiley-Blackwell, Hoboken

Woods SJ, Spriet M, Safra N, Cissell DD and Borjesson DL (2018) Hounsfield units are a useful predictor of pleural effusion cytological type in dogs but not in cats. *Veterinary Radiology & Ultrasound* **59**, 405–407

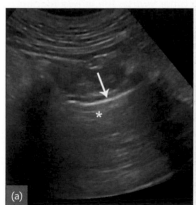 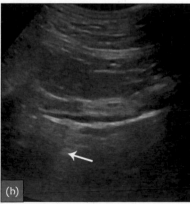 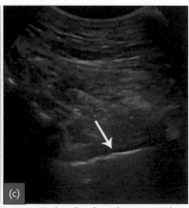

11.46 Intercostal ultrasound images from different locations in the same dog as in Figure 11.42, that developed a pneumothorax following lung lobectomy. (a) Gas (∗) is seen deep to the pleural line (arrowed), between the ribs. On this static image, it is impossible to differentiate free pleural gas from normal air-filled lung. During dynamic imaging, the absence of a glide sign confirmed the presence of pneumothorax. (b) Gas and a B-line (arrowed) are seen deep to the pleural line. If B-lines are identified, then lung is present at that location (B-lines arise from interactions between the sound beam and the pleural surface of the lung). In this image, the pleural line also forms a rougher hyperechoic interface than that produced by the free gas in (a), indicating concurrent pleural or pulmonary changes. (c) The extent of pneumothorax can be estimated by identifying the location of lung points on the body. A lung point is formed where the pulmonary pleura reconnects with the parietal pleura. In this case, identification of the lung point (arrowed) was facilitated by the roughened pulmonary pleura.

Chapter 12

The lungs

Peter Scrivani, Tobias Schwarz and Tiziana Liuti

Diagnostic pulmonary image interpretation is a multistep process that relies on the interpreter having an in-depth knowledge of: the physical capabilities of imaging modalities to capture and display information; pulmonary anatomy, physiology, and pathology; epidemiological principles like those associated with test selection, test accuracy measurements and prior probability of disease. During image evaluation, one of the most fundamental steps for making a diagnosis is determining the anatomical compartment of the lung that is affected by the disease process, especially for widespread diseases. Note that more than one compartment may be affected.

This method of anatomical localization is largely based on the principle that different imaging patterns are discernible when diseases affect different compartments of the lung. Using this principle, interpreters search medical images for familiar signs and patterns to discover which anatomical compartment is abnormal. Once an imaging pattern is identified, interpreters then generate a differential diagnosis (a 'gamut') based on knowing the diseases that affect that part of the lung. This list is then prioritized based on additional information like patient signalment and history, other imaging findings and the results of other clinical tests. The final assessment is a definitive imaging diagnosis, a short list of reasonable differential diagnoses or an acknowledgement that the clinical question is unanswered by the study.

In veterinary medicine, the most common method for determining the anatomical compartment during thoracic radiography may be called the traditional approach. This approach primarily applies to conditions that cause pulmonary opacification and originated in human medicine in the mid twentieth century when radiography was the only common imaging modality used to examine the lungs. This method was based on the hypothesis that discernible radiographic patterns are produced when disease primarily involves the alveoli, bronchi, interstitium or vascular structures. The original 1968 article in veterinary medicine (Suter and Chan, 1968) described the following four patterns of increased pulmonary opacification (Figure 12.1).

- An alveolar pattern is due to the replacement of air in the alveoli by fluid or cells, or the absence of air due to collapse of the alveoli.
- An interstitial pattern is increased thickness of the interstitium due to the influx of fluid, cells or fibres (e.g. collagen) into the connective tissue that supports the blood vessels, lymphatics, bronchi, and alveoli.

- A bronchovascular pattern is increased thickness of the bronchovascular bundle due to the influx of fluid, cells or fibres into airway walls, blood vessels or adventitial sheath that connects these structures. In some cases, it may be possible to subdivide this pattern.
  - A bronchial pattern is increased thickness of the bronchial wall due to the influx of fluid, cells or fibre into the bronchial walls (mucosa to adventitia), smooth muscle hypertrophy or mucus production.
  - A vascular pattern is increased prominence of the pulmonary arteries, veins or both due to increased size, increased number, altered shape or a combination.
- A mixed pattern is present when more than one of the above patterns is simultaneously present in a patient.

From early on, in both human and veterinary medicine, it was understood that this approach was imperfect because most parenchymal lung diseases were not simply confined to only the lung interstitium or the alveolar space; there usually was spread from one compartment to the other, especially as the disease advanced (Felson, 1979; Suter and Lord, 1984). Therefore, to address this important issue, it was emphasized that an 'interstitial lung pattern' was only a descriptive term to relay what was observable in thoracic radiographs and not equivalent to 'interstitial lung disease' as defined by pathologists (Felson, 1979; Suter and Lord, 1984). In other words, these two recognizable radiographic patterns could localize disease to the pulmonary parenchyma but not further discriminate smaller anatomical compartments. In addition, fibrotic and non-fibrotic interstitial diseases could not only affect the parenchymal interstitium, but also produce linear or nodular patterns when involving the other parts of the pulmonary interstitium. With the arrival of computed tomography (CT) in clinical practice, the relationships between signs and patterns observed during X-ray-based medical imaging were better defined for disease involving these anatomical compartments (Figure 12.2):

- Pulmonary parenchyma
- Pulmonary arteries
- Pulmonary veins
- Bronchi (large airways)
- Bronchioles (small airways)
- Peripheral connective tissue.

The *modern approach* to diagnostic pulmonary image interpretation is evolving, builds upon the foundation of the

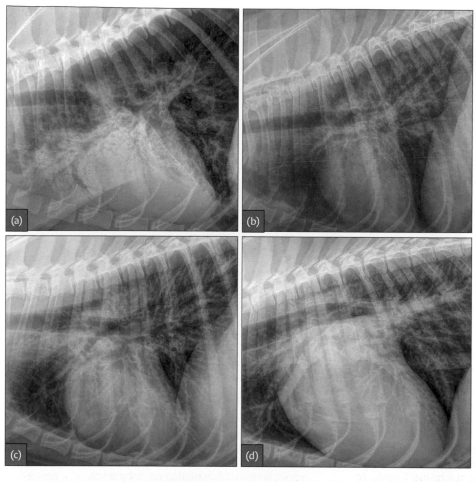

12.1 Lateral thoracic radiographs from four dogs. (a) Alveolar pattern due to pneumonia. (b) Interstitial pattern due to lymphoma. (c) Bronchial pattern due to bronchitis. (d) Vascular pattern due to patent ductus arteriosus.

Bronchovascular bundle	Bronchiolovascular bundle	Lung parenchyma	Peripheral venous bundle
Bronchi	Bronchioles	Alveolar epithelium	Venules and veins
Arteries	Arterioles	Parenchymal interstitium	Lymphatic vessels
Veins*	Lymphatic vessels	Capillaries	Peripheral interstitium
Lymphatic vessels	Bronchovascular interstitium	Air in airspace	
Bronchovascular interstitium	Air in bronchiole lumen		
Air in bronchial lumen			

12.2 Major pulmonary anatomical compartments seen on X-ray-based medical images and component structures. If one considers the larger blood vessels as separate anatomical compartments, then these anatomical compartments are called large airways, small airways, lung parenchyma and peripheral connective tissue. * The pulmonary vein diverges from the bronchoarterial bundle as the structures become more distant to the lung hilus.

traditional approach, and uses terms that apply to both radiography and CT. In people, many of these terms have been standardized (Hansell *et al.*, 2008; El Kaddouri *et al.*, 2021). In dogs and cats, the modern approach differs mostly in the conceptual reorganization of some existing ideas while incorporating novel information that clarifies existing concepts or distinguishes new ones. As with the traditional approach, imaging signs and patterns that localize disease to anatomical compartments, information about lung size, information about disease distribution, and additional imaging and clinical findings are important. The combination of information, rather than focusing on the histological distribution, is emphasized as most helpful for diagnosis. Finally, as with the traditional approach, mixed patterns are possible because lung diseases are complex and often do not conform perfectly to pedagogical constructs. Both approaches are discussed in this chapter: the traditional approach is used extensively when discussing specific diseases because of its widespread familiarity among veterinary surgeons (veterinarians).

Imaging anatomy

The respiratory apparatus is spread across three body parts: head, neck, and thorax. This chapter focuses on lung anatomy but considers it in the framework of the entire respiratory apparatus. The anatomical nomenclature varies with the context and terms often overlap situations, which can be confusing. There are three contexts to consider: clinical, physiological and morphological perspectives (Figure 12.3).

Clinical perspective

The entire respiratory apparatus is divided into three major parts of clinical relevance.

- The upper airway is the passageway from the nostrils to the rima glottidis of the larynx.
  - The rostral part of the laryngeal cavity is included in the upper airway.

Physiological	Clinical		Morphological
Conducting zone	Upper airway		Nasal cavities (and paranasal sinuses)
			Pharynx (nasal and laryngeal parts)
			Laryngeal vestibule (larynx rostral to glottis)
	Lower airway	Large airways	Infraglottic cavity (larynx caudal to glottis)
			Trachea (cervical and thoracic parts)
			Principal bronchi
			Lobar bronchi
			Segmental bronchi
			Bronchi
		Small airways	Bronchioles
			Terminal bronchioles
			Respiratory bronchioles*
Exchange zone	Lungs		Lungs
			Lobes
			Bronchopulmonary segments
			Pulmonary lobules
			Alveolar ducts, alveolar sacs and alveoli

12.3 Comparison of the entire respiratory apparatus from three anatomical perspectives. Structures in bold are the sites of gas exchange between the body and environment; these are generally below the spatial resolution of modern X-ray-based medical imaging equipment and collectively form the lung parenchyma, including the airspace. Technically, the lungs are inclusive of parenchyma, airways and stroma. * Respiratory bronchioles overlap physiological zones as they are involved in both conduction and exchange of gas.

- The lower airway is derived from the embryonic respiratory diverticulum and is the passageway from the rima glottidis to the respiratory bronchioles. The lower airway is subdivided into two parts:
  - The large airway comprises the infraglottic cavity, trachea, and bronchi
  - The small airway comprises the bronchioles.
- The lungs comprise the parenchyma where oxygen and carbon dioxide pass between the blood and the external environment by diffusion.

Physiological perspective

The entire respiratory apparatus is divided into two functional zones.

- The conducting zone comprises the structures that convey air (and blood) to and from the lungs.
  - The penultimate airway in the series, which conducts air and does not participate in gas exchange, is the terminal bronchiole. All downstream structures form the pulmonary acinus.
  - The last and smallest airway, which participates in both conduction and exchange of gas, is the respiratory bronchiole.
- The exchange zone (also called the respiratory zone or lung parenchyma) encompasses the structures that exchange gas between the body and external environment.
  - Gas exchange specifically occurs downstream to the terminal bronchus in the capillaries of the respiratory bronchioles, alveolar ducts, alveolar sacs and alveoli. Therefore, the pulmonary acinus is the largest lung unit where all components participate in gas exchange.
  - The process of delivery of air to this zone is ventilation (V) and the process of delivery of blood to this zone is perfusion (Q). The optimum efficiency

and adequacy of gas exchange is dependent on an equilibrium between air and blood reaching this zone, which is measured using the V:Q ratio. A large or small ratio indicates an imbalance.

Morphological perspective

Organs are either solid (compact) or hollow (tubular) and comprise functional cells and tissues called parenchyma and a supporting framework of cells and tissues called stroma. The lungs are paired, spongy, air-filled organs on both sides of the thoracic cavity that comprise parenchyma, bronchi and stroma. The lungs lie within the thoracic cavity but are neither in the pleural cavities nor the mediastinum.

- The lung parenchyma includes the 'airspace' where gas exchange occurs and all structures that perform gas exchange between the body and external environment (i.e. all structures downstream of the terminal bronchiole).
- The bronchi are a series of progressively smaller branching tubes that conduct air to and from the lungs.
- The lung stroma is the collection of connective tissues, blood vessels, lymphatics and nerves that support the pulmonary parenchyma and bronchi.

Lobar and lobular morphology

Lung morphology is hierarchically organized (Figure 12.4), but the gross appearance of lungs varies between species due to differences in lobation and lobulation (Scrivani et al., 2012). In carnivores, the pulmonary lobes are well developed and distinct, and the pulmonary lobules are not (Figure 12.5; Mclaughlin et al., 1961).

- There are two lungs, left and right. The right lung is about 25% larger.

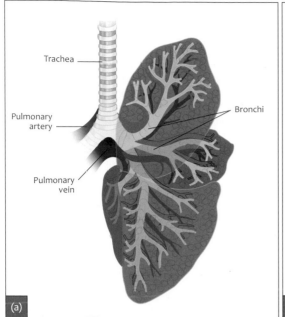

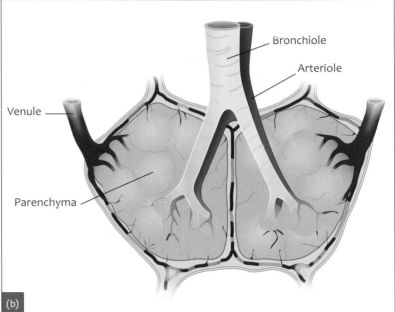

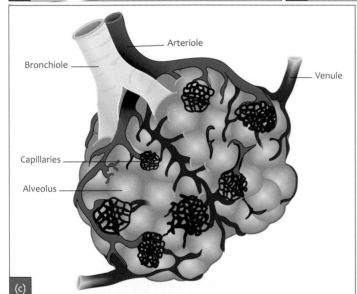

12.4 (a–c) Lung morphology depicting progressively smaller organization. Grossly, the lung is divided into lobes, bronchopulmonary segments and lobules. Carnivore lungs have distinct lobes. The other structures are reflected in the branching pattern of the bronchial tree, but are otherwise unnoticeable when normal. (c) Alveoli are below the spatial resolution of X-ray-based medical imaging: each pixel in a radiograph or CT image represents a summation shadow or average density of several alveoli. The grayscale is more of a representation of the amount of gas within the lung parenchyma than an indication of whether there is an influx of blood, interstitial fluid, cells, or fibre into the alveolar wall or space.
(Redrawn after Lauren D. Sawchyn, DVM, CMI)

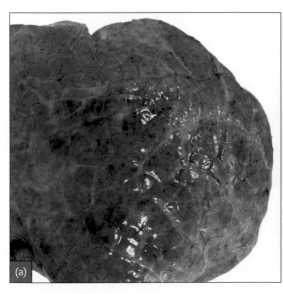

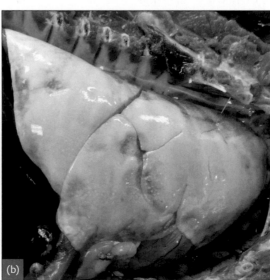

12.5 Normal (a) bovine and (b) canine lungs. Lung morphology varies among species due to differences in lobation and lobulation. Pulmonary lobules are much more prominent in cattle than dogs because cattle have more peripheral lung connective tissue.
(a, Courtesy of Dr. Elena Demeter; b, Courtesy of Dr. Shotaro Nakagun)

- Each lung has a base (near the diaphragm) and apex (near the thoracic inlet), which are connected by the dorsal and ventral margins.
  - The apex of the left lung extends more cranially.
- Each lung has a hilus where the principal bronchus, vessels and nerves pass to or from the lung. Collectively, these structures form the root of the lung.
- Each lung has diaphragmatic, costal (lateral), medial and interlobar surfaces.
  - The junction of the costal and diaphragmatic surfaces forms the basal margin, which extends into the costodiaphragmatic recess.
  - The basal and ventral margins combine to form the acute margin.
  - The medial surface is divided into vertebral and mediastinal parts, and the mediastinal part is indented to accommodate the heart (cardiac impression). The medial surface also has aortic and oesophageal impressions.
- The lungs are divided into six lobes: left cranial (cranial and caudal parts), left caudal, right cranial, right middle, right caudal and accessory lung lobes.
  - In the right lung, the cranial and middle lung lobes diverge to form the cardiac notch, which provides a valuable window for echocardiography and pericardiocentesis. The cardiac notch of the left lung is not as wide and prominent.
  - The right lung has a groove for the caudal vena cava between accessory, middle and caudal lung lobes.
  - The accessory lung lobe has a portion that is ventral to the caudal vena cava, caudal to the heart and cranial to the ventral part of the diaphragm. The accessory lung lobe also has a portion dorsal to the caudal vena cava and cranial to the crura of the diaphragm; when fully inflated, this portion extends dorsally as far as the caudal lung lobes.

- Each lobe is divided into bronchopulmonary segments, which are further divided into pulmonary lobules.
- Each pulmonary lobule is separated by interlobular septa. These septa are connective tissue partitions that are continuous with the connective tissue in the rest of the lung and contain veins and lymphatics that drain the pulmonary lobule. Each pulmonary lobule also is supplied by an arteriole, a bronchiole and lymphatics. The lobular parenchyma between these centrally located structures and the interlobular septa consists of about 3–12 pulmonary acini.
- The pulmonary acini make up the pulmonary parenchyma, where gas exchange occurs between the body and environment.
  - Conceptually, each pulmonary acinus is the part of the lung downstream to a terminal bronchiole (see 'Airways', below).
  - A terminal bronchiole divides into respiratory bronchioles. Conceptually, all structures downstream to a respiratory bronchiole (i.e. alveolar ducts, alveolar sacs, and alveoli) form a primary pulmonary lobule.
  - Each alveolus is a thin-walled sac that forms a blind end to the respiratory tree.

Regarding imaging, part of this organization is more conceptual than forming grossly visible structures. In carnivores, the connective tissue that maintains the structure of the primary and secondary pulmonary lobules is so diminished and haphazard that these structures are often unnoticeable (Mclaughlin *et al.*, 1961). The pulmonary acini and primary pulmonary lobules are usually disregarded, and the secondary pulmonary lobules are simply referred to as pulmonary lobules. The organization of the lungs into lobes, bronchopulmonary segments and pulmonary lobules is maintained in the organization of the airways (Figure 12.6; Scrivani and Percival, 2023).

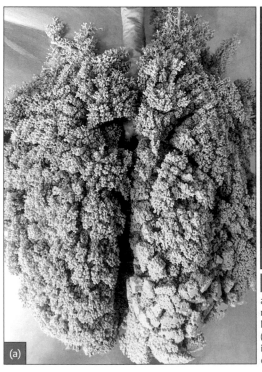

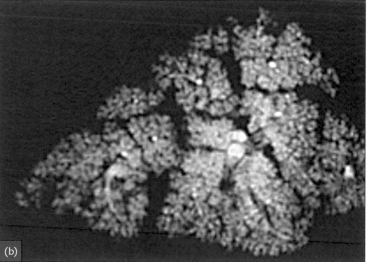

12.6 (a) Dorsal aspect photograph and (b) transverse CT image of a silicone cast of a bronchial tree of a large dog. (a) Blue silicone forms a cast of the lumens of the large airways (trachea and bronchi) and small airways (bronchioles). Notice that the airways maintain the lobular structure even though this is not grossly apparent. (b) The silicone is hyperattenuating compared with air. Notice the lobular structure with the central arteriole (appearing as a black dot) and bronchiole (appearing as a white dot). Studying casts with visual inspection and imaging aids understanding of morphology (Scrivani and Percival, 2023). For example, the pulmonary lobules are easier to appreciate as they are further apart than *in vivo*.

Airways

- Caudal to the thoracic inlet, air is conducted through the thoracic part of the trachea.
- The trachea splits caudally into the left and right principal bronchi at the tracheal bifurcation.
- Before entering a lung lobe, each principal bronchus divides into multiple lobar bronchi.
- Within a lung lobe, each lobar bronchus divides into multiple segmental bronchi.
- Each segmental bronchus divides progressively into smaller bronchi and then into smaller bronchioles (Figure 12.7).
    - Bronchioles (compared with bronchi) have a smaller diameter, lack cartilage and lack glands. Both have smooth muscle and an epithelial lining (mucosa) supported by connective tissue.
- Although not formally listed in *Nomina Anatomica Veterinaria*, the bronchiole entering the pulmonary lobule may be called the 'lobular' bronchiole for descriptive purposes (ICVGAN, 2017; ICVHN, 2017).
- Each 'lobular' bronchiole divides into terminal bronchioles. The terminal bronchiole is not the final airway in the bronchial tree (as suggested by the name) but rather the last one to solely conduct air.
- Each terminal bronchiole divides into respiratory bronchioles, which are involved in both gas conduction and gas exchange. The respiratory bronchioles have alveoli along their walls and deliver air to the exchange surfaces of the lung (i.e. alveolar ducts, alveolar sacs and alveoli).
    - Airflow in the lungs is tidal, meaning that air flows in and out of the alveolus using the same path. However, small openings in the alveolar wall (pores of Kohn) allow for collateral airflow between alveoli.

Blood vessels

Pulmonary blood flow

The pulmonary vasculature permits gas exchange between the body and external environment (Hermanson *et al.*, 2020).

Deoxygenated blood from the right ventricle is delivered to the lungs by two branches of the pulmonic trunk, the left and right pulmonary arteries.

- Clinically, the pulmonic trunk is commonly called the main pulmonary artery.
- As conventional for many viscera, only the artery directly supplying the organ is officially named. Therefore, the term 'pulmonary artery' includes all successive branches to the capillary bed.
- Individual branches frequently are highlighted for explanatory purposes by adding a descriptive modifier. For example, 'lobar' may be used to indicate the branch of the pulmonary artery supplying a single lung lobe, and 'lobular' to indicate the branch supplying a single pulmonary lobule.

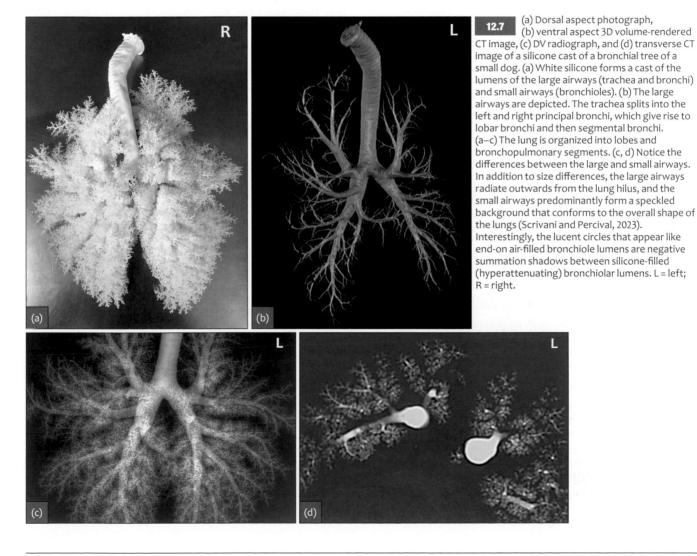

12.7 (a) Dorsal aspect photograph, (b) ventral aspect 3D volume-rendered CT image, (c) DV radiograph, and (d) transverse CT image of a silicone cast of a bronchial tree of a small dog. (a) White silicone forms a cast of the lumens of the large airways (trachea and bronchi) and small airways (bronchioles). (b) The large airways are depicted. The trachea splits into the left and right principal bronchi, which give rise to lobar bronchi and then segmental bronchi. (a–c) The lung is organized into lobes and bronchopulmonary segments. (c, d) Notice the differences between the large and small airways. In addition to size differences, the large airways radiate outwards from the lung hilus, and the small airways predominantly form a speckled background that conforms to the overall shape of the lungs (Scrivani and Percival, 2023). Interestingly, the lucent circles that appear like end-on air-filled bronchiole lumens are negative summation shadows between silicone-filled (hyperattenuating) bronchiolar lumens. L = left; R = right.

- Small-diameter arteries are called arterioles and are the primary site of vascular resistance.
- In dogs, the pulmonary artery continues beyond the alveoli to supply the pleura.

Oxygenated blood returns to the left atrium from the lungs via the pulmonary veins.

- A pulmonary vein is inclusive of the main outflow vessel and all contributing branches: each lung lobe has a least one main outflow vessel.
- Small-diameter veins are called venules.

Bronchial blood flow

The bronchial blood flow provides for nutrient, waste and gas exchange between internal tissues.

Oxygenated blood from the left heart is delivered to the tracheobronchial lymph nodes, peribronchial connective tissue and the bronchial mucous membrane via the bronchial artery.

- In most dogs, the bronchial artery arises from the broncho–oesophageal artery, which arises from the right fifth intercostal artery near its origin from the aorta.
- At the level of the respiratory bronchioles the bronchial artery terminates in a capillary bed that is continuous with that of the pulmonary artery.

Deoxygenated blood returns to the right atrium by bronchial veins.

- Bronchial veins are only present at the lung hilus and empty into the azygos or intercostal vein at the level of T7.

Lymphatic vessels

The lymphatics encompass a series of unnamed thin-walled vessels that convey lymph in the bronchovascular bundle, bronchiolovascular bundle, venous bundle and pleura.

- Lymphatic vessels are absent in the lung parenchyma to facilitate rapid gas exchange. In contrast to lymph, interstitial fluid and plasma are present throughout the lung.
- The pulmonary lymphatic vessels primarily drain into the tracheobronchial lymph nodes, which are near the junction of the trachea and principal bronchi.

Connective tissue and interstitium

The pulmonary interstitium is inextricably linked to the connective tissue supporting the bronchovascular bundles, pulmonary parenchyma and visceral pleura. Therefore, to understand the pulmonary interstitium, it is necessary to understand the structure of connective tissue, which is one of the four basic tissue types distributed throughout the entire body (see Chapter 7).

Connective tissue provides support and protection for the body, forms a pathway for blood vessels, lymphatic vessels, nerves, and airways, and is present in all parts of the lung. It also forms pathways and boundaries to the spread of some diseases (e.g. oedema, suppurative inflammation, neoplasms). Connective tissue consists of cells and an extracellular matrix containing fibres and ground substance.

- A wide variety of cells make connective tissue, including adipocytes, osteocytes, chondrocytes, erythrocytes, leucocytes and fibroblasts. Fibroblasts are the predominant cells making connective tissue in lung.
- Connective tissue fibres are mostly composed of collagen, elastin, or both. Both fibre types contribute to the physical properties of lung (e.g. stiffness and elasticity).
- Ground substance is clear gelatinous extracellular fluid composed of body water, glycosaminoglycans, and proteoglycans, that exists in innumerable gaps or spaces in connective tissue called interstices.
  - Ground substance is called interstitial fluid when in a tissue, lymph when in lymphatic vessel and plasma when in a blood vessel.
- The interstitium is the collection of interstices throughout the body, which are mostly contiguous. In other words, the interstitium is a contiguous fluid-filled space.
  - Throughout most of the body, including the lungs, there is a continuous exchange of nutrients and waste products between the different types of extracellular fluid (i.e. interstitial fluid, lymph, and blood). In the lungs, there also is a continuous exchange of nutrients and waste products between this extracellular fluid and the environment. The volume and composition of the interstitium varies among body structures, including between structures within the lungs.

Connective tissues have different physical properties and functions related to differences in cell types, fibre types, organization of fibres and relative proportions of fibres to ground substance in the matrix. Connective tissue is categorized into two major types based on whether there is proportionally more or less ground substance to fibres: loose connective tissue and dense connective tissue. The latter is further divided based on the orientation of fibres: dense regular connective tissue and dense irregular connective tissue. The lungs comprise a continuum of variably thick strands of loose and dense irregular connective tissue that provide the lobar and lobular structure, overall firmness and elasticity, and pathways for nerves, vessels, and airways. The connective tissue also upholds the pulmonary interstitium, which allows extracellular fluid and gas exchange within the lung, and gas exchange between the lung and external environment.

The pulmonary interstitium exists throughout the lung and is subdivided into three parts, related to the morphological perspective described above. It is important to differentiate the different parts because different fibrotic and non-fibrotic interstitial diseases characteristically affect one or more parts. In addition, a disease may affect different parts at different times, thus producing different imaging findings at different points of the disease. For example, pulmonary oedema in dogs affects different parts of the interstitium (bronchovascular and parenchymal) at different stages of disease (Staub et al., 1967).

- Bronchovascular interstitium surrounds and supports the bronchi, arteries, veins and lymphatic vessels from the lung hilus to the respiratory bronchiole; the interstitium is progressively smaller the further away it is from the lung hilus. It is also called the axial or perivascular interstitium.
- Parenchymal interstitium is situated at the sites of gas exchange and is very thin to allow rapid movement of gas between the body and environment; the alveolar

epithelium and capillary share the same basement membrane. It is also called the acinar or alveolar interstitium.

- Peripheral interstitium extends into the lung from the lung surface, connecting the visceral pleura to the interlobular septa of the pulmonary lobules, and surrounds and supports the veins and lymphatic vessels not associated with the bronchovascular interstitium. In normal carnivores, this connective tissue is thicker near the lung surface but generally thin and haphazard. It is also called the subpleural interstitium.

Bronchovascular bundles

The bronchovascular bundle is an important concept for image interpretation and is the construct formed by the bronchi, pulmonary blood vessels and their surrounding adventitial sheath. This connective tissue sheath provides support and a pathway through the lung for these structures, including the interstitium, linking the lung hilus and visceral pleura. Typically, additional structures such as lymphatic vessels, autonomic nerves and bronchial blood vessels are contained within the fibrous sheath, and extracellular fluid may move between the interstitium and the lumens of lymphatic and blood vessels according to Starling forces.

- The walls of airways and blood vessels are layered. The outer layer of each is the tunica adventitia (tunica externa). Adventitia is loose connective tissue that binds structures together, often blending with the adventitia of adjacent structures (see Chapter 7).
- The external surface of the lungs is covered by visceral pleura, which is another type of loose connective tissue that is organized into a serous membrane (see Chapter 7). The mesenchymal layer of the serous membrane is continuous with the underlying connective tissue that extends deep into the lung.

Near the lung hilus, the pulmonary blood vessels and bronchus form the classic artery–bronchus–vein triad where the pulmonary artery and bronchus are closely apposed; the pulmonary vein is slightly more distant. However, in dogs and cats this arrangement only exists close to the lung hilus where the diameter of the bronchi and pulmonary blood vessels are large. Thereafter, the pulmonary vein takes a separate path to the visceral pleura (Figure 12.8). The bronchus and pulmonary artery remain close together from the hilus to the terminal bronchus. To

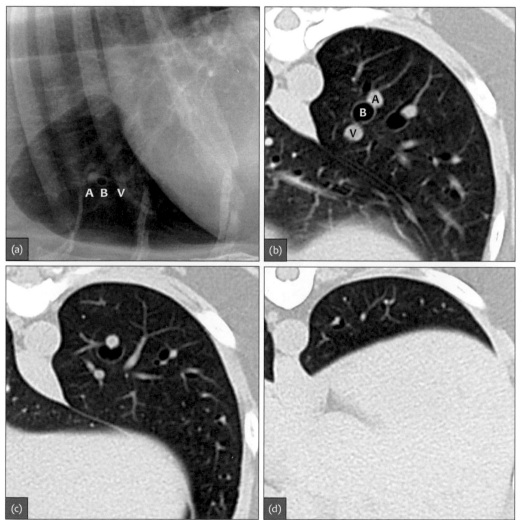

12.8 (a) Lateral thoracic radiograph of a dog and (b-d) sequential transverse CT images of the left caudal lung lobe of another dog; (b) is closest to the lung hilus and (d) is the farthest caudal. The pulmonary artery (A) carries deoxygenated blood (blue) and is closely apposed to the bronchus (B). The pulmonary vein (V) caries oxygenated blood (red) and is further away from the bronchus than the artery. (a, b) Notice the classic artery–bronchus–vein triad, where the pulmonary vein is closest to the heart, is seen only occasionally and typically where the large diameter bronchi and blood vessels are close to the lung hilus. (b-d) Once the lobar bronchi and blood vessels begin branching, the pulmonary vein does not follow the bronchus to the visceral pleura. Blood vessels travel through connective tissue pathways.

relay these anatomical differences, it is helpful to further classify the relationships between the airways, lung parenchyma, blood vessels and other stromal structures as:

- Bronchoarterial bundle: from the lung hilus to the terminal bronchus, especially after the pulmonary vein has diverged. This construct is formed by the bronchi, pulmonary artery and the surrounding fibrous sheath. This structure may be further classified when it is important to specify associations with the large and small airways
- Pulmonary capillary bed: at the site of gas exchange between the body and environment, the pulmonary capillaries are in direct contact with the walls of the alveoli. As a component of the lung parenchyma, the connective tissue sheath is severely reduced to a shared basement membrane between the alveolar epithelium and the capillary endothelium to allow rapid diffusion of gas
- Pulmonary venous bundle: from the interlobular septa of pulmonary lobules to the visceral pleura, the construct formed by the pulmonary vein and its surrounding fibrous sheath (Figure 12.9).

Normal anatomical variation

The imaging appearance of lungs varies with many non-pathological variables including breed conformation, body conditioning, respiratory cycle (inhalation/exhalation), cardiac cycle (systole/diastole), X-ray beam exposure and orientation, and age. Because a vertical X-ray beam is used conventionally in dogs and cats, air/fluid interfaces are not typically observed: a fluid line may be detected when using a horizontal X-ray beam or during cross-sectional imaging (e.g. CT). Age-related changes have been described for the radiographic appearance of the lungs of old dogs, but the importance of this adage was questioned in a recent study that showed dogs undergoing CT had only minimal observable differences; old dogs, however, may have more foci of heterotopic bone and may be more prone to lung lobe collapse than young dogs (Hornby and Lamb, 2017).

During thoracic radiography, both lungs are seen on all views as a summation shadow. However, the 'up' lung is generally better evaluated, because of the tendency of the 'down' lung (gravity-dependent lung) to be less well inflated and the effect this has on differential absorption of the X-ray beam. This phenomenon is often observed

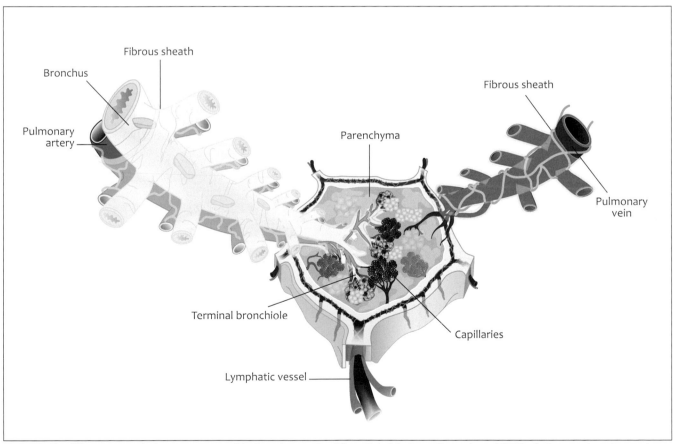

12.9 The different anatomical compartments of the lung that may be differentiated during radiography and CT. The first compartment comprises the pulmonary artery, bronchus and the surrounding adventitial fibrous sheath that extends between the lung hilus to the terminal bronchiole. It conducts air in and out of the body, delivers blood to the parenchyma for oxygenation and may be subdivided by airway size (large and small). The second compartment is the pulmonary parenchyma where gas exchange occurs between the body and environment, it comprises the structures downstream to the terminal bronchioles (the pulmonary acini) and capillaries. The third compartment comprises the pulmonary veins and the surrounding fibrous sheath that extends between the interlobar septa and visceral pleura. In carnivores, these connective tissue pathways for the blood vessels are very thin. The pulmonary veins eventually return to the lung hilus and bring oxygenated blood to the left atrium. Note that the pulmonary interstitium is inextricably related to the connective tissue and is subdivided into the bronchovascular interstitium, parenchymal interstitium and peripheral interstitium.
(Redrawn after Lauren D. Sawchyn, DVM, CMI)

on left and right lateral views, but the caudodorsal lung field is better evaluated on the dorsoventral (DV) view and the cranioventral lung field is better evaluated on the ventrodorsal (VD) view for similar reasons. Abnormalities in the 'up' lung may also be larger and less opaque due to magnification.

Normal bronchioles, capillaries, alveolar septa and supporting connective tissue are not seen on radiographs of dogs and cats (Suter and Lord, 1974). Therefore, the opacity of normal lungs is typically determined by the ratio of gas and blood within the lungs (Figure 12.10). However, because radiographs are planar images, conditions affecting the pleural cavities, mediastinum, pericardium/heart, and thoracic boundaries will produce positive and negative summation shadows that contribute to the observed opacity of the lungs.

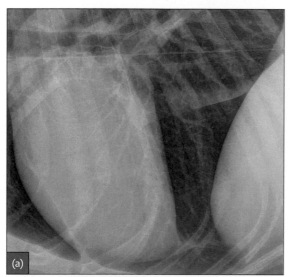

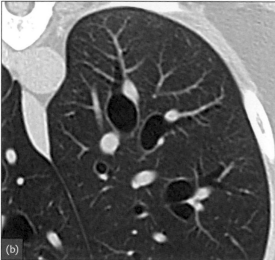

12.10 (a) Lateral thoracic radiograph of an adult dog and (b) transverse thoracic CT image of another adult dog. During radiography, normal lungs have homogeneous background opacity that is a dark grey: the only soft tissue opacity seen in the lungs is due to the pulmonary blood vessels. In general, the normal airway walls are too thin to be detected. Occasionally, the bronchial walls are mineralized. This opacity is normal when thin and linear, and not a pattern of disease. During CT, normal lungs have a similar appearance, but the bronchial walls are visible and generally thinner than adjacent blood vessels. From the lung hilus, the pulmonary blood vessels branch numerous times and may be traced to the periphery of the lung. These branches normally have a progressively smaller diameter that tapers towards the periphery. In addition, the airways branch and the walls form corresponding line pairs (tram lines) or rings that progressively taper or become smaller towards the periphery.

Lung lobes

- The lungs should extend cranially to the first rib pair.
- All lung lobes (Figure 12.11), except for the right cranial and left cranial (cranial part) lung lobes, contact the diaphragm.
- The right cranial and right caudal lung lobes contact each other dorsally; the same is true for the left cranial (cranial part) and left caudal lung lobes.
- The right middle and left cranial (caudal part) lung lobes are ventral to the carina, mostly at the same level as the heart.
- The accessory lung lobe is caudal to the heart, between the left caudal and right caudal lung lobes, and encircles the caudal vena cava. On lateral views, the location is usually described as within the triangle formed by the heart, caudal vena cava, and cupula of the diaphragm. However, the normal accessory lobe extends dorsal to the caudal vena cava.

Pulmonary blood vessels

- Near the lung hilus, the pulmonary blood vessels form a 'classical triad' of artery–bronchus–vein.
  - The artery and vein are on opposite sides of the airway, and the veins are either most ventral or closest to the median plane ('veins are ventral; veins are central').
  - From the lung hilus to the capillary bed, the pulmonary artery is always in close contact with the bronchus. Once the airway terminates, the pulmonary artery continues to the visceral pleura.
  - When seeing the 'classic triad,' the pulmonary vein is slightly further away from the bronchus than the artery. The pulmonary vein is in close contact with the bronchus and artery near the hilus and diverges away from these structures towards the lung periphery.
- Pulmonary blood vessels should be widest near the lung hilus with branching and tapering towards the periphery. At a given level, the diameters of the pulmonary artery and pulmonary vein are about the same, or the pulmonary vein is slightly larger.
- On DV and VD thoracic radiographs, the pulmonary artery diameter should not be larger than the width of the ninth rib where the two summate with each other.
- On lateral thoracic radiographs, the pulmonary vein diameter should not be larger than the width of the dorsal third of the fourth rib (Figure 12.12).
- Normal bronchial arteries and veins are not typically seen.
- End-on blood vessels may be mistaken for nodules, especially when enlarged or near the lung hilus.

Bronchi

- Normal bronchi are typically not seen, and their location is usually surmised by identifying the adjacent pulmonary artery and vein on either side.
- In some dogs, but not cats, the bronchial walls may be partially mineralized. These bronchial walls appear as thin linear mineral opacities.
- On lateral views, it may be possible to differentiate some lobar bronchi based on the branching pattern. The lobar bronchus to the left cranial lung lobe arises as a short stalk off the left principal bronchus that divides into branches for the cranial and caudal parts. The lobar bronchi to the right cranial and right middle lobes arise from the right principal bronchus but are separate stalks (Figure 12.13).

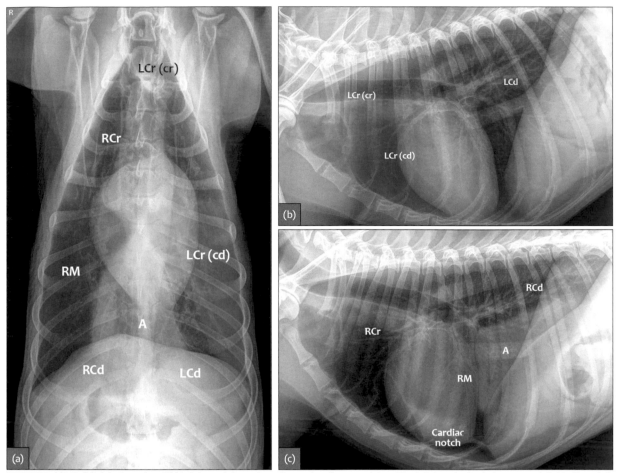

12.11 (a) VD, (b) right lateral and (c) left lateral thoracic radiographs of a normal dog. The left lung is shaded green and divided into left cranial (LCr) and left caudal (LCd) lung lobes. The left cranial lung lobe is subdivided into cranial (cr) and caudal (cd) parts. The right lung is mostly shaded orange, but the accessory lung lobe (A) is yellow. The right lung is divided into right cranial (RCr), right caudal (RCd), and right middle (RM) lung lobes.

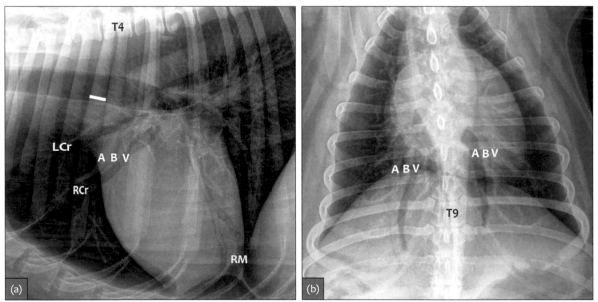

12.12 (a) Left lateral and (b) DV thoracic radiographs of a normal dog. The pulmonary arteries (blue) carry deoxygenated blood from the right heart to the lungs and the pulmonary veins (red) carry oxygenated blood from the lungs to the left heart. The classic triad of artery (A), bronchus (B) and vein (V) can be differentiated in certain locations. (a) On the lateral view, they form distinct opacities in the left cranial (LCr) and right cranial (RCr) lung lobes. In the other lung lobes, they summate with each other (purple). The diameter of the pulmonary veins where they summate with the fourth rib should not be greater than the width of the dorsal third of that rib (white line). (b) On the DV view, the artery, bronchus and vein are differentiated in the left caudal and right caudal lung lobes. The pulmonary artery diameter should not be greater than the width of the ninth rib (yellow) where they summate. Many additional blood vessels are visible in the lungs, but it is impossible to consistently accurately identify them. T4/9 = fourth/ninth thoracic vertebra.

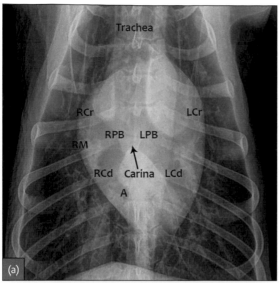

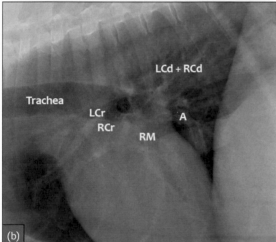

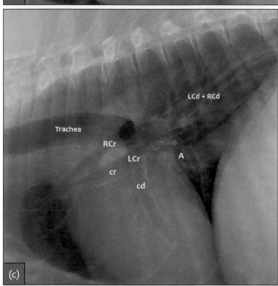

12.13 (a) VD, (b) left lateral and (c) right lateral thoracic radiographs of a normal dog. The trachea divides into the right (RPB) and left (LPB) principal bronchi. The principal bronchi divide into lobar bronchi, which supply the right cranial (RCr), right middle (RM), right caudal (RCd), left cranial (LCr) and left caudal (LCd) lung lobes. The RCd lobar bronchus sends a branch to the accessory (A) lung lobe. The LCr lobar bronchus divides into cranial (cr) and caudal (cd) parts. The carina is a soft tissue structure resembling a keel, located between the RPB and LPB. On lateral views (b, c), a round negative summation shadow produced by the tracheal bifurcation denotes the approximate location of the carina. (b) The RCr and RM lobar bronchi are separate tubes. (c) The LCr lobar bronchus splits into cr and cd branches.

Interpretative principles

Diagnostic pulmonary image interpretation relies on evaluation of the:

- Opacity of the lung
- Overall lung size
- Macroscopic distribution of disease within the lung
- Presence or absence of miscellaneous signs that may prioritize the differential diagnosis.

Pulmonary opacification

Pulmonary opacification simply means that the lungs are more opaque (whiter) or hyperattenuating compared with normal. During thoracic radiography, pulmonary opacification may be detected due to positive summation shadows with abnormalities of the pleural cavities, mediastinum, pericardium/heart or thoracic boundaries. Pulmonary opacification attributed to abnormal lung conditions occurs when there is a decreased ratio of gas to soft tissue in the lungs due to one or more of the following:

- Hypoventilation: reduced gas volume in the pulmonary parenchyma (e.g. incomplete inhalation, tracheal collapse, brachycephalic obstructive airway syndrome, fibrotic lung disease)
- Hyperperfusion: increased blood volume in the lung (e.g. fluid overload, left-to-right shunt, inflammation)
- Influx of fluid, fibre, or cells into the lungs (e.g. pneumonia, pulmonary oedema, neoplasm, fibrotic lung disease).

Different imaging signs and patterns associated with pulmonary opacification help localize disease to anatomical compartments (Figure 12.14).

Anatomical compartment*	Some localizing imaging signs and patterns
Lung parenchyma	Ground-glass opacity
	Consolidation
	Pulmonary necrosis
	Pulmonary masses/nodules/micronodules
	Airspace nodules
	Atelectasis (collapse)
Large airway (bronchial)	Radiating thick tram lines and rings (large diameter)
	Bronchial mineralization
	Bronchiectasis
	Bronchial narrowing (widespread or localized)
	Intraluminal bronchial obstruction (partial or complete)
	Loss of bronchial wall integrity (collapse or rupture)
	Bronchial nodule or mass
Small airway (bronchiolar)	Non-radiating thick tram lines and rings (small diameter)
	Centrilobular nodules and micronodules
	Tree-in-bud
	Bronchiolectasis
Peripheral connective tissue	Stromal bands
	Coarse reticular pattern
	Nodules (perilobular, subpleural, pleural)

12.14 Relating anatomical compartments to pulmonary opacification findings observed during X-ray-based medical imaging. Some signs are detectable only during CT. * Excluding pulmonary arteries and veins.

Parenchymal opacification patterns

These descriptive patterns localize disease to the alveolar epithelium, pulmonary capillaries, parenchymal interstitium and airspace, without further differentiation. Parenchymal opacification also may be called airspace opacification when specifically referring to filling of the alveolar spaces with material that attenuates the X-ray beam more than normal lung parenchyma.

- Ground-glass opacity: the airspace retains some gas, and the pulmonary opacification appears hazy, foggy, and unstructured or comprising fine lines (Figure 12.15). Notably, the pulmonary blood vessels (and bronchial walls) are visible through the abnormal opacity (Figure 12.16).
  - This description of ground-glass opacity is essentially equivalent to the description of an unstructured interstitial pattern in the traditional approach.
- Consolidation: the airspace is void of air (solid lung) and the pulmonary opacification is unstructured with border effacement of pulmonary blood vessels and bronchial walls (Figure 12.17). Additional signs might be observed but are not required to recognize consolidation (Figure 12.18).
  - Border effacement: the creation of an imaging silhouette that occurs when adjacent structures in the image (not necessarily adjacent in the body) attenuate the X-ray beam to the same degree, making it impossible to distinguish the border between structures.
- Air bronchograms: air-filled bronchial lumens surrounded by consolidated lung. If the adjacent blood vessels or bronchial walls are visible (even if just barely so), then it is not an air bronchogram.
- Air alveolograms: air-filled alveoli appearing as small gas opacities surrounded by airless (consolidated) lung (The alveolar equivalent of air bronchograms).
- Lobar sign: lung consolidation that extends to the periphery of the lobe will have an abrupt delineated border when adjacent to normally aerated lung.
- This description of consolidation is essentially equivalent to the description of an alveolar pattern in the traditional approach.
- Pulmonary masses/nodules/micronodules (see 'Nodular opacification patterns', below).
- Airspace nodules (see 'Nodular opacification patterns', below).
- Atelectasis (collapse) (see 'Decreased size', below).

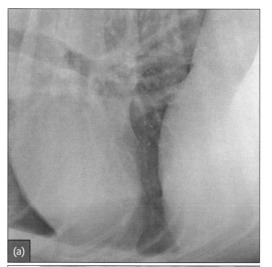

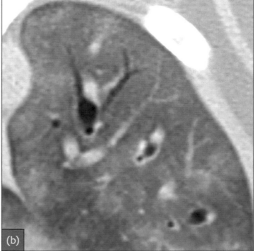

12.16 (a) Lateral thoracic radiograph and (b) transverse thoracic CT image (lung window) depicting ground-glass opacity (unstructured interstitial pattern) that affects both lungs. There is widespread unstructured (foggy) parenchymal opacification with blurring of the pulmonary blood vessels and bronchial walls. Some air remains in the airspace.

12.15 'Walking through the forest in fog' can be used as an analogy to better understand parenchymal opacification. Two parenchymal opacity patterns, ground-glass opacity and consolidation, relate to how much air remains in the airspace. In this analogy, tree branches represent pulmonary blood vessels and fog-filled air represents the lung parenchyma. Notice that certain areas may have more fog, and the edges of the fog may be discernible, but the fog is unstructured (i.e. does not form linear or nodular shapes). In the near distance, the trees have clearly visible branches that divide and taper as they extend away from the trunk. This description is like looking at pulmonary blood vessels in a normally expanded and aerated lung. In the mid distance, the tree branches remain visible, but the margins are fuzzy due to the fog, and it may be difficult to see some of the fine twigs at the periphery of the tree. This description is like looking at pulmonary blood vessels when there is ground-glass opacity (unstructured interstitial pattern). In the far distance, the fog completely obscures the branches of the tree (border effacement). This description is like looking at pulmonary blood vessels when there is lung consolidation (alveolar pattern).

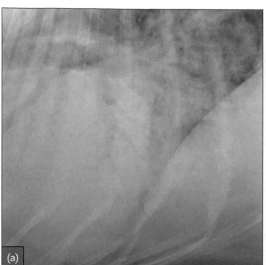
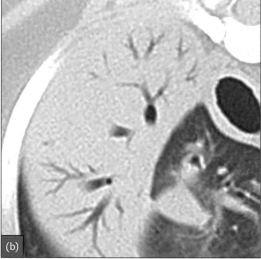

12.17 (a) Lateral thoracic radiograph and (b) transverse thoracic CT image (lung window) depicting lung consolidation (alveolar pattern). Notice the unstructured parenchymal opacification with border effacement of the pulmonary blood vessels and bronchial walls. No air remains in the affected airspace – the affected lung is solid. Air bronchograms and lobar signs also are present.

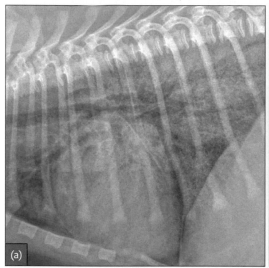
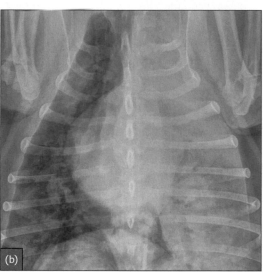

12.18 (a) Lateral and (b) VD thoracic radiographs of different adult dogs with parenchymal opacification. A defining feature of lung consolidation (*versus* ground-glass opacity) is border effacement of the pulmonary blood vessels. (a) There is diffuse parenchymal opacification with mixed appearances. The cranioventral lung field has a pattern of ground-glass opacity (unstructured interstitial pattern) because the margins of the pulmonary blood vessels are blurred but visible. The caudodorsal lung field has a pattern of consolidation (alveolar pattern) because there is border effacement of the pulmonary blood vessels. The presence of air bronchograms also indicates lung consolidation, but it is not a required feature. (b) The entire left lung has a pattern of consolidation without air bronchograms in the left cranial lung lobe and with air bronchograms in the left caudal lung lobe. There also is a lobar sign between the left caudal and accessory lung lobes.

Linear opacification patterns

These patterns localize disease to the bronchi, bronchioles, pulmonary arteries, pulmonary veins, bronchovascular interstitium and peripheral connective tissue (including the peripheral interstitium). Further differentiation is possible. Abnormalities of tubular structures, like airways and blood vessels, are associated with differences in overall diameter, wall thickness, wall integrity, lumen diameter and lumen contents. Abnormalities of the connective tissue typically produce variably thick soft tissue bands that conform to existing connective tissue pathways and constructs.

Some of the listed signs and patterns are associated with pulmonary opacification only occasionally but are included because of a similar anatomical localization.

Large airway signs and patterns:

- Bronchial pattern: diffuse increased bronchial wall thickness that produces thick, wide-gauge, rings and tram lines that radiate outwards from the lung hilus (Figure 12.19). Typically, the bronchial lumens have a gas opacity that contrasts with the internal layer of the bronchial wall. Increased wall thickness may be due to any combination of increased thickness of the mucosa, submucosa, muscularis and adventitia (including the bronchovascular interstitium).
- Bronchial wall mineralization: diffuse increased opacity of the bronchial wall with normal bronchial wall thickness (Figure 12.20). Commonly an age-related change of minor consequence in dogs, but occasionally a sign of metastatic calcification (any cause of hypercalcaemia, hyperphosphataemia, or both). Bronchial mineralization also may be more prominent in chondrodystrophic animals due to early cartilaginous degeneration and is often of minor consequence.
- Bronchial nodule or mass: regional increased bronchial wall thickness producing a bronchocentric mass, which might extend into the bronchial lumen or compress adjacent lung parenchyma. Solitary or multiple nodules are possible.

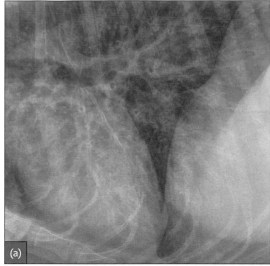

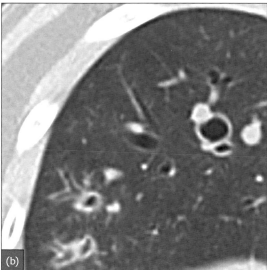

12.19 (a) Lateral thoracic radiograph and (b) transverse thoracic CT image (lung window) of different dogs with a bronchial pattern. Note the bronchial walls that produce thick rings and tram lines that radiate outwards from the lung hilus.

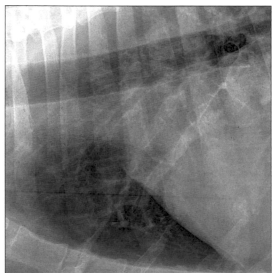

12.20 Close-up lateral thoracic radiograph of an adult dog with bronchial wall mineralization; this finding may be normal or degenerative and of minor consequence or a sign of disease (e.g. causes of metastatic calcification). Notice the thin linear opacities that are parallel to and more opaque than the pulmonary blood vessels.

- Bronchial rupture: regional interruption of the bronchial wall is an uncommon sign associated with trauma. Gas may be seen dissecting through the bronchovascular interstitium, possibly leading to pneumomediastinum or pneumothorax.
- Intraluminal bronchial obstruction: abnormal narrowing of the bronchial lumen due to material within the lumen (e.g. foreign body, mucus plug) (Figure 12.21). Secondary parenchymal opacification or hyperlucency also is possible when airflow to the airspace is altered (e.g. obstructive air trapping, obstructive atelectasis).
- Bronchiectasis: irreversible increased overall lumen diameters of the bronchi (bronchial dilatation) that predisposes the patient to infection due to excess mucus and disrupted mucociliary apparatus function. Bronchial wall thickness may be thinner than normal or moderately diffusely thick depending on whether there is concurrent inflammation. Typically, the affected bronchi lack downstream tapering and branches of the bronchial tree, rather than only the lobar bronchi, are involved. Bronchial lumens may have a gas or fluid opacity. Air-filled bronchial lumens produce tram lines and rings (Figure 12.22). Fluid-filled bronchial lumens produce broad soft tissue bands that may radiate outward from the lung hilus when viewed 'side on' or appear nodular when viewed 'end-on' (Figure 12.23).

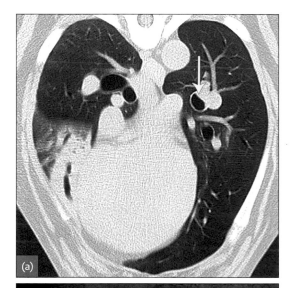

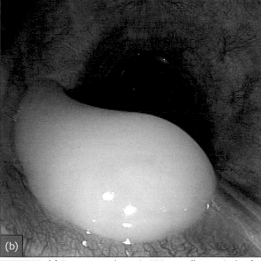

12.21 (a) Transverse thoracic CT image (lung window) and (b) endoscopic image of the bronchi of a dog with a mucus plug in the lumen of a bronchus (arrowed).

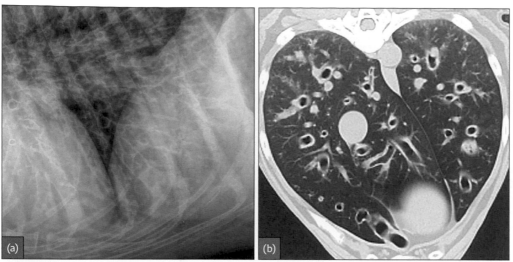

12.22 (a) Close-up lateral thoracic radiograph and (b) transverse thoracic CT image (lung window) of an adult dog with bronchiectasis. Notice that the bronchi have increased overall diameter, thick walls and lack of tapering. Also notice that the thick lines radiate outwards from the lung hilus, and most lumens are gas-filled, but a few are seen on the radiograph as fluid-filled (especially ventrally).

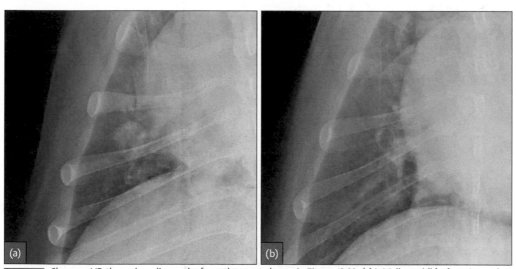

12.23 Close-up VD thoracic radiographs from the same dog as in Figure 12.22. (a) initially and (b) after six weeks of treatment. (a) The enlarged bronchial lumen is fluid-filled and viewed end-on, appearing as a nodule. (b) The bronchial lumen is now air-filled.

Bronchial shape may be cylindrical or saccular.
- On CT, a bronchoarterial ratio greater than 2.0 is suggestive of bronchiectasis in dogs (Cannon *et al.*, 2009).
- Widespread bronchial lumen narrowing: widespread reduced lumen diameter due to wall weakness (e.g. chondromalacia causing dynamic or static collapse), smooth muscle contraction (e.g. bronchoconstriction (Basher *et al.*, 2019)) or as a component of pulmonary hypoplasia (a congenital developmental anomaly) (Figure 12.24).
- Localized bronchial lumen narrowing: localized abnormal narrowing of the bronchial lumen diameter. Commonly interchangeably called bronchial stricture or stenosis to indicate narrowing of a tubular structure (e.g. bronchus, blood vessel) although there is a subtle difference.
  - Stricture: usually applied when the cause of the narrowing is due to something external to the lumen and usually involves all wall layers. Also applied to widespread narrowing of a tubular structure, usually seen as a congenital condition (e.g. tracheobronchial hypoplasia).

- Stenosis: usually applied when the cause of the narrowing is internal; may be eccentric and often does not involve all wall layers (e.g. mucosal mass, embolus).

Small airway signs and patterns:
- Bronchiolar pattern: increased bronchiolar wall thickness, producing thick, narrow-gauge rings and tram lines that do not radiate outward from the lung hilus. Two distinct signs may be seen when the bronchiole lumens are filled with fluid or soft tissue (Figure 12.25):
  - Centrilobular micronodules (see 'Nodular opacification patterns', below)
  - Tree-in-bud sign: a linear branching pattern with micronodules (Figure 12.26).
- Bronchiolectasis: increased overall diameter and increased lumen diameter of the bronchioles (bronchiolar dilatation) usually secondary to fibrosis or inflammatory airway disease. The bronchiole wall is usually thin or not seen (Figure 12.27).

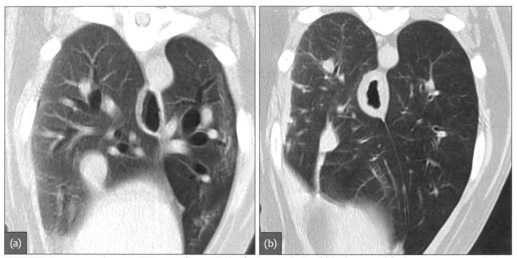

12.24 Transverse thoracic CT images (lung window) of an adult dog (a) before and (b) after intravenous administration of contrast material. (a) Normal bronchial and oesophageal morphology. (b) The dog developed severe diffuse bronchial constriction and oesophageal oedema as a severe adverse reaction to the contrast medium. The bronchi have severely reduced overall diameter and lumen diameter and normal wall thickness. The oesophageal wall is diffusely thick with a smaller lumen diameter and unchanged overall diameter.

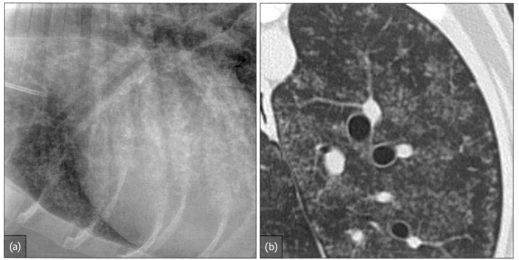

12.25 (a) Lateral thoracic radiograph and (b) transverse thoracic CT image (lung window) depicting a bronchiolar pattern. Fluid, cells or fibre are accumulated in and around the bronchiolovascular bundles (small airways). Notice that the overall pattern appears speckled and any small-gauge tram lines do not radiate outwards from the lung hilus. On CT, the abnormal bronchioles are seen in short-axis and can appear nodular, especially when the lumens are hyperattenuating. This is referred to as a centrilobular distribution when the abnormal opacity is centred in the pulmonary lobule. Notice that the hyperattenuating foci do not extend all the way to the periphery because the airways do not extend to the visceral surface.

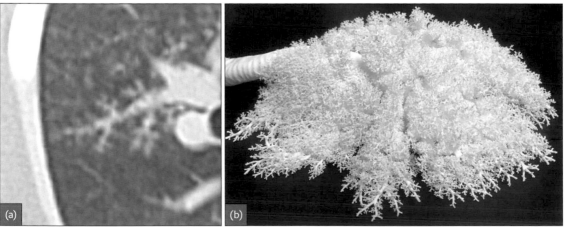

12.26 (a) Close-up transverse thoracic CT image (lung window) of a dog with a tree-in-bud pattern indicating small-airway (bronchiolar) disease. (b) Left aspect photograph of a silicone cast of a bronchial tree of a small dog demonstrating how filling of the bronchiolar lumens can produce a tree-in-bud pattern.

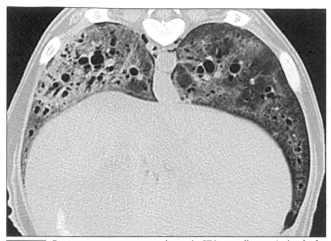

12.27 Post-mortem transverse thoracic CT image (lung window) of a dog with bronchiolectasis related to extensive pulmonary fibrosis due to chronic interstitial pneumonia. Notice the bronchiolar dilatation with gas-filled lumens.

Blood vessels:

- Vascular patterns: any increase in the number or size of the pulmonary blood vessels can lead to pulmonary opacification. Abnormal vessels may also be tortuous or terminate abruptly (lack of downstream tapering). A widespread increase in blood vessel size is usually due to factors associated with increases in pulmonary or systemic blood pressure and volume. Regional blood vessel changes may be due to disturbances by a mass (e.g. granuloma, haematoma, abscess, neoplasm) or wall malformation (e.g. aneurysm, post-stenotic dilatation) (see Chapter 9).
  - Pulmonary artery enlargement is detected on DV thoracic radiographs when the pulmonary artery diameter is larger than the ninth rib width where the two summate with each other (Figure 12.28).

- Pulmonary venous enlargement is detected on lateral thoracic radiographs when the pulmonary vein (where it summates with the fourth rib) is wider that than the dorsal third of that rib.
- Increased number and size of pulmonary blood vessels due to pulmonary over-circulation, pulmonary venous congestion or vascular malformation (Figure 12.29).
- On cross-sectional and angiographic studies, stricture, stenosis or intraluminal blockage may be observed although this does not typically produce pulmonary opacification unless there are secondary changes.

Peripheral connective tissue:

- Stromal bands: increased thickness of the peripheral interstitium producing structured linear opacities that typically arise from the visceral pleura and extend deep into the lung parenchyma. Likely associated with pleural and pulmonary fibrosis and may distort lung morphology (Figure 12.30).
- Coarse reticular pattern: pulmonary stromal bands that are polygonal due to associations with the interlobular septa of pulmonary lobules (perilobular distribution) (Figure 12.31).

Nodular opacification patterns

Pulmonary nodular opacifications are classified by differences in size, opacity and distribution. These patterns are based on seeing a rounded opacity, primarily associated with the pulmonary interstitium, that are typically neither linear nor angular. Note that bronchial masses are mostly considered separately.

The proposed thresholds to classify pulmonary nodules based on size are arbitrary 'rules of thumb' given the wide range of body sizes encountered in normal dogs; it is helpful to simply consider the rounded opacities as big, small, and very small.

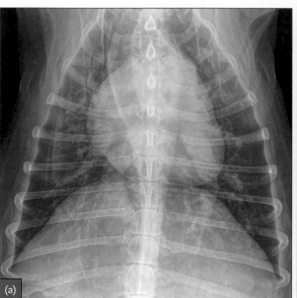

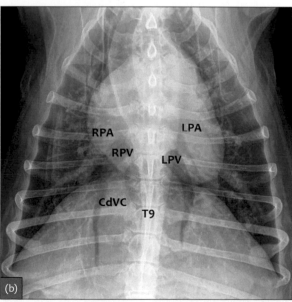

12.28 (a) Plain and (b) annotated DV thoracic radiograph of a dog with enlargement of the right heart, pulmonic trunk and left pulmonary artery due to heartworm infestation. Deoxygenated blood (blue) is present in the right pulmonary artery (RPA), left pulmonary artery (LPA) and caudal vena cava (CdVC). Oxygenated blood (red) is present in the right pulmonary vein (RPV) and left pulmonary vein (LPV). The LPA is enlarged: notice that the LPA diameter is wider than the ninth rib (yellow) where they summate. T9 = ninth thoracic vertebra.

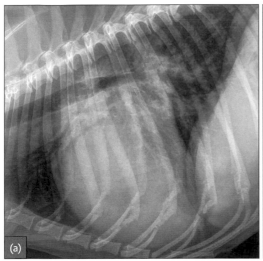

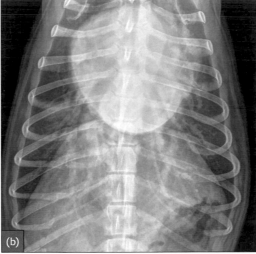

12.29 (a) Right lateral and (b) DV thoracic radiographs of a dog with severe left heart enlargement. There is caudodorsal-to-diffuse pulmonary opacification due to pulmonary venous congestion and early cardiogenic pulmonary oedema. Note the increased number and size of the pulmonary veins.

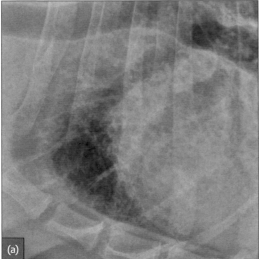

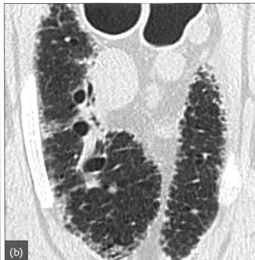

12.30 (a) Lateral thoracic radiograph and (b) transverse thoracic CT image (lung window) depicting pulmonary stromal bands due to increased thickness of the peripheral connective tissue (peripheral interstitium) that is worst near the visceral pleura and extends deep into the lung.

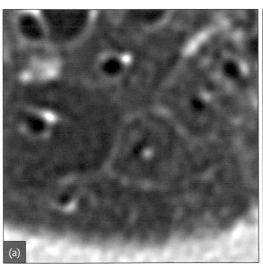

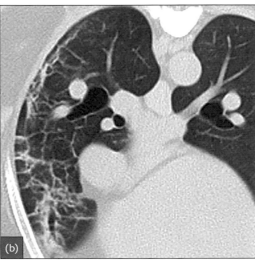

12.31 Transverse thoracic CT images (lung window) of two dogs with coarse reticular patterns due to increased thickness of the peripheral connective tissue (peripheral interstitium) surrounding the pulmonary lobules (i.e. interlobular septa). (a) Notice the central ('lobular') bronchiole and arteriole. (b) Stromal bands are visible.

- Mass: An area of pulmonary opacification larger than 3 cm in any direction (Figure 12.32).
- Nodule: An area of pulmonary opacification between 3 mm and 3 cm in all directions (Figure 12.33).
- Micronodule: An area of pulmonary opacification smaller than 3 mm in all directions (Figure 12.34).

A mass that forms a nodular opacification also may produce signs of displacement or compression of adjacent structures when sufficiently large. A mass that is more infiltrative may produce a nodular opacification that is not coupled to signs of mass effect.

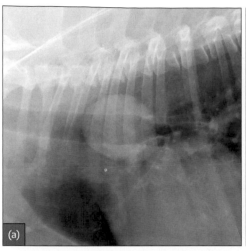

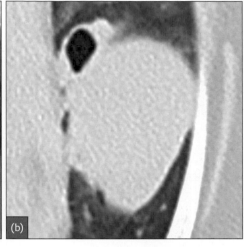

12.32 Close-up (a) lateral thoracic radiograph and (b) transverse thoracic CT image (lung window) depicting a solitary pulmonary mass. Note the mass is not bronchocentric.

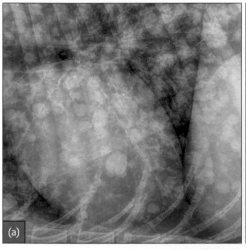

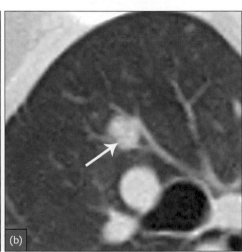

12.33 (a) Lateral thoracic radiograph of a dog depicting multiple pulmonary nodules (nodular lung pattern) and (b) transverse thoracic CT image (lung window) of another dog depicting a solitary lung nodule (arrowed).

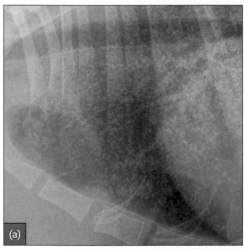

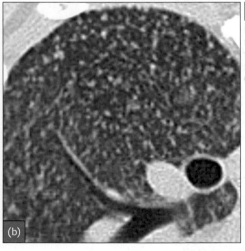

12.34 (a) Lateral thoracic radiograph and (b) transverse thoracic CT image (lung window) of a dog depicting micronodules. (b) Notice that the tiny nodules extend to the lung periphery suggesting a haematogenous spread (miliary pattern).

Opaque nodular structures also may be characterized by differences in opacity or attenuation (Figure 12.35):

- Solid: a circumscribed area of pulmonary opacification with border effacement of adjacent bronchial walls and blood vessels
  - May be calcified or hyperattenuating (e.g. when non-calcified material is inhaled)
- Subsolid
  - Ground-glass nodule: a circumscribed area of pulmonary opacification whereby the bronchial and vascular margins remain visible
  - Part-solid: A ground-glass nodule with a solid component.

Nodular structures occasionally may be characterized by differences in distribution, especially during CT:

- Pulmonary mass: typically a focal or multifocal distribution. When large enough, a mass may conform

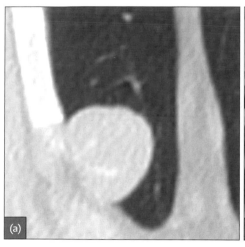
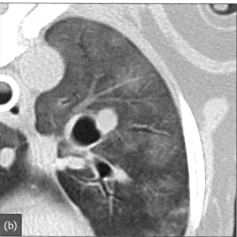

12.35 Close-up transverse thoracic CT images (lung window) of two adult dogs showing different nodule attenuations. (a) An undiagnosed solitary discrete circumscribed lung nodule that is solid. (b) A metastatic mammary carcinoma (confirmed by post mortem examination) that produced multiple indistinct ground-glass nodules as well as widespread ground-glass opacity.

to the shape of a lung lobe. Multiple abnormalities may coalesce or summate with each other. A solitary mass may be bronchocentric, depending on whether it arose near or far from a bronchus. Some masses may grow around a bronchus and produce air bronchograms when the bronchial lumen retains gas. Pulmonary masses that arise near the visceral pleura may be difficult to differentiate from masses that arise from the thoracic body wall, diaphragm or mediastinum. A solitary lung mass may be due to a cyst, haematoma, abscess, neoplasm or granuloma. In dogs and cats, a primary bronchial or pulmonary neoplasm is one of the most common causes of a solitary lung mass

- A mass of bronchial origin is typically bronchocentric
- A mass of pulmonary origin is either bronchocentric or not
- Airspace nodules: multiple small ill-defined nodular areas of consolidation centred on a bronchiole (Figure 12.36)
- Pulmonary nodules: small, relatively well defined, round or oval, pulmonary parenchymal abnormalities that are surrounded by pulmonary parenchyma, visceral pleura or both
  - Solitary pulmonary nodule
  - Multiple pulmonary nodules ('Nodular lung pattern') are most commonly due to infectious or neoplastic metastasis, but may be due to other conditions (e.g. trauma, inflammatory granulomatous lung diseases)
    - Random pulmonary nodules or micronodules: nodular opacities distributed throughout the lungs without preference for specific anatomical locations (e.g. cancer metastasis). Some abnormalities may extend to the periphery of the lung due to spread via a haematogenous route. Miliary pattern is another descriptive term for innumerable small (less than 3 mm) nodular opacities that are disseminated throughout the lungs, especially when they extend to the lung periphery
    - Centrilobular pulmonary nodules or micronodules: nodular opacities associated with the centre of pulmonary lobules; commonly indicates disease of the small airways (bronchioles). From a wide perspective, the nodules tend to produce a speckled appearance

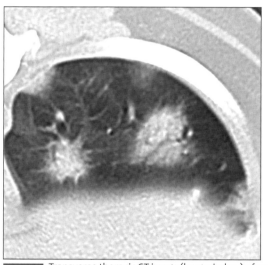

12.36 Transverse thoracic CT image (lung window) of an adult dog with airspace nodules due to histologically confirmed pyogranulomatous and necrotizing bronchointerstitial pneumonia with oedema (cause undetermined). Notice that the granulomas are discrete, irregularly margined and centred on bronchioles.

and typically spare the lung periphery because the airways do not extend that far
- Perilymphatic pulmonary nodules or micronodules: nodular opacities that follow lymphatic vessels and are typically located subpleurally or along pleural fissures, interlobular septa, or bronchovascular bundles. Note that pulmonary lymph nodes are rarely present in dogs
- Ossifying pulmonary metaplasia: a benign condition of minor consequence producing hyperattenuating micronodules due to heterotrophic bone formation. The micronodules are often angled, distinct from blood vessels and airways, and concentrated closer to the visceral pleura.

Widespread pulmonary opacification overview

- Parenchymal opacification patterns.
- Linear opacification patterns.
- Nodular opacification patterns.

Pulmonary hyperlucency

Pulmonary hyperlucency simply means that the lungs are less opaque (blacker) or hypoattenuating compared with normal. The distribution of hyperlucency may be widespread in one or both lungs, confined to a lobe, or focal. Different imaging signs and patterns associated with pulmonary hyperlucency also can help localize disease to anatomical compartments. During radiography, the lungs also may have reduced opacity due to negative summation shadows with abnormalities in the pleural cavities, mediastinum, pericardium/heart, and thoracic boundaries.

Widespread parenchymal hyperlucency

The affected lungs are diffusely less opaque due to an increased ratio of gas to soft tissue. The pulmonary blood vessels typically extend to the periphery of the thoracic cavity and may be abnormally small (Figure 12.37).

- Hyperinflation: an increased volume of gas in the lungs due to:
  - Physiological changes: deep breath, exercising, positive pressure ventilation
  - Emphysema: alveolar wall destruction with irreversibly enlarged airspaces downstream to the terminal bronchiole

- Air trapping: abnormal air retention within the lung downstream to a partial (typical) or complete obstruction.
- Hypoperfusion: a decreased volume of blood (e.g. hypovolaemia, decreased cardiac output).

Solitary and multiple lung hyperlucencies

- Bleb: a small gas accumulation within the visceral pleura or subpleural lung (Reed, 1997; Hansell *et al.*, 2008). Often described as a small bulla.
- Bulla: an area of the airspace that is larger than 1 cm and circumscribed by a thin (<1 mm) or absent wall.
  - 'Pneumatocoele' is another term for a thin-walled, gas-filled space in the lung that is often temporary and frequently due to trauma. If fluid-filled (e.g. haematocoele), then the abnormality will appear as a nodular opacification.
- Cavity (cavitation): a gas-filled space within an area of pulmonary consolidation, mass or nodule (Figure 12.38). The wall of the cavity is typically thick, fluid level might be observed within the abnormal space, and the cavity may enlarge or resolve over time.

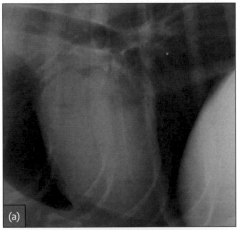
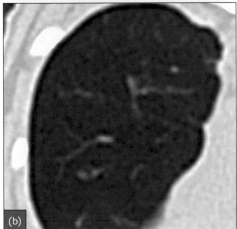

12.37 (a) Lateral thoracic radiograph of an adult dog and (b) transverse thoracic CT image of another adult dog. During radiography and CT, hyperlucent lungs have a homogeneous background opacity that is very dark. Hyperlucency may be due to (a) reduced blood volume in the lungs, increased air volume in the lungs, or (b) both. (b) Note the paucity of pulmonary blood vessels in the image: the pulmonary blood vessels are thin and spread further apart by the hyperinflated lung.

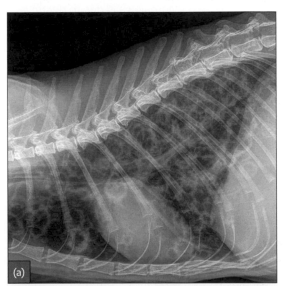
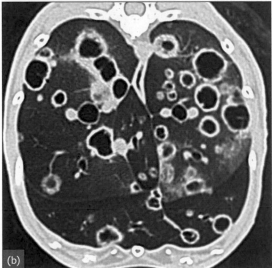

12.38 (a) Lateral thoracic radiograph and (b) transverse thoracic CT image (lung window) of a cat with multiple cavitary nodules due to anaplastic bronchogenic carcinoma. Notice the gas-filled space within the thick-walled nodules.

- Typically, the gas-filled space forms because of expulsion of necrotic material via the bronchial tree in association with a neoplasm or abscess. However, the causes of pulmonary cavities are broad and include infarction and other types of infectious or non-infectious inflammation. Cavitation is often acquired but may be congenital.
  - A pseudocavity has the appearance of a cavity but the low attenuation is due to normal or focal emphysematous lung, or normal or ectatic bronchi.
- Vesicular gas pattern: multiple small gas opacities in a region of widespread lung consolidation. May be seen with lung lobe torsion, severe bacterial infections and infarctions including pulmonary embolus and lung lobe torsion.
- Cyst: any round circumscribed space in the lung parenchyma surrounded by a membrane of variable thickness (typically thin) and may be filled with gas or fluid.
  - The definition of a cyst is contextual. In pathology, the membrane of a true cyst is specifically lined by epithelium. A cyst detected during imaging may or may not be equivalent to a cyst detected during histology (Figure 12.39).
- Honeycombing: numerous medium-sized air-filled cysts with variably thick fibrous walls due to destroyed pulmonary acinar architecture and pulmonary fibrosis.
- Traction bronchiectasis and traction bronchiolectasis: irregular enlargement of the airway lumens caused by fibrotic lung disease producing retraction; can resemble parenchymal abnormalities (i.e. honeycombing).
- Bronchovascular interstitial emphysema (Macklin effect): pneumomediastinum may arise from blunt trauma that causes alveolar rupture. Escaped gas dissects through the adventitial sheath of the bronchovascular bundles into the mediastinum.
- Absent blood vessels (Westermark sign): territorial hyperlucency of a lung lobe secondary to pulmonary embolus causing collapse of blood vessels downstream of the occlusion (see Figure 12.44ai).

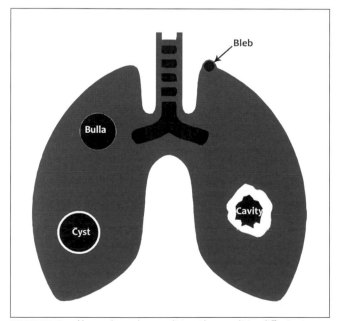

12.39 Focal lucent lung abnormalities. Abnormalities differ in size, location and wall thickness. These abnormalities are drawn with a gas-filled centre. Sometimes the lumen may be filled with fluid or a combination of gas and fluid.

Overall lung size

Overall lung size may vary due to normal inhalation and exhalation, technical complications associated with image acquisition, or because of disease affecting the lungs directly (e.g. fibrosis) or indirectly (e.g. pneumothorax). Therefore, assessing the overall size of the lungs and lung lobes and potential causes are a vital consideration during pulmonary image interpretation.

In normal animals, pulmonary size is primarily a reflection of how much gas is within the alveolar spaces (i.e. the airspace) and changes within a physical range due to changes that occur during respiration. The normal range is different under some circumstances, like exercise. Acquiring images during peak inhalation is a method to standardize this variability, but some abnormal conditions are best detected during exhalation (e.g. air trapping).

In abnormal animals, pulmonary size also is primarily a reflection of the size of the airspace (normal, increased or decreased) but also may be a result of space-occupying disease arising from the lung stroma. For example, the airspaces may be expanded and filled with any combination of gas, fluid, fibre or cells, or incompletely expanded due to several conditions (see also 'Types', below). A large mass arising from the stroma could increase overall lung or lung lobe size.

Normal or increased size

Pulmonary expansion is present when the lungs have a normal or increased size because the alveolar spaces are filled with a normal or increased amount of gas, fluid, fibre or cells (Figure 12.40). Therefore, pulmonary expansion is associated with normal and abnormal conditions. The measure of lung expandability is pulmonary compliance, which relates pressure changes and volume changes to quantify lung stiffness and elasticity.

Normal lung size is generally determined based on clinical experience and knowledge of topographical thoracic anatomy, such as the normal location of interlobar fissures. The degree of lung inflation also is partly assessed by looking at anatomical features such as:

- The angle formed between the vertebral column and diaphragm
- The distance between the heart and diaphragm
- Whether the lungs extend cranially to the first pair of ribs
- The distance between the lung margin and thoracic boundaries
- Whether the heart is in the midline
- Whether the left cranial lung lobe is the most cranial lung lobe.

Increased overall lung size may refer to one or both lungs or one or more lung lobes.

- Increased overall lung size is recognized by a flat diaphragm, barrel-shaped rib cage, and ribs more parallel to each other and more perpendicular to the vertebral column.
- Increased overall lobe size is recognized when lung lobe margins are convex and bulging or there is a mass effect (displacement of structures away from the abnormality).

Opacity (attenuation): Although opacity and size may be independent variables, pulmonary expansion may influence parenchymal opacification. Therefore, the assessment of parenchymal opacification must always consider the

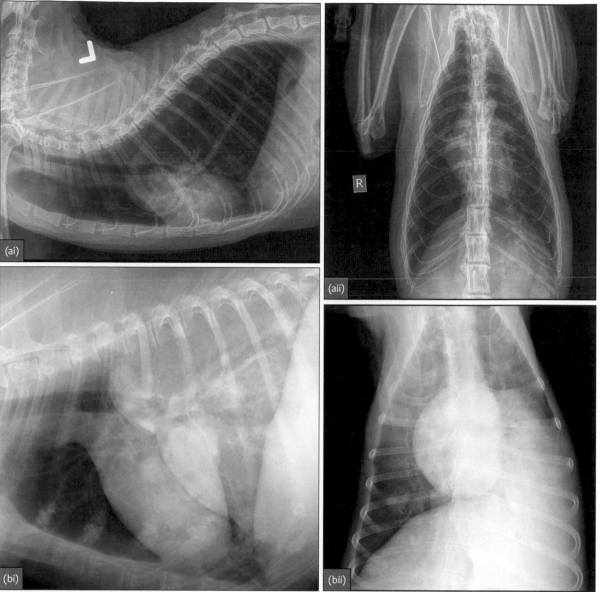

12.40 (ai) Lateral and (aii) VD thoracic radiographs of an adult cat with bilateral lung hyperinflation and (bi) Lateral and (bii) VD thoracic radiographs of a dog with a large lung mass. The normal size of the lungs is assessed by evaluating the thoracic boundaries (body wall including the ribs, diaphragm and sternum), lobar margins and the mediastinum. (a) Both lungs are enlarged and hyperlucent. The lung hyperinflation causes expansion of the rib cage, flattening of the diaphragm, and rounding of the lung margins. (b) The dog has a large lung mass in the left caudal lung lobe. The lobe is hyperexpanded with overall increased size and a caudal mediastinal shift to the right. The opaque lobe also has convex margins (bulging surface) indicating that a mass is likely present.

degree of pulmonary expansion to determine whether lung pathology is likely to be present or not. Expanded lung may have a normal, decreased, or increased opacity.

- Normal lung size without pulmonary opacification generally indicates that the lungs are normal or that there is disease that is undetected (the imaging tests are insensitive).
- Normal or increased lung size with pulmonary opacification always indicates the present of pulmonary disease:
  - Neoplasm
  - Pneumonia
  - Eosinophilic bronchopneumopathy
  - Fluid overload.
- Normal lung size with decreased opacity of the lung usually indicates hypovolaemia due to any cause, a technical complication (especially in thin animals), or very mild hyperinflation or emphysema.

- Increased lung size with decreased opacity of the lung generally indicates hyperinflation due to any cause:
  - Congenital
  - Obstructive air trapping
  - Feline asthma
  - Overinflation (e.g. during positive pressure ventilation); may mask some diseases
  - Compensatory hyperinflation (following removal or collapse of another lung or lobe).

Decreased size

Abnormally small lung size is rarely due to pulmonary hypoplasia (a congenital developmental anomaly) or incomplete lung expansion due to the lung never inflating at birth (anectasis). It is commonly due to lost gas volume in a previously expanded lung (atelectasis or collapse) (Figure 12.41). Note that the terms atelectasis and collapse are synonyms, although collapse is used more commonly when lung size is

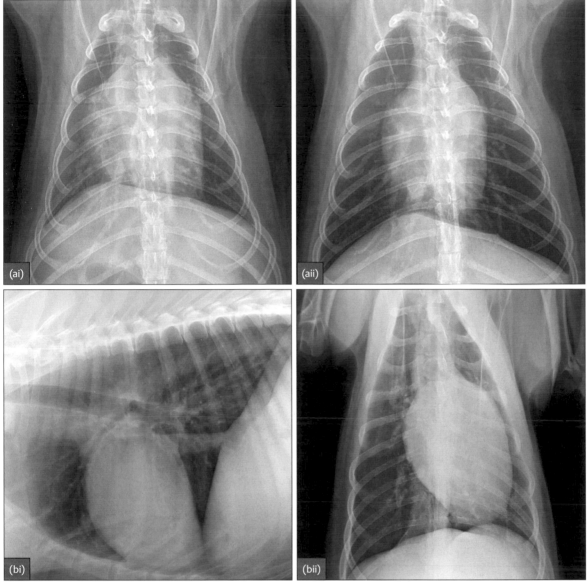

12.41 (a) VD thoracic radiographs of an adult dog acquired during (ai) exhalation and (aii) inhalation. Notice the lungs are smaller during exhalation, which gives the illusion of diffuse parenchymal opacification and cardiomegaly. (bi) Lateral and (bii) orthogonal thoracic radiographs of an adult dog with mild relaxation atelectasis associated with recumbent positioning. Note the mediastinal shift towards the side of lung collapse, and ipsilateral rib crowding, cranial displacement of the left diaphragmatic crus and mild pulmonary opacification.

severely reduced. Modifiers also may be used to convey information about severity (e.g. partial or complete collapse), shape (plate-like, rounded), and distribution (whole lung, lobar, segmental) of atelectasis. Atelectasis may be:

- An incidental technical complication (e.g. incomplete inhalation during image acquisition) of minor consequence
- A cause for misinterpretation due to obscuring other signs of disease or creating spurious signs of disease such as pulmonary opacification or cardiac silhouette enlargement
- The most important sign that lung disease is present
- A condition that contributes to the development of hypoxia during anaesthesia or disease
  - For example, atelectasis-related hypoxia during general anaesthesia is not only due to poor lung ventilation, but also disproportional lung perfusion because hypoxic pulmonary vasoconstriction may be ineffective during general anaesthesia (Lennon and Murray, 1996). The lack of normal physiological

shunting of blood away from hypoxic lung produces a V:Q mismatch with deoxygenated blood entering the systemic circulation (a physiological right-to-left shunt).

Decreased lung size is detected mostly by observing what happens to adjacent structures when there is loss of lung volume. Some examples include (Reed, 1997):

- Mediastinal shift towards the side of collapse (unless tension pneumothorax is present, and the mediastinal shift is in the opposite direction)
- Rib crowding
- Crowding and reorientation of pulmonary blood vessels
- Compensatory hyperinflation of other lung lobes
- Cardiac rotation
- Bronchial rearrangement
- Cranial displacement of diaphragm
- Rounded pulmonary margins
- Displacement of interlobar fissures
- Changed location of abnormal structures.

Opacity (attenuation): Atelectasis is associated with either normal or increased opacity of the affected lung (Figure 12.42).

- Atelectasis with normal parenchymal opacity: parenchymal opacity is normal because there is a proportional decrease in both gas and blood due to hypoxic pulmonary vasoconstriction (a normal physiological process whereby blood is shunted away from poorly oxygenated portions of the lung so there is a match between ventilation and perfusion).
- Atelectasis with parenchymal opacification: increased parenchymal opacity occurs when there is a decreased ratio of gas to blood in the affected lung (collapsed lung may be otherwise normal) or when there is proportionally more loss of gas volume concurrent with the influx of fluid, cells, or fibre (concurrent lung disease is present). The appearance of the opacity is identical to what was described for parenchymal opacification.
  - Atelectasis with ground-glass opacity: the airspace contains some gas.
  - Atelectasis with consolidation: the airspace is totally, or nearly totally, void of gas.

Types: There are various ways to classify the different types of atelectasis and sometimes the distinction is unclear because of overlapping factors (Winegardner *et al.*, 2008). For example, space-occupying disease can compress the lung (compressive atelectasis), allow it to recoil under its inherent elasticity (relaxation atelectasis), or both. Commonly, six types of atelectasis are defined: resorptive, adhesive, compressive, passive, cicatrization and gravity-dependent. Synonyms are common. In the following list, the different types of atelectasis are categorized based on the four different mechanisms that disrupt lung inflation.

- Lung does not expand due to reduced total lung capacity (Figure 12.43a). Called compressive atelectasis or restrictive atelectasis.
  - Thoracic cage disease (e.g. pectus excavatum).
  - Space-occupying lesion.
  - Restrictive pleuritis.
  - Obesity hypoventilation ('Pickwickian syndrome').
- Lung does not expand due to the unopposed tendency for lung to recoil due to inherent elasticity. Called passive atelectasis or relaxation atelectasis. In some classifications, the first three listed conditions are presented as types of compressive atelectasis (especially when the expansion of the pleural cavity is large).
  - Pleural fluid (Figure 12.43b).
  - Pneumothorax.
  - Diaphragmatic hernia of abdominal fat or viscera, or diaphragmatic dysfunction.
  - Exhalation/shallow breathing.
  - 100% oxygen (gas is absorbed faster than it is replaced).
  - Gravity. This special condition, characterized by reduced alveolar volume and increased perfusion, is also called gravity-dependent atelectasis, and may have a more complex mechanism.
- Lung is not expanded due to absorption of alveolar gas without replacement due to airway obstruction. Called resorptive atelectasis or obstructive atelectasis (Figure 12.43c). In all other forms of atelectasis, the airway is at least partially patent.
  - Infectious bronchitis or pneumonia (airway plugging).
  - Mucus plugging (e.g. asthma).
  - Ciliary dyskinesia.
  - Foreign body.
  - Neoplasm.
  - Bronchial constriction.
- Reduced lung compliance (increased stiffness and decreased volume).
  - Localized or generalized fibrotic lung disease. Called cicatrization atelectasis (Figure 12.43d).
    - Radiation fibrosis.
    - Idiopathic fibrotic lung disease.
    - Chronic pneumonia.
  - Surfactant deficiency (adhesive atelectasis). Lungs do not expand due to lumen surfaces of alveoli sticking as a result of surfactant abnormality.
    - Neonatal respiratory distress syndrome.
    - Acute respiratory distress syndrome.
    - Pulmonary embolus (Figure 12.44).

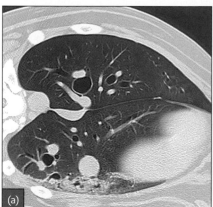 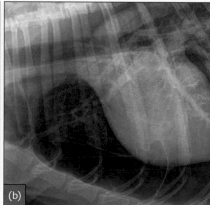 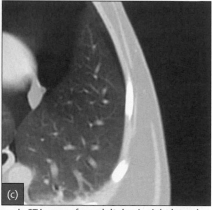

12.42 Atelectatic lungs have reduced size with normal or increased opacity. (a) Transverse thoracic CT image of an adult dog in right lateral recumbency: the image is displayed as acquired (i.e. dorsal is to the left of the image and right is to the bottom of the image). Notice pulmonary opacification and reduced lung volume in the gravity-dependent portion of the right lung. (b) Close-up lateral thoracic radiograph of an adult dog with relaxation atelectasis due to normotensive (simple) pneumothorax. Notice the normal opacity of the lung. The loss of gas is compensated by hypoxic pulmonary vasoconstriction, which is a normal physiological process whereby blood is shunted away from poorly ventilated regions of the lung. (c) Close-up transverse thoracic CT image of an adult dog with relaxation atelectasis due to normotensive pneumothorax. The image was acquired in dorsal recumbency and is displayed as acquired (i.e. dorsal is to the bottom of the image and left is to the left of the image). Notice the lung lobe is small and retracted away from the parietal pleura. The gravity-dependent portion of the lung (dorsal) has increased opacity and increased blood flow (note the blood vessels have a larger diameter and the parenchyma has an increased opacity). The ventral portion of the lung is better ventilated but has less perfusion. Perfusion of poorly ventilated lung and ventilation of poorly perfused lung leads to a physiological left-to-right shunt (V:Q mismatch), which can produce hypoxaemia, especially in anaesthetized patients when hypoxic pulmonary vasoconstriction is less effective.

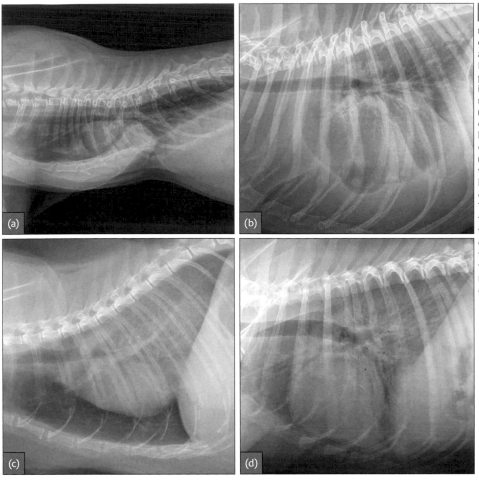

12.43 Reduced lung size due to different pathogenic mechanisms. (a) Lateral thoracic radiograph of a cat with compressive (restrictive) atelectasis due to pectus excavatum. (b) Lateral thoracic radiograph of a dog with passive (relaxation) atelectasis due to fluid in both pleural cavities. (c) Lateral thoracic radiograph of a cat with resorptive (obstructive) atelectasis due to a neoplasm obstructing the lumen of the lobar bronchus to one of the caudal lung lobes causing the heart to deviate dorsolaterally. (d) Lateral thoracic radiograph of a dog with cicatrization atelectasis because the lung is stiff and cannot expand (poor compliance) due to fibrotic lung disease. The opacity of the affected lung will vary from normal (e.g. in hypoxic pulmonary vasoconstriction) to increased. Increased opacity may be due to reduced air volume in the lung; the infiltration of fluid, cells or fibre into the lungs; summation of pleural, mediastinal, cardiac or thoracic boundary disease; or a combination.

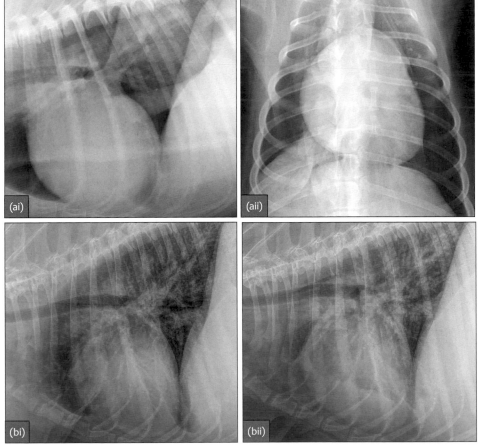

12.44 The radiographic diagnosis of pulmonary embolus with infarction is challenging because most patients have normal radiographs, signs are variable and are absent in the acute phase. Signs include localized areas of hyperlucency due to decreased perfusion (Westermark sign), parenchymal consolidation by haemorrhage and oedema, non-specific areas of atelectasis, cavitation (most specific sign but late occurring) and pleural fluid. (a) Orthogonal thoracic radiographs of an adult dog with emboli in the right middle, right caudal and left caudal lung lobes (confirmed by post-mortem examination). Notice the wedge-shaped region of consolidation in the right caudal lung lobe. (ai) Notice the absence of pulmonary blood vessels summating with the heart. (aii) Notice the reduced number of pulmonary blood vessels in the left caudal lung lobe. (b) Lateral thoracic radiographs of a dog with pulmonary embolism (confirmed by post-mortem examination). The images were obtained (bi) prior to and (bii) after the dog developed clinical signs. (bii) The only new finding is diffuse atelectasis, which is presumed to be a result of a surfactant deficiency. Notice the reduced lung size, especially the retraction of the ventral lung margin away from the sternum, and diffuse ground-glass opacity. Adhesive atelectasis is a type of cicatrization atelectasis.

Disease distribution

Distribution refers to the spread of a disease condition through the body. The spread may be distant or local (confined to a single organ or an area within an organ). Diseases that arise within in the lungs tend to be distributed locally and uncommonly spread to distant sites except for regional lymph nodes (i.e. tracheobronchial lymph nodes); lung–digit syndrome in cats and systemic blastomycosis are two of the notable exceptions. Conversely, the lungs are a common site of distant spread (e.g. neoplastic or infectious metastasis) from lesions that arise elsewhere in the body or systemically (e.g. systemic inflammatory response syndrome, lymphoma). During imaging, pulmonary distributions specifically describe the macroscopic or gross spread of the disease because that is what is observable. There are several terms used to describe distribution; these terms may be used independently or in combination.

Widespread disease

Widespread disease indicates that the disease is distributed over a large area of lung and should be modified to specify which anatomical compartment is affected by the disease process. For example, there is a big difference between widespread bronchial disease, widespread pulmonary artery disease, and widespread lung parenchymal disease. Although the following two terms are used interchangeably, a subtle distinction about widespread distributions can be made (Figure 12.45).

- Diffuse: a widespread distribution whereby all parts of the affected anatomical compartment are abnormal.
  - Uniform: all parts of the anatomical compartment are affected to the same degree.
  - Non-uniform: different parts of the anatomical compartment are affected by different degrees of severity (minimal-to-severe).
- Generalized: a widespread distribution of disease whereby the entire lung is affected but normal tissue is interspersed between abnormalities. This is commonly seen with widespread pulmonary metastasis.
  - Generalized random: generalized disease that does not have a predilection for a certain anatomical location.
  - Disseminated: used to describe a widespread distribution whereby the abnormalities are innumerable small nodules and dispersed over a broad area (like sowing seed).

Widespread disease may affect one (unilateral) or both (bilateral) lungs. Widespread disease affecting both lungs may be further described as:

- Bilateral symmetrical: the abnormalities in the right and left lungs appear like mirror images
- Bilateral asymmetrical: the abnormalities in the right and left lungs have different shape, location, or severity (Figure 12.46).

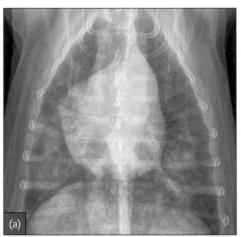
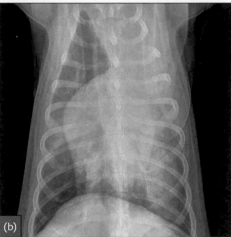

12.46 (a) DV and (b) VD thoracic radiographs of two dogs with widespread non-uniform bilateral lung disease. (a) The spread of disease may be symmetrical, whereby the distribution is comparable in both lungs and roughly forms a mirror image in each lung. (b) Alternatively, the distribution may be asymmetrical when comparing left and right lungs.

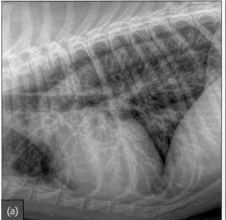
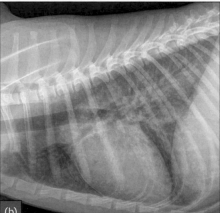
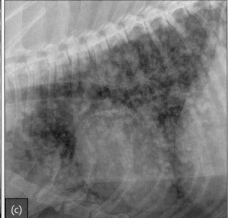

12.45 Lateral thoracic radiographs of three adult dogs with widespread distribution of disease in both lungs. (a) Uniform diffuse bronchial (large airway) disease. (b) Non-uniform diffuse parenchymal disease. (c) Multiple pulmonary nodules with a generalized random distribution; notice the normal lung between nodules.

Lung fields

During radiography, especially for pulmonary parenchymal diseases, the distribution of disease may be restricted to a lung field, which is a simple useful subdivision of the lungs that is clinically meaningful. This is particularly true for bilateral disease as unilateral disease can often be more precisely localized (e.g. right cranial lung lobe is more specific than cranioventral lung field). The distribution of disease within a lung field also can vary (e.g. locally extensive, patchy, diffuse).

The term 'lung field' implies that the lesion is in the lung. If that localization is uncertain, then 'thorax' is a better descriptor (e.g. caudodorsal lung field has a different implication than caudodorsal thorax). There are two methods for defining five lung fields (Figure 12.47):

- Lung fields defined as concentric zones (Suter and Lord, 1984)
  - Central lung field (perihilar): this distribution refers to the area of the lung surrounding the lung hilus, typically sparing the periphery (Figure 12.48)
  - Middle lung field: this distribution refers to the area of the lung between the central and peripheral zones

- Peripheral lung field: this distribution classically refers to the area of the lung adjacent to the thoracic boundaries (i.e. body wall/rib cage, vertebral column, sternum, thoracic inlet and diaphragm). On cross-sectional imaging, peripheral also may be used to describe disease that is primarily associated with the perimeter of the lung lobes (in contrast to bronchocentric)
- Lung fields defined as groups of lung lobes
  - Cranioventral lung field: this distribution roughly conforms to the location of the left cranial, right cranial and right middle lung lobes (Figure 12.49)
  - Caudodorsal lung field: this distribution roughly conforms to the location of the left caudal, right caudal and accessory lung lobes (Figure 12.50).

On radiographs, note that the cranioventral lung field extends into the caudal part of the thorax and the caudodorsal lung field extends into the ventral part of the thorax. This leads to overlap of lung fields on the DV and VD views. The definition of these lung fields is based on an obliquely oriented line referable to the gross anatomy (Figure 12.51).

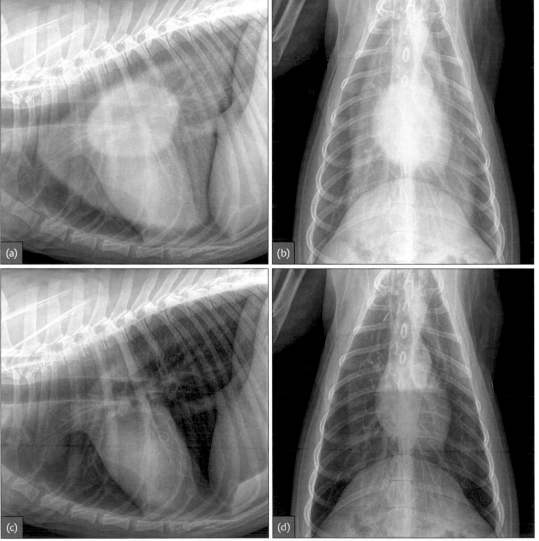

12.47 Orthogonal thoracic radiographs showing two methods for defining lung fields. There are five lung fields. (a, b) Lung fields defined as concentric zones: central or perihilar (bright yellow), middle (medium yellow), and peripheral (light yellow) lung fields. (c, d) Lung fields defined as groups of lung lobes: cranioventral (blue) and caudodorsal (red) lung fields. On DV and VD views, the cranioventral and caudodorsal lung fields overlap (purple).

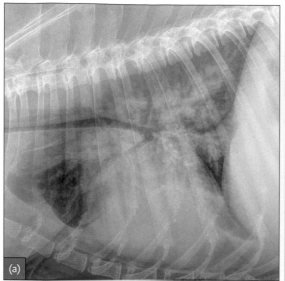
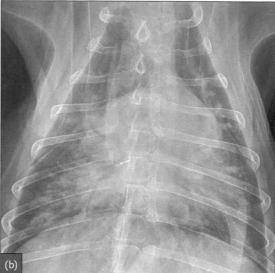

12.48

(a, b) Orthogonal thoracic radiographs of a mature dog depicting a perihilar distribution of parenchymal lung disease, attributed to lung trauma associated with cardiopulmonary resuscitation.

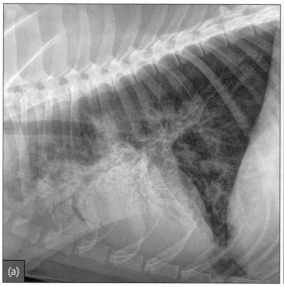
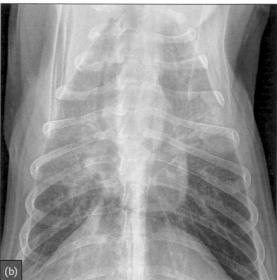

12.49

(a, b) Orthogonal thoracic radiographs of a mature dog depicting a cranioventral distribution of parenchymal lung disease.

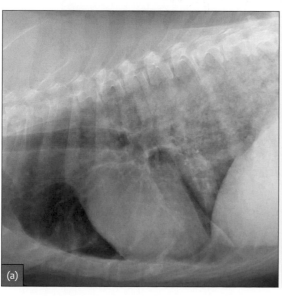
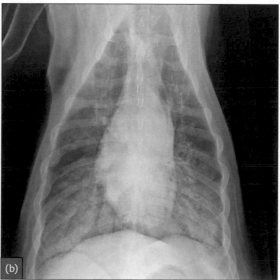

12.50

(a, b) Orthogonal thoracic radiographs of a mature dog depicting a caudodorsal distribution of parenchymal lung disease.

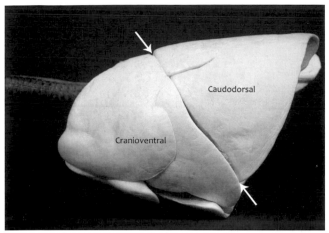

12.51 Left aspect photograph of preserved inflated canine lungs. There are two types of pleural fissures seen in this photograph: inconstant (accessory pleural fissure) and constant (interlobar fissure). Notice the small accessory pleural fissure in the craniodorsal aspect of the left caudal lung lobe. Constant pleural fissures reliably divide the lungs into exact lobes. Notice the interlobar fissure (arrowed) between the left cranial and left caudal lung lobes, which corresponds to the division of the lungs into cranioventral and caudodorsal lung fields. Using this definition, no caudoventral nor craniodorsal lung field exists. On DV and VD thoracic radiographs, the two lung fields summate with each other at the level of the heart: a lateral view is needed to determine whether a summation shadow is in the cranioventral or caudodorsal lung field.

Additional modifiers

The distribution of disease may be described relative to lobar anatomy. It is most helpful to specify the affected lung lobe, but there are some useful modifiers.

- Lobar: the distribution of disease is widespread within a lung lobe (Figure 12.52).
- Multilobar: the distribution of disease involves multiple lung lobes.
- Sublobar: the distribution of disease is within part of a lung lobe. The location may be further described (e.g. ventral tip, central) (Figure 12.53).
- Bronchocentric: disease conspicuously centred on the bronchovascular bundle. The abnormality may arise from the bronchial wall, bronchovascular interstitium ('peribronchial cuffing'), adjacent pulmonary parenchyma, or in combination. In this distribution, the products of disease tend to be concentrated in the centre of lung lobes with sparing of the periphery (central lobar or central lung) (Figure 12.54).
- Peripheral lobar or peripheral lung: disease concentrated near the visceral pleura or thoracic boundaries (Figure 12.54).

Number and margination:

- Solitary: a single abnormality. Single lesions often are described as locally extensive (patch) when uncircumscribed or invading adjacent tissues. Single lesions also are often described as regional or focal.
- Multiple: more than one abnormality. Multiple lesions often are described as multifocal, or patchy when uncircumscribed. These lesions typically are interspersed by normal tissue but may coalesce.
- Circumscribed means that an abnormality has defined boundaries with adjacent tissues. Local extension into adjacent tissues may or may not be present. This term should be differentiated from distinct, which means recognizably different, and discrete, which means both separate and distinct.

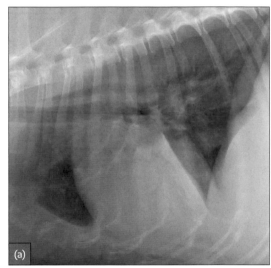

(a)

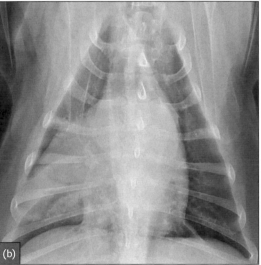

(b)

12.52 (a, b) Orthogonal thoracic radiographs of a mature dog depicting a lobar distribution of parenchymal lung disease. The right middle lung lobe is expanded and consolidated (lobar consolidation). Also notice the lobar signs, air bronchograms and border effacement of the adjacent part of the cardiac silhouette.

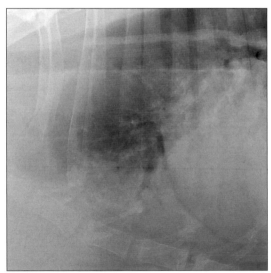

12.53 Lateral thoracic radiograph of a mature dog depicting a sublobar (locally extensive) distribution of parenchymal lung disease in the ventral periphery of the lobe (sublobar consolidation).

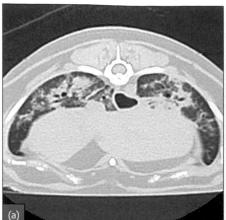
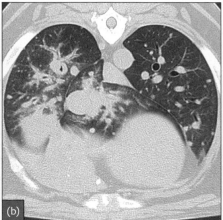
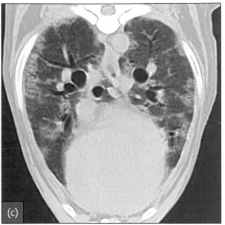

12.54 (a) Transverse thoracic CT image (lung window) depicting a generalized central lung (bronchocentric) distribution of disease. (b) Transverse thoracic CT image (lung window) of an adult dog with histologically confirmed spread of carcinoma along the bronchovascular bundle. A bronchocentric distribution may be observed with diseases of the bronchovascular bundle or adjacent lung parenchyma. (c) Transverse thoracic CT image (lung window) depicting a predominantly peripheral distribution of lung disease.

- Uncircumscribed means that an abnormality has poorly delineated boundaries due to the diffusion or accumulation of fluid, cells or fibre into adjacent tissues. This term should be differentiated from indistinct, which means not clearly seen.

Miscellaneous imaging signs

Innumerable idiosyncratic imaging signs of lung disease exist and are extremely helpful for making certain diagnoses beyond what already has been described. For example, herniation of the lung through the thoracic inlet may be seen with dynamic tracheal collapse. Herniation of the lung through a defect in the thoracic body wall may be seen with trauma. Lung lobe torsion may produce a combination of some or all the following signs: increased lung lobe size, lobar consolidation, peripheral lobar consolidation with central small gas opacities, abnormally positioned bronchi, focally narrowed bronchi and lack of vascular enhancement with contrast material (Figure 12.55; Benavides *et al.*, 2019; Belmudes *et al.*, 2021). Knowledge of these countless signs is important and largely acquired through clinical experience, awareness of the medical literature, and continued education.

Quantification of disease severity

Disease severity may be characterized quantitatively or qualitatively using several variables, including extent of disease spread, how much gas is displaced from the lungs and size of the abnormality. Often the assessment is subjective, which can be problematic when undefined terms (e.g. mild, large) have a unique meaning to different people or in different contexts, or are used inconsistently. Nonetheless, assessment of severity provides essential information to the receiver of the imaging report and may help prioritize the differential diagnosis or offer prognostic information. In addition, when serial studies are performed, changes in disease severity may offer information about disease progression or response to treatment. There are several different methods to convey information about severity and the ways vary with the context (e.g. it is more customary to conclude a 'large' lung mass versus a 'severe' lung mass):

- Small, medium, large
- Mild, moderate, severe
- Extent of disease spread
- Extent of interrupted function.

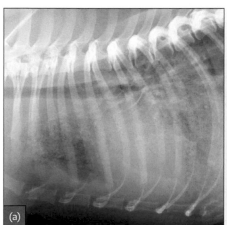
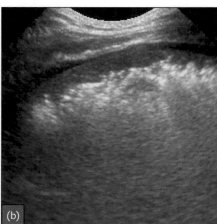
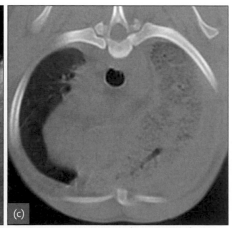

12.55 (a) Lateral thoracic radiograph, (b) thoracic ultrasound image (intercostal window) and (c) transverse thoracic CT image (lung window) of a dog with a lung lobe torsion. The left cranial lung lobe is enlarged and consolidated with innumerable small centrally located gas opacities (vesicular pattern). In (b) and (c) the consolidated edge of the lung lobe forms a distinct peripheral band. Additionally, there is bilateral pleural fluid.

Integration

Diagnostic pulmonary image interpretation requires one to assimilate all the above information when evaluating an imaging examination to make a diagnosis. In addition, it is important to incorporate ancillary information such as signalment, history, lab results and non-pulmonary imaging signs. For example, patients with lung lobe torsion frequently also have concurrent pleural fluid and certain dog breeds are predisposed (e.g. Pugs, sight hounds). Patients with cardiogenic pulmonary oedema commonly also have left heart enlargement. The result of the evaluation should be a definitive diagnosis, a short prioritized differential diagnosis, or an acknowledgement that the clinical question is unanswered by the study.

When the results of an imaging study strongly indicate a particular disease, then that disease should be established as the imaging diagnosis or explicitly included in the differential diagnosis. It is also helpful to quantify the confidence at which patterns are detected or not, and the results of the evaluation for being positive or negative for a specific disease: indeterminate (questionable, possible), probable, or definitive. Avoid hedging (be confident that something is indeterminate or definitive). Imaging signs of lung disease, however, are commonly generic, indicating only that lung disease is present, but not the cause. This information is helpful because it can rule out pleural or cardiac disease as the cause of clinical signs, but additional examination (e.g. histology, genetic testing, infectious agent testing) is needed to determine the type of lung disease. In this situation, because the number of possible causes is large, it may be best to state the anatomical compartment(s) affected by the disease process and prioritize only the category of disease that is most likely (e.g. inflammatory disease, infectious disease, neoplastic disease, trauma). This information may guide patient management more meaningfully than providing a long or incomplete list of specific diseases.

The following is an incomplete list of imaging patterns, which integrates the information in the above sections, and associated diagnoses. Keep in mind that diseases that can affect multiple anatomical compartments can produce different imaging patterns depending on which anatomical compartments are affected at a given time; these diseases should not be considered to have a single appearance. Some diseases also have varied appearances due to unique host/agent reactions. Finally, there are some diseases that may not be associated with a specific anatomical compartment because all components of the affected lung or lobe are involved (e.g. lung lobe torsion).

Parenchymal patterns

Ground-glass opacity and consolidation are typically better descriptors of parenchymal disease severity (i.e. how much gas remains in the lung parenchyma) than descriptors of anatomical localization within the pulmonary parenchyma which may be used during histology; each pixel in the image is the sum or average of multiple alveoli (Suter and Lord, 1984; Scrivani, 2009).

- Cranioventral parenchymal opacification with pulmonary expansion is commonly associated with aspiration pneumonia, bronchopneumonia, haemorrhage and neoplasia.
    - The differential diagnosis for lobar and sublobar distributions is similar.
- Caudodorsal parenchymal opacification with pulmonary expansion is commonly associated with cardiogenic pulmonary oedema (i.e. left-sided congestive heart failure), non-cardiogenic pulmonary oedema (e.g. toxin inhalation, electrocution, near drowning, upper airway obstruction, vasculitis, neurogenic causes, disseminated intravascular coagulation, acute respiratory distress syndrome, systemic inflammatory disease), neoplasia (especially lymphoma), infectious cause and non-infectious inflammatory causes.
    - A caudodorsal distribution may spread to become diffuse when the disease is more severe. In these circumstances, the descriptor caudodorsal-to-diffuse may be used to indicate it is a diffuse distribution with a greater severity caudodorsally. The same differential diagnosis applies.
    - Cardiogenic pulmonary oedema tends to be symmetrical, but may be asymmetrical and typically worse in the right lung (Diana et al., 2009).
- Perihilar parenchymal opacification with pulmonary expansion is classically associated with cardiogenic pulmonary oedema but may be due to other causes. A true perihilar distribution of lung disease should be differentiated from a positive summation shadow caused by an enlarged left atrium and regional restrictive atelectasis (caused by left atrial enlargement).
- Patchy parenchymal opacification with pulmonary expansion is commonly associated with infectious causes (e.g. blastomycosis, canine influenza, atypical pneumonia, parasitic pneumonia, pneumocystis carinii), non-infectious inflammatory causes (e.g. eosinophilic bronchopneumopathy), neoplastic causes, and traumatic or non-traumatic (e.g. rodenticide toxicity) haemorrhage.
- Bronchocentric parenchymal opacification with pulmonary expansion is often associated with inflammatory and neoplastic causes.
- Atelectasis: see 'Overall lung size' (above) for conditions associated with atelectasis. It is not always possible to differentiate the types of atelectasis or determine the underlying cause. The chronicity of atelectasis may help prioritize the differential diagnosis. For example, atelectasis that develops acutely during anaesthesia is more likely to be due to relaxation atelectasis and atelectasis that develops due to radiation fibrosis is more likely to be chronic and repeatable on serial examinations. The distribution also helps prioritize the differential diagnosis. For example, regional atelectasis is more likely to be due to such conditions as bronchial foreign body and radiation fibrosis, and diffuse atelectasis is more likely due to such conditions as incomplete inhalation, bilateral pleural cavity disease and some types of fibrotic lung disease.

Linear patterns

Linear patterns are due to diseases that produce the infiltration of fluid, cells or fibre into the bronchovascular bundle, bronchiolovascular bundle or peripheral connective tissue (i.e. oedema, inflammatory diseases, infectious diseases, neoplastic diseases, and fibrotic lung disease). Note that tram lines and thick opaque rings do not differentiate involvement of the bronchial walls (bronchiolar walls) versus the bronchovascular interstitium, and most of the diseases that produce these patterns tend to have a widespread distribution, but the distribution can be regional.

- Bronchial diseases include all causes of infectious bronchitis (bacterial, viral, parasitic), allergic bronchitis, immune-mediated bronchitis (e.g. feline asthma,

eosinophilic bronchopneumopathy), neoplastic spread along the lymphatics, and early left-sided congestive heart failure ('cardiogenic asthma').
- Bronchiolar diseases affect the tissues in and/or around the small airway (bronchiolar) walls including infectious, non-infectious inflammatory and neoplastic causes.
  - These diseases may be either primary or a secondary extension of large airway disease.
- Peripheral connective tissue diseases include infectious causes, non-infectious inflammatory causes, neoplastic causes and several types of fibrotic lung disease.
- Vascular patterns are commonly due to pulmonary hypertension (pulmonary artery enlargement and increased tortuosity, heartworm disease), pulmonary venous congestion (left-sided congestive heart failure) or pulmonary over-circulation (patent ductus arteriosus, fluid overload).

Nodular patterns

See 'Nodular opacification patterns' (above).

Bronchial diseases

Canine chronic bronchitis

Chronic bronchitis is an inflammatory disease of the airways. Animals usually present with a history of chronic harsh cough (more than 2 months) and exercise intolerance. Typically middle-aged to older small-breed dogs are predisposed, but the disease is also common in large breeds. Tracheal sensitivity may be present on clinical examination and inspiratory crackles and expiratory wheezes may be identified on auscultation. Heart rate is usually normal to low and a pronounced sinus arrhythmia may be present. Diagnosis of chronic bronchitis in the dog and cat is usually one of exclusion. Other conditions such as infectious airway disease, structural airway disease (collapse, bronchiectasis) and neoplasia must be ruled out.

This chronic condition is never completely cured but can be controlled by a combination of medical therapy, weight loss and environmental changes (reduced smoke, pollutants, heat, etc.). When poorly controlled, bronchitis may result in irreversible bronchiectasis and even pulmonary hypertension (secondary to chronic hypoxia and/or vascular remodelling).

Radiography

Radiographic findings include:

- Presence of a bronchial pattern
- Increase in the non-vascular linear markings and peribronchial infiltration (peribronchial cuffing)
- Thick bronchial walls and increased numbers of visible bronchial walls are reportedly the most reliable evidence of canine chronic bronchitis on radiographs
- Bronchi containing exudate may appear as solid structures and may be confused with vessels or even nodules when seen end-on
- There may be right-sided cardiomegaly in dogs with chronic airway disease that develop pulmonary hypertension and/or cor pulmonale.

Radiographic abnormalities might not be present. Normal thoracic radiographs do not rule out chronic bronchitis.

Computed tomography

CT findings include:

- Increased visibility of the bronchial markings
- Thick bronchial walls. Attempts have been made to characterize the bronchial wall thickness, but currently it remains a subjective evaluation.

Canine acute bronchitis

Thoracic radiographs in cases of acute bronchitis are indicated mainly to rule out other diseases or complications, especially if clinical signs are severe or prolonged. Many animals with acute bronchitis show no radiographic change. Acute bronchitis may appear as a bronchial pattern irrespective of the cause and radiographic findings are similar to those seen in canine chronic bronchitis (see above).

Feline chronic lower airway disease

Feline chronic lower airway disease encompasses a multitude of small airway diseases in the cat including feline asthma. Inflammation of the airways leads to a reversible obstruction to airflow (functional obstruction) and hence air trapping. The obstruction is due to a combination of bronchoconstriction, bronchial wall oedema and submucosal gland hypertrophy.

Clinical signs vary from chronic coughing and wheezing to severe respiratory distress. The condition can affect cats of any age with Siamese appearing to have an increased incidence. Hyper-responsive airways and reversible airflow obstruction lead to a reduced airway lumen diameter and increased airway resistance. The condition can be extremely severe in presentation and care should be taken when handling dyspnoeic cats.

Radiography

Radiographs may be normal. The severity of the radiographic signs may not correlate with the clinical signs. Findings include the following:

- Classically peribronchial cuffing is identified, although a variety of bronchial (Figure 12.56), interstitial and alveolar lung patterns may be observed
- Excessive mucus production and accumulation in the bronchial lumen may give the impression of pulmonary nodules if seen end-on
- Obstruction of larger airways can cause alveolar infiltrates, consolidation or atelectasis
- In particular, right middle lung lobe collapse (Figure 12.57) is a common sequel to severe feline chronic lower airway disease
- Evidence of air trapping and hyperinflation (Figure 12.58; see also Figure 12.110) may be seen: flattened diaphragm and hyperlucent lungs (variable depending on the lung pattern present)
- Severe coughing may produce rib fractures in the cat and on occasion multiple fractures at differing stages of healing may be identified (see Figure 12.110).

Computed tomography

CT findings include:

- Thick bronchial walls with increased attenuation (Figure 12.59)

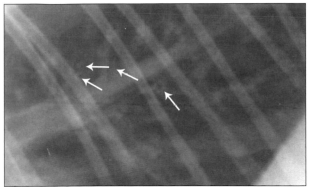

12.56 Close-up of a lateral thoracic radiograph of an 8-year-old Domestic Shorthaired cat with prominent bronchial wall thickening. 'Doughnuts' (arrowed) are visible throughout the lungs.

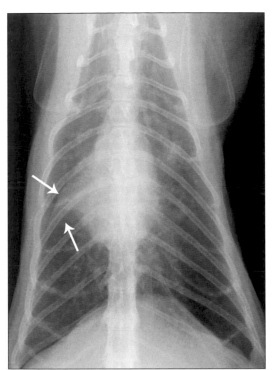

12.57 VD thoracic radiograph of a Siamese cat with chronic lower airway disease. The right middle lung lobe is collapsed and consolidated and is seen as a triangular soft tissue opacity on the right side adjacent to the cardiac silhouette (arrowed).

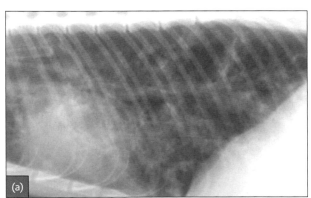

12.58 (a) Close-up of a lateral thoracic radiograph of a 15-month-old Domestic Shorthaired cat with chronic lower airway disease. The bronchial walls are thick throughout both lungs and in areas where the lumen is filled with mucus they resemble pulmonary nodules when seen end-on (especially visible in the caudoventral thorax). The lungs are hyperinflated as shown by the flattened diaphragm and ribs that are more widely spaced than normal. (continues) ▶

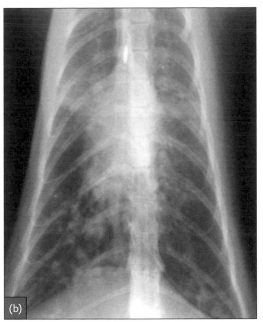

12.58 (continued) (b) Close-up of a VD thoracic radiograph of a 15-month-old Domestic Shorthaired cat with chronic lower airway disease. The bronchial walls are thick throughout both lungs and in areas where the lumen is filled with mucus they resemble pulmonary nodules when seen end-on (especially visible in the right caudal lung lobe). The lungs are hyperinflated as shown by the flattened diaphragm and ribs that are more widely spaced than normal.

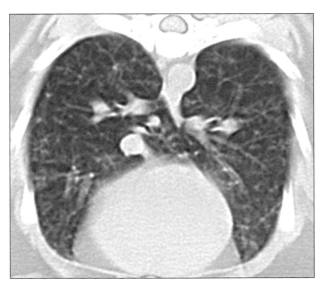

12.59 Transverse CT image (lung window) of the lung of an 8-year-old Domestic Shorthaired cat with markedly thick bronchial walls visible throughout both lungs.

- Nodular non-enhancing hyperattenuating areas representing mucus-filled bronchi
- Hyperattenuating lung in areas of consolidation or atelectasis
- Generally hypoattenuating lungs due to hyperinflation (see Figure 12.112).

Bronchiectasis

The word bronchiectasis was derived from the Greek words 'bronchos' meaning bronchus and 'ectasis' meaning extension. Bronchiectasis is irreversible bronchial dilatation often with accumulation of pulmonary secretions. It can be focal or disseminated and it is uncommon in dogs and rare in cats. In cats, a predisposition in older males has been described.

It can occur as a sequel to long-standing infectious or inflammatory pulmonary disease, secondary to airway obstruction or smoke inhalation, as a complication of radiation-induced pneumonitis or in association with primary ciliary dyskinesia. Also, it has been noted that halothane dilates airways by blocking baseline vagal tone.

Bronchial secretions accumulate in the dilated bronchi and predispose the patient to recurrent airway and pulmonary infections. Dogs with bronchiectasis are commonly presented with a history of chronic productive coughing and recurring pneumonia that initially responds to antibiotics.

Radiography

Changes may be localized or generalized (see Figure 12.111).

- The bronchial lumen is wide and uneven (Figure 12.60). This may be saccular or, more commonly, cylindrical (also known as tubular) dilatation. Cystic and varicose forms have also been described but are rarely identified. Saccular bronchiectases have round drop-like saccules filled with secretions at the end of normal bronchi (Figure 12.61). Cylindrical bronchiectases are dilated bronchi with a fairly even lumen and little diameter change as they subdivide. Each bronchus is club-like and occluded distally.

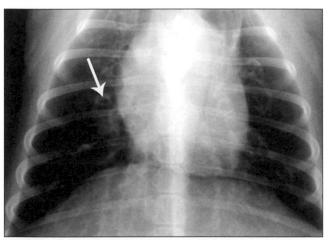

12.60 Close-up of a DV thoracic radiograph of a 7-year-old Fox Terrier. The dilated bronchi are visible in longitudinal section and end-on (arrowed).

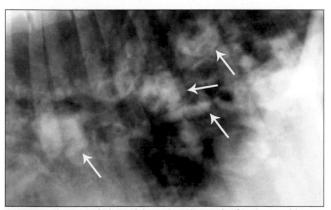

12.61 Close-up of a lateral thoracic radiograph of an 8-year-old mixed-breed dog with saccular bronchiectasis. The bronchi are dilated and filled (partially or fully) with secretions (arrowed) and should not be confused with pulmonary nodules.

- There may be thickened bronchial walls.
- The dilated bronchial lumen may be visualized further into the periphery than normal, e.g. in the ventral areas of the lung fields.
- Bronchi filled with secretions/exudate may appear as nodular opacities when seen end-on.
- In saccular bronchiectasis many of the bronchi distal to the saccular dilatations are obliterated or filled with an exudate. Occasionally, after secondary infection, the saccules may form localized abscesses.
- Often there are multiple regions of lung consolidation due to accompanying pneumonia.
- Development of bronchogenic cysts secondary to bronchiectasis has been described in the dog.

Thoracic radiography may not be sensitive for the diagnosis of bronchiectasis in cats.

Computed tomography

CT findings include:

- Dilated airways: 'tramline' and 'ring'/'doughnut' appearance of the bronchi (when the lumen is air filled) that are significantly wider than the adjacent vessels, mostly due to increased lumen diameter
- Clusters of dilated bronchi in more severely affected areas
- Dilated medium-sized bronchi may extend almost to the pleura
- Thick bronchial walls and obstructed lumens (e.g. from mucus plugs)
- There may be lung consolidation.

Primary ciliary dyskinesia

Primary ciliary dyskinesia (PCD), also known as immotile cilia syndrome, is a diverse group of inherited structural and functional abnormalities of the respiratory tract and other cilia, which results in recurrent respiratory tract infections in the dog. More specifically, PCD is an inherited defect in microtubule formation, affecting cilia of the respiratory and urogenital tracts and the auditory system.

Typically PCD is diagnosed in young purebred animals, with a reported higher incidence in the Bichon Frise. The condition may be seen in mixed-breed dogs and also in cats.

There is a relatively high prevalence of respiratory disease and the phenotype is almost identical to PCD in humans. The respiratory manifestations include chronic rhinitis, bronchitis and severe pneumonia with or without bronchiectasis. Affected animals are presented with recurrent chronic nasal discharge, productive cough, respiratory distress and exercise intolerance. Additional findings are infertility, hydrocephalus and hearing loss.

Assessment of deficient mucociliary transport is initially performed with nuclear scintigraphy. Transmission electron microscopy of nasal or bronchial respiratory epithelium or seminal samples confirms the diagnosis.

Radiography

The findings are variable and include signs of bronchitis and pneumonia with or without bronchiectasis (Figure 12.62).

Computed tomography

Feline PCD has been reported in a 2.5-year-old cat with morphological alterations in the ultrastructure of oviductal

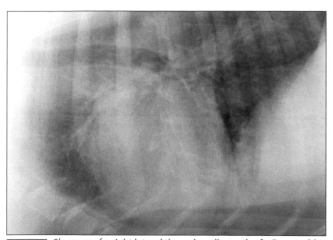

12.62 Close-up of a right lateral thoracic radiograph of a 5-year-old Rottweiler with bronchiectasis and ventral bronchopneumonia (seen over the diaphragm) consistent with PCD.

cilia. CT findings were consistent with early lesions of bronchiectasis. Foci of thick pleurae and interstitial enlargement were also observed.

Scintigraphy

To perform a scintigraphic study (see Chapter 5) a droplet of 99mTc-MAA is deposited in the caudal aspect of the trachea. The diagnosis is confirmed by the absence of movement of the radiopharmaceutical droplet throughout the scintigraphic study (Figure 12.63). Droplet movement always indicates normal ciliary function (i.e. this test produces no false-negative results).

Findings include the following:

* False-positive results (no droplet movement) may occur if the droplet is deposited in an ulcerated area of the trachea, in an area of thick mucus or inside the endotracheal tube

* Occasionally the droplet may move initially, then come to a stop; this happens most commonly because the droplet comes in contact with the end of the endotracheal tube or because it encounters an area of exudate, mucus or ulceration.

Kartagener's syndrome

Kartagener's syndrome is an uncommon congenital condition that has been reported in several breeds of dogs. It is a subset of PCD characterized by situs inversus, rhinosinusitis and bronchiectasis.

Bronchial collapse

Bronchial collapse may occur concurrently with tracheal collapse (see Chapter 10). Usually animals are presented with a history of chronic non-productive cough or respiratory difficulty. The condition is more common in dogs (especially small and toy breeds) than in cats. The disease is caused by progressive bronchial cartilage degeneration and results in a dynamic bronchial obstruction. Changes may occur in the principal bronchi and/or the more peripheral smaller airways. The remainder of this discussion refers to principal bronchial collapse. The gold standard for diagnosis of this condition is fibreoptic bronchoscopy. However, radiographic and fluoroscopic examinations provide a preliminary two-dimensional (2D) evaluation and dynamic CT may provide a non-invasive alternative to bronchoscopy.

Radiography

Radiographic findings include:

* Narrowed lumen of principal or lobar bronchi near the carina. This may be demonstrated better on a lateral thoracic radiograph acquired during expiration
* Lungs are usually normal.

Fluoroscopic and bronchoscopic examination are usually required for evaluation of intrathoracic airway collapse.

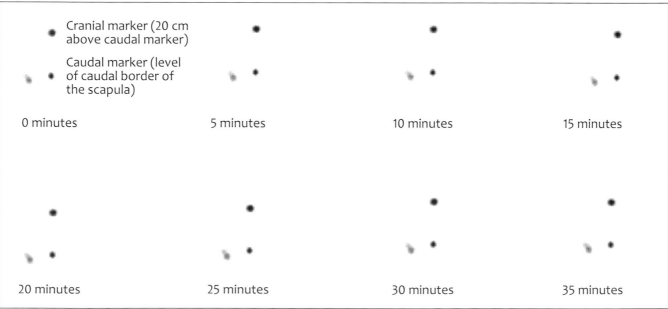

Cranial marker (20 cm above caudal marker)

Caudal marker (level of caudal border of the scapula)

| 0 minutes | 5 minutes | 10 minutes | 15 minutes |
| 20 minutes | 25 minutes | 30 minutes | 35 minutes |

12.63 Composite mucociliary radionuclide scans of a 1-year-old Golden Retriever with PCD and a history of recurrent pneumonia. The two static foci of radioactivity to the right of each image represent external markers positioned at the caudal border of the scapula and 20 cm cranial to it. The images are dorsal views obtained at 0, 5, 10, 15, 20, 25, 30 and 35 minutes after deposition of a small droplet of ^{99m}Tc-MAA just cranial to the carina. The radioactive droplet is at the level of the caudal external marker in the top left image (time 0) and remains at the same location throughout the duration of the study, indicating lack of mucociliary function.

Fluoroscopy

Fluoroscopy allows dynamic examination of bronchial lumen changes and associated tracheal collapse. The patient can remain conscious for evaluation and can also be assessed during an induced cough. It is surpassed by fibre-optic bronchoscopy as fluoroscopy remains a 2D study.

Computed tomography

CT allows identification of the narrowed or collapsed bronchus. Other causes of narrowing such as external compression or intraluminal material can be excluded. Dynamic CT may provide real-time assessment of collapse.

Bronchial foreign body

A variety of foreign bodies may be inhaled, for example plant awns, toys, pebbles, bones, peanuts, dental calculus and even teeth.

The foreign body may cause complete or incomplete morphological bronchial obstruction and hence a wide spectrum of radiographic changes (see Chapter 1). Smooth foreign bodies (metal, marbles, pebbles) do not cause irritation, but usually cause obstruction. These do not usually pass beyond the carina. Irritant foreign bodies (such as seeds or grass awns with rough surfaces) may cause intense focal bronchial irritation with or without obstruction.

Bronchial foreign bodies should be considered in animals with an acute onset of respiratory signs progressing to chronic cough. Animals with laryngeal paralysis are more likely to aspirate material. Eventually pneumonia, bronchiectasis and even pulmonary abscessation may result. Identification of the underlying cause can be a diagnostic challenge.

Radiography

The foreign body will be visible if it is contrasted by gas or soft tissue. No radiographic changes may be seen in the early stages if the foreign body is not contrasted and collateral ventilation is maintained.

- Obstructive atelectasis: complete blockage of a principal bronchus with loss of ventilation causes lobar atelectasis and a resultant increase in opacity and a mediastinal shift towards the affected lobe. Pleural effusion may be seen around the collapsed lobe.
- Complete blockage of a smaller bronchus with collateral ventilation maintained may cause no radiographic changes, or focal consolidations due to infection and trapped secretions, especially along a bronchus (Figure 12.64).
- Obstructive air trapping: incomplete obstruction with 'check valve' effect appears as a hyperlucency and volume gain (mediastinal shift away from the lesion). It is important to acquire both end-expiratory and end-inspiratory radiographs to aid diagnosis.
- An irritant non-obstructing foreign body causes a focal interstitial opacity with central radiolucency and increased bronchial pattern (Figure 12.65), resulting from focal pneumonia. Over time more severe pneumonia, bronchiectasis and lung abscessation are seen.

Hypertrophic osteopathy associated with a bronchial foreign body has been reported in a dog.

Migrating grass awns may initially present as a spontaneous pneumothorax and later as a paralumbar abscess or draining tract with adjacent spondylitis.

Computed tomography

CT is more sensitive than radiography in the detection of bronchial foreign bodies (Figure 12.65). Secondary pulmonary changes, bronchiectasis and pleural effusion may also be seen and the severity assessed more accurately.

Bronchial neoplasia

Bronchial tumours are a type of primary pulmonary tumour. Primary pulmonary tumours are uncommon in dogs and cats. Most primary lung tumours arising from the bronchial epithelium are carcinomas. Cytology and histopathology can provide the definitive diagnosis. Bronchoalveolar carcinoma, for example, has the unique characteristic of extension along the airways and alveolar septa with occasional projections into the alveolar lumen.

The clinical signs of animals with bronchial tumours vary. Chronic cough unresponsive to antibiotics, exercise intolerance, tachypnoea and overt respiratory distress may be seen in dogs. Cats may be presented with signs including anorexia, weight loss, lethargy, tachypnoea, dyspnoea and non-productive cough.

Regional lymph nodes, the pleura and other organs should be assessed for metastatic disease. CT is particularly useful in this respect and should be considered when surgical resection is contemplated.

Radiography

Radiographic findings include:

- Canine bronchoalveolar carcinoma (Figure 12.66; see also Figures 12.73 and 12.106). A varied radiographic appearance has been reported. Solitary nodules, multiple non-circumscribed interstitial nodules, diffuse opacities or alveolar consolidation may be seen (see Figures 12.105 and 12.107)
- Feline bronchoalveolar carcinoma. Three main patterns have been described: mixed bronchoalveolar pattern, ill-defined alveolar mass and mass with cavitation. All cats have a coexisting bronchial pattern. Cavitation is common, suggesting a tendency for the tumour to form necrotic centres. Mineralization should increase the degree of suspicion for neoplasia. Beware: neoplasia may mimic severe feline chronic lower airway disease.

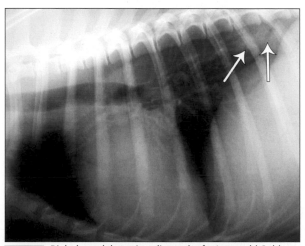

12.64 Right lateral thoracic radiograph of a 4-year-old Golden Retriever with a grass awn in the right caudal lobar bronchus. Note the focal interstitial to alveolar infiltrate in the tip of the caudodorsal lung field (arrowed).

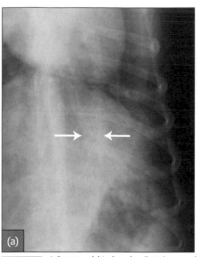
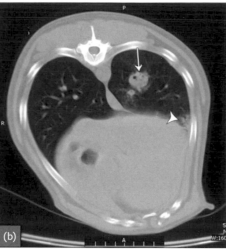
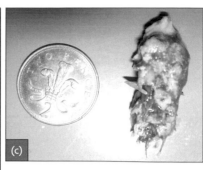

12.65 A 3-year-old Labrador Retriever with a bronchial foreign body. (a) Close-up of a DV thoracic radiograph showing a focal interstitial opacity in the left caudal lung lobe (between the arrows). (b) Transverse lung CT image showing a dilated left caudal lobar bronchus containing hyperattenuating material compatible with a foreign body (arrowed). No enhancement of the material was seen. Note also the hyperattenuating ventral tip of the left caudal lung lobe (arrowhead) compatible with aspiration pneumonia. (c) A grass awn was removed from the left caudal lobar bronchus. (Courtesy of S. Niessen)

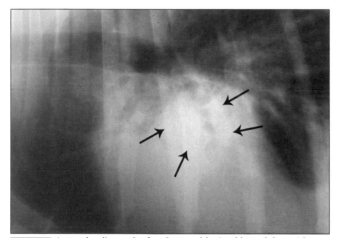

12.66 Lateral radiograph of an 8-year-old mixed-breed dog with a chronic cough and weight loss. There is a focal alveolar pattern surrounding a bronchus (arrowed). The bronchus has an irregular outline. The final diagnosis was bronchoalveolar carcinoma.

Enlarged tracheobronchial lymph nodes may also be identified; these are suggestive of metastatic disease. Pleural effusion may be seen and pleural metastases have been reported.

Computed tomography

CT is more sensitive than radiography for the detection of small lesions. It allows excellent assessment of the location and course of the tumour, the presence of tissue within the bronchial lumen, cavitation and necrosis, mineralization, etc.

The CT appearance of bronchial neoplasms (Figure 12.67) is variable. CT-guided biopsy may be performed. CT is extremely useful for surgical planning. It may detect enlarged regional lymph nodes suggestive of metastasis and thus assist with tumour staging.

Magnetic resonance imaging

The use of thoracic magnetic resonance imaging (MRI) is experimental in lung cancer diagnosis and treatment in humans. It has the potential to provide more accurate information on tumour extension/margins before surgical resection.

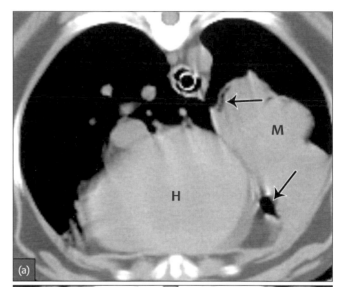
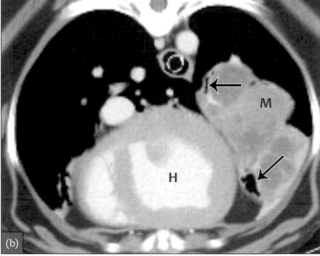

12.67 Transverse CT images (soft tissue window) of an 8-year-old Beagle with a bronchoalveolar carcinoma, (a) before and (b) after intravenous contrast medium administration. Both images were acquired at the level of the heart (H). A large mass (M) in the left lung compresses and distorts a bronchus (arrowed). (b) Contrast medium administration reveals multiple non-enhancing cystic or necrotic regions.

Bronchial rupture

Bronchial rupture is uncommon; tracheal rupture is more common. Usually the rupture occurs within 1–4 cm of the tracheal bifurcation. The most common causes are:

- Blunt trauma to the neck and/or thorax
- Chronic cough
- Venepuncture resulting in bronchial rupture and resultant fatal tension pneumothorax has been reported in a kitten.
- Traumatic avulsion of the left principal bronchus has also been reported in a cat
- Foreign body.

Bronchial rupture will usually result in pneumomediastinum and/or pneumothorax (less common), depending on the location and orientation of the tear. Free gas commonly tracks along the bronchial adventitia into the mediastinum.

Radiography

Radiographic findings include:

- Pneumomediastinum, normotensive (simple) pneumothorax or tension pneumothorax
- In cases of tracheal rupture, tracheal discontinuity may be identified on survey radiographs; bronchoscopy is more helpful for identification of bronchial rupture.

Computed tomography

Tracheobronchoscopy is usually performed, but CT may be useful when tracheobronchoscopy fails to identify the location of the rupture. CT is able to localize small peribronchial gas pockets suggestive of bronchial rupture.

Bronchiolitis obliterans with organizing pneumonia

Bronchiolitis obliterans with organizing pneumonia (BOOP) is a rare inflammatory condition in the cat and dog and is a multifactorial disease. The characteristic pathohistological finding is granulated tissue plugs within the lumen of small airways, which extend into the alveolar ducts and alveoli. Definitive diagnosis relies on lung biopsy. In humans BOOP may be secondary to a interstitial pneumonia. A few case reports exist in dogs, and CT and open or keyhole lung biopsy have been used successfully for diagnosis.

Radiography

Various combinations of bronchial, interstitial and alveolar patterns may be seen radiographically. One case report in the dog describes a diffuse interstitial pattern in both lungs. Commonly, patchy areas of alveolar pattern and thick bronchial walls are seen. The radiographic changes are non-specific.

Computed tomography

CT has been reported as a sensitive technique for this condition. One canine case report describes bilateral asymmetrical areas of lung consolidation and bronchial dilatation.

Bronchial microlithiasis

Miliary broncholithiasis is a rare sequel to inflammatory bronchial disease reported in cats. Inspissated mucopurulent plugs with calcified concretions are found throughout the bronchi. It can lead to obstructive resorption atelectasis and compensatory emphysema.

Radiography

Radiographic findings include:

- Small mineralized opacities contained within the bronchi, scattered throughout the lungs (Figure 12.68)
- Atelectasis of obstructed lobes/areas is possible
- Compensatory hyperinflation and emphysema.

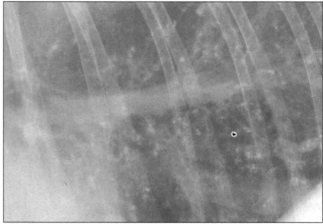

12.68 Close-up of a lateral thoracic radiograph of a cat. Multiple mineralized opacities are visible throughout the lungs consistent with bronchial microlithiasis.

Broncho-oesophageal fistula

Broncho-oesophageal fistulae may be congenital or acquired. The latter may occur secondary to trauma or an oesophageal or bronchial foreign body. The result of the condition is usually recurring aspiration pneumonia and hence cough. Definitive diagnosis is by oesophagography (see Chapters 1 and 10), although the fistula may occasionally be recognized on endoscopic examination.

Radiography

Radiographic findings include:

- Recurrent focal pneumonia
- Occasionally gas distension of the oesophagus.

Congenital bronchial anomalies

Congenital bronchial anomalies are uncommon but have been reported in the dog and cat.

Bronchial cartilage dysplasia, causing congenital lobar bullous emphysema, has been reported in dogs. Lung hyperlucency, mediastinal shift and flattening of the diaphragm are identified radiographically.

Bronchial dysgenesis has been reported in a cat. Thoracic radiographs showed hyperinflation of the right lung and atelectasis or agenesis of the left lung. Bronchial dysgenesis was identified in all but the right caudal lung lobe.

Lung diseases

Solid pulmonary masses

A pulmonary mass is a fluid, soft tissue or mineralized structure replacing, compressing or displacing the air-filled portion of the lung. The clinical implications rest on the assessment of benignity or malignancy (Figure 12.69). It can be difficult to differentiate between various types of lung masses solely on imaging features; however, a prioritized differential diagnosis can be created based on imaging characteristics described below and other factors, such as:

- Age
- Species and breed
- Geographical area the animal lives in and travel history
- Additional diagnostic tests.

Cystic masses are discussed separately (see 'Cysts', below).

- Metastatic disease
- Primary lung tumour
- Granuloma
- Abscess
- Cyst
- Fluid-filled bulla
- Mucus-filled bronchus
- Haematoma

12.69　Differential diagnosis of pulmonary nodule/mass.

Radiography

Radiographically a pulmonary mass is evident as a discrete opacity, surrounded by (more) lucent lung.

***Expansile mass* versus *infiltrative lesion*:** Most pulmonary masses are expansile, and displace rather than contain major airway structures (Figure 12.70). Common features of such masses are:

- Bronchial deviation
- Absence of air bronchograms.

However, some lung masses are infiltrative and can contain and occlude bronchi (Figures 12.71 and 12.72). Both types of mass can result in bronchial obstruction and subsequently, pulmonary atelectasis or secondary haemorrhage and infection that can result in:

- A large area of alveolar lung disease with air bronchograms and lobar sign
- Border effacement between mass and adjacent secondary lung changes making size assessment difficult.

Features of alveolar lung pattern can therefore be suggestive of a mass in some circumstances, but they are not sufficient for assessment of the growth pattern.

Classical Röntgen signs of pulmonary masses:
- Size.
  - A lesion up to 3 cm is termed a nodule.
  - A lesion larger than 3 cm is termed a mass.
- Shape.
  - Usually round (equal growth into each direction).
  - Other shapes are possible and are commonly seen at lung margins.

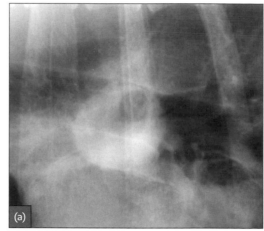

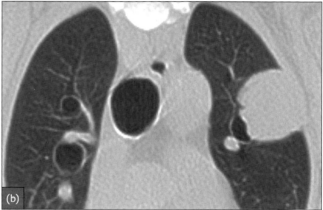

12.70　(a) Central close-up of a right lateral thoracic radiograph of a 12-year-old German Shepherd Dog with a pulmonary carcinoma. The mass slightly deviates the air-filled left cranial lobar bronchus but does not give rise to an air bronchogram. This indicates it has an expansile rather than infiltrative nature. (b) The corresponding CT image confirms how the mass abuts but does not encroach the bronchus. (Courtesy of Lobo Jarrett)

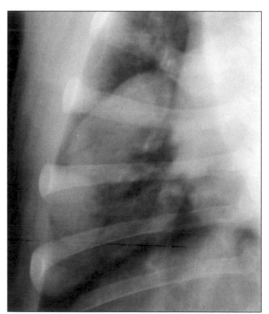

12.71　Close-up of a DV thoracic radiograph of a dog with a histiocytic sarcoma in the right middle lung lobe. The mass occupies a large portion of the lobe giving rise to a lobar sign cranially and caudally and does contain air bronchograms. This is consistent with an infiltrative lesion encroaching airways.

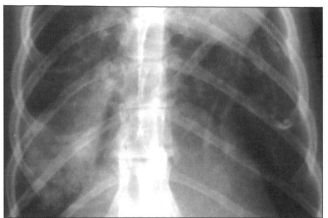

12.72 Caudal close-up of a VD thoracic radiograph of a 12-year-old Domestic Shorthaired cat with nasal and pulmonary lymphoma. Notice the increased opacity with an alveolar pattern (air bronchogram) supportive of an infiltrative process. Radiographically evident pulmonary involvement in feline lymphoma is extremely rare.

- Opacity.
  - Usually soft tissue opacity.
  - Central lucency in cavitated lesions.
  - May see mineralized centre due to dystrophic mineralization.
- Location.
  - Random.
  - Some diseases extend from lymph nodes into adjacent perihilar lung tissue (lymphomatoid granulomatosis).
- Number.
  - Solitary or multiple.

Neoplasia: A primary pulmonary neoplasm typically presents as a solitary nodule (Figure 12.73) or mass (see Figures 12.70a, 12.71 and 12.74).

- May be accompanied by additional, smaller nodules, representing metastasis.
- Occasionally concurrent cranial mediastinal or tracheobronchial lymphadenopathy and/or pleural effusion are radiographically visible.

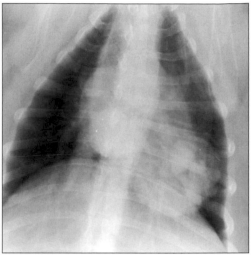

12.74 VD thoracic radiograph of an 8-year-old Rottweiler with pulmonary adenocarcinoma. There is a soft tissue mass in the left caudal lung lobe. Note the border effacement between the mass and the heart.

- A small solitary nodule is equally likely to be metastatic or a primary neoplasm. The larger the nodule is, the more likely it is primary neoplasia.
- Pulmonary neoplasia can also manifest as diffuse parenchymal disease:
  - Interstitial, peribronchial infiltration or a patchy alveolar pattern are possible (interstitial pattern in canine lymphoma, see Figure 12.203a)
  - May be caused by complications of the neoplastic disease, such as inflammation, infection, or haemorrhage
  - Lobar consolidation occurs if a lung lobe is completely infiltrated, or the lobar bronchus is obstructed by the mass (Figure 12.75). Examples:
    - Lymphomatoid granulomatosis (a rare primary pulmonary angiodestructive neoplasm seen mainly in young to middle-aged dogs). Lung lobe typically has an increased volume, resulting in convex, bulging borders

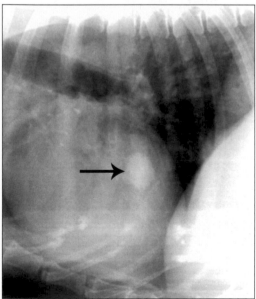

12.73 Left lateral thoracic radiograph of a 12-year-old mixed-breed dog with primary bronchoalveolar carcinoma. A solitary soft tissue nodule is seen in the right middle lung lobe (arrowed).

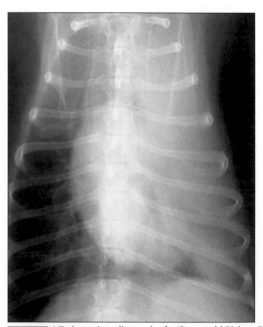

12.75 VD thoracic radiograph of a 12-year-old Bichon Frise with primary pulmonary carcinoma. The entire left cranial lung lobe is consolidated and enlarged.

- Bronchogenic carcinoma may also occlude a bronchus, causing atelectasis, and thus loss of volume and concave margins
- A lung tumour may become cavitated, and uncommonly is mineralized. No correlation has been found between the radiographic pattern and the histological diagnosis.

Species differences

Mineralization of lung tumours
- Cats: Central mineralization of primary pulmonary neoplasia is common (Figure 12.76).
- Dogs: Central mineralization is rare.

Pulmonary infiltration of lymphoma
- Cats: Very rarely any radiographically evident lung lesion in lymphoma (see Figure 12.72).
- Dogs: Commonly causes diffuse unstructured interstitial lung pattern, but very rarely nodules or masses.

Pulmonary metastasis
- Cats: Often poorly marginated, irregularly shaped (see Figure 12.88).
- Dogs: Usually well defined round nodules (see Figure 12.87).

Primary pulmonary neoplasia and digital metastasis in cats
The digits are a predilection site for metastasis from feline primary pulmonary neoplasia. This has been reported in:
- Pulmonary adenocarcinoma
- Pulmonary squamous cell carcinoma
- Bronchogenic carcinoma.

Older cats are usually presented for digital swelling and lameness and are free of respiratory signs. Skeletal metastases of lung tumours in dogs occasionally occur in the axial skeleton and long bones proximal to stifle and elbow but have not been reported in digits.

Primary digital neoplasia and pulmonary metastasis in dogs
The most diagnosed digital neoplasms in dogs are:
- Squamous cell carcinoma
- Subungual melanoma (Figure 12.77).

Melanoma has a high rate of lung metastasis. Dogs or cats with digital swelling and lameness warrant examination for neoplastic lung disease.

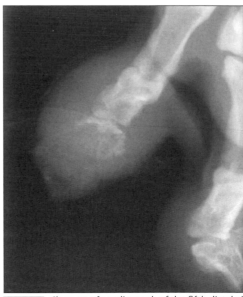

12.77 Close-up of a radiograph of the fifth distal phalanx (P3) of the right manus of a 9-year-old Rottweiler with digital pain. Notice the soft tissue swelling and extensive osteolysis of P3 (histological diagnosis: subungual melanoma). Digital neoplasia is associated with pulmonary primary (cats) or metastatic (dogs) neoplasia and thoracic radiographs should be obtained routinely.

Abscess:
- A mass that typically has a thick wall with an irregular inner surface.
- May be cavitary if it contains gas due either to gas-producing bacteria or to connection with airways (Figure 12.78).
- May be surrounded by consolidated lung or may be well demarcated and surrounded by normal lung.
- Horizontal beam radiographs may demonstrate a fluid-gas interface.
- Not commonly associated with pleural effusion.

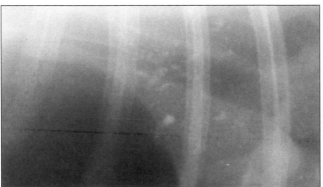

12.76 Craniodorsal close-up of a right lateral thoracic radiograph of a 10-year-old Domestic Shorthaired cat with a primary lung lobe tumour in the left cranial lobe. There are multiple small mineralizations in the dorsal part of the cranioventral lung field. A VD view confirmed their location within the left cranial lung lobe. Such soft tissue mineralization is not uncommon in primary lung lobe tumours in cats and is a relatively specific sign for them.

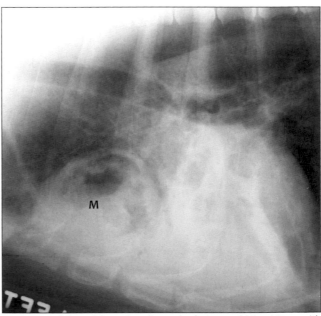

12.78 Left lateral thoracic radiograph of a 1-year-old Great Dane with suppurative pneumonia. An abscess is seen as a cavitary mass (M) in the right cranial lung lobe. The centrally present gas delineates a thick wall with irregular inner surface. The caudally adjacent right middle lung is increased in opacity with an alveolar pattern (air bronchograms, lobar sign) consistent with pneumonia.

Granulomas:

* Comprise localized inflammation with aggregation of macrophages to isolate infectious agents or foreign material that cannot be eliminated otherwise.
* Nodules/confluent nodules/amorphous masses (Figure 12.79).
* Poorly defined margins when active, more sharply marginated when resolving.
* Often in association with tracheobronchial and/or cranial mediastinal lymphadenopathy and with a bronchointerstitial pulmonary pattern.
* May become cavitated (most common in Paragonimus fluke infection).
* May become mineralized (especially histoplasmosis granulomas).
* Foreign body granulomas differ from other granulomas: they are usually solitary and larger than most other granulomas and tracheobronchial lymphadenopathy is absent. May develop into an abscess, if secondarily infected.
* Pulmonary infiltration with eosinophilia (PIE) can manifest with single or multiple pulmonary nodule(s)/mass(es) (also known as eosinophilic granulomas), varying in size from 2 to over 10 cm, in addition to more commonly seen peribronchial changes. Tracheobronchial lymphadenopathy is a consistent feature (Figure 12.80).

Haematoma:

* While pulmonary haemorrhage often presents as patchy areas of interstitial or alveolar disease, a haematoma may appear as a round to oval, well circumscribed soft tissue opacity and may contain air.
* Typically associated with lung contusions and pneumothorax. Will be suspected based on the history of trauma.
* Can be differentiated from other masses by follow-up radiographs that will show a decrease in its size within several days.

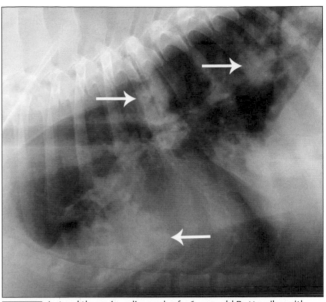

12.80 Lateral thoracic radiograph of a 6-year-old Rottweiler with pulmonary infiltration and eosinophilia. There is increased lung opacity with a mixed bronchial and alveolar pattern. Note the nodular component (arrowed) caused by the formation of granuloma.

Contrast studies:

* Are not often indicated.
* An oesophagram can be helpful in differentiating a pulmonary mass from an oesophageal lesion or a hiatal hernia (Figure 12.81).
* Bronchography can outline mass effect, lobar location and relation to bronchial system of a mass (Figure 12.82). The technique has been superseded by less invasive techniques (e.g. CT).

Ultrasonography

A pulmonary mass is typically identified on thoracic radiographs. If there is not much aerated lung present between the mass and the thoracic wall, thoracic ultrasonography may be helpful to:

* Confirm pulmonary origin of an intrathoracic mass
* Differentiate between a soft tissue and a fluid-filled lesion
* Perform ultrasound-guided fine-needle aspiration for cytology.

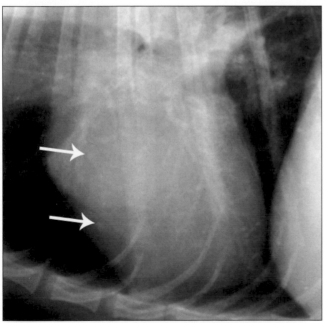

12.79 Close-up of a lateral thoracic radiograph of a 3-year-old mixed-breed dog with granulomatous fungal pneumonia (same dog as in Figure 12.94). There are multiple small soft tissue nodules throughout the lungs (arrowed). There is also tracheobronchial lymphadenopathy, evident by the increased opacity dorsal to the heart base.

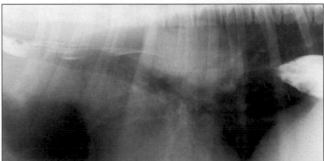

12.81 Close-up of a lateral oesophagram of a 14-year-old Boxer with a perihilar mass. Barium outlines the oesophageal mucosa cranial and caudal to the mass with a normal pattern (bolus caudal to the mass). The oesophagus appears deviated and compressed but not invaded by the mass, making an oesophageal lesion unlikely. Final diagnosis: bronchial adenocarcinoma.
(Courtesy of the University of Pennsylvania)

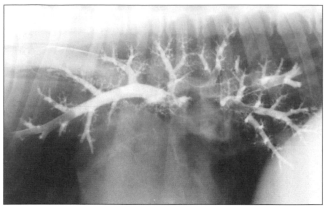

12.82 Close-up bronchogram of the left lung of an 8-year-old English Springer Spaniel with bronchial adenocarcinoma arising from the left principal bronchus. Survey radiographs showed a hilar soft tissue mass. The contrast study demonstrates the central filling defect owing to the mass and residual patency allowing filling of peripheral bronchi with contrast medium.
(Courtesy of the University of Pennsylvania)

Neoplasia:

- Typically appears as a round, hypoechoic mass, but can have a variable appearance, depending on the presence of central necrosis, cavitations and trapped gas (Figure 12.83).
- The deep margin of the mass is often smooth, in contrast to inflammatory lesions.
- It usually arises in the interstitium and displaces surrounding lung tissue. As a result, no fluid-filled bronchi or normal branching vessels are seen within the mass. Inflammatory and infiltrative lesions may show fluid bronchograms and encroached vessels.
- A sterile abscess as a complication of tumour necrosis is indistinguishable from a septic abscess.

Abscess:

- Usually appears as a mass with a cavitated centre and thick walls with irregular internal margins (Figure 12.84).

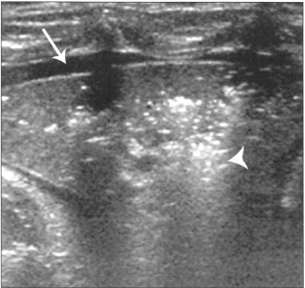

12.83 Thoracic linear-transducer ultrasound image of a 5-year-old Domestic Shorthaired cat with a primary lung tumour. The affected lung lobe has lost its normal reflectivity and appears with the echogenicity of soft tissue. Residual amounts of trapped air are hyperechoic and cause dirty shadowing distally (arrowhead). There is a small amount of anechoic pleural effusion (arrowed).

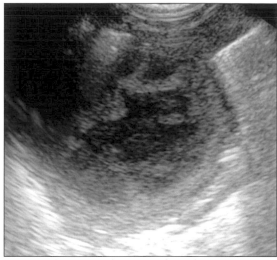

12.84 Thoracic curvilinear transducer ultrasound image of a 2-year-old Weimaraner with a lung abscess. Adjacent to the visceral pleural margin, there is a round mass with a thick echoic capsule with irregular internal margins and a hypoechoic core. The hyperechoic area around the mass represents normal aerated lung.

- Contents may be anechoic, hypoechoic or echogenic, and often move with gravity to the dependent side. Internal septations possible.
- May contain gas in addition to the fluid, indicating communication with a bronchus or anaerobic infection.
- When an abscess is suspected, an underlying foreign body should be considered. Most foreign bodies will create a clean acoustic shadow within the mass.

Computed tomography

Computed tomography is very helpful to confirm the pulmonary origin of a mass seen on radiographs and to determine its extension and involvement of surrounding structures more accurately, especially when surgical resection is considered (see Figures 12.70b, 12.85 and 12.86; see also Chapter 3).

- CT may confirm the presence of a solid mass that is unclear on radiographs due to summation of adjacent alveolar infiltrate (representing secondary oedema, inflammation or extension) with the mass.
- CT enables detection of smaller nodules than radiography and may reveal additional lesions such as metastatic disease and lymphadenopathy.
- CT can be very helpful to obtain a guided aspirate of a lesion, when the presence of aerated lung peripheral to the lesion prevents an ultrasound-guided biopsy. While pneumothorax and haemorrhage are commonly seen complications of this procedure, these are rarely clinically evident or significant.

Magnetic resonance imaging

- Very few publications describe lung mass MRI in veterinary medicine.
- In human medicine, breath-hold techniques enable lung nodules of 5 mm to be detected. A three-dimensional (3D) gradient echo sequence is preferred for imaging lung parenchyma to minimize phase artefacts from cardiac motion.

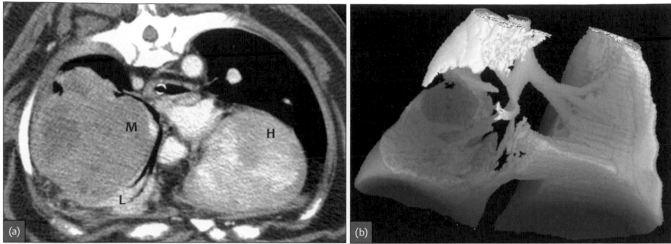

12.85 (a) Post-contrast transverse thoracic CT image at a level immediately caudal to the carina of a 7-year-old Bulldog with a primary pulmonary carcinoma. A large soft tissue mass (M) displaces the heart (H) and major blood vessels towards the left, deviating and compressing the right middle lung lobe (L) and its bronchus. There is heterogeneous mild enhancement of the mass with rim enhancement and strong enhancement of the collapsed lung. (b) Ventral aspect three-dimensional reconstruction with air-filled spaces in white. A large void in the right lung corresponds to the tumour and atelectatic lung tissue.

(b Courtesy of Jennifer Kinns)

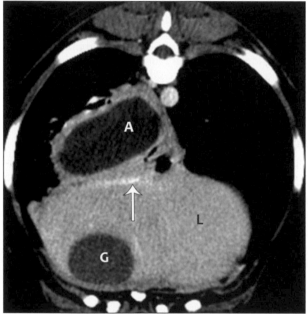

12.86 Post-contrast transverse caudal-thoracic CT image of a 2-year-old Cocker Spaniel with a lung abscess. The right caudal lung lobe has a hypoattenuating mass (A) with a thick, mildly enhancing capsule. The liver (L) and hypoattenuating gallbladder (G) are seen ventrally. Note the complete flattening of the contrast-enhanced caudal vena cava (arrowed) due to compression by the mass.

Metastatic lung disease

Radiography is commonly used to detect lung metastasis in cases of known or suspected primary neoplasia anywhere in the body. Since radiography is such a simple, fast, non-invasive and inexpensive test, examining patients with a relatively low risk of neoplasia is still useful if other complex, time-consuming, invasive and expensive diagnostic tests or interventions are anticipated. Most pulmonary metastases manifest as lung nodules. These need to be differentiated from benign nodular lesions (granulomas, incidental osteoma) and end-on vessels.

Radiography

- Thoracic radiography has a relatively low sensitivity to pulmonary metastasis because a pulmonary soft tissue nodule must be 3 to 5 mm in size to be visible. Nodules smaller than this may be visible if multiple nodules summate with each other, or if the nodule is mineralized.
- Pulmonary metastases rarely mineralize. A clearly visible nodule smaller than 3–5 mm most likely represents an end-on vessel or a non-neoplastic mineralized nodule (heterotopic bone, granuloma).
- Nodules are more detectable when surrounded by well inflated lucent lung, with maximal contrast between the lesion and normal lung. Inspiratory, opposite lateral views are therefore essential, since on each view the lung on the dependent side is incompletely inflated, and metastasis in that lung could be missed.
- Nodules identified on one or both lateral views might not be visible on DV and VD views. This should not lead to the lesion mistakenly being dismissed.
- When a nodule summates with the lungs, extrapulmonary locations such as skin (mass, nipple, tick) and mediastinum should be ruled out by evaluating an orthogonal view and by careful examination of the body wall of the patient. An extrapulmonary location should be suspected if a nodule or mass has high opacity. This is a summation phenomenon due to the increased contrast provided by the surrounding air outside the body.
- While identification of a nodule on two orthogonal views confirms the intrapulmonary location of a lesion with high degree of certainty, it is often impossible to see a nodule on both views.

The purpose of acquiring opposite lateral thoracic radiographs is to enhance detection of pulmonary nodules. If a nodule is seen only on one view, this should not lead to dismissal of a lesion.

- The most characteristic radiographic appearance of pulmonary metastasis is the presence of well defined soft tissue opacity nodules of variable size, randomly distributed throughout the lungs (Figure 12.87).
- Other manifestations:
  - Ill-defined nodules (particularly in cats) (Figure 12.88)
  - Unstructured interstitial lung pattern
  - Lung consolidation (coalescing nodules, infiltrative lesion)
  - Miliary nodular pattern (many small metastases of 2–3 mm in diameter spread throughout the lung).
- Mesenchymal tumours, which spread primarily via the blood, tend to produce a low number of well defined metastases while epithelial tumours, which spread primarily via the lymphatic vessels, often produce large numbers of relatively small, ill-defined nodules. However, this is only a general rule.
- Radiographic patterns described for several tumour types:
  - Haemangiosarcoma commonly produces poorly defined small coalescing nodules (Figure 12.89) or, less commonly, well circumscribed nodules or an alveolar infiltrate secondary to haemorrhage

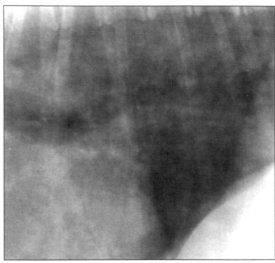

12.89 Caudodorsal close-up of a lateral thoracic radiograph of a 10-year-old Papillon with pulmonary metastasis from a splenic haemangiosarcoma. There are multiple poorly defined small coalescing nodules spread throughout the lungs.

- Transitional cell carcinoma commonly produces a diffuse interstitial pattern or nodular interstitial pattern
- Mammary gland neoplasia in dogs produces well defined nodule(s), ill-defined nodules or miliary nodules. Pulmonary alveolar septal metastasis is a rare form of mammary tumour spread described in dogs, where lungs are diffusely infiltrated by carcinoma predominantly in arteries and small capillaries of the alveolar septae. It results in a wide range of radiographic manifestations, but commonly an unstructured interstitial pattern
- Mammary gland neoplasia in cats produces ill-defined nodules, a diffuse pulmonary pattern or, less commonly, well defined nodules.

Contrast studies: Not indicated.

Ultrasonography

As for solid pulmonary masses (see above), it may be possible to image a peripheral metastatic nodule and obtain an ultrasound-guided aspirate of the lesion (Figure 12.90).

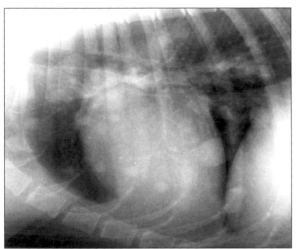

12.87 Lateral thoracic radiograph of a 4-year-old Rottweiler with pulmonary metastasis from an unidentified primary neoplasm. Both lungs have numerous, round, relatively well marginated, randomly distributed, soft tissue nodules of variable size.

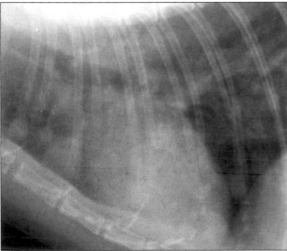

12.88 Close-up of a lateral thoracic radiograph of a 12-year-old Domestic Longhaired cat with metastatic pulmonary neoplasia. Compared with the dog in Figure 12.87, the nodules are ill defined and not round. This is a relatively common appearance of metastatic nodules in cats.

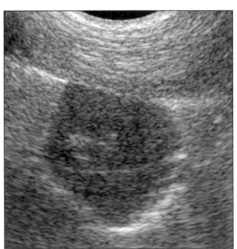

12.90 Thoracic curvilinear transducer ultrasound image of a 9-year-old Boxer with a neuroendocrine heart base tumour and pulmonary metastasis. The metastatic nodule is round and hypoechoic, with a small hyperechoic core and smooth margins surrounded by hyperechoic aerated lung.

Computed tomography

- CT is the preferred imaging modality for pulmonary metastasis in human medicine.
- CT is more sensitive than radiography for identifying pulmonary metastasis. Nodules as small as 1 mm may be seen with standard techniques, and sub-millimetre lesions with high-resolution CT techniques (Figures 12.91 and 12.92). CT also identifies more nodules than radiography (see also Chapter 3).

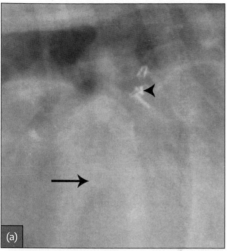

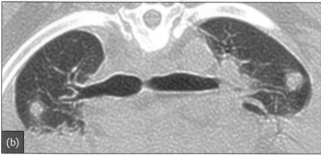

12.91 (a) Central close-up of a right lateral thoracic radiograph of a 9-year-old mixed-breed dog acquired 3 months after removal of the right middle lung lobe with a pulmonary carcinoma. Notice the surgical staples (arrowhead) and a faintly visible nodular opacity (arrowed). The opposite lateral view was normal. (b) High-resolution thoracic CT image at the level of the tracheal bifurcation. There is a soft tissue nodule in each cranial lung lobe (diameter: right, 6 mm; left, 9 mm) and atelectasis related to ventral recumbency. CT can detect more and smaller nodules.

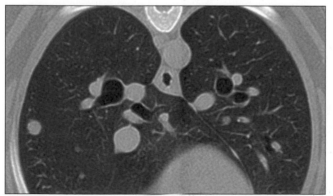

12.92 High-resolution transverse thoracic CT image at the level of the accessory lung lobe of a 7-year-old mixed-breed dog with anal sac adenocarcinoma and pulmonary metastasis. Multiple small (1–4 mm) nodules are visible throughout the lungs. Nodules in the lung periphery are easily identified, whereas more central lesions must be distinguished from normal blood vessels with slice-by-slice comparison. Such nodules appear like granulomatous soft tissue nodules (see Figure 12.94) and must be evaluated in context with clinical history and disease progression.

Ditzels – little things that *might* matter

The ability to observe very small lung lesions with CT poses new challenges for interpretation and prognostication because the importance of these findings is usually unknown. These commonly seen findings are informally called ditzels and appear as small (1–2 mm) nodules. These findings are potentially important and there is currently no reliable way to determine whether they are malignant or benign non-invasively and instantaneously.

Procedural recommendations for ditzels:

- Small, mineralized lesions are unlikely to be neoplastic (Figure 12.93)
- Consider granulomatous lesions in patients living in areas where fungal diseases are endemic (Figure 12.94)
- Consider the primary disease and likelihood of metastasis (see Figures 12.91, 12.92 and 12.95)
- Search for occult primary neoplasia elsewhere in body
- Consider follow-up CT to monitor progression of lesion
- Consider peripheral lymph node aspiration and imaging-guided fine-needle lung aspiration if feasible.

- Metastases are more commonly located in the peripheral lung, in a subpleural location, making these lesions more difficult to detect radiographically, but easier to distinguish from vessels on a CT image. Nodules can be distinguished from vessels by the fact that they are not continuous with a vascular structure on adjacent slices (see Figure 12.92).
- CT can document unusual spread of metastatic disease such as peribronchial infiltrate (Figure 12.96) parenchymal bands, subpleural interstitial thickening, subpleural lines, irregular perfusion and ground-glass opacity (Figure 12.97).

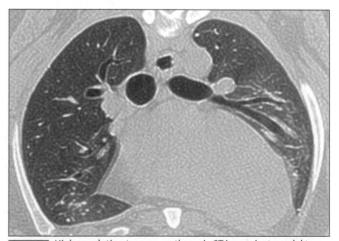

12.93 High-resolution transverse thoracic CT image just caudal to the carina of a 9-year-old Labrador Retriever with a nasal adenocarcinoma. There are numerous, small (1 mm), mineralized ditzels throughout the lungs. These are incidental osteoma and not neoplastic metastases. Nasal neoplasia rarely metastasizes to the lungs and pulmonary metastases only very rarely mineralize.

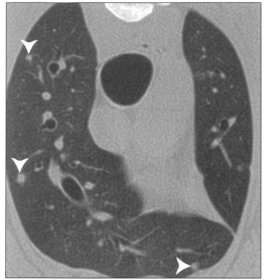

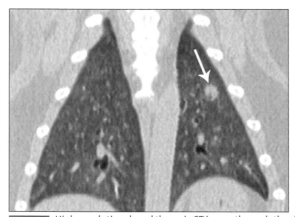

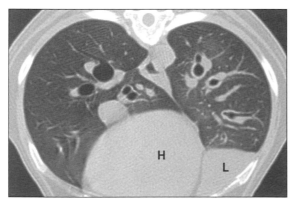

12.94 High-resolution transverse thoracic CT image at the level of the aortic arch of the same dog as in Figure 12.79 with granulomatous pneumonia. Note the soft tissue nodules in the peripheral lung (arrowheads). These can be differentiated from blood vessels by their larger size in the peripheral lung, and by evaluating contiguous images (blood vessels can be followed cranially and caudally).

12.95 High-resolution dorsal thoracic CT image through the dorsal part of the lungs of a 13-year-old West Highland White Terrier with idiopathic pulmonary fibrosis. In the cranial aspect of the left lung, there is a small (4 mm) soft tissue nodule (arrowed) including a lucent bronchus. Because the nodule encroaches a bronchus, it is an unlikely candidate for metastasis. A follow-up investigation showed no progression of the lesion.

12.96 High-resolution transverse thoracic CT image at the level of the accessory lung lobe of an 11-year-old Bichon Frisé with an anaplastic carcinoma in the left cranial lung lobe causing complete consolidation of that lobe (L) and deviation of the heart (H). No lung nodule was detected, but the bronchial walls were thick in the left caudal lung lobe (compare with right). Subsequent investigation confirmed neoplastic peribronchial infiltrate.

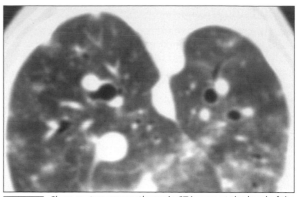

12.97 Close-up transverse thoracic CT image at the level of the accessory lung lobe of an 11-year-old Cairn Terrier with adrenal carcinoma and pulmonary carcinosis with widespread infarction of pulmonary capillaries and tributary lung tissue. Notice the multiple small wedge-shaped subpleural lesions with pleural retraction and ill-defined parenchymal lesions consistent with infarction, and ventral areas of ground-glass opacity, which is a non-specific finding.

Scintigraphy:

- Can be of value in patients with thyroid neoplasia because a primary neoplasm may arise in the mediastinum at the level of or cranial to the heart. Even small metastatic lung nodules can have visible increased radiopharmaceutical uptake.
- Very useful technique to detect bone metastasis secondary to pulmonary or other neoplasia.

Gas- or fluid-containing pulmonary lesions
Bullae and blebs

Bullae are gross air accumulations within the lung parenchyma formed by the loss or breakdown of alveolar walls. Bullae may also be known as pneumatocoeles and the two terms may be used interchangeably. Some authors and medical texts consider pneumatocoele a specific term for a large pulmonary bulla. Bullae are not true cysts because they lack an epithelial lining. The bulla wall is created by connective lung tissue and visceral pleura, and this defines the bulla type (Figure 12.98). Pulmonary bullae can also be classified according to their origin as:

- Congenital bullae: see 'Congenital lobar emphysema', below
- Traumatic bullae: the result of blunt thoracic trauma causing sudden rise in intrathoracic pressure. Air cannot be exhaled due to reflexive epiglottic closure (diving reflex) leading to lung laceration. Chronic lung diseases with chronic cough can also weaken pulmonary parenchyma and lead to lung laceration
- Idiopathic bullae: occur in combination with spontaneous pneumothorax, without known cause of gas accumulation.

Blebs are intrapleural gas accumulations that arise when air escapes the pulmonary parenchyma and gets trapped between the internal and external layer of the visceral pleura (Figure 12.99). Some sources define a bleb as a small bulla.

- Often located at lung apices.
- Usually a sequel to parenchymal bullous disease of any origin.
- More difficult to detect radiographically.
- More prone to rupture and to create pneumothorax.

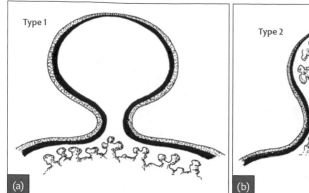
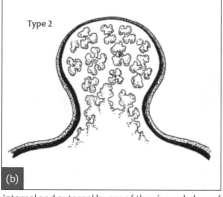
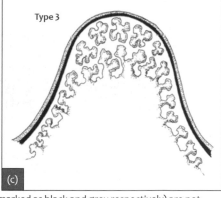

12.98 Different types of pulmonary bullae. The internal and external layers of the visceral pleura (marked as black and grey respectively) are not dissected by bullae but can be herniated in different ways. (a) A type 1 bulla is a round gas accumulation within herniated visceral pleura with a small isthmus to the pulmonary parenchyma. They are usually found at lung apices. These bullae macroscopically resemble blebs, except blebs are usually not spherical. (b) A type 2 bulla arises from subpleural parenchyma and contains emphysematous lung tissue connected to the pulmonary parenchyma with a wider neck. (c) A type 3 bulla is a usually a large gas pocket without emphysematous lung tissue deep in the pulmonary parenchyma and may involve more broad-based deviation of the visceral pleura.
(Reprinted from Lipscomb VJ et al. (2003) with permission)

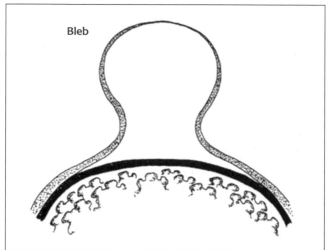

12.99 Pulmonary bleb. The internal and external layers of the visceral pleura (marked as black and grey respectively) are dissected by a gas pocket that has escaped from the pulmonary parenchyma.
(Reprinted from Lipscomb VJ et al. (2003) with permission)

Cysts

Pulmonary cystic lesions are fluid- or air-filled lesions surrounded by a thin wall of respiratory epithelium. The histological composition of the cyst wall determines the cyst type:

- Pulmonary cysts are formed from alveolar epithelium with no remnant of a bronchial wall on histopathology
- Bronchogenic cysts are dilated bronchioles or bronchi that have a bronchial wall remnant on histopathology.

Cavitating lung lesions

Cavitating lung lesions may be defined as soft tissue masses with a fluid- or gas-filled centre. They may develop from an apparently solid nodule or mass, as the centre of the solid structure can liquefy due to a necrotic process. On occasion, a neoplasm may grow around a bronchus thus incorporating the bronchus into the mass; therefore it is important to distinguish air within a bronchus that is in a mass from a cavitating lung lesion. The clinical signs vary with the underlying disease. In radiographs, cavitating

lesions can usually only be identified if they are air-filled, whereas ultrasonographically, cavitating lesions can usually only be identified if they are fluid-filled. In CT, both fluid- and gas-filled cavitations can be observed.

Radiography

Gas-filled pulmonary lesions (blebs and bullae): These are best seen when they are surrounded by more opaque lung tissue, which is best achieved with:

- An expiratory-phase radiograph
- The dependent side lung on laterally recumbent radiograph (obtain both lateral views).

Pneumothorax and bullae/blebs

A search for pulmonary bullae/blebs is a common procedure to identify the cause of pneumothorax.

- Pneumothorax can hinder or promote visibility of a bulla, depending on the amount of free air, degree of collapse and location of bulla. Pre- and post-thoracocentesis radiographs are recommended.
- Ruptured bullae/blebs tend to collapse. Identified bullae/blebs are suggestive of the general cause of pneumothorax (ruptured lung tissue) but the currently leaking collapsed bullae/blebs may not be visible.
- Superficial blebs are more prone to rupture than deep parenchymal bullae. This should be weighted in the decision making for conservative/surgical treatment of pneumothorax. It may not be safe to release a patient with a large bleb despite successful drainage of pneumothorax.

- Typical radiographic features of bullae/blebs are:
  - Radiolucent structure with an absent or barely perceptible wall (Figure 12.100)
  - Bullae are usually round and within lung parenchyma
  - Blebs are often ovoid and always peripheral (Figure 12.101).
- Secondarily infected or haemorrhagic bullae may appear as a circular soft tissue opacity with areas of

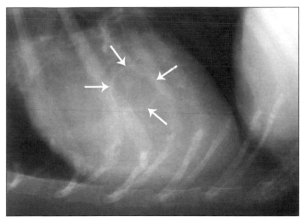

12.100 Close-up of a lateral thoracic radiograph of a 10-year-old Labrador Retriever. Notice the round gas opacity surrounded by a very thin opaque wall (arrowed) that summates with the cardiac silhouette. This bulla was an incidental finding.

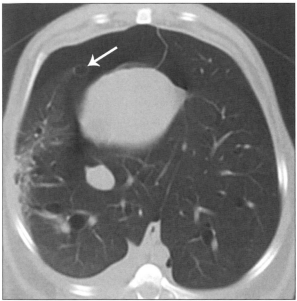

12.101 Transverse thoracic CT (dorsal recumbency, lung window) of a 7-year-old Poodle with spontaneous pneumothorax. Notice both pleural cavities are expanded and gas-filled (worse on the right side). A bleb or small bulla (arrowed) is seen at the ventral tip of the right caudal lung lobe. The increased opacity of the lung parenchyma adjacent to the body wall is attributed to atelectasis.

hyperlucency and may mimic a cavitating lung lesion or a soft tissue mass (Figure 12.102).
- Horizontal beam radiography can help in outlining a fluid line in cysts or in infected bullae.

Fluid-filled pulmonary lesions:
- Similar opacity to solid masses, hence difficult to differentiate.
- Fluid-filled cysts are often ovoid (see Figure 12.102), whereas metastatic lung nodules are usually round.
- Follow-up radiographs may show reduction in size and/ or gas accumulation (fluid drainage) and help in differentiating them from solid masses (equal or increased size).

Pulmonary lesions containing fluid and gas:
- Assessment of the location, number, size and shape of gas opacity allows further characterization of the lesion (Figures 12.103 and 12.104).

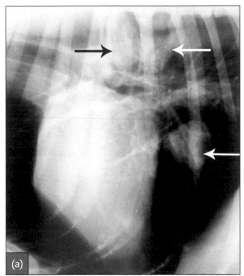

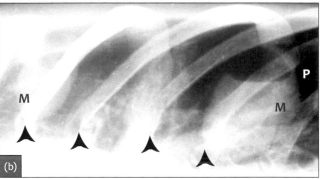

12.102 (a) Close-up of a lateral thoracic radiograph (vertical beam) of a dog that was involved in a road traffic accident 24 hours previously. A sternal dislocation, pneumothorax and multiple ovoid pulmonary soft tissue masses (arrowed) are identified, which could be related to trauma or an unrelated illness. (b) Close-up of a VD thoracic radiograph of the non-dependent hemithorax obtained with a horizontal beam. Beside the serial rib fractures (arrowheads) and free pleural gas (P) in the most elevated part of the thorax, two of the previously seen masses (M) are also visible with a straight fluid–gas interface and a thin smoothly outlined wall. These findings are most consistent with blood- and gas-filled bullae, haemopneumatocoeles.

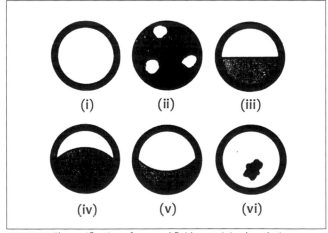

12.103 The typification of gas- and fluid-containing lung lesions according to gas location and fluid–gas interface. In vertical beam radiography, (i) one large central gas lucency is more likely to indicate a cyst, large abscess or bulla; (ii) Several small, irregularly shaped and distributed gas lucencies are more suggestive of neoplasia, foreign body or gas-producing bacteria. In horizontal beam radiography, (iii) low-viscosity fluid tends to create a straight interface with gas, whereas (iv and v) high-viscosity fluid tends to create a convex or concave margin and (vi) gas within solid lesions creates no interface. (Adapted from Silverman et al. (1976) with permission)

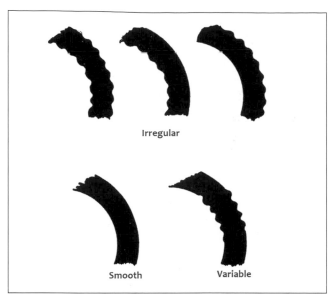

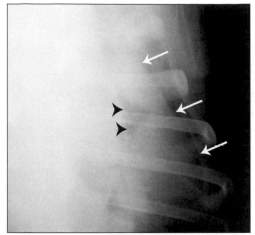

12.104 The typification of gas-containing lung lesions according to their wall characteristics. The wall can be regular or irregular on either or both sides or have various combinations of the two. Smooth-walled lesions are most likely bullae or cysts, whereas irregular margins are a result of tissue necrosis and infection and are commonly seen with abscesses and neoplasms (cavitating lesions). In lesions that contain fluid and gas, these features can only be applied to horizontal beam radiographs.
(Adapted from Silverman *et al.* (1976) with permission)

- Cavitated abscesses are most likely to have thick irregular walls (see Figure 12.78) and less likely to have thin and smooth walls (Figure 12.105).
- Cavitated neoplasms may contain amorphously shaped air bubbles (Figure 12.106).
- Cavitated parasitic granulomas are commonly seen with paragonimiasis infection (Figure 12.107).

Other imaging techniques

- CT is a more sensitive diagnostic imaging modality for detection of bullae and blebs (Figures 12.108 and 12.109).
- Ultrasonography and CT are sensitive techniques to characterize fluid-filled lesions (see Figures 12.84, 12.85 and 12.86).

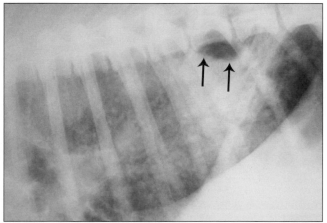

12.105 Close-up of a lateral (standing/horizontal) thoracic radiograph of a 4-year-old Great Dane with extreme dyspnoea and cough. In the caudodorsal lung field, there is a cavitating lung abscess with a horizontal fluid line (arrowed) separating fluid from gas. The lungs have an alveolar lung pattern with a diffuse increase in soft tissue opacity.

12.106 Close-up of a DV thoracic radiograph of an 11-year-old mixed-breed dog with a chronic productive cough. The left cranial lung lobe (caudal part) has a severe increase in soft tissue opacity with retraction of the lobe edge from the thoracic wall (arrowed). There is an irregularly shaped gas opacity eccentrically positioned within the lung lobe (arrowheads), which represents a cavitated centre. This was confirmed to be bronchogenic carcinoma with central necrosis.

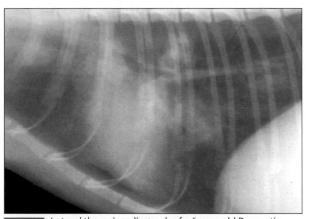

12.107 Lateral thoracic radiograph of a 6-year-old Domestic Shorthaired cat with *Paragonimus kellikotti* fluke infection. Notice the multiple pulmonary soft tissue nodules containing irregular small central air bubbles. This is a classical radiographic feature of paragonimiasis in dogs and cats.

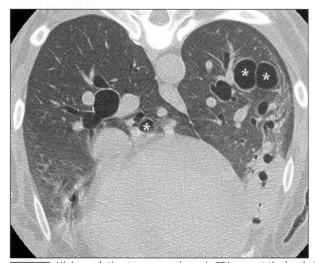

12.108 High-resolution transverse thoracic CT image at the level of the accessory lung lobe of a 16-year-old Standard Poodle with numerous pulmonary bullae (*) in both lungs. Slice-by-slice image analysis is necessary to rule out bronchiectasis. These relatively small bullae would be difficult to identify radiographically. The interpretation of the relevance of such small lesions can only be made in light of the clinical history of the patient. There is ventral hypostatic lung collapse.

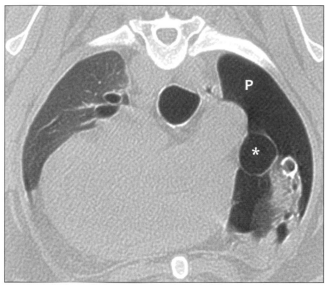

12.109 High-resolution transverse thoracic CT image at the level of the aortic arch of an 8-year-old Golden Retriever with spontaneous left-sided pneumothorax (P). CT enabled identification of a leaking type 1 bulla (*) in the left cranial lung lobe. A thoracocentesis drain is seen in cross-section adjacent to the collapsed left lung.

- Ultrasonography can only be used for peripheral lung lesions but offers easy guidance for fine-needle aspiration.
- CT is indicated for deeper lesions with the option of CT-guided fine-needle aspiration.

Pulmonary emphysema

Pulmonary emphysema is characterized by an abnormal increase in size of the alveolar airspaces due to destruction of alveolar walls.

- Bronchiolar obstruction with valve mechanism (dynamic collapse):
  - Inspired air enters the pulmonary parenchyma but is unable to escape even with forced expiration (air trapping)
  - Increased expiratory intra-alveolar pressure leads to laceration of alveolar walls and bulla formation.
- Usually confined to lung periphery.
- Clinically manifesting lung emphysema is rare in dogs and cats.
- It is important not to confuse air trapping with forced inspiration or pneumothorax.

Congenital lobar emphysema

- A rare congenital bronchial cartilage abnormality or bronchial plug in puppies that leads to dynamic airway collapse and air trapping.
- Usually only one lung or lobe affected.
- Tension collapse of other lobes.
- Reported in dogs and cats, most commonly in small-breed dogs.

Acquired pulmonary emphysema

- Obstructive bronchiolar disease (chronic bronchitis, feline asthma, bronchial neoplasia, bronchial foreign body) can lead to dynamic airway collapse and air trapping.

- Chronic compensatory hyperinflation has been reported to cause lobar emphysema.
- Mild changes commonly seen in cats with feline asthma.
- Marked changes are rarely seen in dogs or cats.
- Changes are usually bilateral.

Radiography

- Radiographs should be acquired during full inspiration and full expiration. Typically, the lungs are well inflated with a gas opacity. Emphysema is confirmed when there is minimal difference between the position of the diaphragm or the degree of pulmonary opacification during inspiration and expiration.
- A horizontal beam DV or VD radiograph can be useful, as the dependent lung lobe does not collapse with lobar emphysema.
- Signs of pulmonary hyperinflation on expiratory radiographs (Figures 12.110 and 12.111; see also Chapter 8):
  - Hyperlucent, enlarged lungs
  - Scant but visible vascular markings
  - Caudally displaced, flattened diaphragm
  - Transverse rib position
  - Chronic rib fractures.
- With lobar emphysema:
  - Mediastinal shift away from affected lung lobes and compression of unaffected lung lobes
  - Herniation of affected lung lobes into contralateral hemithorax
  - No collapse of affected lung in dependent position on lateral radiograph.

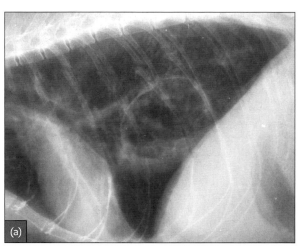

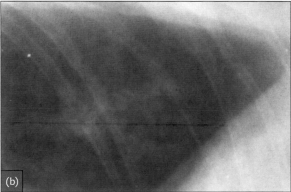

12.110 (a) Expiratory lateral thoracic radiograph of a cat with feline asthma. Notice the small size of cardiovascular structures, generalized bronchial pattern, large bulla and multiple non-union rib fractures. (b) Caudodorsal close-up of the same radiograph reveals hyperlucent peripheral lung fields consistent with air-trapping and emphysema.

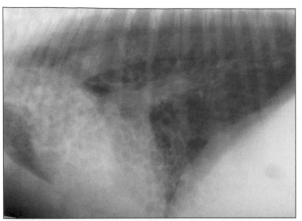

12.111 Lateral thoracic radiograph of a 5-month-old Australian Cattle Dog with chronic bronchopneumonia. Both lungs have multiple distended tortuous bronchi and gas pockets, consistent with bronchiectasis and bullous emphysema.

Other imaging techniques

- Ventilation/perfusion lung scintigraphy to establish V:Q mismatch.
- Pulmonary angiography to establish lack of regional blood flow.
- CT to detect small emphysematous lung areas (Figure 12.112).

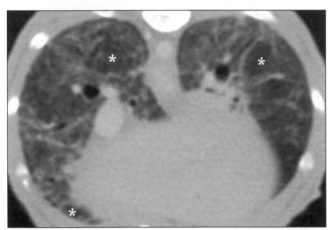

12.112 High-resolution transverse thoracic CT image at the level of the accessory lung lobe of a 16-year-old cat with chronic lower airway disease. Both lungs have multiple soft tissue septae consistent with fibrotic changes and focal areas of pulmonary hyperlucency consistent with emphysema (*).

Lung lobe torsion

Lung lobe torsion is an uncommon condition in small animals, but it is potentially life-threatening and requires surgery in most cases.

- Rotation of a lung lobe occurs around its axis, usually close to the hilus or rarely also in the middle of a lobe, leading to twisting and occlusion of the bronchovascular structures.
- Venous return and lymphatic drainage from the lung lobe are compromised, whereas arterial supply is preserved initially to some degree due to the stronger muscular arterial walls. However, this is less prominent in the lungs than in other organs because there is less difference in blood pressure between arteries and veins in the pulmonary circulation compared with the systemic circulation.

- This leads to venous congestion, pulmonary oedema, sequestration of blood within the twisted lung lobe and eventually lung lobe necrosis.
- Blood and fluid enter the alveoli and bronchi.

Air can be trapped within the twisted lung lobe due to incomplete bronchial obstruction with a one-way valve effect. Pulmonary emphysema can develop because of increased alveolar pressure, alveolar or bronchial tears; pneumothorax or pneumomediastinum can result from bronchial tears.

Decreased lymphatic drainage, as well as increased interstitial and hydrostatic pressure within the affected lung lobe, leads to production of pleural effusion.

- The effusion initially presents as a transudate.
- It later becomes haemorrhagic or suppurative.
- Necrosis or fibrosis in the later stages of the disease lead to a decrease in lung lobe volume.

Large-breed dogs with deep and narrow chests, particularly Afghan hounds, are predisposed. Small chondrodystrophic dogs with round chests, in particular Pugs, have also been described with spontaneous lung lobe torsion. Other small breeds of dogs and cats are more commonly reported to have an underlying condition that leads to the lung lobe torsion.

Underlying diseases are characterized by collapse of a lung lobe, which is also suspended in either pleural fluid or air, leading to increased lung lobe mobility. Pleural effusion, pneumothorax, trauma with compression of the thoracic cavity and partial collapse of a lung lobe, but also pneumonia and surgical manipulation, are predisposing conditions. In Pugs, a bronchial cartilage dysplasia has been proposed to cause some hilar instability leading to lobar torsion. The shape of the rib cage has also been proposed to promote lung lobe torsion; however, this does not explain, why other small brachycephalic dog breeds with similar anatomical features have a much lower risk of lung lobe torsion.

The most affected lung lobes are:

- Right middle lung lobe (most common in deep-chested dogs)
- Left cranial lung lobe, the entire lobe or the cranial part (most common in small, chondrodystrophic breeds).

All other lung lobes can be affected, and more than one lung lobe can be affected. Recurring lung lobe torsion has been described but is unusual.

Radiography

Pleural effusion is a consistent finding in patients with lung lobe torsion. The pleural effusion can be:

- Bilaterally symmetrical
- Asymmetrical
- Unilateral and centred around the affected lung lobe (Figure 12.113).

In most cases pleural effusion is the consequence rather than the cause of the lung lobe torsion, and therefore it may be absent very early on in the disease process. However, this very early stage is rarely observed.

A mediastinal shift with displacement of the cardiac silhouette is sometimes present (Figure 12.114), usually away from the affected lung lobe, but can be towards a lung lobe with chronic torsion. The trachea can be dorsally deviated or have some degree of axial rotation at the level of the carina, caused by the abnormal position of the twisted lung lobe. This is best seen on a lateral radiograph (Figure 12.115).

Consolidation of the affected lung lobe is evident as an alveolar pattern with effacement of the pulmonary vasculature. The unaffected lung lobes are relatively normal.

- The affected lobe is enlarged and has rounded borders due to congestion.
- Small air bronchograms or scattered gas lucencies throughout the affected lung lobe (air alveolograms, vesicular gas pattern) result in a foamy appearance of the lung.
- Gas bubbles can also be gathered in 'clusters' (Figure 12.116).

Less commonly, the lung lobe is uniformly opacified without evidence of air bronchograms, as air bronchograms usually disappear after a few days, when the air is replaced by blood or fluid. In chronic cases there is a loss of volume in the twisted lung lobe.

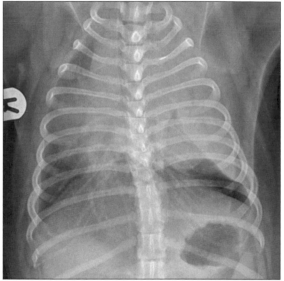

12.114 DV thoracic radiograph of an 18-month-old Pug with a left cranial lung lobe torsion. The left cranial lung lobe is consolidated with a central vesicular pattern, extends abnormally far caudally, and causes a right shift of the cardiac silhouette.

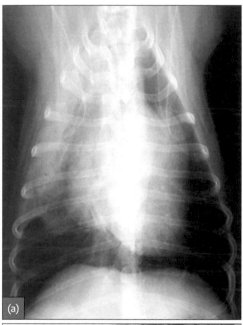
(a)

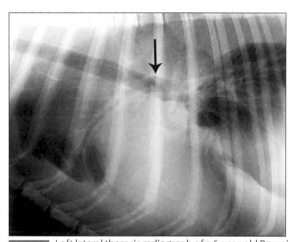

12.115 Left lateral thoracic radiograph of a 6-year-old Borzoi with left cranial lung lobe torsion. There is moderate pleural effusion. The carina is axially rotated, resulting in dorsal displacement of the right cranial lobar bronchus (arrowed); a bronchus to the left cranial lung lobe is not visible. The increased opacity dorsal to the carina represents the consolidated left cranial lung lobe.

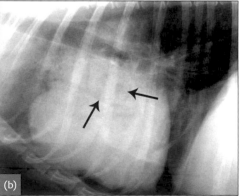
(b)

12.113 An 8-year-old Jack Russell Terrier with right middle lung lobe torsion. (a) VD thoracic radiograph. Pleural fluid is present in the right cranial thorax, centred around the right middle and right cranial lung lobes. The right middle lung lobe is rounded and contains some air with a vesicular pattern. The cardiac silhouette is misshapen due to a previous pericardectomy. (b) Right lateral thoracic radiograph. In the cranioventral thorax, the lung has an increased opacity with air alveolograms. The right middle lobar bronchus is very narrow close to the carina and turns sharply cranially instead of caudoventrally (arrowed), a sign consistent with lung lobe torsion.

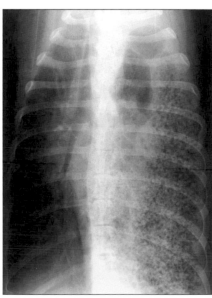

12.116 DV thoracic radiograph of a 6-year-old Akita Inu with a left caudal lung lobe torsion. The left caudal lung lobe is enlarged, causing a right mediastinal shift, and contains multiple small air bubbles (vesicular pattern).

The lobar bronchus to the affected lung lobe is visible only over a short distance and is blunted, narrowed or ends abruptly close to the carina.

- Air-filled bronchi running in an abnormal direction (inverted air bronchograms) indicate an abnormal position of a lung lobe (see Figure 12.113b).
- Blood vessels in an abnormal position are rarely observed due to the consolidation of the lung lobe.
- The adjacent aerated lung lobes are displaced towards the centre of the thorax, evident by a change in direction of the blood vessels and bronchi, as well as the pleural fissure lines.
- Rupture of a bronchus can lead to pneumomediastinum or pneumothorax.

The change in shape or orientation of the affected lung lobe is best seen after removal of the pleural fluid. In the presence of large amounts of pleural effusion, radiographs should be repeated after drainage of the pleural fluid. In addition, horizontal beam radiographs can provide valuable information by shifting the pleural fluid.

Ultrasonography

This can be helpful in patients with inconclusive radiographic findings and may give additional information about the presence of a lung lobe torsion and/or underlying disease. Ultrasonography can be performed in the non-sedated patient in a standing position or in ventral recumbency, which is tolerated even by dyspnoeic patients.

Ultrasonographic findings include (Figure 12.117):

- Pleural effusion, particularly around the twisted and congested lung lobe. The pleural fluid can be anechoic to cellular, depending on the haemorrhagic component of the fluid
- Enlarged, consolidated lung lobe, which is either hypoechoic or isoechoic to solid organs like the liver ('hepatization'), with rounded borders
- In chronic torsions, the lung lobe may be smaller and retracted towards the hilus
- Foci of gas trapped within the centre of the lobe, recognized as hyperechoic foci with reverberation artefacts. The periphery of the lobe may appear as a consolidated band. If a large amount of gas is trapped within the twisted lung lobe, the whole lobe is hyperechoic with many reverberation artefacts

- Linear hypoechoic structures without blood flow and with a hyperechoic wall, representing fluid-filled bronchi (fluid bronchograms)
- Abnormal course or shape of fluid bronchograms
- Abnormal position of the affected lung lobe, dorsal to the base of the heart, with the tip pointing up, or pointing cranially.

Care should be taken to assess the thoracic cavity and especially the cranial mediastinum for associated problems, such as mediastinal lymphadenopathy or other masses, which are obscured radiographically by the pleural effusion but may be an underlying problem, leading to the pleural effusion and consequent lung lobe torsion.

Doppler examination: Doppler (colour or power Doppler) examination can be very helpful to determine whether a consolidated lung lobe is twisted, or if it is filled with fluid or cellular infiltrates (pneumonia, neoplasia). In a lung lobe torsion, typical Doppler findings include:

- Absence of venous blood flow
- Absence of, or reduced, arterial blood flow.

However, Doppler examination is hampered by artefacts produced by the motion of the lung lobe in the pleural effusion, due to the usually increased respiratory rate.

Computed tomography

This is the diagnostic method of choice, other than exploratory thoracotomy, for patients with unclear or inconclusive radiographic and ultrasonographic findings. It requires at least sedation, but it is diagnostic in almost all cases of lung lobe torsion, and in addition allows surveying for underlying diseases, such as lung or cranial mediastinal masses.

CT findings (Figures 12.118 and 12.119) are like radiographic findings; however, the position and patency of each bronchus can be better assessed.

- All bronchi should be followed from the carina into their respective lung lobes. This is best achieved on images reformatted in various planes, according to the position of the bronchus to be evaluated. The bronchus to a twisted lung lobe is blunted, ends abruptly or is narrowed considerably and changes its direction. Using virtual bronchoscopy, a fish-mouth-like opening of the twisted bronchus can sometimes be observed.

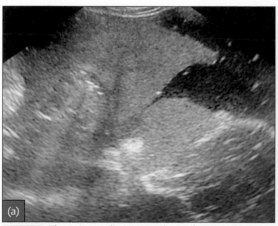
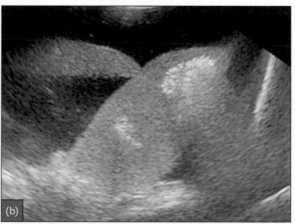

12.117 Thoracic curvilinear transducer ultrasound images of the same dog as in Figure 12.115. Left oblique (intercostal) window, craniodorsal is to the left. (a) There is a large volume of anechoic pleural fluid and consolidation of both parts of the left cranial lung lobe with an abnormally dorsal location. (b) A slightly more caudal image, showing the periphery of the twisted left cranial lung lobe. There are large pockets of trapped gas present within the lung lobe, seen as hyperechoic areas with distal reverberation artefacts.

- In animals with chronic pleural effusion, consolidated lung parenchyma can be best differentiated from pleural effusion after administration of intravenous contrast medium; non-aerated collapsed lung will strongly contrast-enhance. Lung that has undergone torsion often has a compromised blood supply and will either show very poor contrast enhancement or only enhancement of the visceral pleura. This usually allows differentiation of pleural fluid and non-aerated lung, as well as between collapsed lung and lung that has undergone torsion. Twisted lung also contains trapped gas in the alveolar spaces, leading to a vesicular pattern.
- It can be very difficult to differentiate a collapsed lung lobe from a chronically twisted lung lobe, as both may have lost volume and collapsed lung lobes are also slightly dorsally rotated in the presence of large amounts of pleural effusion. It is helpful in these cases to scan the patient in dorsal and ventral or lateral recumbency to direct the pleural effusion away from the lung lobe. After ventilating the lungs for a few minutes, the lung lobe should be reassessed for degree of reinflation, position and shape of the bronchus. Failure to inflate in the non-dependent position is a sign of lung lobe torsion or other bronchial obstruction.
- An abnormal course of pulmonary blood vessels can also be seen; this is best observed after intravenous administration of an iodinated contrast medium.

Lung herniation

A hernia is the displacement of a structure through a defective anatomical boundary.

Mediastinal lung herniation is displacement of lung through the mediastinum and into the opposite pleural cavity. It should be differentiated from a mediastinal shift, which is displacement of the lung and mediastinum away from midline without a defect in the mediastinum (the displaced lung does not enter a pleural cavity). A mediastinal shift is commonly seen in dogs and cats with lung masses and unilateral hyperinflation or emphysematous changes. Affected lung lobes push the mediastinal structures and heart away from the midline. It is usually reversible if the increased lung volume can be reduced. In patients with lung removal or lobectomy or lung collapse, the remaining lungs will compensate by expanding to occupy the vacant space in the thoracic cavity. A mediastinal shift also may occur towards the side of lung collapse.

Cervical or thoracic wall lung herniation of the lung lobes is very rarely seen in dogs and cats. It can occur due to interruption of the thoracic boundaries (e.g. thoracic inlet, thoracic body wall) with sudden intrathoracic pressure changes resulting from trauma or chronic coughing. Caudal lung herniation through a defect in the diaphragm typically does not occur.

Imaging findings

- Mediastinal shift (Figure 12.120): marked mediastinal displacement towards the contralateral hemithorax due to lung expansion.
- Cervical or thoracic wall lung herniation (Figures 12.121 and 12.122):
  - Protrusion of a lung lobe outside the thoracic boundaries, often with dynamic appearance consistent with respiratory phase
  - Possible concurrent signs of thoracic trauma (e.g. rib fractures, pneumothorax).

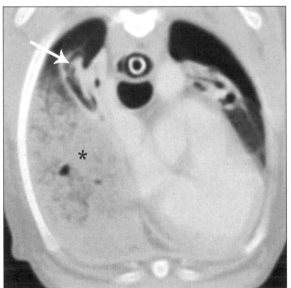

12.118 Transverse thoracic CT image at the level of the aortic root of the same dog as in Figure 12.113. There is a left mediastinal shift and free gas in the dorsal pleural spaces. The twisted right middle lung lobe is enlarged and partially consolidated with multiple gas pockets (*). The right cranial lung lobe is completely collapsed (arrowed) and dorsally displaced by the enlarged right middle lung lobe.

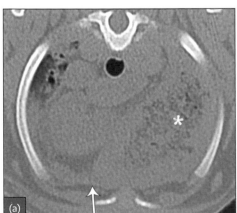
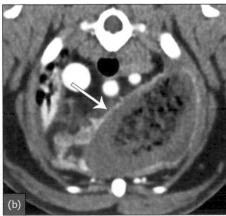
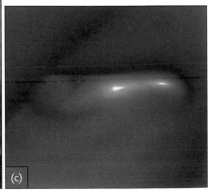

12.119 (a, b) Transverse thoracic CT images at the level of the cranial mediastinum of a Pug with left cranial lung lobe torsion, the same dog as in Figure 12.114. (a) High-resolution lung CT image showing the enlarged consolidated left cranial lung lobe with central vesicular gas pattern (*) and mediastinal shift towards the right hemithorax (arrowed). (b) Post-contrast CT image showing contrast enhancement only of the pleural layer (arrowed). (c) Virtual bronchoscopy CT image of the left cranial lobar bronchus with a view of the tapered lumen near the torsion site with a fish-mouth appearance.

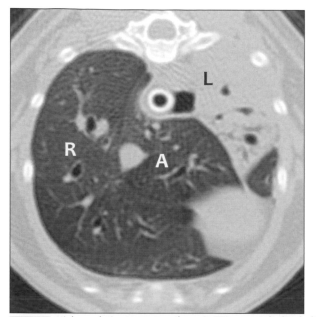

12.120 High-resolution transverse thoracic CT image at the level of the accessory lung lobe of an 11-year-old Domestic Shorthaired cat with a primary lung lobe tumour, leading to bronchial obstruction and collapse of the left caudal lung lobe (L). The compensatory hyperinflation of the right lung leads to mediastinal shift with movement of the right caudal (R) and accessory (A) lung lobes towards the left hemithorax.

Predominantly alveolar lung diseases

The term alveolar disease in this chapter is used for lung parenchymal diseases in which alveolar radiographic pattern (lung consolidation) is a predominant feature. Some types of pneumonia that do not produce a predominantly alveolar pattern are also included in this section.

Diagnosis of specific alveolar lung diseases is challenging because:

- Most alveolar diseases also affect other components of the lung, e.g. interstitium and bronchi. Very few diseases affect only the alveolar spaces (e.g. pulmonary alveolar proteinosis)
- There is a wide overlap in radiographic changes seen with the different alveolar diseases.

A meaningful diagnostic approach to alveolar lung diseases therefore includes:

- Consideration of history and results of other tests
- Temporal assessment of disease: different diseases may vary in speed of onset and resolution (Figures 12.123 and 12.124)
- Localization of pathology: different diseases often differ in preferential locations (Figure 12.125).

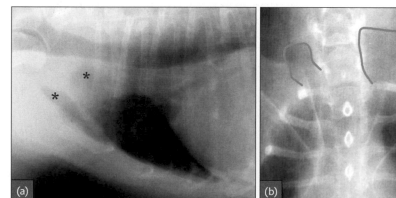
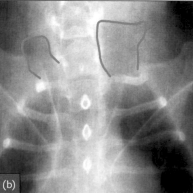
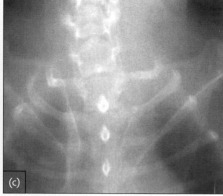

12.121 (a) Expiratory lateral thoracic radiograph of a 9-year-old Yorkshire Terrier with intrathoracic tracheal collapse. The intrathoracic trachea is mildly narrowed. Cranial to the thoracic inlet, both cranial lung lobes protrude into the caudal neck (∗). Only the left cranial lung lobe normally protrudes cranial to the thoracic inlet, and usually not during expiration. (b) Expiratory VD fluoroscopic image of the thoracic inlet, demonstrating the cervical herniation of both cranial lung lobes (outlined). (c) Inspiratory VD fluoroscopic image showing the cranial lung margins within the thoracic boundaries. This is cervical lung herniation, secondary to expiratory intrathoracic tracheal collapse and associated pressure changes.

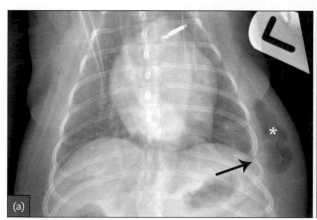
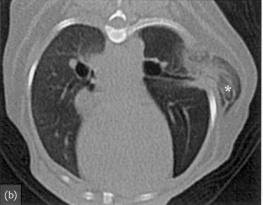

12.122 (a) DV thoracic radiograph and (b) transverse thoracic CT image at the level of the 7th intercostal space of an 8-year-old Pomeranian dog with chronic mitral valve disease and an old fracture of the left 7th rib (arrowed). There is herniation of a large part of the left caudal lung lobe through the 7th intercostal space into the external layers of the thoracic wall, consistent with intercostal lung herniation (∗).

Disease	Onset within	Resolution following treatment within
Acute alveolar diseases		
Oedema	Hours	Hours
Haemorrhage	Minutes	Days
Pneumonia	Hours to days	Days to weeks
Aspiration	Minutes	Days to weeks
Chronic alveolar diseases		
Pneumonia	Days	Weeks to months
Granulomatous diseases	Weeks	Months to never
Neoplasia	Weeks	Weeks to never (depending on tumour type and treatment)

12.123 Onset and resolution of different alveolar lung diseases.

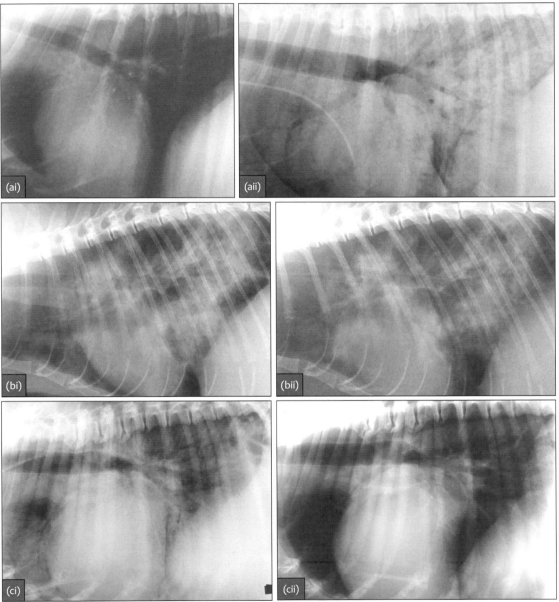

12.124 (ai) Lateral thoracic radiograph of a Labrador Retriever with pancreatitis. The thorax is normal. (aii) Lateral thoracic radiograph taken 48 hours later. Note the severe diffuse alveolar pattern, which has developed rapidly following aspiration of gastric fluid. The acute progression of the changes is helpful in producing a differential diagnosis list. (bi) Lateral thoracic radiograph of a 6-year-old Maine Coon cat presented with chronic cough and dyspnoea. There are multiple areas of ill-defined soft tissue opacity in several lung lobes. The presumptive diagnosis was pneumonia, possibly granulomatous or atypical in origin. Open lung biopsy showed chronic inflammatory changes. (bii) Lateral thoracic radiograph following treatment with antibiotics for 3 weeks. There is no change in the lung lesions. Histopathological examination post mortem confirmed diffuse pulmonary adenocarcinoma. (ci) Lateral thoracic radiograph of an Irish Wolfhound with widespread pulmonary oedema secondary to dilated cardiomyopathy. (cii) Lateral thoracic radiograph taken 72 hours later following treatment with diuretics. Note the resolution of the oedema, in contrast to the lack of progression seen in (b).
((b) Courtesy of Cambridge Veterinary School)

Disease	Preferential lung location
Bacterial pneumonia	• Ventral lung areas • Right middle lobe • Both cranial lobes
Pneumocystis carinii infection	• Caudal and middle lobes
Hypostatic atelectasis	• Right middle lobe • Lung periphery • Dependent lung
Resorption atelectasis secondary to bronchial obstruction (plugging) in feline asthma	• Right middle lobe
Resorption atelectasis secondary to chronic obstructive bronchial foreign body	• Caudal lobes
Atelectasis secondary to pleural effusion	• Right middle lobe
Neoplasia	• Caudal lobes
Contusion	• Ipsilateral to trauma
Haemorrhage	• Random • Location of penetrating injury
Lung lobe torsion	• Right middle lobe (deep-chested dogs) • Left cranial lobe (barrel-chested dogs)
Canine cardiogenic pulmonary oedema	• Perihilar • Symmetrical or slightly more in right caudal lobe
Canine non-cardiogenic pulmonary oedema	• Caudodorsal aspect of caudal lobes (bilateral) • Right caudal lobe often more affected
Feline pulmonary oedema	• Random
Pulmonary emboli and infarcts	• Lung periphery
Acute respiratory distress syndrome	• Random
Metastatic neoplasia	• Random
Angiostrongylus vasorum infection	• Lung periphery

12.125 Preferential location of different alveolar lung diseases.

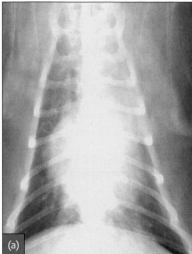
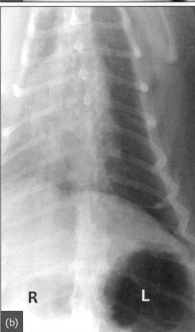

12.126 (a) VD thoracic radiograph (vertical beam orientation) of a 13-year-old Domestic Shorthaired cat obtained after the cat was under general anaesthesia in left lateral recumbency for 20 minutes. The left cranial lung lobe is collapsed with mild cardiac shift towards the left. (b) Immediate repeat VD thoracic radiograph with the cat in right lateral recumbency (horizontal beam orientation). The non-dependent left lung is now well aerated whereas the dependent right middle and caudal lobes are atelectatic under the weight of the heart (hypostatic lung collapse). L = left; R = right.

Atelectasis (collapse)

The Greek word ατελεκτασία stands for non-expansion of a terminal space. As a medical term, atelectasis is defined as an acute or chronic collapse or airless state of the whole lung or parts of it, caused by congenital or acquired conditions. This broad definition is synonymous with collapse and both terms are used in this book in this sense.

In the normal lung, surfactant maintains lung compliance and alveolar stability. The negative pleural pressure and surfactant prevent elastic recoil and lung lobe collapse. If either of these is missing, then the lung may collapse. There are different types of atelectasis:

- Passive atelectasis (Figures 12.126 and 12.127):
  - Occurs if extra-alveolar pressure moderately increases
  - Condition is non-obstructive: If pressure normalizes, reinflation is possible
  - Mild to moderate loss of volume and recoil
  - A common form is hypostatic collapse: dependent lung portion collapses under weight of non-dependent structures (particularly heart) if full lung capacity is not used. This is a physiological process
  - Examples: Mild pleural effusion or pneumothorax, prolonged unchanged recumbency (especially if anaesthetized)

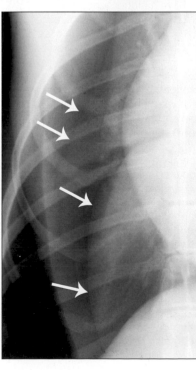

12.127 DV thoracic radiograph of a greyhound with a simple pneumothorax following trauma. There is passive collapse of all the lung lobes. Note how the collapsed lobes maintain their shape and collapse to a similar degree (arrowed). There is an increase in opacity within the atelectatic lung due to reduced aeration.

- Compression atelectasis (Figure 12.128)
  - Occurs if extra-alveolar pressure exceeds atmospheric pressure
  - Condition is non-obstructive: If pressure normalizes, reinflation is possible
  - Considerable loss of lung volume beyond recoil
  - Examples: Tension pneumothorax, large pleural effusion, large thoracic mass
- Resorption atelectasis (Figures 12.129 and 12.130)
  - Occurs if gas enters alveoli at a slower rate than it is removed
  - May be either obstructive or non-obstructive
  - Non-obstructive form: If oxygen replaces nitrogen as the predominant alveolar gas. Oxygen diffuses more readily into bloodstream leading to reduction in alveolar volume. This is a physiological process
  - Obstructive form: Resorption of alveolar gas following total bronchial obstruction
  - Examples: Supplemented oxygen inhalation (non-obstructive); bronchial foreign body, mass, plug (obstructive)
- Adhesive atelectasis
  - Occurs due to lack or destruction of surfactant. Surfactant normally diminishes surface tension allowing alveoli to inflate
  - Condition is non-obstructive: Major airways remain patent
  - Examples: Congenital atelectasis, pneumonia, acute respiratory distress syndrome (ARDS)
- Cicatrization atelectasis (Figure 12.131)
  - Occurs if fibrosis and scar formation of lung tissue reduces lung compliance
  - Condition is non-obstructive: Major airways remain patent
  - Examples: Idiopathic pulmonary fibrosis, chronic pneumonia, adhesive pleuritis.

The degree and location of lung collapse depends on many factors, including:

- Pleural surface area:lung volume ratio:
  - Lobes/lung areas with a relatively large surface area and small volume have a higher tendency to collapse, e.g. right middle lobe, lobe apices
- The caudal lobes have a low pleural surface area:lung volume ratio and more collateral ventilation, so are unlikely to collapse
- Collateral ventilation:
  - Term used to describe aeration of the alveoli other than by direct airway connections
  - Major factor in preventing lobar collapse and allowing pulmonary reinflation after pneumonia. Also explains why a lobe may not collapse distal to a complete bronchial obstruction
  - Gas exchange occurs between lung segments via small pores and channels and airway anastomoses
  - 'Check valve' effect of pores of Kohn allows reinflation of collapsed lung areas during inspiration and prevents air escape during expiration
  - Collateral ventilation is particularly effective with large pressure differences, e.g. during coughing
  - But is ineffective with:
    - Small pressure differences
    - Pulmonary exudate and secretions obliterating pores and alveoli
    - High pleural surface:lung volume ratio
  - Collateral ventilation also promotes spread of infection throughout a lobe

- Gravitational effects:
  - Dependent lung areas always have a higher tendency to collapse
  - Non-physiological recumbency during medical procedures can put additional weight on dependent lungs (e.g. from heart, mediastinal structures) and promote collapse
- Tidal volume:
  - Reduced activity, particularly under sedation/anaesthesia and during prolonged medical procedures reduces airspace volume needed and promotes collapse
- Inhaled gases:
  - Oxygen supplementation promotes resorption atelectasis.

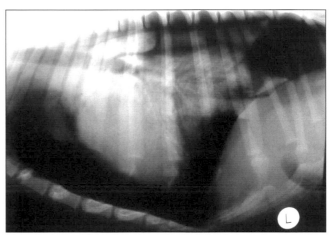

12.128 Lateral thoracic radiograph of a skeletally immature dog with a tension pneumothorax caused by a road traffic accident. The lung lobes are significantly reduced in size and are almost as opaque as other soft tissue structures in the image, indicating compression atelectasis.

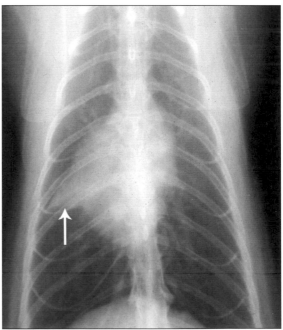

12.129 VD thoracic radiograph of a cat with chronic bronchial disease. The right middle lung lobe is collapsed and has an alveolar pattern (arrowed) probably due to obstruction of the bronchus (plug formation) and resorption of air from the affected lobe and a mild shift of the cardiac silhouette towards the right hemithorax. This is an example of obstructive resorption atelectasis, commonly seen in the right middle or cranial lobes in cats with bronchial disease.

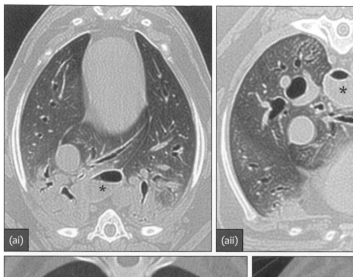

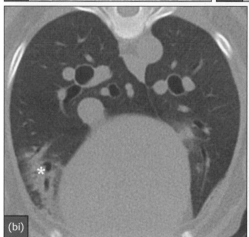

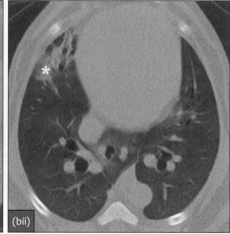

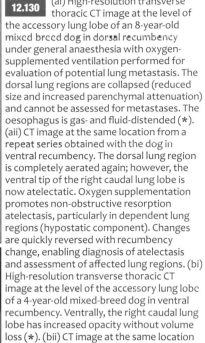

12.130 (ai) High-resolution transverse thoracic CT image at the level of the accessory lung lobe of an 8-year-old mixed breed dog in dorsal recumbency under general anaesthesia with oxygen-supplemented ventilation performed for evaluation of potential lung metastasis. The dorsal lung regions are collapsed (reduced size and increased parenchymal attenuation) and cannot be assessed for metastases. The oesophagus is gas- and fluid-distended (∗). (aii) CT image at the same location from a repeat series obtained with the dog in ventral recumbency. The dorsal lung region is completely aerated again; however, the ventral tip of the right caudal lung lobe is now atelectatic. Oxygen supplementation promotes non-obstructive resorption atelectasis, particularly in dependent lung regions (hypostatic component). Changes are quickly reversed with recumbency change, enabling diagnosis of atelectasis and assessment of affected lung regions. (bi) High-resolution transverse thoracic CT image at the level of the accessory lung lobe of a 4-year-old mixed-breed dog in ventral recumbency. Ventrally, the right caudal lung lobe has increased opacity without volume loss (∗). (bii) CT image at the same location from a repeat series obtained with the dog in dorsal recumbency. The area of lung opacification is unchanged. The final diagnosis was bacterial bronchopneumonia.

Radiography and CT findings: Radiographic and CT findings (see Figures 12.126–12.131) include:

- Affected lung volume is reduced
- Increased opacity with alveolar pattern
- Affected lung is triangular with broad base and apex to periphery
- Mediastinal shift and cranial displacement of the ipsilateral diaphragmatic crus on the DV or VD view
- Unaffected lobes may hyperinflate to compensate (non-specific sign)
- Narrowing of intercostal spaces on the affected side
- Displacement of interlobar fissures may be seen due to displacement of lobes adjacent to the atelectatic lobe
- Thin parts of the lung lobes are preferentially affected. Atelectasis is most common in the right middle lung lobe and ventral and cranial parts of the lungs
- In cases of chronic pleural effusion, fibrosis of the lung and pleura may prevent lung re-expansion following drainage. The atelectatic lung remains reduced in size and in some cases rounded
- Atelectasis of the right middle lobe is often present in cases of feline bronchial disease; other radiographic changes may be present.

Ultrasonography:

- Only gas-free lung directly adjacent to thoracic wall allows ultrasonographic assessment.
- Ultrasonography is, therefore, a good method for further investigation of lung that is radiographically collapsed or consolidated.

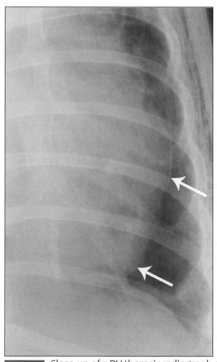

12.131 Close-up of a DV thoracic radiograph of an English Springer Spaniel following thoracocentesis (causing subcutaneous emphysema) for a chronic pyothorax. There is an iatrogenic pneumothorax, which contrasts with the pleural surface of the left caudal lung lobe. The lung has lost its normal shape and is rounded with increased opacity and thick pleura (arrowed). There is cicatrization atelectasis due to the thick pleura preventing lung re-expansion.

- Induction of hypostatic lung collapse is also useful to further investigate or allow ultrasound-guided fine-needle aspiration of a soft tissue lung lesion in proximity to the lung margin.
- Ultrasonographic technique:
  - Position animal with affected lung in dependent position for several minutes prior to scanning
  - Scan from underneath table (an echocardiology table is helpful) or rotate patient and scan immediately before reinflation occurs.

Ultrasonographic findings include (see also Chapter 2):

- Highly echogenic lung tissue
- Dispersed residual gas pockets
- Usually, no fluid bronchograms
- Reduced volume of affected lobe
- Sharp pointed or triangular margins are retained
- There is a gradual increase in reverberation in non-dependent position with physiological collapse, but not with pathophysiological collapse, consolidation or mass.

Relevance of atelectasis in the diagnostic imaging work-up: Atelectasis is a very common phenomenon that can occur within minutes of animal positioning during diagnostic imaging procedures. It is useful to be able to:

- Differentiate atelectasis from non-atelectatic alveolar lung diseases. The lobar shape and position, mediastinal and diaphragmatic shift should be evaluated. Lung volume is reduced in atelectasis, and normal or increased in non-collapsing alveolar diseases
- Differentiate between physiological and pathophysiological forms of atelectasis:
  - Progression and resolution of collapse: rapid onset and resolution in physiological collapse; chronic, non-reversible collapse in pathological forms of atelectasis
  - Gravitational effects. Obtain and assess radiographs in opposite recumbency and/or with manual inflation. Pathological collapse does not resolve in non-dependent position or inflated state
  - Tidal volume and inhaled gases. The patient should be assessed without general anaesthesia, sedation, prolonged recumbency or oxygen supplementation which all promote physiological atelectasis
- Avoid/reverse physiological atelectasis for radiographic/CT assessment of relevant lung areas (see Figures 12.126 and 12.130):
  - Prolonged unchanged recumbency prior to anaesthesia or sedation should be avoided
  - If the animal is anaesthetized, it should be positioned in ventral recumbency as soon as possible following induction
  - DV or VD radiographic views should be taken prior to lateral views
  - The recumbency of the patient can be reversed to assess affected lung areas
  - The lungs should be manually inflated
- Promote hypostatic lung collapse for pulmonary ultrasonography (see above).

Pulmonary oedema

Pulmonary oedema is defined as a pathological extra-vascular fluid accumulation in the lungs originating from pulmonary vessels. Direct aspiration is treated as a separate entity in this book. Oedema develops if interstitial fluid production exceeds the capacity of the pulmonary lymphatic drainage. Increased fluid accumulates initially within the interstitium and then extends into the alveolar spaces. There are four main mechanisms for its development:

- Permeability oedema:
  - Increased vascular permeability due to alveolar/capillary wall damage
  - High protein content oedema fluid
  - Normal vascular pressure
- Hydrostatic oedema:
  - Increased microvascular pressure
  - Low protein content oedema fluid
  - Volume overload of pulmonary vascular bed:
    - Left heart disease
    - Left-to-right shunt
    - Anuric renal failure
    - Excessive intravenous fluid therapy (hyperhydration). Commonly seen in cats
- Reduced capillary plasma oncotic pressure:
  - Due to severe hypoalbuminaemia
  - Low protein content oedema fluid
  - Rarely leads to pulmonary oedema in dogs and cats
  - Contributing factor with intravenous fluid therapy (haemodilution)
- Reduced lymphatic drainage:
  - Most likely due to neoplasia
  - Rarely leads to pulmonary oedema in dogs and cats.

In most diseases, there is a combination of mechanisms, with permeability and hydrostatic oedema as the most important factors (mixed oedema). Because of the clinical implications pulmonary oedema is often classified as cardiogenic or non-cardiogenic.

Cardiogenic pulmonary oedema (congestive heart failure): Primarily hydrostatic oedema is seen. It is one of the pathological processes in left-sided heart failure and occurs primarily because of increased vascular pressure due to backward left heart failure:

- With mitral regurgitation there is an increased volume of blood within the left ventricle and left atrium
- Elevated left atrial pressure causes increased pressure within the pulmonary veins
- This results in increased interstitial fluid production, which, if lymphatic drainage capacity is exceeded, leads to pulmonary oedema.

Aetiology includes:

- Mitral valve disease. Most common cause in small-breed dogs (myxomatous mitral valve degeneration)
- Cardiomyopathies. Common cause in large-breed dogs (dilated cardiomyopathy) and most common cause in cats (all forms)
- Left-to-right shunts (patent ductus arteriosus, ventricular septal defect)
- High-output states (hyperthyroidism, anaemia, etc.) (rare).

Cardiovascular diseases causing pressure overload (aortic stenosis, systemic hypertension) do not commonly induce left-sided heart failure.

Radiography: Findings with untreated hydrostatic pulmonary oedema (Figure 12.132) include:

- Initially an unstructured interstitial pattern, progressing to an alveolar pattern
- Pulmonary vascular distention, particularly venous (inconsistently seen)
- Left-sided cardiomegaly common in cardiogenic oedema
- Normal heart size in hyperhydration, some left heart diseases (bacterial endocarditis, chordae tendinae rupture, myocarditis), traumatic chordae tendinae rupture and mitral valve prolapse
- Gas-distended stomach from aerophagia if very dyspnoeic
- Right caudal lung lobe may be more severely affected than other lobes
- Individual lung lobes may be affected if their pulmonary vein is obstructed (e.g. with some cases of cor triatriatum sinister and anomalous pulmonary venous drainage)
- Oedema is labile and may change distribution within lungs with alteration in the animal's position.

Species differences

- In dogs, changes are centred on the perihilar region but extend to the periphery of the caudal lung lobes as severity increases. Ventral and peripheral areas are relatively spared, possibly due to greater lymphatic drainage than hilar regions. The changes are often symmetrical.
- In cats, expanding patchy alveolar lung areas are randomly located.

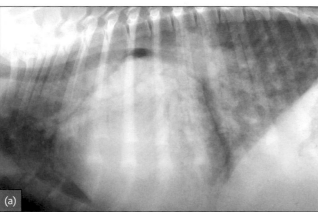

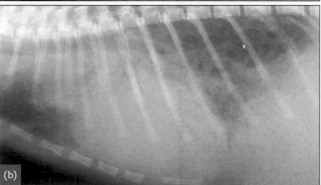

12.132 (a) Lateral thoracic radiograph of a 4-month-old German Shepherd Dog puppy with a patent ductus arteriosus (left-to-right shunting) and congestive heart failure. Note the typical perihilar distribution of the pulmonary oedema and enlargement of the pulmonary veins and arteries and cardiac silhouette. (b) Lateral thoracic radiograph of a kitten with a patent ductus arteriosus and pulmonary oedema. Pulmonary oedema in cats is more variable in distribution than in dogs.
(a, Courtesy of Cambridge Veterinary School)

Cardiogenic or hyperhydration-induced pulmonary oedema responds within a few hours to diuretic treatment (see Figure 12.124c). Imaging findings include:

- Pulmonary vessels return to a normal size
- Resolution of alveolar pattern
- Disappearance of interstitial pattern as a sign of complete oedema resolution.

Resolution of lung opacity does not always correlate well with normalization of vascular size. The administration of a diuretic, such as frusemide, may reduce pulmonary venous size before lung pattern resolution.

Other imaging techniques: Echocardiography may be used to identify the cause of the heart disease and assess cardiac function. CT shows soft tissue opacification of the lungs with a perivascular distribution (Figure 12.133).

Non-cardiogenic pulmonary oedema: This is primarily a permeability oedema. It is uncommon in dogs and rare in cats. There are three main aetiological subtypes:

- Neurogenic pulmonary oedema (Figures 12.134 and 12.135):
    - Working dogs undertaking strenuous exercise are the most affected. Male Swedish Drevers are over-represented with a familial trait
    - Head injuries and other causes of raised intracranial pressure
    - Seizures
    - Electric cord bite injury causing electric shock; mostly seen in young dogs
- Pulmonary oedema secondary to decreased interstitial tissue pressure (Figures 12.136 and 12.137):
    - Rare sequel to laryngeal paralysis or other forms of laryngeal obstruction or compression. Bulldogs are over-represented due to their high incidence of upper airway disease
    - Re-expansion pulmonary oedema is a rare sequel to rapid pleural draining of fluid or air. Occurs within 1–2 hours of re-expansion and resolves over a few days

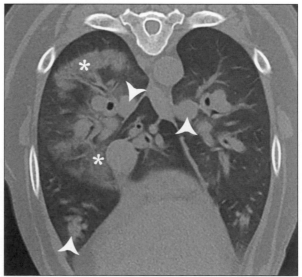

12.133 High-resolution transverse CT image of the caudal thorax of a 9-year-old Dalmatian with hypertrophic cardiomyopathy and secondary severe cardiogenic pulmonary oedema. Note the perivascular distribution of lung opacification (*) and pulmonary venous distention (arrowheads).

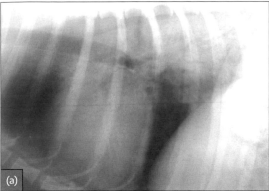

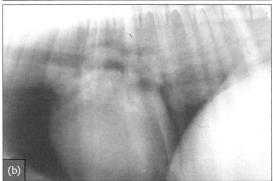

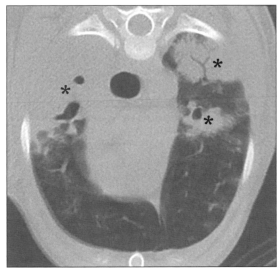

12.136 High-resolution transverse CT image of the mid-thorax of a 3-month-old Border Terrier with marked laryngeal oedema and secondary severe pulmonary oedema in the dorsal and caudal aspects of the lungs (∗). Note the perivascular distribution.

12.134 (a) Lateral thoracic radiograph of a 4-year-old mixed-breed dog with neurogenic pulmonary oedema following electrocution due to biting an electric cord. Notice the caudodorsal alveolar lung pattern, consistent with a non-cardiogenic form of pulmonary oedema. (b) Lateral thoracic radiograph of a dog with a history of strangulation. There is a caudodorsal interstitial to alveolar lung pattern.

- Pulmonary oedema due to direct toxic effects on capillary endothelium and alveolar epithelium
  - Severe viral or bacterial infection
  - Toxic inhalants: smoke, sulphur dioxide, toxic gases
  - Vascular toxins: snake venoms, endotoxins, kerosene
  - Vasoactive substances: kinins, prostaglandins, allergens

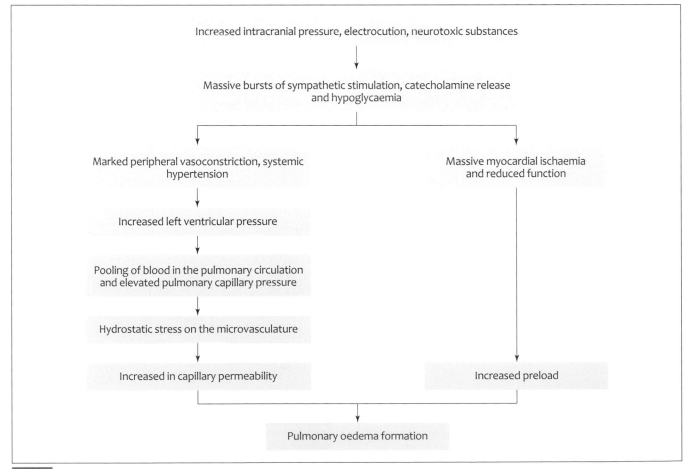

12.135 Suspected pathophysiology of neurogenic pulmonary oedema.

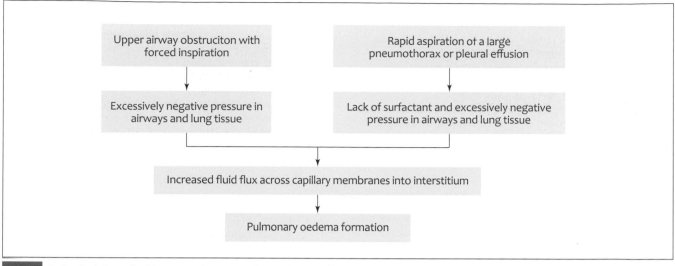

12.137 Pathophysiology of pulmonary oedema secondary to decreased interstitial tissue pressure.

- ARDS, fat embolism, uraemia
- Lung trauma
- Aspiration of acidic gastric content
- Hyperosmolar effect of aspirated salt water or ionic iodinated contrast media.

Radiography: Radiographic findings include:
- Increased lung opacity with predominantly alveolar pattern (see Figure 12.134)
- May be unstructured interstitial lung pattern in mild/early form
- Distribution:
  - Caudodorsal lung field
  - Additional perihilar location common, cranioventral rare
  - Diffuse in severe cases
  - Lung periphery in early/mild cases
  - Right lung usually more severely affected
- Rarely, complete lobar opacification with air bronchograms occurs (in contrast to pneumonia)
- In case of upper airway obstruction:
  - Dilated intrathoracic trachea

- Scalloping of intercostal spaces or small inspiratory volume
- Direct evidence of upper airway obstruction
- Gas-distended stomach (non-specific feature of dyspnoea).

Other imaging techniques: Head CT or MRI may be useful in patients with neurological signs. Respiratory CT may be used to differentiate pulmonary oedema from other alveolar diseases and identify upper airway obstruction. Laryngotracheal ultrasonography (echolaryngiography) allows assessment of upper airways. This technique does not require sedation or anaesthesia. It may show laryngeal paralysis or laryngeal masses/swelling; it is particularly useful in cases of laryngeal masses in cats and allows guided biopsy. Echocardiography may be used to rule out cardiogenic oedema.

Near drowning

Near drowning is defined as survival (at least temporarily) following asphyxia and/or aspiration while submerged in fluid and usually comes with a history of submersion (Figure 12.138).

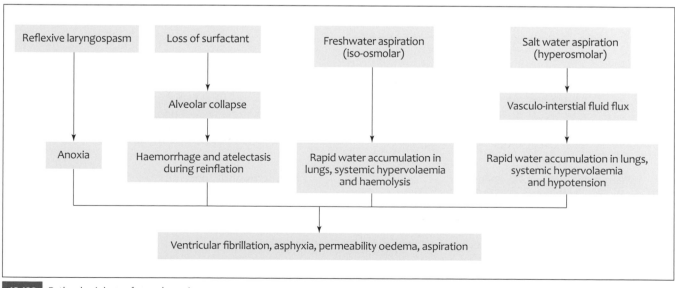

12.138 Pathophysiology of near drowning.

Radiography: Radiographic findings include (Figure 12.139):

- Increased lung opacity, preferentially caudal lobes
- Diffuse interstitial pattern to complete consolidation
- Right lung often more severely affected
- Sand bronchograms possible with submersion in sandy-bottomed rivers.

Radiographic abnormalities commonly occur or worsen between 3 and 24 hours post submersion. If radiographic abnormalities do not clear within 48 hours, secondary pneumonia should be suspected.

Smoke inhalation

This diagnosis is based upon history of exposure to fire or smoke (Figure 12.140). There is no breed, age or sex predisposition. There is a seasonal bias with increased incidence in winter months. Smoke inhalation results in a variety of pulmonary abnormalities:

- Clinical signs include stupor, coma, respiratory distress, coughing, epistaxis, ataxia, weakness, ptyalism, and ocular irritation

- Evidence of burns or smoke contamination of the skin
- Most animals have evidence of respiratory disease on clinical examination with a peak within 24 hours
- Cyanosis or hyperaemic mucous membranes may be present in some cases
- Secondary bronchopneumonia or ARDS is possible.

Radiography: There may be no radiographic abnormality (in approximately 25% of reported cases). Radiographic changes may not appear until 16–24 hours after insult (Figure 12.141). A reduced luminal gas column is seen with laryngeal oedema.

Species differences
- Dogs:
  - Random distribution
  - Alveolar pattern most common.
- Cats:
  - Predilection for cranial or middle lobes
  - Diffuse interstitial pattern or focal alveolar opacities.

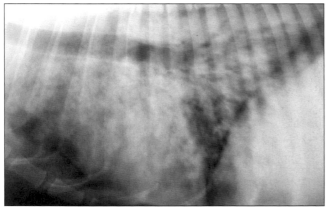

12.139 Lateral thoracic radiograph of a dog obtained 8 hours after a near-drowning accident in a river. The dog was able to walk home and became severely dyspnoeic several hours later. The lungs have a diffuse patchy alveolar pattern and slight dyspnoea-related movement blur.

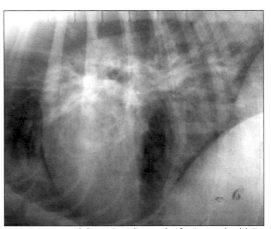

12.141 Lateral thoracic radiograph of a 6-month-old German Shepherd Dog that was rescued from a fire. The lungs have a patchy alveolar pattern, worse caudodorsally, consistent with smoke inhalation.

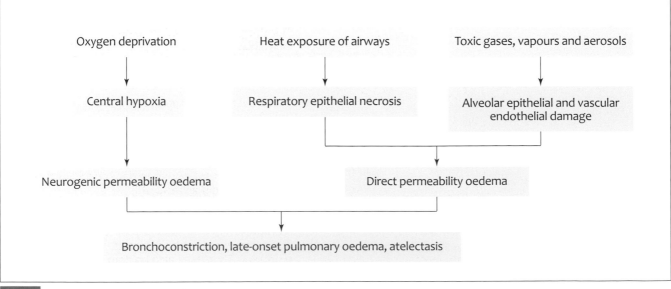

12.140 Pathophysiology of smoke inhalation.

Acute respiratory distress syndrome

ARDS is a human term defined as acute fulminating respiratory failure resulting from a variety of diseases leading to diffuse lung injury. It may also be called adult respiratory distress syndrome or shock lung.

ARDS is a subgroup of non-cardiogenic oedema. It is part of the systemic inflammatory response, leading to increased vascular permeability, pulmonary hypertension and airway constriction and obstruction. Inciting factors may be pulmonary (e.g. smoke inhalation, bacterial pneumonia) or non-pulmonary (e.g. endotoxaemia, pancreatitis, trauma, paraquat and other toxicities, fat embolism).

Histologically, ARDS is characterized by alveolar inflammation, oedema, haemorrhage, necrosis with formation of hyaline membranes or vascular congestion in conjunction with type 2 alveolar cell proliferation or interstitial fibrosis.

Clinical signs are acute onset of severe and progressive respiratory distress; in some cases signs are associated with an underlying cause (e.g. vomiting, trauma etc). Progressive tachypnoea and dyspnoea are seen in most animals with altered lung sounds.

Commonly reported underlying causes in dogs are:

- Bacterial pneumonia (which may be secondary to smoke inhalation or parasitic pneumonia)
- Sepsis and aspiration pneumonia
- Ventilator-acquired pneumonia
- Lung lobe torsion
- Non-pulmonary causes: gastric torsion, splenic torsion, trauma, laryngeal obstruction, pancreatitis, parvovirus infection, uraemia, disseminated intravascular coagulation (DIC), snake venom, drug toxicity
- Hyperoxia due to high inspired oxygen concentration (may result in lung injury similar to ARDS).

ARDS is possibly more common in younger dogs; no sex predisposition is reported. A familial form is suspected in young Dalmatians (<1 year old), some of which also have renal aplasia or hydrocephalus.

Radiography:

- May be normal in initial 24 hours.
- Diffuse interstitial ± alveolar lung pattern, affecting all lobes, is most common (Figure 12.142). Increasing severity with time, with air bronchograms visible by 36 hours after onset of lung injury.
- Opacities relatively slow to change due to high protein content of fluid within alveoli.
- Bilateral distribution.
- Pneumothorax and pneumomediastinum may occur in later stages.
- Radiographic signs associated with underlying cause may be present.
- In the familial form, pneumomediastinum and gastro-oesophageal intussusception are seen in the late stages of the disease. Radiographic changes are mixed alveolar, interstitial and peribronchial patterns.

Other imaging techniques: Abdominal ultrasonography or CT may identify source of sepsis.

Uraemic pneumonitis

Histopathological changes are like those of ARDS and uraemic pneumonitis may be part of this syndrome. The high protein content of the oedema fluid suggests permeability oedema due to toxic lung damage. Other factors are

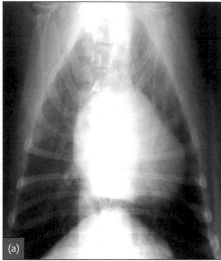

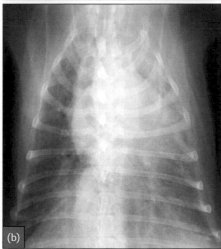

12.142 (a) VD thoracic radiograph of a 6-year-old Bernese Mountain Dog obtained 1 day after a road traffic accident resulting in multiple pelvic fractures and hindlimb injuries. The thorax is normal. (b) A repeat radiograph obtained 4 days later. There is progressive pulmonary opacification, particularly in the left lung, with a partial alveolar pattern. The dog had developed progressive systemic disease characterized by hyperthermia, immune-mediated haemolytic anaemia, erlichiosis, lymphadenopathy and metabolic acidosis, and was euthanized with a clinical diagnosis of ARDS.

also likely to play a role, e.g. reduced oncotic pressure and cardiovascular effects.

Clinical signs are related to severe renal disease (polyuria, polydipsia, anorexia, etc.) plus respiratory signs associated with oedema. Uraemic pneumonitis should be differentiated from other renal-induced respiratory diseases:

- Volume overload pulmonary oedema
- Thromboembolic disease.

Radiography:

- Pulmonary oedema within caudodorsal lobes may be associated with ARDS or non-cardiogenic oedema due to fluid overload (Figure 12.143).
- Abdominal radiographs may contain evidence of underlying renal disease.
- In cases of renal secondary hyperparathyroidism, mineralization of the blood vessels or myocardium may be present. There may also be demineralization of the skeleton.
- Chronic uraemia may lead to degeneration and calcification of connective tissue.

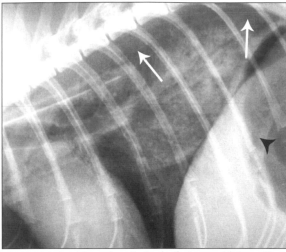

12.143 Lateral thoracic radiograph of a 5-year-old Domestic Shorthaired cat with terminal chronic renal failure. There is increased opacity with a partial alveolar pattern in the caudal lung lobes, aortic (arrowed) and gastric rugal (arrowhead) mineralization and gas distension of the stomach suggesting dyspnoea. Post-mortem examination confirmed chronic renal failure with extensive metastatic mineralization and uraemic pneumonitis.

Other imaging techniques:
- Renal ultrasonography is indicated to identify structural renal changes.
- Scintigraphy allows measurement of the glomerular filtration rate and quantification of severity of the renal disease.

Anomalous systemic arterial supply to the lungs

This is a congenital abnormality with an anomalous systemic arterial blood supply to the dorsal aspect of the caudal lung lobes (Figure 12.144).

- The condition is also called pulmonary sequestration.
- It results in reduced respiratory function of affected areas.
- It is visible in CT images in caudodorsal lung areas.
- It has been reported in dogs in 2.5% of a study population (Shimbo and Takiguchi, 2021).
- In humans, it can be associated with haemoptysis; not identified in affected dogs.
- It is most relevant for surgical planning to avoid interoperative systemic arterial bleeding.

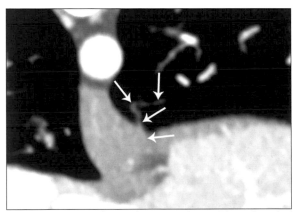

12.144 CT image of anomalous systemic arterial supply to the lung in a 3-year-old mixed-breed dog. A small vessel (arrowed) arising from a branch of the left gastric artery is supplying a small caudodorso-medial area in the left caudal lung lobe. Such vessels are occasionally seen in dogs and are incidental, except for surgical planning purposes.

Pulmonary vascular embolic events and lung infarction

Pulmonary arterial embolism can occur in dogs and cats due to:

- Thromboembolic disease
- Iatrogenic foreign material embolism and thrombosis, e.g. coil occlusion of patent ductus arteriosus and accidentally dislodged coils into pulmonary arteries, broken off intravascular catheter material
- Fat/bone marrow embolism due to trauma or bone marrow compressive surgery
- Septic emboli (vegetative endocarditis)
- Neoplastic vascular emboli
- High heartworm burden or broken off parts during attempted extraction.

Pulmonary venous embolism is uncommon in dogs and cats. Infarction is an uncommon sequel to embolic disease because:

- The lungs have an extensive collateral circulation
- Occlusion of central vessels results in ischaemia rather than infarction
- Infarcts typically occur in the lung periphery.

Consequences of infarction depend upon the size and the amount of lung affected:

- Small numbers of emboli may cause no clinical or radiographic changes (e.g. transient fat emboli seen during total hip replacement surgery)
- Large numbers of emboli can result in severe respiratory distress due to ventilation of non-perfused lung.

Infarction is reported more commonly in dogs than cats. Reported predisposing causes for infarction include amyloidosis, pancreatitis, immune-mediated haemolytic anaemia, hyperadrenocorticism, dirofilariasis, neoplasia (thromboembolism) and surgical intervention with bone marrow compression (fat embolism). Renal disease is the most commonly identified underlying cause. Clinical signs include acute onset dyspnoea. Septic emboli may lead to multiple abscessation or pneumonia. Neoplastic emboli may lead to atypical metastatic tumour seeding.

Radiography: Lungs are radiographically normal in most cases. Findings may include (Figures 12.145, 12.146, 12.147 and 12.148):

- Hyperlucent portion of lung with attenuation of vessel if pulmonary thromboembolism (PTE) occurs without infarction
- Distribution:
  - Caudodorsal lung fields most common, especially at costodiaphragmatic recess
  - A focal area of peripheral alveolar or interstitial lung pattern with a wedge shape (base towards hilus in large infarcts, apex towards hilus in small infarcts) is highly suggestive of infarction but is rare. The increased opacity extends to the pleural surface. Rarely, in severe cases, it may affect the entire lobe
  - Small areas of alveolar disease affecting multiple lobes (right lung more than left and caudal more than cranial) are the most common radiographic abnormality seen

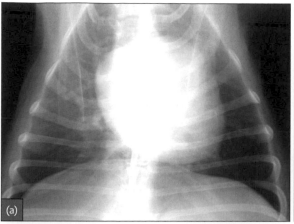

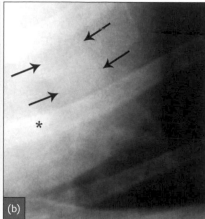

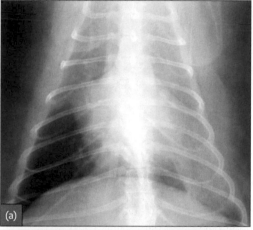

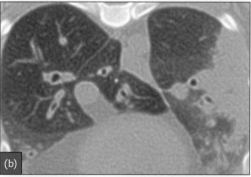

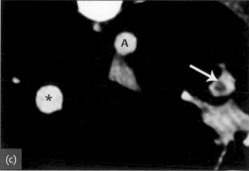

12.145 (a) A VD thoracic radiograph of an 8-year-old Irish Setter with sudden onset of dyspnoea. The left caudal lung lobe appears hyperlucent and less vascularized. (b) Close-up of the left caudal lung lobe. The lobar artery (between arrows) is distended cranial to and disappears at the level of the 9th rib (✱). These are classical, albeit rare, signs of pulmonary thrombo-embolism: a thrombus-distended pulmonary artery and tributary oligaemia.

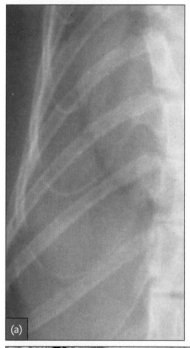

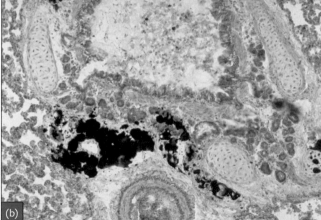

12.146 A 6-year-old Domestic Shorthaired cat with sudden onset of severe dyspnoea. (a) VD thoracic radiograph. There is increased opacity with a partial alveolar pattern in the left caudal lung lobe at the level of the costodiaphragmatic recess. (b) High-resolution transverse thoracic CT image at the level of the accessory lung lobe. The left caudal lung lobe has a wedge-shaped peripheral consolidation consistent with infarction. (c) A close-up of a pulmonary CT angiogram at the same level demonstrates contrast medium within the caudal vena cava (✱) and aorta (A) and a large filling defect (dark core) in the left caudal lobar pulmonary artery (arrowed) indicating an occlusive thrombus.

12.147 (a) Close-up of the right caudal lung lobe on a VD thoracic radiograph of a 1-year-old Domestic Shorthaired cat that had sustained a sudden respiratory arrest when an intramedullary pin was advanced into the humerus for a fracture repair. The radiograph was obtained during the resuscitation attempts, which ultimately failed. There is increased lung opacity with an alveolar pattern at the level of the right costodiaphragmatic recess. (b) Microscopic examination of the lungs (Oil Red O with Mayer's haemulum stain) confirmed a massive shower of occlusive fat emboli (stained red) throughout the pulmonary capillary bed and pulmonary fat embolism was established as the cause of death.
(Reprinted from Schwarz et al. (2001) with permission)

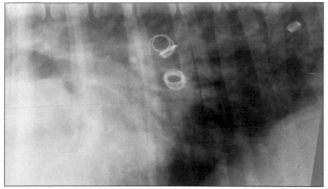

12.148 Caudal close-up of a lateral thoracic radiograph of a 4-year-old Labrador Retriever with a patent ductus arteriosus and left-to-right shunt, obtained during a coil embolization procedure. Three metallic coils have been dislodged into the caudal lung lobe arteries. Coils designed for human infants are commonly used in dogs, which typically have a wider ductus arteriosus. Due to the well developed collateral circulation, dislodged coils are usually of no clinical consequence. The ductus arteriosus was eventually successfully occluded.

- May see absence or attenuation of pulmonary artery, but may be obscured by the alveolar infiltrate
- Mild to moderate pleural fluid is often present
- Iatrogenically dislodged foreign bodies are usually in caudal lobar arteries
- Cardiac changes are uncommon but may include right ventricular or pulmonary artery enlargement
- In some cases, signs associated with underlying disease are seen.

Contrast studies: Selective pulmonary arteriography may be used. Infarction shows failure of opacification or filling defects within the affected blood vessels. Requires general anaesthesia and ideally fluoroscopy.

Other imaging techniques:
- Echocardiography allows diagnosis of:
  - Pulmonic trunk (main pulmonary artery) thrombosis
  - Pulmonic valve insufficiency or tricuspid regurgitation secondary to pulmonary hypertension (Doppler echocardiography)
  - Embolic showers during bone marrow compressing surgery (e.g. total hip replacement) (monitoring device).
- CT (Figure 12.149; see also Figure 12.146):
  - High-resolution lung CT is used to identify pulmonary infarction and neoplastic subpleural infiltrate
  - CT angiography can be used to identify vascular emboli.
- Scintigraphic ventilation and perfusion scans (see Chapter 5): a normal ventilation scan with a deficit in the perfusion scan is diagnostic for pulmonary thromboembolism.

Pulmonary haemorrhage

Most cases are associated with coagulopathies or trauma. Rodenticide poisoning (coumarin derivatives) is the most common cause of severe pulmonary haemorrhage; outdoor cats and dogs are at risk. Other causes include:

- DIC
- Trauma
- *Angiostrongylus* infection (dogs)
- Other coagulopathies
- Neoplasia (usually mass-related signs predominate).

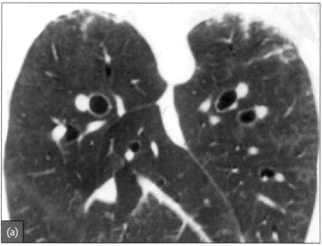
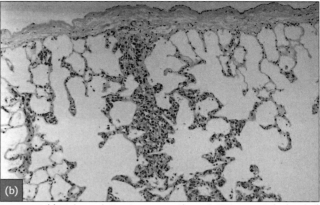

12.149 (a) High-resolution transverse thoracic CT image at the level of the accessory lung lobe of an 8-year-old Hungarian Vizsla with pyrexia and carcinomatous infiltrate in a peripheral lymph node. The dorsal aspects of both caudal lung lobes have a frond-like subpleural infiltrate. (b) Microscopic examination of one corresponding lung area (H&E stain) reveals a matching neoplastic capillary and interstitial subpleural infiltrate. Final diagnosis on post-mortem examination was adrenal carcinoma and pulmonary carcinosis.
(Reprinted from Johnson *et al.* (2004) with permission)

Clinical signs include:

- Generalized blood loss (weakness, bruising, haematochezia, haematuria)
- Respiratory bleeding (cough, dyspnoea, haemoptysis)
- Upper airway obstruction.

Thoracic changes may include haemorrhage of the mediastinum, pleura and tracheobronchial airways.

Radiography: Radiographic abnormalities include:
- Generalized patchy interstitial/alveolar pattern with random distribution
- Possible pleural or mediastinal haemorrhage
- Tracheal narrowing due to submucosal/mucosal haemorrhage or extratracheal haematoma with narrowing of tracheal lumen – often generalized.

The combination of tracheal narrowing with pleural and mediastinal fluid and lung changes is suggestive of anticoagulant toxicity (Figure 12.150). Thoracic changes due to coumarin toxicity should resolve within 1–5 days of starting therapy. Haemorrhage due to *Angiostrongylus vasorum* infection usually also has radiographic changes of parasitic pneumonia. The pattern is classically peripherally distributed.

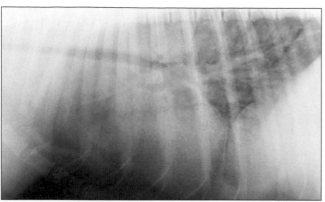

12.150 Lateral thoracic radiograph of a Labrador Retriever with coagulopathy due to warfarin toxicity. Note the tracheal narrowing, pleural fluid and partial alveolar lung pattern. This combination is highly suggestive of coumarin toxicity.
(Courtesy of Cambridge Veterinary School)

Pulmonary contusion and laceration

Blunt external thoracic trauma is the most common cause of traumatic lung changes in dogs and cats, commonly seen in road traffic accidents and with high-rise syndrome (Figure 12.151).

Blunt internal thoracic trauma (barotrauma) is a relatively common cause of lung laceration in cats; for example, following iatrogenic manual or automated hyperinflation of lungs during anaesthesia. It can cause pneumomediastinum, pneumo- or haemothorax, but does not cause widespread contusion.

Perforating lung injuries are uncommon in dogs or cats:

- External: bite, gunshot, stab wound, iatrogenic laceration during fine-needle lung aspiration or biopsy
- Internal: intubation injury, penetrating bronchial or oesophageal foreign body or instrument.

Perforating lung injuries can cause pneumomediastinum, pneumo- or haemothorax; there is usually a local area of pulmonary haemorrhage.

Radiography: Radiographic findings include (Figure 12.152):

- Contusion:
  - Consolidated lung lobe(s), usually ipsilateral to impact
  - Patchy alveolar opacity in mild or resolving contusion
  - Rounded lung margins
  - Enlarged lobes causing mediastinal shift
- Rib fractures and thoracic body wall swelling
- Traumatic gas- or blood-filled bullae (pneumato- and haematocoeles)
- Free pleural or mediastinal gas or fluid.

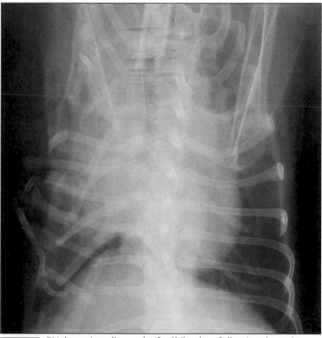

12.152 DV thoracic radiograph of a Chihuahua following thoracic trauma. There are multiple right rib fractures. The right lung is consolidated and causes a cardiac shift towards the left. Lung contusion is usually adjacent to the site of blunt impact.
(Courtesy of Cambridge Veterinary School)

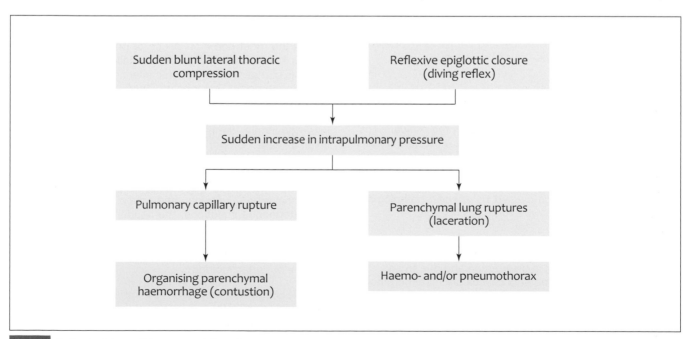

12.151 Pathophysiology of blunt external thoracic trauma.

Contrast studies: These should be used if necessary for confirmation of a suspect diaphragmatic hernia (in cases of trauma). Positive-contrast gastrointestinal studies or peritoneography may be used to identify loss of diaphragmatic integrity.

Other imaging techniques: Abdominal radiography or CT should be performed in cases of suspected trauma. Thoracic ultrasonography may be used to differentiate mediastinal fluid from mediastinal masses and for evaluation of diaphragmatic integrity. Thoracic CT is generally more sensitive for trauma and can better characterize the type and extent of injuries.

Pulmonary alveolar microlithiasis (pumice stone lung)

This is a condition with widespread mineralized concretion within the alveolar lumen reported in humans, dogs and other animals. Inflammatory changes may be present. The aetiology is unknown.

Despite its marked radiographic manifestation at an early stage, the clinical onset is insidious and progresses very slowly. Cardiorespiratory signs range from completely absent or harsh lung sounds to pulmonary insufficiency and cor pulmonale. The term 'pumice stone lung' relates to the post-mortem appearance of the lung, which is stone hard and requires a saw for sectioning.

Radiography: There is marked widespread micronodular mineralization in all lung lobes, tapering towards the lung periphery (Figure 12.153). There is slow progression of radiographic signs over time. Differential diagnoses should include:

- Incidental pulmonary osteoma and mineralized granulomas, which are fewer and bigger (2–4 mm)
- Bronchial microlithiasis is seen in cats. Concretions are intrabronchial, fewer and larger (2–4 mm) (see 'Bronchial microlithiasis', above)
- Metastatic mineralization due to neoplastic, metabolic (hyperadrenocorticism) or inflammatory conditions (uraemic pneumonitis) usually result in an interstitial lung pattern
- Incompletely resorbed barium aspiration is usually more localized (ventral: right middle and cranial lung lobes).

Pneumonia

Pneumonia is inflammation of the alveolar parenchyma, and the term has been used to describe acute and exudative inflammation. Regardless of the aetiology, the clinical signs and radiographic features of pneumonia are often similar. In this chapter pneumonias are classified first according to the initial site of involvement and the spread of infection, which can be documented radiographically. The characteristic radiographic findings caused by specific pathological agents are discussed following this classification.

- Bronchopneumonia originates at the bronchoalveolar junction. Often acute in onset and infectious in origin. Usually, cranioventral in distribution and due to an aerogenous origin. Bacterial causes are most common, often secondary to other lung insult, and result in suppurative pneumonia.
- Lobar pneumonia: the entire lobe is affected, usually due to fulminating bronchopneumonia, less commonly due to a tracheobronchial foreign body.

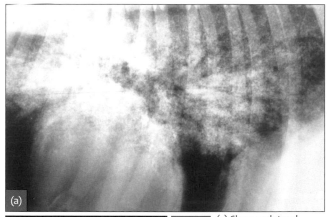

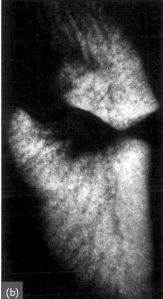

12.153 (a) Close-up lateral thoracic radiograph of a 10-year-old Labrador Retriever with pulmonary alveolar microlithiasis. The dog had harsh lung sounds but otherwise no cardiorespiratory abnormality. Notice the widespread micronodular mineralization, which is most pronounced in the perihilar region. (b) Post-mortem radiograph of the right lung. The lung was solidly mineralized and had to be sectioned with a saw. Cause of euthanasia was severe chronic hip and elbow arthritis and unrelated to cardiorespiratory disease.
(Reproduced from O'Neill *et al.* (2006) with permission)

- Interstitial pneumonia: huge variety of causes and probably under-recognized. Predominantly interstitial pattern with viral infection and chronic inflammatory diseases.

Non-specific canine bacterial pneumonia

This is the most common cause of pneumonia and often develops as a secondary infection following primary lung insult (e.g. haemorrhage, viral infection). Research suggests a complex relationship between viral respiratory disease, environmental factors and developmental of bacterial infection in dogs. In cats, bacterial pneumonia is less commonly identified than inflammatory feline bronchial disease. Bronchopneumonia is the most common manifestation and is thought to be due to an aerogenous infection. The cranial and middle lung lobes are preferentially affected due to the inherent vulnerability of the bronchoalveolar junction and gravitational effects. In haematogenous infections, the caudal lung lobes may be more severely affected. Involvement of the entire lobe is often seen as extensive collateral ventilation allows rapid spread of infection (lobar pneumonia). Clinical signs are variable but often include:

- Soft cough with increased respiratory effort
- Anorexia and lethargy
- Pyrexia is variably present
- Clinical signs of an underlying cause, e.g. regurgitation, dysphagia.

Animals with impaired immune systems or mucociliary clearance (e.g. ciliary dyskinesia) are predisposed. Irish Wolfhounds and brachycephalic dogs are also predisposed.

Radiography: A three-view study is very useful to assess all lung areas and differentiate alveolar disease from collapse. In cases of collapse, the lung volume will decrease with associated mediastinal shift visible on the VD view, while in pneumonia, the lung volume will be preserved. The radiographs may be normal (or just have an interstitial pattern) in the early stages. Changes often start in the tip of the lobes. Findings include:

- Alveolar pattern, often affecting the entire lobe (lobar pneumonia) (Figure 12.154)
- Ventral location is most common
- Patchy peribronchial areas in bronchopneumonia (Figure 12.155)
- Predominately cranial and middle lobes affected
- Asymmetrical distribution is common
- Variable bronchial component but normally present (Figures 12.155 and 12.156)

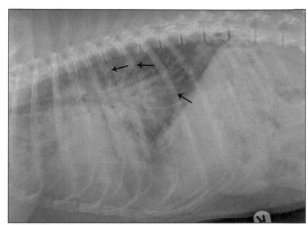

12.155 Lateral thoracic radiograph of a 6-year-old Labrador Retriever with severe cough and lethargy. Note the severe alveolar pattern obliterating the cardiac silhouette and extending to the cranial and caudal lung lobes; also note the peribronchial component with increased peribronchial infiltrate (arrowed). Bronchopneumonia was diagnosed on bronchoalveolar lavage.

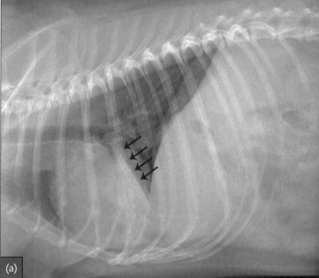

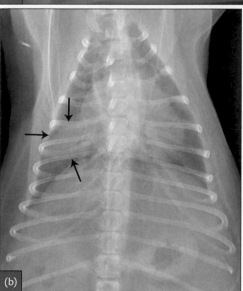

12.154 (a) Lateral and (b) DV thoracic radiographs of a 5-year-old crossbreed dog with cough and pyrexia. Note the lobar sign, air bronchogram and consolidation of the right middle lung lobe (arrowed). Bacterial pneumonia was diagnosed on bronchoalveolar lavage.

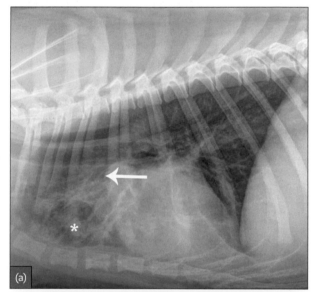

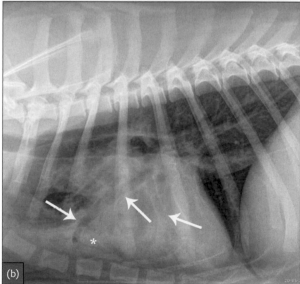

12.156 (a) Left and (b) right lateral thoracic radiographs of a 6-year-old Bernese Mountain Dog with severe coughing. Note the cranioventral alveolar pattern (*) with peribronchial infiltrate and bronchiectasis (arrowed); bronchopneumonia and bronchiectasis were diagnosed.

- In bacterial pneumonia, secondary to haematogenous infection, there may be a generalized miliary or nodular pattern or septic infarction
- Small volume of pleural fluid or thick pleurae in severe cases
- After recovery, a mild bronchial pattern often remains
- Abscess formation with a cavitating lung lesion is occasionally seen
- If there is necrosis of the lung, spontaneous pneumothorax may occur
- Ciliary dyskinesia often results in bronchiectasis, and situs inversus may be seen (right-to-left transposition of thoracic and abdominal viscera).

Other imaging techniques:

Ciliary dyskinesia: Scintigraphy to demonstrate lack of mucociliary clearance.

Lung consolidation: For lung consolidation (and abscessation) thoracic ultrasonography may be used. Findings include:

- Homogeneous, mid to low echogenic lung with often small areas of gas with reverberation artefacts (Figure 12.157)
- The lung may be mildly enlarged with rounded borders as seen with lung lobe torsion
- Fluid bronchograms may be seen with branching anechoic fluid-filled bronchi. Doppler ultrasonography helps differentiate fluid bronchograms from blood vessels
- Abscesses may be identified.

Aspirates can be obtained for culture and sensitivity. It should be noted that consolidated lung may mimic the appearance of the liver, especially when large fluid bronchograms are present. Care should be taken not to misdiagnose liver herniation. CT (high-resolution, contrast-enhanced) may be used for the diagnosis of lung abscessation, interstitial pneumonia and differentiation from other lung diseases (Figures 12.158 and 12.159).

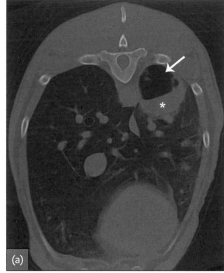

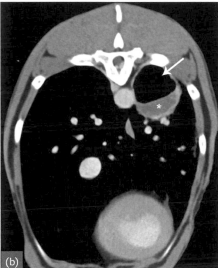

12.158 (a) High-resolution lung window and (b) post-contrast transverse thoracic CT images of a 3-year-old Golden Retriever with a lung abscess. Note the gas-filled cavity in the dorsal aspect of the left caudal lung lobe (arrowed) and the non-enhancing fluid (∗).

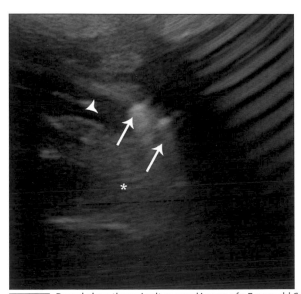

12.157 Dorsal plane thoracic ultrasound image of a 7-year-old Golden Retriever with lobar pneumonia. Note the consolidated right middle lung lobe (∗) with gas bubble and associated reverberation artefact (arrowed); also note the tubular structure (arrowhead) representing a bronchus.

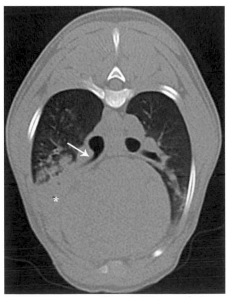

12.159 Transverse thoracic CT image of a 7-year-old crossbreed dog with lobar pneumonia (high-resolution lung window). Note the right middle bronchus (arrowed) and the consolidated right middle lung lobe (∗).

Non-specific feline pneumonia

Pneumonia occurs less commonly in cats than in dogs. Clinical signs include coughing, increased tracheal sensitivity, dyspnoea and tachypnoea. Coughing may be absent. Males are possibly predisposed. A variety of infectious agents have been recorded but the most common are *Pasteurella multocida*, *Escherichia coli*, *Klebsiella pneumoniae*, *Bordetella bronchiseptica*, *Salmonella* spp., and eugonic fermenter-4 infection.

Radiography: Radiographic findings include:

* May have a granular appearance in the early stages with peribronchial spread
* Bronchial pattern in combination with alveolar disease is most common
* Right middle and cranial lobes most affected, often lobar signs (Figure 12.160)
* Nodular pattern may be seen with toxoplasmosis, mycoplasmosis, cryptococcosis and eugonic fermenter-4 infection (Figure 12.161)
* *Pasteurella* infection often causes abscessation.

Aspiration pneumonia

This is caused by pulmonary intake of large particles or fluid. Aspiration of small quantities of oral contents is common and does not cause problems if there are normal respiratory defence mechanisms. Barium is commonly

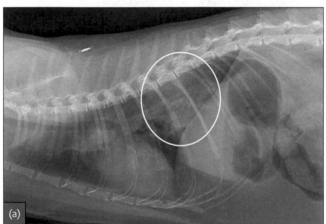
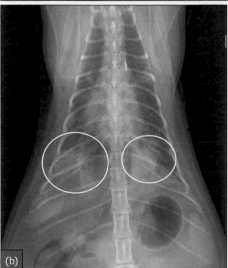

12.160 (a) Lateral and (b) DV thoracic radiographs of a 4-year-old Domestic Shorthaired cat with mycoplasmosis. Note the patchy alveolar pattern in the right and left caudal lung lobes with lobar sign (circled).

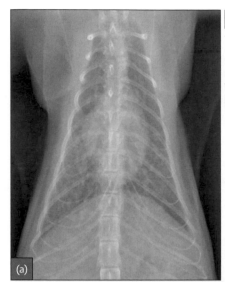

12.161 (a) DV and (b) lateral thoracic radiographs of an 8 year old Domestic Shorthaired cat with mycoplasmosis. Note the widespread nodular pattern involving both lungs.

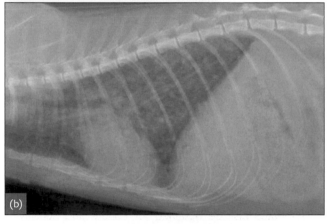

aspirated if orally fed for alimentary contrast studies; small to medium amounts are well tolerated by animals, but resorption by tributary lymph nodes can take months to years.

With defective mucociliary clearance, immunodeficiency or aspiration of large quantities of infective material, aspiration pneumonia may develop. Gastric contents cause chemical damage to the airways and resultant airway constriction and oedema. This may be followed by secondary bacterial infection and development of ARDS. Airway obstruction or constriction may occur.

Aspiration usually affects the cranioventral aspect of the lungs unless the animal aspirated while anaesthetized or recumbent, when any part of the lung may be affected. Aspiration is common with any condition causing mega-oesophagus or dysphagia and occurs most often in the right middle lobe. Clinical signs include:

* Acute dyspnoea within 2 hours of aspiration; may be longer if particulate material, e.g. food
* Coughing, tachypnoea, wheezing and cyanosis.

Chronic tracheobronchial foreign bodies may lead to lobar pneumonia, due to occlusion of the bronchus and secondary bacterial infection.

* Caudal and middle lobes are most affected.
* Grass awns are the commonest inhaled foreign body in dogs, usually in summer/autumn.
* Large-breed and working dogs are predisposed.
* Clinical signs of acute onset coughing after running in vegetation.

Radiography: Radiographs are normal in the initial stages but develop abnormalities within 12–36 hours. In cases of particulate aspiration, radiographic changes may take longer to appear and disappear. The gravity-dependent lung at the time of aspiration is predominantly affected. Cranioventral parts of the cranial and middle lobes are most affected, often with lobar opacification (Figures 12.162 and 12.163). Signs of the underlying condition may be seen, especially with oesophageal disease (Figure 12.164). A combination of aspiration pneumonia, mega-oesophagus and cranial mediastinal mass may be seen in thymoma and may be reversible if the tumour can be treated successfully.

Other imaging techniques:

- Barium contrast oesophagraphy to identify oesophageal diseases causing aspiration. Barium aspiration may further aggravate lung disease.
- Fluoroscopic barium contrast study to demonstrate the functional abnormalities of swallowing.
- Thoracic CT for bronchial obstruction and bronchiectasis (Figure 12.165).
- Head CT or MRI for suspected central nervous cause of reduced gag reflex.

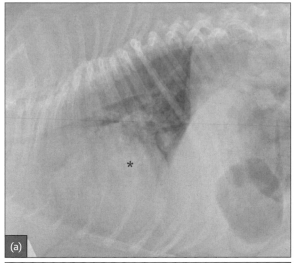

(a)

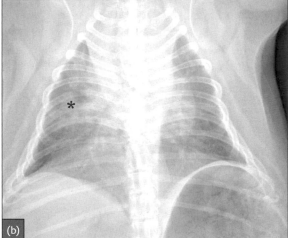

(b)

12.163 (a) Lateral and (b) DV thoracic radiographs of a 3-year-old French Bulldog with aspiration pneumonia. Note the ill-defined alveolar pattern (∗) with air bronchogram involving the right middle lung lobe.

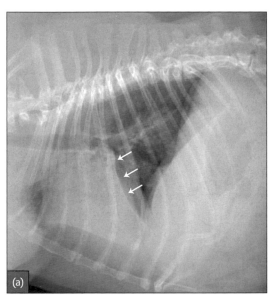

(a)

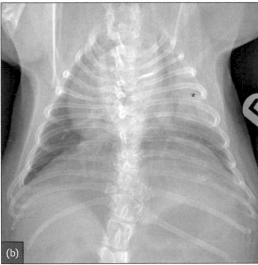

(b)

12.162 (a) Lateral and (b) DV thoracic radiographs of a 5-year-old English Bulldog with aspiration pneumonia. Note the consolidation (∗) with air bronchogram of the left cranial lung lobe and the lobar sign (arrowed).

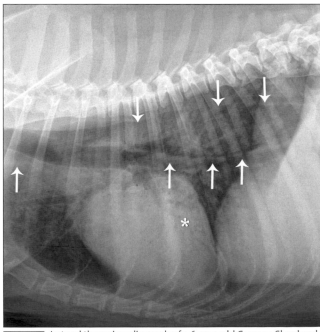

12.164 Lateral thoracic radiograph of a 6-year-old German Shepherd Dog with megaoesophagus and aspiration pneumonia. Note the generalized oesophageal enlargement with gas distension (arrowed) and the cranioventral alveolar pattern (∗).

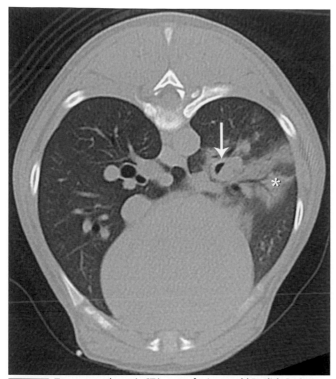

12.165 Transverse thoracic CT image of a 4-year-old English Springer Spaniel with a bronchial foreign body (grass awn) (high-resolution lung window). Note the distended and fluid filled bronchus (arrowed) and consolidation (*) secondary to the foreign body pneumonia induced.

Canine leptospiral pneumonia

Clinical signs relate to acute renal failure rather than pulmonary involvement.

Radiography: A mild to severe unstructured or finely structured interstitial pattern is seen, most noticeable in the caudodorsal lung field, or disseminated patchy opacities (Figure 12.166). In severe cases there may be a generalized increase in opacity in all lobes.

Other imaging techniques: Renal ultrasonography may be used to demonstrate increased renal cortical echogenicity, subcapsular fluid and an echogenic medullary band.

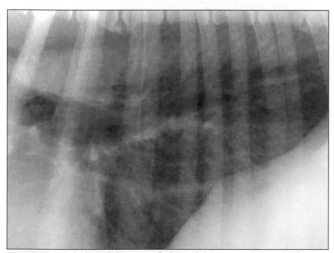

12.166 Caudodorsal close-up of a lateral thoracic radiograph of a dog with leptospiral pneumonia. There is a mild increase in lung opacity with a fine-structured interstitial pattern, typical of mild or early-phase leptospirosis.

Mycoplasmal pneumonia

Mycoplasma spp. are small bacteria that are part of the normal oral flora in dogs and cats. Among other bacteria, *Mycoplasma* may be involved in lower airway and lung disease. Immunodeficient or otherwise compromised animals are predisposed to mycoplasmal disease.

Radiography: A diffuse bronchointerstitial pattern is seen (Figure 12.167; see also Figures 12.160 and 12.161). An alveolar component is less common.

Viral pneumonia

Common pneumonia-inducing viruses include:

- Dogs: canine distemper virus, canine adenovirus 2, canine parainfluenza
- Cats: feline calicivirus.

Young, unvaccinated or immunocompromised animals are most affected. Clinical signs include pyrexia, coughing and oculonasal discharge. Thoracic involvement with feline coronavirus infection, which causes feline infectious peritonitis, usually presents as pleural effusion rather than lung disease.

Radiography: Radiographic findings include:

- Radiographs may be normal
- Mild diffuse interstitial lung pattern, often in the caudodorsal lung field (Figure 12.168)
- In severe cases, an alveolar lung pattern
- Peribronchial cuffing, if there is secondary bacterial infection; the radiographic signs resemble those seen with bacterial and aspiration pneumonia.

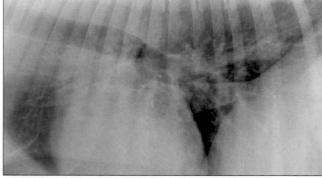

12.167 Lateral thoracic radiograph of a 9-year-old mixed-breed dog with mycoplasmal pneumonia. There is a diffuse bronchointerstitial lung pattern throughout the lungs.

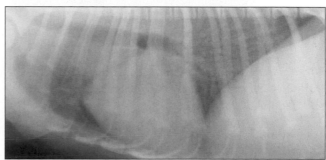

12.168 Lateral thoracic radiograph of a 7-month-old Chihuahua with canine distemper virus infection. There is a diffuse increase in lung opacity with an interstitial pattern, more pronounced caudodorsally. This feature is representative of an early viral stage of pneumonia. Bacterial secondary infection will add a patchy alveolar pattern with a random or ventral distribution.
(Courtesy of the University of California Davis)

Fungal pneumonia

Dimorphic fungi (fungi that can exist as mould or yeast) have a relatively well defined geographical distribution due to their specific growth requirements (Figure 12.169). Species include:

- *Histoplasma capsulatum*
- *Blastomyces dermatitidis*
- *Coccidioides immitis*.

Yeast species, e.g. *Cryptococcus neoformans*, have a worldwide distribution. Infection occurs due to inhalation of fungal particles in most cases. Dimorphic fungi convert from the mycelial to the parasitic phase at body temperature and can cause primary infection in the lungs and mediastinal lymph nodes. Failure of the immune system to contain infection can lead to disseminated disease.

Histoplasmosis: This is caused by *Histoplasma capsulatum*. It affects dogs and cats, most commonly less than 4 years old. In dogs there is usually gastrointestinal involvement; in cats there is usually pulmonary involvement. The fungus requires a humid environment and has a wide distribution throughout temperate and tropical regions of the world; in the USA it is found in the drainage system of the Ohio, Missouri and Mississippi rivers (midwestern states).

Clinical signs are often absent, but may include coughing, dyspnoea, weight loss, lethargy and fluctuating fever. Thoracic radiographic findings (Figure 12.170) include:

- Active phase: diffuse interstitial lung pattern and/or areas of coalescing opacities
- Chronic/healed phase: numerous 2–4 mm soft tissue or mineralized nodules; tracheobronchial lymphadenopathy and mineralization

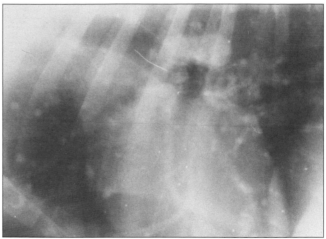

12.170 Lateral thoracic radiograph of a dog with chronic inactive histoplasmosis. The lungs have numerous small, randomly distributed, mineralized nodules (calcified granulomas). The left tracheobronchial lymph node is moderately enlarged and mineralized.

- Disseminated form: polyostotic aggressive bone lesions are the most obvious radiographic feature.

Blastomycosis: This is caused by *Blastomyces dermatitidis*. It is common in dogs and uncommon in cats; most often seen in animals less than 4 years old. It is endemic in south-eastern and eastern parts of the USA and south-eastern Canada.

Routes of infection and primary focus include:

- Direct skin inoculation
- Inhalation and primary pulmonary form
- Dissemination to abdomen, skeleton and central nervous system is possible.

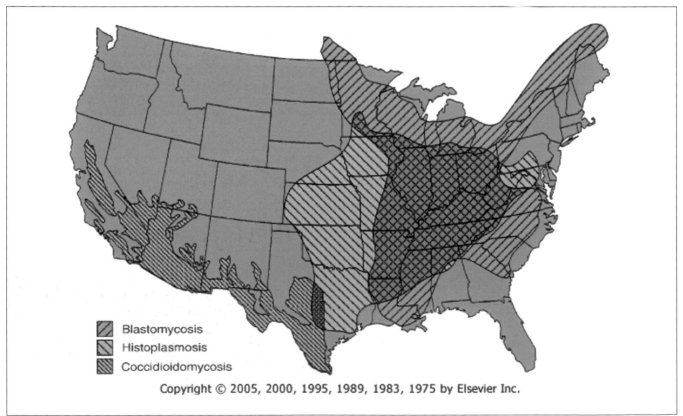

Blastomycosis
Histoplasmosis
Coccidioidomycosis

Copyright © 2005, 2000, 1995, 1989, 1983, 1975 by Elsevier Inc.

12.169 Major endemic areas for blastomycosis, coccidioidomycosis and histoplasmosis in the USA.
(Reproduced from Wolf and Troy (1989) with permission)

Clinical signs of the primary pulmonary form include dyspnoea, tachypnoea, coughing, fever, anorexia and weight loss. Thoracic radiographic findings are highly variable (Figure 12.171) and include:

- Active phase:
  - Miliary or mixed patterns
  - Focal lung nodule/mass/consolidation
  - Pleural effusion
  - Tracheobronchial lymphadenopathy is common
- Chronic/healed phase: tracheobronchial lymphadenopathy possible; numerous non-mineralized nodules
- Disseminated form: polyostotic aggressive bone lesions are the most obvious radiographic feature.

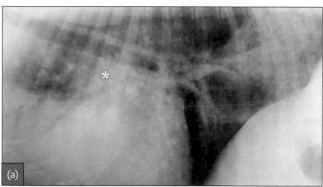

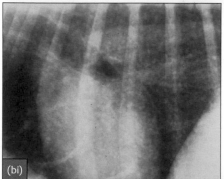

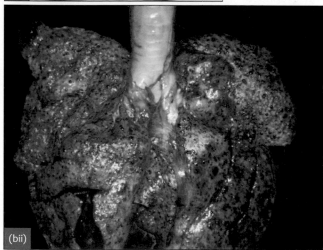

12.171 (a) Lateral thoracic radiograph of a 3-year-old Golden Retriever with active pulmonary blastomycosis. There is alveolar disease cranioventrally and caudodorsally, numerous 2–4 mm soft tissue nodules throughout the lung, and a mild dorsal deviation of the thoracic trachea and an associated soft tissue opacity (*) suggestive of cranial mediastinal lymphadenopathy. (bi) Lateral thoracic radiograph of a dog with active diffuse pulmonary blastomycosis. There is a miliary pattern throughout the lungs created by many small soft tissue nodules. (bii) Corresponding post-mortem photograph with multiple small pulmonary granulomas.
((a) Courtesy of the University of California Davis; (b) Courtesy of the University of Pennsylvania)

Coccidioidomycosis: This is caused by *Coccidioides immitis*. It is common in dogs and rare in cats. The fungus requires semi-arid conditions and is endemic in southwest and western regions of the USA, and widespread in parts of Mexico, Central and South America.

Routes of infection and primary focus include:

- Direct skin inoculation (very rare)
- Inhalation and primary pulmonary form
- Dissemination to abdomen, skeleton and central nervous system is possible.

The primary pulmonary form often has no clinical signs (subclinical and self-limiting). There may be a mild cough and fever, partial anorexia and weight loss. Thoracic radiographic findings (Figure 12.172) include:

- Active phase: interstitial lung pattern; tracheobronchial lymphadenopathy is possible
- Chronic/healed phase: disseminated, ill-defined soft tissue nodules; tracheobronchial lymphadenopathy is uncommon
- Disseminated form: polyostotic aggressive bone lesions are the most obvious radiographic feature.

Cryptococcosis: Caused by the yeast *Cryptococcus neoformans*. It is common in cats and uncommon in dogs. It has a worldwide distribution.

Routes of infection and primary focus include:

- Inhalation and primary nasal form in cats
- May extend to central nervous system and cause neurological disease
- Primary or secondary lung infection is possible.

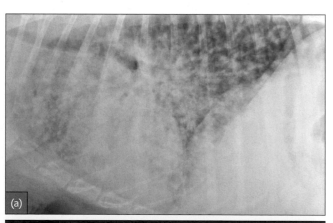

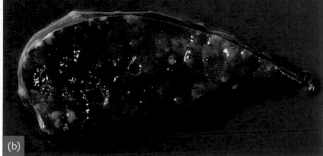

12.172 (a) Lateral thoracic radiograph of a 2-year-old Rottweiler with pulmonary coccidioidomycosis. There is a diffuse pattern of poorly circumscribed nodules throughout the lungs and tracheobronchial lymphadenopathy, causing deviation of the caudal trachea. (b) Post-mortem photograph of a lung section that demonstrates disseminated fungal granulomas.
(Courtesy of the University of California Davis)

Thoracic radiographic findings (Figure 12.173) include:

- Multiple nodules or small masses throughout the lungs
- Lung consolidation and pleural effusion are possible.

Aspergillosis: Caused by *Aspergillus* spp. It is common in dogs and rare in cats; the disseminated form is rare in both. German Shepherd Dog bitches are predisposed to the disseminated form. Aspergillosis has a worldwide distribution. Routes of infection and primary focus include:

- Inhalation and primary nasal form with *Aspergillus fumigatus*; usually restricted to nose
- Inhalation and usually primary pulmonary form with *A. terreus* and *A. deflectus*; haematogenous spread to other organs is possible.

Disseminated aspergillosis causes a variety of non-specific clinical signs, often including signs of spinal disease (discospondylitis). Thoracic radiographic findings are usually less important than other organ changes and include:

- Non-specific interstitial lung pattern
- Soft tissue nodules throughout the lungs.

Pneumocystosis: *Pneumocystis carinii* is a ubiquitous saprophytic fungus that is present within the alveoli in normal animals. Clinical signs are seen in immunocompromised dogs and include dyspnoea, weight loss and exercise intolerance. Young Cavalier King Charles Spaniels and Miniature Dachshunds are predisposed. Naturally occurring clinical disease in cats has not been reported, but it may be caused experimentally with infection and concurrent glucocorticoid therapy. Radiographic findings (Figure 12.174) include:

- Usually, a widespread interstitial and peribronchial pattern, progressing to a bilateral alveolar lung pattern (most severe in the middle lobes), which is symmetrical
- May affect all lung lobes and be severe, but cranioventral lobes may be less severely affected
- Patchy distribution is less common
- Bronchiectasis, pneumothorax, cavitating lesions and emphysema have also been reported but are uncommon presentations.

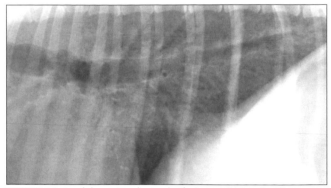

12.174 Lateral thoracic radiograph of a 1-year-old Cavalier King Charles Spaniel with *Pneumocystis carinii* infection. There is a generalized interstitial pattern with mildly thick bronchi. The generalized nature of the changes in a young dog is unusual but in combination with the breed is highly suggestive of pneumocystosis.

Parasitic pneumonia

Toxoplasmosis: *Toxoplasma gondii* is a protozoon with a worldwide distribution. Cats and other felidae are the only definitive host; they may also serve as intermediate hosts. Clinical toxoplasmosis occurs during the intermediate phase. Cats and dogs may be affected; cats are most commonly infected and have non-specific multiorgan signs. Respiratory involvement is common in acute disease.

Thoracic radiographic findings (Figure 12.175) include:

- Diffuse interstitial and patchy alveolar infiltrate
- Random distribution of changes.

Heartworm disease: This is caused by *Dirofilaria immitis*, a filarial nematode that resides primarily in the pulmonary arteries. It has a worldwide distribution in temperate and tropical climates, including most of the USA, Central and South America, Japan, Australia and southern Europe.

Clinical signs include exercise intolerance, weight loss, coughing and, in severe cases, right-sided heart failure and dyspnoea. It is a predisposing factor for pulmonary thromboembolism. Heartworm disease is common in dogs and less common in cats.

Radiographic findings (Figure 12.176) include:

- Patchy to extensive alveolar pattern, worst in the caudal lobes in severe cases

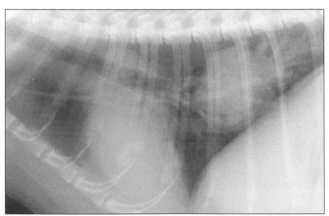

12.173 Lateral thoracic radiograph of a 10-year-old Domestic Shorthaired cat with pulmonary cryptococcosis. There is a large caudodorsal soft tissue mass (granuloma) and moderate tracheobronchial lymphadenopathy.
(Courtesy of the University of California Davis)

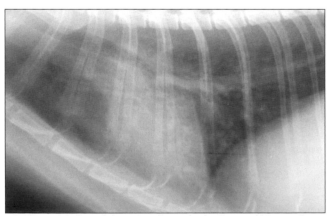

12.175 Right lateral thoracic radiograph of a 10-year-old Domestic Shorthaired cat with pulmonary toxoplasmosis. There are patchy areas of alveolar lung pattern forming summation shadows with the heart. The opposite lateral radiograph revealed right middle lung lobe collapse.

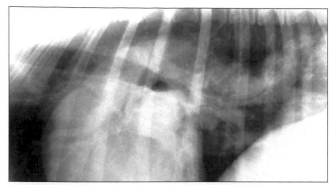

12.176 Lateral thoracic radiograph of a dog with dirofilariasis. There is a widespread increase in lung opacity, caused by enlarged, tortuous pulmonary arteries, and oedematous and granulomatous reactive lung.

- Changes have a periarterial distribution
- Enlarged and tortuous arteries (caudal in most cases but also often in the cranial lobes)
- Right-sided heart enlargement
- Pulmonary granulomas present in some cases.

Echocardiography may demonstrate *D. immitis* worms within the right ventricle or pulmonic trunk in some cases. The worms typically appear as thin, parallel linear echogenicities, or as an echogenic mass in severe cases. Signs of pulmonary hypertension with right ventricular hypertrophy may be seen.

Angiostrongylosis (French heartworm disease): *Angiostrongylus vasorum* is a metastrongylid parasite of dogs and foxes. The adult worm lives in the pulmonic trunk, the right side of the heart or the pulmonary arteries. It is most reported in the southern UK and southern Europe; it is rarely diagnosed in the USA.

There are two main clinical syndromes:

- Respiratory disease due to an inflammatory response to the eggs and migrating larvae
- Haemorrhagic diathesis, possibly due to antigenic factors secreted by the parasite.

The disease is more common in young dogs, with Cavalier King Charles Spaniels and Staffordshire Bull Terriers possibly over-represented. Clinical signs include coughing, dyspnoea, ecchymotic haemorrhage, haemoptysis, haematomas, gastrointestinal bleeding, vomiting, diarrhoea and neurological disease.

Radiographic findings (Figure 12.177) include:

- Diffuse bronchial and interstitial pattern initially (5 weeks after infection)
- Patchy alveolar pattern with peripheral distribution, preferentially affecting the caudodorsal lung field. Maximal changes 7–9 weeks after infection. May have lobar opacification. Bronchial changes present in most cases
- Small volume of pleural fluid in some cases
- Mild hazy interstitial pattern remains following treatment
- Cardiovascular changes are uncommon.

Paragonimiasis: Caused by the lung fluke *Paragonimus kellicotti*. It is endemic around the Great Lakes, and in midwestern and southern parts of the USA. Transmission occurs via a crayfish as the intermediate host. Adult flukes reside in pulmonary cysts and cause lung

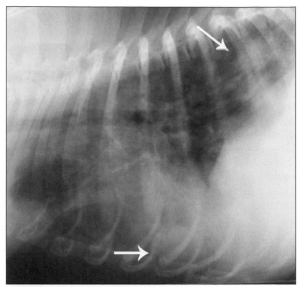

12.177 Lateral thoracic radiograph of a Staffordshire Bull Terrier with *Angiostrongylus vasorum* infection. Note the peripheral distribution of the pulmonary lesions (arrowed), which is commonly seen in angiostrongylosis.

pathology. Clinical signs may be absent. When present, signs include coughing, wheezing and acute dyspnoea with pneumothorax.

Radiographic findings are relatively specific:

- Solitary or multiple ill-defined nodular opacities
- Lesions are often cavitated and contain gas pockets
- Peribronchial or interstitial infiltrate.

Verminous pneumonia: Collective term for pneumonia induced by worms residing in or migrating through the lower airways:

- *Capillaria aerophila* is a small lungworm that resides in the upper airways and bronchi of dogs and cats
- *Aelurostrongylus abstrusus* is a small lungworm that resides in the bronchioli of cats
- *Filaroides hirthi* is a small lungworm that resides in the terminal bronchioli and alveoli of dogs
- *Oslerus osleri* is a worm that resides in the trachea and major bronchi of dogs
- *Crenosoma vulpis* is a worm that resides in the trachea, bronchi and bronchioles of dogs.

Clinical signs of lungworms may be absent or those of bronchopneumonia.

Toxocara canis, *Ancylostoma caninum* and *Strongyloides stercoralis* are intestinal parasites in dogs that undergo pulmonary migration. With heavy infection, transient pulmonary signs are possible.

Radiographic findings (Figure 12.178) include:

- Patchy bronchointerstitial and/or alveolar pattern
- Miliary or nodular pattern (*Filaroides hirthi*, *Aelurostrongylus abstrusus*)
- Tracheobronchial abnormalities (*Oslerus osleri*).

Allergic pneumonia

Eosinophilic bronchopneumopathy: Eosinophilic bronchopneumopathy (pulmonary infiltrate with eosinophilia (PIE)) is a manifestation of immunological hypersensitivity.

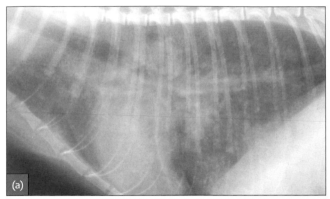

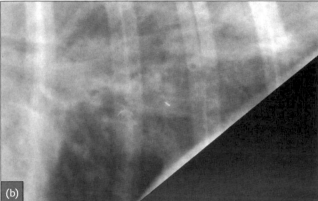

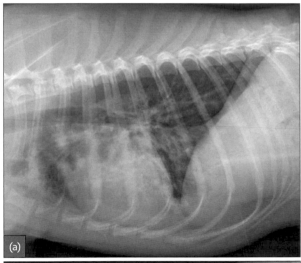

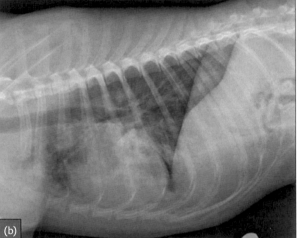

12.178 (a) Lateral thoracic radiograph of a 7-month-old Domestic Shorthaired cat with an *Aelurostrongylus abstrusus* infection in the small airways. There is a bronchointerstitial infiltrate with peribronchial thickening throughout the lungs. (b) Caudodorsal close-up of a lateral thoracic radiograph of a 2-year-old Cavalier King Charles Spaniel with a *Filaroides hirthi* infection. There is a bronchointerstitial pattern with bronchial thickening.

The underlying cause is not found in most cases. It usually occurs in young adult or middle-aged dogs. Siberian Huskies and Alaskan Malamutes are possibly predisposed. The main clinical sign is coughing, but signs may include dyspnoea, exercise intolerance and nasal discharge.

Radiography: Radiographic findings include:

- Bronchointerstitial pattern in most cases, with or without bronchiectasis (Figures 12.179 and 12.180)
- Less commonly, nodules and pulmonary masses are seen
- Patchy alveolar pattern and lobar consolidation are seen in severe cases
- Distribution is similar to bronchopneumonia, but it is often diffuse and tends to affect the caudal lobes.

Other imaging techniques: CT can be used to assess peribronchial infiltrates and masses (Figure 12.181). CT is also useful to localize solid areas for ultrasound-guided fine-needle aspiration and to guide for bronchoalveolar lavage.

Other non-infectious pneumonia

Inhalation pneumonia: This is caused by intake of noxious gases, fumes, aerosols and vapours. It is rare in dogs and cats. Smoke inhalation is a specific form of inhalation pneumonia (see 'Smoke inhalation', above). Usually, inhalation pneumonia is a result of inhalation of non-infectious toxic substances, such as acute inhalation of carpet cleaner or chronic exposure to silicate dusts. Silicate pneumoconiosis is a rare disease in dogs exposed to silicate dusts, resulting in chronic coughing.

12.179 (a) Right lateral and (b) left lateral thoracic radiographs of a 5-year-old crossbreed dog with eosinophilic bronchopneumopathy. In the cranial thorax, note the patchy lung pattern and the thick peribronchial infiltrate.

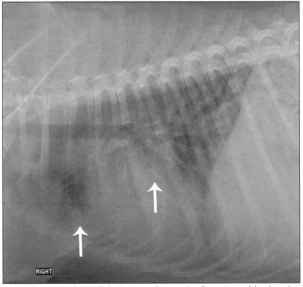

12.180 Right lateral thoracic radiograph of a 4-year-old Labrador Retriever with an early stage of eosinophilic bronchopneumopathy. Note the increased peribronchial thickening and peribronchial infiltrate (arrowed).

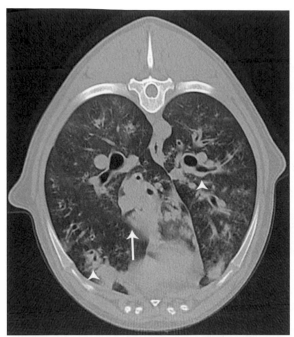

12.181 Transverse thoracic CT image of a 7-year-old Golden Retriever with eosinophilic bronchopneumopathy (high-resolution lung window). Note the increased peribronchial thickening (arrowheads) and the mass-like lesion formed at the level of the accessory lung lobe (arrowed).

Radiographic findings include:

- Predominantly interstitial or bronchointerstitial pattern (Figure 12.182)
- Tracheobronchial lymphadenopathy with silicosis
- Smoke inhalation (see above).

Lipid (lipoid) pneumonia: Exogenous lipid pneumonia is most often reported in cats. It is due to oil aspiration following forced oral oil administration (e.g. liquid paraffin for constipation or hairballs) or the aspiration of milk. There is no cough reflex with mineral oil aspiration. There may be a varying degree of respiratory compromise and the animal may be febrile, anorexic and depressed. The severity of the lung changes depend upon the type and amount of oil aspirated:

- Most vegetable oils are reportedly non-irritant
- Animal and some vegetable oils are hydrolyzed by pulmonary lipases and invoke an acute inflammatory response and necrosis

- Mineral oils act as foreign bodies and provoke a granulomatous reaction
- Macrophages transport lipids through the lungs, where they can persist for years.

Endogenous lipid pneumonia is occasionally seen in cats and rarely in dogs. The pathogenesis of this condition is uncertain:

- Stressor on alveolar membrane (airway obstruction, toxic inhalants or disturbed lipid metabolism)
- Pulmonary cell wall breakdown and alveolar type II cell proliferation
- Overproduction of cholesterol-containing surfactant that is phagocytosed but not removed by macrophages.

In addition, endogenous lipid pneumonia may be associated with pulmonary neoplasia (see 'Pulmonary neoplasia', below). In these cases, lipid pneumonia may affect the clinical signs, staging, treatment and monitoring of pulmonary neoplasia.

Radiography: Radiographic findings include:

- Diffuse interstitial lung pattern in mild cases or as a late change (can persist for several years)
- Poorly circumscribed alveolar opacities in severe cases (Figure 12.183)
- Consolidation peripheral to a bronchial obstruction (endogenous form)
- Lung masses of variable size and shape (endogenous form associated with neoplasia) (Figure 12.184a)
- Cavitated lung lesions with granulation (mineral oil aspiration)
- Chronic changes that do not resolve with standard antimicrobial treatment.

Other imaging techniques: On CT, endogenous lipid pneumonia can appear as a patchy interstitial pattern or a fluid-filled or soft tissue lung mass (Figure 12.184b). Definitive diagnosis requires a cytological examination or histopathology to demonstrate intra-alveolar lipid deposition.

Thoracic mycobacterial and other granulomatous diseases: Mycobacterial infection of the thorax has been described in dogs and in cats. Pulmonary tuberculosis is usually acquired as an aerogenous infection. Clinical signs are variable but there is often weight loss, chronic coughing and dyspnoea if there is a large volume of pleural fluid.

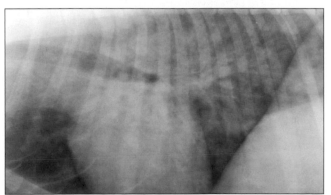

12.182 Lateral thoracic radiograph of a 6-month-old Afghan Hound that developed acute dyspnoea after being doused in chlorinated carpet cleaner. Both lungs have a widespread interstitial to alveolar pattern. The preferential caudodorsal distribution is a hallmark of inhalation pneumonitis.

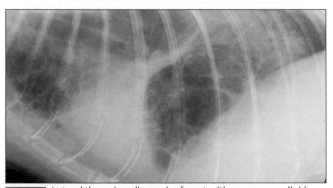

12.183 Lateral thoracic radiograph of a cat with exogeneous lipid pneumonia. The cat had been medicated with liquid paraffin for constipation. Note the right middle lung lobe collapse, caudodorsal alveolar opacity and bronchiectasis, and cavitating lesions throughout the ventral lungs. The generalized interstitial pattern could be related to lipid transport without removal by pulmonary macrophages.

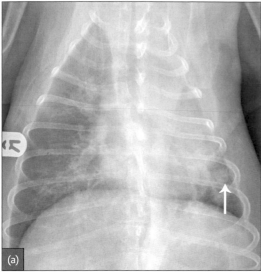

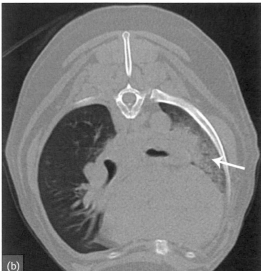

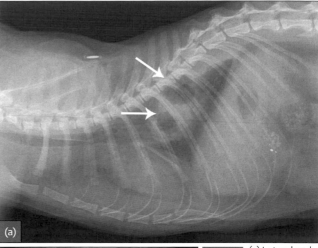

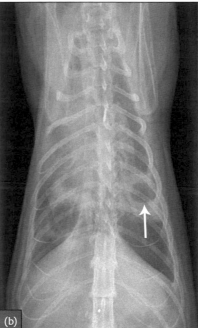

12.185 (a) Lateral and (b) DV thoracic radiographs of a Domestic Shorthaired cat with mycobacteriosis. Note the large cavitated lesions (arrowed) surrounded by a patchy increased lung opacity in the caudodorsal lung field.

12.184 (a) DV thoracic radiograph of a 12-year-old Springer Spaniel with a lung carcinoma in the left cranial lung lobe and endogenous lipid pneumonia. (b) Transverse thoracic CT image of the same dog (high-resolution lung window). Note the ground-glass opacity in the left cranial lung lobe (arrowed). On FNA the neoplasia was confirmed in association with lipid pneumonia.

In cats, mycobacterial disease is recognized with increasing frequency and is a worldwide veterinary health concern. The most identified species are *Mycobacterium microti* and *Mycobacterium bovis*. Clinical presentation is variable and depends on route of infection and degree of dissemination of the disease. Historically it was an alimentary disease; however, cutaneous disease acquired from prey species now predominates. Definitive diagnosis is difficult, and the disease is likely to be underdiagnosed. Thoracic abnormalities are most commonly detected but signs of systemic disease may also be seen (a combination of pulmonary infiltration, lymphadenomegaly and organomegaly).

Radiography: Radiographic findings include:
- Multiple patchy areas of ill-defined soft tissue opacity (Figure 12.185)
- Usually, involvement of multiple lung lobes and an asymmetrical distribution
- Primary foci often occur initially within the dorsal aspect of the lobes

- Spread of infection follows the bronchial tree
- May appear nodular but nodules are poorly marginated
- *Actinomyces*, *Nocardia* and mycobacterial infections often have similar radiographic findings, with intrathoracic lymphadenopathy, pleural fluid (may be localized) and nodules, pulmonary masses or lobar consolidation. Multiple nodules are more common in mycobacterial and Nocardia infections. Nodules or masses may cavitate
- Mineralization of the lymph nodes or granulomas in some cases of mycobacterial infection
- Periosteal reaction on the ribs and sternebrae may be seen in cases of *Actinomyces* infection
- Bone lesions have been described in mycobacteriosis in cats.

Other imaging techniques: Ultrasonography allows identification of enlarged sternal lymph nodes and guided fine-needle aspiration. In addition, CT allows complete assessment of the thorax and bony structures (Figures 12.186 and 12.187).

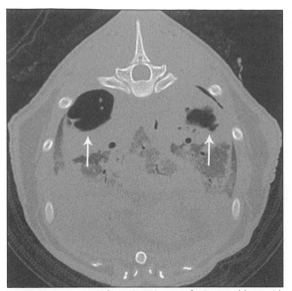

12.186 Transverse thoracic CT image of a 6-year-old cat with mycobacteriosis (high-resolution lung window). Note the increased lung opacity and cavitated lesions (arrowed) in the caudodorsal lung field.

Pulmonary neoplasia

Neoplasms may produce an alveolar pattern due to extension of the tumour into the alvooli, bronchial obstruction or inflammatory reaction to the tumour. An alveolar pattern may be seen with both primary and, less commonly, secondary pulmonary neoplasia (metastasis). Neoplastic alveolar disease is chronic and does not resolve with standard antimicrobial treatment. Its relatively slow development helps differentiate it from the more common acute alveolar diseases.

Primary lung neoplasms usually affect a single lobe but frequently cause lobar consolidation either due to obstruction of a bronchus or direct invasion of the lobe. Air bronchograms are uncommon, in contrast to acute alveolar disease, as the bronchi are often filled by tumour tissue or displaced by it. Lymphoma and some bronchoalveolar tumours grow around the airways, so may result in air bronchograms (Figure 12.188).

In cats, generalized or multifocal alveolar disease may be seen with primary and metastatic tumours. Neoplasia should be suspected if there is enlargement of an affected lobe, particularly in older animals.

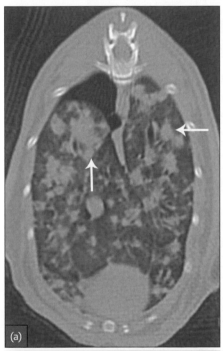

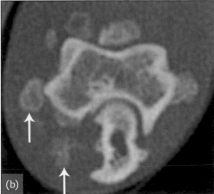

12.187 (a) Transverse thoracic CT image of a cat with mycobacteriosis (high-resolution lung window). Note the disseminated and patchy interstitial pattern scattered throughout the lungs (arrowed) and the small amount of pneumothorax dorsal to the right caudal lung lobe. (b) Transverse thoracic CT image of the same cat at the level of the elbow. Note the large amount of periarticular new bone formation (arrowed).

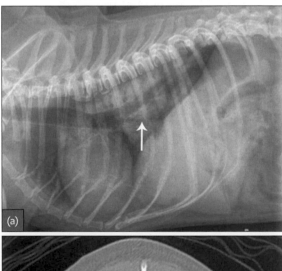

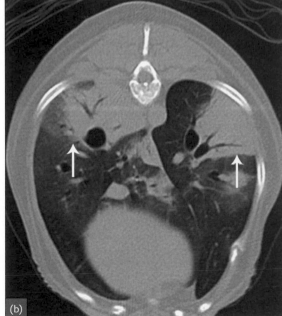

12.188 (a) Lateral thoracic radiograph of a 10-year-old West Highland White Terrier with FNA-confirmed lung lymphoma. Note the alveolar pattern involving the caudal lung lobes (arrowed).
(b) Transverse thoracic CT image of the same dog (high-resolution lung window): note the caudodorsal distribution of the alveolar pattern.

Radiography

Radiographic findings include:

- Primary lung tumours (especially carcinomas) in dogs are commonly solitary and in the caudal lobes (Figures 12.189 and 12.190)
- The most common findings of intrathoracic histiocytic sarcoma in dogs are lymphadenopathy and pulmonary masses (Tsai *et al.*, 2012; Barrett *et al.*, 2014). The tumours are frequently large and located in the entire or ventral aspect of the right middle or left cranial lung lobes. Internal air bronchograms are seen in about half of the tumours
- Haemangiosarcoma (see Figure 12.89)
- Feline bronchoalveolar carcinoma results in a mixed bronchoalveolar pattern (Figures 12.191 and 12.192), ill-defined alveolar masses and cavitated masses. These are seen in combination with bronchiectasis or other bronchial abnormalities, an interstitial component of lung opacity, or a generalized or focal mass
- Metastasis generally produces randomly distributed nodules, but in cats may cause focal consolidation or patchy alveolar opacities (often mammary or other carcinoma)

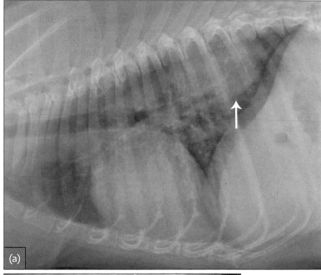

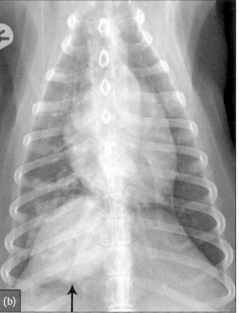

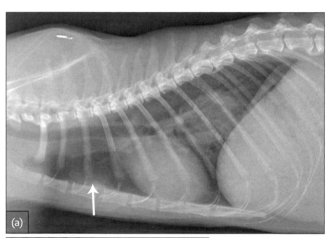

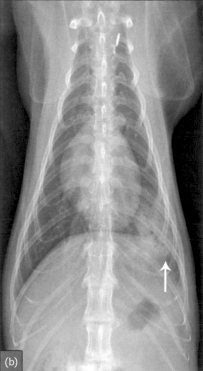

12.189 (a) Lateral and (b) DV thoracic radiographs of a 12-year-old Siamese cat with lung carcinoma. (a) Note the enlarged sternal lymph node (arrowed). (b) Note the ill-defined and patchy alveolar pattern in the left caudal lung lobe (arrowed).

12.190 (a) Lateral radiograph of a 10-year-old crossbreed dog with pulmonary histiocytic sarcoma. (b) DV thoracic radiograph of a 10-year-old crossbreed dog with pulmonary histiocytic sarcoma. Note the well defined lung mass (arrowed) in the right caudal lung lobe.

- A small amount of pleural effusion is commonly associated with pulmonary neoplasia (Figure 12.192):
  - Usually caused by the prevention of normal lymphatic lung drainage
  - May contain malignant cells (malignant effusion)
  - May be most severe around lesion.

Other imaging techniques

Ultrasonography is useful in pulmonary neoplasia both to identify and to characterize the lesion, as well as to guide sampling for definitive diagnosis (Figure 12.193):

- Neoplastic masses may have a wide variety of appearances but are often solid and homogeneous
- An increase in lobar size and rounding of lobar borders are common findings
- Doppler ultrasonography is useful to identify vascularity within a mass

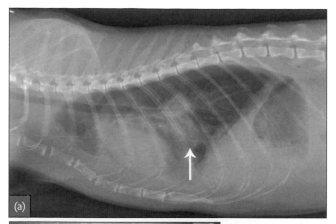

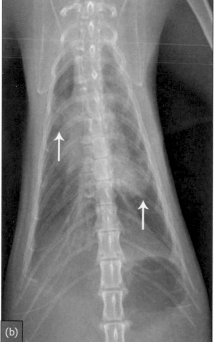

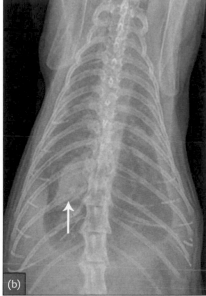

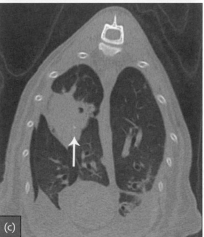

12.191 10-year-old Domestic Shorthaired cat with bronchoalveolar carcinoma. (a) The lateral view demonstrates ill-defined and patchy peribronchial pattern (arrowed).(b) The DV view shows areas of alveolar pattern in the left caudal and right cranial lung lobes (arrowed). Note also the small volume of pleural effusion.

12.192 (continued) A 14-year-old Domestic Shorthaired cat with bronchoalveolar carcinoma. (b) DV thoracic radiograph. Note the ill-defined and patchy peribronchial pattern with areas of alveolar pattern and lung consolidation (arrowed). Note also the large amount of pleural effusion and retraction of the lung lobes from the rib cage. (c) Transverse CT image (high-resolution lung window). Note the lung consolidation and the dystrophic mineralization within the lung mass (arrowed).

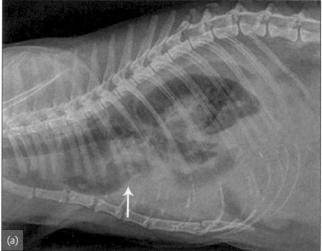

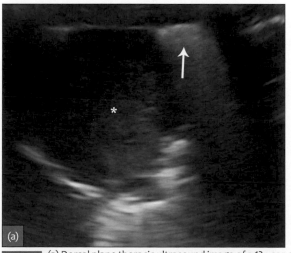

12.192 A 14-year-old Domestic Shorthaired cat with bronchoalveolar carcinoma. (a) Lateral thoracic radiograph. Note the ill-defined and patchy peribronchial pattern with areas of alveolar pattern and lung consolidation (arrowed). Note also the large amount of pleural effusion and retraction of the lung lobes from the rib cage. (continues) ▶

12.193 (a) Dorsal plane thoracic ultrasound image of a 12-year-old Domestic Longhaired cat with lung carcinoma. Note the consolidated right caudal lung lobe (*) with reverberation artefact arising from the normal and adjacent lung (arrowed). (continues) ▶

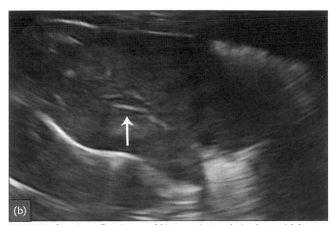

12.193 (continued) A 12-year-old Domestic Longhaired cat with lung carcinoma. (b) Longitudinal plane image: note the bronchus within the consolidated right caudal lung lobe (arrowed).

- Neoplasms may be more likely to have smooth regular margins at their junction with the normal lung, in comparison with non-neoplastic consolidation where the junction may be irregularly marginated
- Gas or mineralized foci may be seen within the mass. Necrotic centres may also be identified as more hypo- or anechoic regions.

CT and MRI allow identification of pulmonary masses. CT is preferred as it is faster and allows better assessment of the airways; it also allows assessment of the tracheobronchial lymph nodes (Figure 12.194).

Predominantly interstitial lung diseases

The pulmonary interstitium consists of the subserosal lung capsule (peripheral connective tissue) and a network of fibroblasts, collagen and elastic fibres covering the alveolar membranes (lung parenchyma), airways and vessels (bronchovascular bundles). Normal dogs and cats lack identifiable interstitial septae between lung lobules. The interstitium has a trophic and immunoprotective function, provides a mechanical framework for the alveoli, airways and vessels, and is responsible for the elastic recoil of the lung. Diseases that affect the interstitium often change pulmonary compliance.

- Destruction of the elastic fibre network results in abnormally high compliance, e.g. emphysema, causing distended airspaces in inspiration and expiration.
- Interstitial proliferation results in an abnormally low compliance, e.g. interstitial fibrosis, resulting in incompletely distended airspaces during inspiration.

The major types of pulmonary interstitial disease are:

- Fluid accumulation causing interstitial oedema
- Infiltration with inflammatory or neoplastic cells
- Chronic conditions causing collagen deposition, fibrosis and mineralization.

All these conditions can lead to thick alveolar walls and peribronchial tissues that result in overall increased opacity of the lungs and blurring of the fine vascular structures. Primarily interstitial lung diseases may be localized or diffuse, with systemic diseases often associated with diffuse pulmonary involvement. Interstitial disease can progress to an alveolar pattern if the alveoli become fluid filled, such as in acute interstitial pneumonia or secondary pneumonia, or if the alveolar walls become thick enough to compress the alveolar sac. Identification of an interstitial pattern can help to determine the nature of the disease process. The interstitial pulmonary pattern is a common and often non-specific radiographic sign.

The interstitial pattern must first be differentiated from age-associated changes and physiological causes such as hypoinflation and obesity. Once the pattern is determined to be significant, a list of differential diagnoses of disease can be formulated. An interstitial pattern is a stage in many disease processes and the temporal aspect needs to be considered in the radiographic interpretation.

All these remarks refer to unstructured or fine-structured interstitial pattern. Nodular pattern, which is also a form of interstitial pattern, is discussed above (see 'Solid pulmonary masses', above).

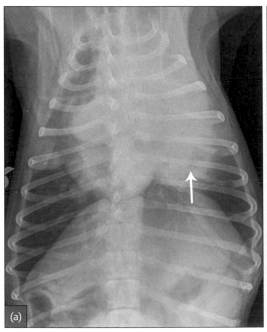
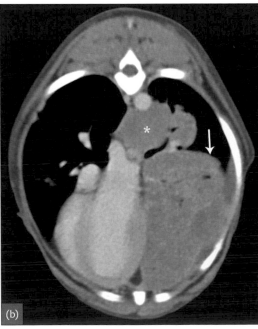

12.194 (a) Lateral thoracic radiograph of a 15-year-old Schnauzer with lung carcinoma: note the consolidation of the left cranial lung lobe (arrowed). (b) Transverse thoracic CT image of the same dog (high-resolution lung window): note the lung consolidation (arrowed) and the enlarged tracheobronchial lymph node (*).

Interstitial oedema

Under normal conditions, there is fluid flux from the pulmonary capillaries through small gaps between endothelial cells into the interstitium and drainage from the interstitial space by lymphatic vessels. Increased interstitial fluid accumulation (oedema) occurs due to one or more of the following:

- Increased microvascular hydrostatic pressure
- Reduced capillary oncotic pressure
- Increased vascular permeability
- Reduced lymphatic drainage.

The pulmonary lymphatics can increase their drainage capacity 3–10 fold in an acute situation to prevent oedema from occurring. If this flow is exceeded, fluid starts to accumulate, initially in the interstices surrounding the vessels and lymphatics. The largest amount of fluid tends to gather around the pulmonary arteries.

The interstitial space can expand up to twice its normal volume. When the pressure In the expanded perivascular interstitial space rises to a level similar to that in the alveolar interstitium, forward flow decreases and the alveolar interstitium starts to expand causing the alveolar wall to become thick. Eventually the alveolar walls cannot withstand the pressure, and gaps or ruptures form in the alveolar epithelium. Filling of the alveoli with fluid is the alveolar stage of pulmonary oedema.

Radiography: Interstitial oedema (Figure 12.195) can only be recognized radiographically if it does not summate with any alveolar opacities, and should be expected in the:

- Early stage of developing pulmonary oedema
- Late stage in the resolution of pulmonary oedema
- Less affected area of an oedematous lung.

Radiographic features may include:

- Mild increase in lung opacity
- First- and second-branch pulmonary blood vessels are visible, but edges become indistinct and bronchi may become more prominent
- A 'ground glass' pattern (fine, granular soft tissue opacity)
- Generally homogeneous, may become patchy as it progresses to alveolar oedema
- Interstitial pulmonary pattern in the perihilar region or right caudal lung lobe
- Patchy interstitial to alveolar pattern diffusely or peripherally (cats)
- Rapid progression or resolution of disease on repeat radiographs.

Additional radiographic findings may help to determine the cause of interstitial oedema (see 'Pulmonary oedema', above).

Interstitial pneumonia

Interstitial pneumonia (see also 'Pneumonia', above) is caused by infiltration of inflammatory cells into the alveolar walls (sparing the airways) or by toxic exposure. The original inflammatory or toxic insult may arise from the bloodstream or may be carried by aerosol, resulting in acute damage to the alveolar membranes. Several different aetiologies (viral, bacterial, parasitic, fungal, toxic) may result in pneumonia manifesting as an interstitial pattern.

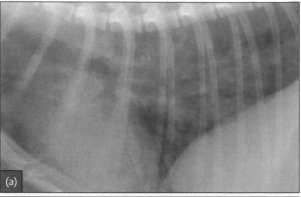

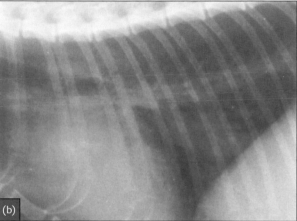

12.195 (a) Lateral thoracic radiograph of a cat with hypertrophic cardiomyopathy and cardiogenic interstitial pulmonary oedema. There is cardiomegaly, pulmonary vascular distension, a small amount of pleural effusion and a diffuse interstitial pattern throughout the lungs, most pronounced in the perihilar region. (b) A repeat radiograph 12 hours after initiation of diuretic treatment reveals persistent cardiomegaly, normal sized pulmonary blood vessels, resolution of pleural effusion and lung opacification, and better lung inflation. Prompt resolution of radiographic signs after diuresis is a hallmark of cardiogenic pulmonary oedema.

Interstitial pneumonias are divided into acute and chronic, with some degree of overlap, and may present at either stage:

- Acute pneumonia is often caused by infectious agents and is self-limiting. It does not always cause a radiographic interstitial pattern
- Chronic interstitial pneumonia begins with an acute phase, followed by an ongoing idiopathic or toxic inflammatory process. The final stage is development of fibrosis, which may reduce gas exchange due to increased thickness of the alveolar wall. Infectious causes of interstitial pneumonia do not usually lead to significant or progressive fibrosis.

Radiography: Radiographic findings (Figure 12.196; see also Figures 12.166 and 12.168) include:

- Diffuse increase in opacity with poor definition of vessels and bronchi
- Unstructured or fine-structured interstitial pattern
- Occasionally, an alveolar pattern in the acute phase
- Often begins in lung periphery
- Less uniform than interstitial oedema
- Tracheal distension with increased respiratory effort
- Acute viral interstitial pneumonia, such as with distemper virus infection, is often complicated by secondary bacterial infection by the time of

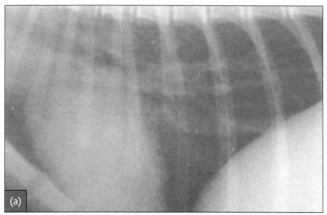

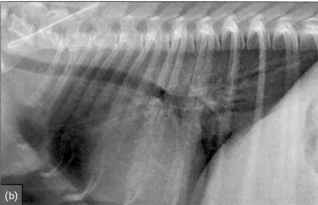

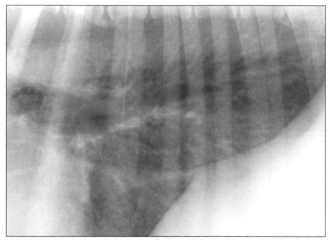

12.197 Caudodorsal close-up of a lateral thoracic radiograph of a 5-year-old German Shepherd Dog with marked dyspnoea. The caudodorsal lung field has a fine-structured interstitial pattern. The histological diagnosis was pulmonary fibrosis of unknown aetiology.

- Overlap of the diaphragmatic and cardiac silhouettes
- Minimal change between inspiratory and expiratory radiographs
- Stable radiographic appearance or gradual progression over time
- Pleural fissure lines due to pleural fibrosis.

Idiopathic pulmonary fibrosis: Idiopathic pulmonary fibrosis (IPF) is a chronic progressive fibrosis of the lung interstitium in older terrier breed dogs. It is particularly common in West Highland White and Cairn Terriers. It shares many features to a similarly named condition in humans. A similar but not identical condition has been reported in cats.

Affected animals suffer from progressive exercise intolerance, coughing and dyspnoea, and have marked inspiratory crackles on auscultation.

Radiography: Findings in canine IPF (Figure 12.198) include:

- Diffuse interstitial infiltrate in all lung lobes
- Right heart enlargement
- Hepatomegaly of unclear origin. Hepatic congestion due to right heart failure is usually not present. It has been proposed that this is hypoxia-related
- Often concurrent partial tracheal collapse.

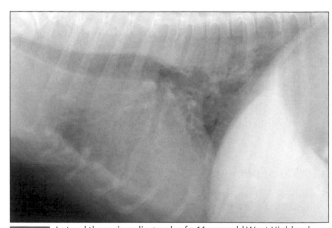

12.198 Lateral thoracic radiograph of a 14-year-old West Highland White Terrier with IPF. Notice the general increase in lung opacity with an interstitial pattern, partial tracheal collapse and dyspnoea-related gas distension of the stomach (aerophagia). There is mild right cardiac and marked hepatic (not included in image) enlargement, features commonly seen in terrier breed dogs with IPF.

12.196 (a) Lateral thoracic radiograph of a kitten with acute interstitial pneumonia secondary to feline leukaemia virus infection. The fine vascular structures are blurred yet still visible, and there is an overall increase in lung opacity. Acute viral pneumonia typically presents with radiographically normal lungs or interstitial lung pattern as in this case. (b) Lateral thoracic radiograph of a 2-year-old Border Terrier with interstitial pneumonia with cultured *Bordetella bronchiseptica*. There is a diffuse unstructured interstitial lung pattern, worse caudodorsally.

radiography, resulting in a mixed interstitial to alveolar or bronchial pattern
- Caudodorsal or peribronchial distribution of interstitial pattern may indicate an inhaled agent or toxin (toxic gases or vapours).

Interstitial fibrosis

Interstitial fibrosis is the end-stage of a variety of pulmonary diseases with irreversible alterations to the collagen-supporting structures of the interstitium. The original insult may be infectious, inflammatory or idiopathic in nature and often is not determined. Acute infectious pneumonias and cardiogenic pulmonary oedema usually do not result in chronic fibrosis. Pulmonary fibrosis can occur focally, or secondary to an abscess, infarction or trauma but this is usually insufficient to cause respiratory compromise. Consequences of pulmonary fibrosis are a decrease in functioning lung tissue, compliance and tidal volume.

Radiography: Radiographic findings (Figure 12.197) include:

- Diffuse unstructured or fine-structured interstitial pattern
- In severe cases of decreased lung compliance ('stiff lung'), the thoracic volume may be small and the trachea enlarged on inspiratory radiographs:
  - Lumbodiaphragmatic recess at the tenth thoracic vertebra

Radiographic signs are non-specific and all differentials for interstitial lung pattern apply. The age and breed of the patient should be considered when making a diagnosis, which often requires ruling out other lung diseases. Feline IPF is often seen radiographically as patchy interstitial lung opacities and bullous emphysema (Figure 12.199).

High-resolution lung computed tomography: Findings in canine IPF (Figure 12.200) include:

- Ground-glass opacity of some or all lung lobes
- Parenchymal bands of lung consolidation
- Crazy-paving pattern of areas of lung opacity
- Subpleural and peribronchial consolidations
- Mild traction bronchiectasis.

CT findings in feline IPF (Figure 12.201) include:

- Ground-glass opacity of some or all lung lobes
- Subpleural consolidations
- Parenchymal bands
- Bullous emphysema.

Radiation-induced lung fibrosis

Radiation damage to the lung from accidental exposure is rare. However, with radiation therapy for thoracic wall neoplasia and prolonged fluoroscopic and interventional procedures becoming more common, radiation damage to focal areas of the lung may be encountered.

Radiation damage depends on dose and irradiated volume. Clinical signs are expected when more than 25% of both lungs are exposed. The lung is one of the most sensitive tissues with a late response to radiation:

- After a latent period of 1 to 6 months, acute pneumonitis develops, causing interstitial oedema and inflammation and capillary congestion
- Chronic inflammation leads to pulmonary fibrosis 2–24 months after the exposure to radiation. These changes are permanent and static.

Radiation pneumonitis may cause clinical signs such as respiratory distress, decreased exercise tolerance and cough. These should improve as the inflammatory phase subsides. Radiographic changes are visible 2–3 weeks before the onset of clinical signs.

Radiography: Radiographs are initially normal. At 1–2 months post irradiation, an alveolar pattern is seen (acute pneumonitis) (Figure 12.202). In later stages (2–24 months post exposure) there is:

- Diffuse interstitial pattern (whole body exposure)
- Focal homogeneous interstitial or alveolar pattern near site of radiation therapy or imaging
- Bronchiectasis
- Cicatrization atelectasis (scar formation) with chronic fibrosis.

Dipyridylium derivate intoxication

Dipyridylium (paraquat, diquat, morfamquat) derivates are used as desiccant and defoliant herbicides. Paraquat is one of the most used herbicides worldwide and is highly toxic to animals and humans. It reacts with oxygen to form oxygen free radicals, which are extremely damaging to the lungs. Contamination is usually via oral ingestion and has a vascular distribution with an affinity for the lungs. The

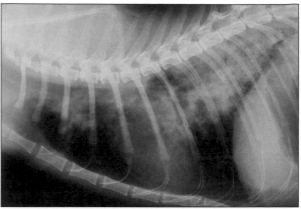

12.199 Lateral thoracic radiograph of a 10-year-old Siamese cat with idiopathic pulmonary fibrosis. There are patchy areas of interstitial to alveolar lung opacity and interspersed hyperlucent areas, consistent with emphysema.

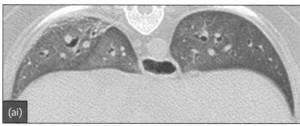

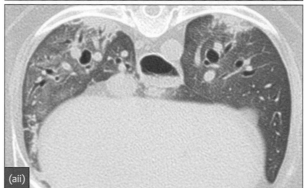

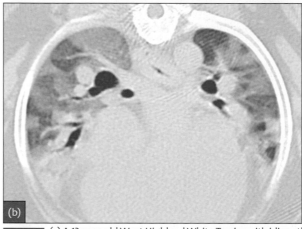

12.200 (a) A 12-year-old West Highland White Terrier with idiopathic pulmonary fibrosis. (ai) High-resolution transverse lung CT image at the level of the caudal thorax. There is a mild generalized increase in lung opacity (ground-glass opacity) and small subpleural fibrotic infiltrate in the right caudal lung lobe. The oesophagus is mildly distended with gas. (aii) On a slightly more cranial image, there is hyperattenuating infiltrate in the dorsal portions of both caudal lung lobes and subpleural bands. Patches of ground-glass opacity are present in the right lung. These changes are consistent with fibrosis. (b) High-resolution transverse lung CT image of an 8-year-old West Highland White Terrier with idiopathic pulmonary fibrosis at the level of the left cardiac atrium. There is a mosaic lung pattern, with haphazardly arranged lung areas of different density.

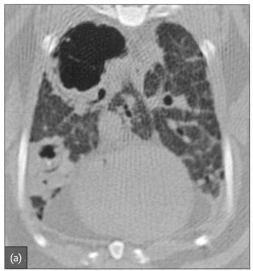

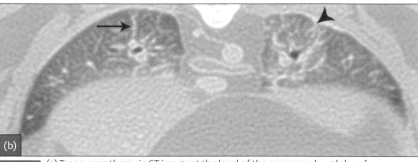

12.201 (a) Transverse thoracic CT image at the level of the accessory lung lobe of an 8-year-old Siamese cat with pulmonary fibrosis. There are parenchymal bands, areas of consolidation and bullous emphysema throughout the lungs. (b) High-resolution transverse lung CT image at the level of the caudal thorax of an 11-year-old obese Domestic Shorthaired cat with fibrotic lung changes. Notice the ground-glass opacity of the lung, a small subpleural consolidation (arrowhead) and bands of soft tissue originating from the pleural surface (arrowed).

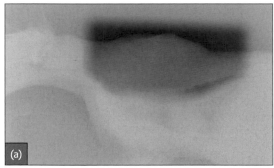

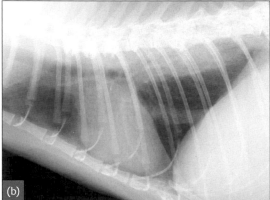

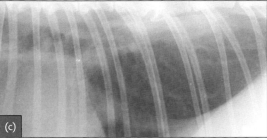

12.202 (a) Radiation treatment planning lateral port image, acquired with cobalt photons, of a 9-year-old Domestic Longhaired cat with a non-resectable interscapular fibrosarcoma. The beam field includes the dorsal aspect of the caudodorsal lung field. (b) Lateral thoracic radiograph obtained 1 month after completion of radiation therapy demonstrates a sharply delineated area of alveolar opacity in the exposed lung, consistent with acute radiation pneumonitis. (c) Caudodorsal close-up of a lateral thoracic radiograph obtained 6 months after radiation. The affected area is now slightly reduced in size and of mixed interstitial–alveolar pattern. These findings are consistent with radiation-induced chronic lung fibrosis and are permanent.
(Courtesy of Donald Thrall)

underlying mechanism of damage to the alveolar epithelial cells is necrosis and oedema, with subsequent inflammation and fibrosis of the alveolar septal walls. The clinical course is progressive respiratory and renal failure.

Radiography: Radiographic findings depend on the stage of disease (see 'Interstitial fibrosis', above):

- Acutely there may be no radiographic change
- Progressive diffuse interstitial pattern
- Cicatrization atelectasis (scar formation)
- Pleural fibrosis causes fissure lines
- Pneumomediastinum.

Interstitial neoplastic infiltrate

In dogs and cats, primary lung neoplasia and metastatic neoplasia can both cause diffuse interstitial patterns. Diffuse pulmonary neoplasia is more commonly metastatic than primary, and more common in cats than dogs. Secondary oedema, infection, infarction, fibrosis and necrosis may accompany neoplastic disease and complicate radiographic diagnosis.

Multicentric lymphoma: This is the most common canine interstitial lung tumour; it rarely affects the lungs of cats. It usually also affects other non-thoracic organs (multicentric). The neoplastic cells accumulate in the interstitium and lymphatic system. The presence of pulmonary lymphoma infiltrate does not correlate with survival or remission. In dogs with multicentric lymphoma, there is thoracic involvement (lymphadenopathy and/or pulmonary infiltrate) in approximately 70% of cases. Thoracic radiographs are indicated in staging lymphoma.

Alveolar septal metastases: These are common in anaplastic mammary carcinoma and less common in salivary or pulmonary carcinoma or transitional cell carcinoma of the urinary bladder. Metastatic spread to the interstitium of the lung occurs via the lymphatic system and microvasculature. Neoplastic cells infiltrate the alveolar septal walls, making them thick, and may cause thrombosis of small vessels.

Diffuse primary bronchoalveolar carcinoma: This is an uncommon primary lung neoplasm that spreads along airways and alveolar interstitium.

Haemangiosarcoma: Metastases in pulmonary capillaries can cause a diffuse fine-structured interstitial pattern.

Radiography:

Multicentric lymphoma: Radiographic findings include:

* Diffuse unstructured or fine-structured interstitial pattern is most common (Figure 12.203ai; see also Figure 12.72). This is often described as reticular, honeycomb or micronodular
* Most apparent in caudodorsal and perihilar lung fields
* Thick bronchial walls (neoplastic lymphatic infiltrate)
* The pulmonary blood vessels are generally clearly visible despite the interstitial pattern
* May develop within days and regress similarly quickly with chemotherapy
* Very rarely, a nodular pattern or large masses can occur
* Additional common findings are pleural effusion, intrathoracic lymphadenopathy and a wide mediastinum.

An interstitial pattern with lymphadenopathy is very suggestive of lymphoma, with the other main differential being fungal pneumonia. Differential diagnoses of other rapidly appearing interstitial infiltrates are:

* Oedema
* Infection
* Haemorrhage due to trauma or DIC
* Metastatic disease.

Alveolar septal metastases and bronchoalveolar carcinoma: Radiographic findings are not specific (see Figure 12.191) but may include:

* Diffuse interstitial disease with occasional alveolar infiltrates or ill-defined nodules
* Hyperlucent lung areas (regional embolic oligaemia)
* Peribronchial cuffing (filling of lymphatics with tumour cells)
* Thick pleura
* Mild pleural effusion
* Sternal lymphadenopathy.

Computed tomography:

Multicentric lymphoma: CT findings (Figure 12.203) include:

* Ground-glass opacity that may be more prominent in the caudal lung lobes
* Enlarged sternal, cranial mediastinal and tracheobronchial lymph nodes.

Alveolar septal metastases: CT provides exceptional detail of the lung and is very useful for diagnosis and staging of radiographically occult neoplastic disease. Imaging findings in dogs may include:

* Normal pleura
* Subpleural zone
  * Subpleural lines due to interstitial infiltrate and fibrosis (see Figure 12.149)
  * Subpleural wedge-shaped interstitial thickening (base parallel to the pleura) caused by neoplastic infiltration and fibrosis
  * Patches of ground-glass opacity caused by tumour cells, necrosis and haemorrhage
  * Subpleural emphysema, due to small airway obstruction by fibrosis
  * Mosaic perfusion: patchy hyperattenuating and hypoattenuating areas with small pulmonary

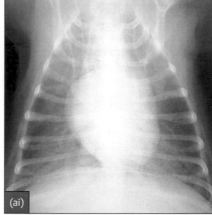

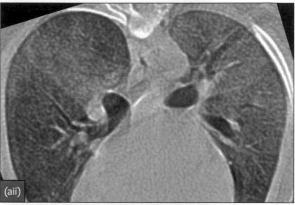

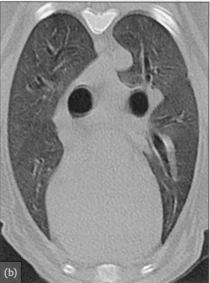

12.203 (a) A dog with systemic lymphoma. (ai) VD thoracic radiograph showing diffuse fine-structured interstitial infiltrate. (aii) High resolution transverse thoracic CT image at the level caudal to the carina demonstrating a diffuse ground-glass opacity throughout the lungs. (b) Transverse thoracic CT image of a 5-year-old Cocker Spaniel with multicentric lymphoma. There is diffuse interstitial lung infiltration resulting in a ground-glass opacity and tracheobronchial lymphadenopathy.

  arteries, due to altered perfusion patterns secondary to neoplastic embolization
  * Distortion of architecture
  * Small nodules
  * Areas of consolidation
* Peribronchial zone
  * Peribronchovascular interstitial thickening due to tumour nodules or atelectasis
  * Small nodules
  * Areas of consolidation.

Interstitial mineralization

Mineralization of lung tissues may be dystrophic, metastatic or idiopathic. Calcium and other minerals are concentrated in the mitochondria of the cell or in vesicles in the extracellular space. Minerals are deposited as non crystalline calcium phosphate (dystrophic), calcium carbonate salts (metastatic) or hydroxyapatite crystals (dystrophic and metastatic).

Dystrophic mineralization: This occurs in damaged or necrotic lung tissue in dogs with normal serum calcium, and with diseases of calcium metabolism, secondary to parasitic or fungal granulomas (histoplasmosis), abscessation, neoplasia or metabolic disease (hyperadrenocorticism). Diffuse inflammatory lesions that result in fibrosis, such as chronic uraemia, can also have a component of mineralization. Heterotopic bone (pulmonary osteoma) is a form of dystrophic mineralization. Small islands of bone matrix are deposited in the pulmonary parenchyma and mineralize. This is commonly seen in older dogs as an incidental finding of minor consequence. Bronchial walls commonly mineralize in dogs, but not normally in cats. Osteosarcoma occasionally forms mineralized osteoid pulmonary metastases.

Hyperadrenocorticism (Cushing's disease): This causes dystrophic mineralization of soft tissues, including skin, stomach, arteries, skeletal muscle and kidneys. Cortisol alters glucose production in the liver and has catabolic effects. Proteins formed in relation to these processes are altered and may result in increased calcium binding to the organic matrix. The lungs are one of the most frequently mineralized tissues at microscopic level; radiographically evident macroscopic mineralization is rare. Serum calcium levels are generally within normal limits.

If the degree of mineralization is severe, dogs may experience significant respiratory distress and become oxygen dependent. This hypoxaemia may be due to impaired gas diffusion across mineralized alveolar walls.

Metastatic mineralization: This is caused by altered serum calcium and phosphorous levels with deposition of minerals in the normal tissues. Causes of hypercalcaemia include primary and secondary hyperparathyroidism, hypervitaminosis D, lymphoma, cholecalciferol rodenticide toxicity and disseminated bone cancer such as multiple myeloma. Tumours (e.g. apocrine gland anal sac adenocarcinoma) can also produce a parathormone-like hormone, which causes hypercalcaemia as a paraneoplastic syndrome. Most instances of metastatic mineralization in the lung are visible only at the microscopic level.

Idiopathic mineralization: This includes pulmonary alveolar microlithiasis and bronchiolar microlithiasis.

Iatrogenic mineralization: This includes mineralization secondary to barium aspiration.

Radiography: Interstitial lung mineralization can manifest as:

- Lung with normal appearance
- Small nodular mineralizations (heterotopic bone)
- Central or peripheral mineralization of masses (Figure 12.204)
- Unstructured interstitial lung pattern with or without mineralized appearance (Figure 12.205)
- Diffuse marked mineralization (alveolar microlithiasis, barium resorption) (Figure 12.206; see also Figure 12.153).

Hyperadrenocorticism: Radiographic findings in dogs with hyperadrenocorticism are often mild and can be partially caused by artefact. The obesity of cushingoid dogs means that a high kVp setting is required to obtain the radiographs, which reduces image contrast (scatter, high penetration, Compton-related low image contrast). Low image contrast can mimic interstitial lung pattern. Body condition should, therefore, be considered when diagnosing interstitial disease.

Common radiographic findings in the lungs (see Figures 12.205 and 12.207) include:

- Mineralization is difficult to see radiographically and usually causes an unstructured interstitial pattern
- Marked bronchial mineralization, most pronounced in caudodorsal lung field due to increased volume of lung in that area
- May progress to alveolar pattern with air bronchograms
- Interstitial pattern does not resolve with diuresis (as opposed to oedema).

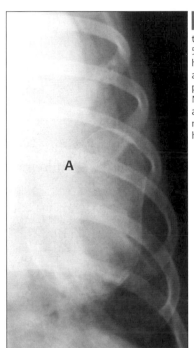

12.204 Left caudal close-up of a VD thoracic radiograph of a 5-year-old Irish Setter with heartworm disease and an associated calcified pulmonary haematoma. Notice the distended left lobar artery (A) and the egg-shell mineralization of the haematoma.

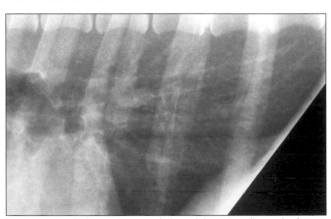

12.205 Caudodorsal close-up of a lateral thoracic radiograph of a 5-year-old Dachshund with hyperadrenocorticism. Diffuse interstitial and bronchial mineralization result in a bronchointerstitial pattern. The bronchi and pulmonary parenchyma have a subtle mineral opacity. In most cases interstitial mineralization is insufficient to cause a mineral opacity and the interstitial opacity is often mistaken for interstitial oedema. Persistent interstitial lung pattern despite diuretic treatment in hyperadrenocorticoid dogs should prompt consideration of mineralization or fibrosis as possible causes.

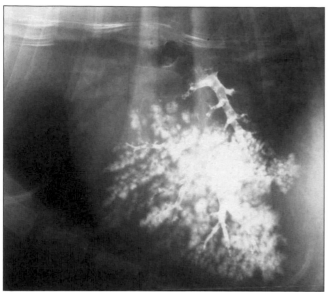

12.206 Lateral oesophagram of a 9-year-old Labrador Retriever obtained after oral administration of a barium sulphate suspension. The oesophagus is normal but barium was aspirated into the right middle and left caudal lung lobes.

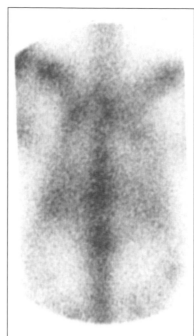

12.208 Dorsal thoracic scintigram of a dog obtained about 2 hours after intravenous injection of a bone-binding diphosphonate compound. Notice the diffuse radiopharmaceutical uptake in the lungs compared with the photopenic abdomen. Differentials for this uptake include hyperadrenocorticism, heterotopic bone formation, diffuse pulmonary metastases and recently performed lung scintigraphy.

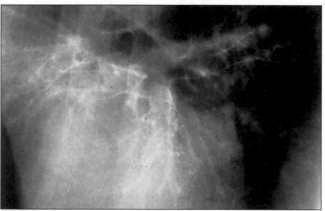

12.207 Close-up of a lateral thoracic radiograph of a 9-year-old Standard Poodle with hyperadrenocorticism causing excessive widespread bronchial mineralization. Increased lung opacity results from bronchi that are more opaque, but not thicker, than normal (bronchial pattern).

(Reprinted from Schwarz et al. (2000) with permission)

Computed tomography: CT is very sensitive to changes in density and is more sensitive than radiography for diagnosing pulmonary mineralization (see Figure 12.93). The Hounsfield units (HU) can be measured and compared to normal values of soft tissue and mineral to determine the presence of mineralization. Soft tissue is usually 30–60 HU, and mineralized tissue is greater. CT is also useful in patients with hyperadrenocorticism to identify pituitary or adrenal masses.

Scintigraphy: Pulmonary mineralization can be diagnosed using nuclear scintigraphy. ^{99m}Technetium-methylene diphosphonate (MDP) can be injected intravenously, as for a bone scan. At the 2-hour time point, the pulmonary parenchyma will show increased uptake of radiopharmaceutical due to binding with the hydroxyapatite crystals in the interstitium, which are similar to those in bone (Figure 12.208). This may be a useful technique if the dog has a mild interstitial pattern, and it is unclear whether it is due to pulmonary oedema or diffuse mineralization.

Acknowledgement

The authors and editors gratefully acknowledge the contributions of the following authors to this chapter in the first edition of this manual: Victoria Johnson, Wilfried Maï, Panagiotis Mantis, Fraser McConnell, Federica Morandi, Robert O'Brien, Yael Porat-Mosenco, Gabriela Seiler, Emma Tobin and Allison Zwingenberger.

References and further reading

Adams WM and Dubielzig R (1978) Diffuse pulmonary alveolar septal metastases from mammary carcinoma in the dog. *Journal of the American Veterinary Radiology Society* **19**, 161–167

Anderson GI (1987) Pulmonary cavitary lesions in the dog. *Journal of the American Animal Hospital Association* **23**, 89–94

Au JJ, Weisman DL, Stefanacci JD and Palmisano MP (2006) Use of computed tomography for evaluation of lung lesions associated with a spontaneous pneumothorax in dogs: 12 cases (1999–2002). *Journal of the American Veterinary Medical Association* **228**, 733–737

Ballegeer EA, Forrest LJ and Stepien RL (2002) Radiographic appearance of bronchoalveolar carcinoma in nine cats. *Veterinary Radiology & Ultrasound* **43**, 267–271

Barr FJ, Gibbs C and Brown PJ (1986) The radiological features of primary lung tumours in the dog: a review of thirty-six cases. *Journal of Small Animal Practice* **27**, 493–505

Barrett LE, Pollard RE, Zwingenberger A, Zierenberg-Ripoll A and Skorupski KA (2014) Radiographic characterization of primary lung tumors in 74 dogs. *Veterinary Radiology & Ultrasound* **55**, 480–487

Barthez PY, Hornof WJ, Theon AP, Craychee TJ and Morgan JP (1994) Receiver operating characteristic curve analysis of the performance of various radiographic protocols when screening dogs for pulmonary metastases. *Journal of the American Veterinary Medical Association* **204**, 237–240

Basher KL, Porter IR and Martin-Flores M (2019) Severe (grade IV) hypersensitivity to iodinated contrast agent in an anesthetized dog. *Canadian Veterinary Journal* **60**, 766–769

Baumann D and Flückiger M (2001) Radiographic findings in the thorax of dogs with leptospiral infection. *Veterinary Radiology & Ultrasound* **42**, 305–307

Belmudes A, Gory G, Cauvin E et al. (2021) Lung lobe torsion in 15 dogs: Peripheral band sign on ultrasound. *Veterinary Radiology & Ultrasound* **62**, 116–125

Benavides KL, Rozanski EA, Oura TJ (2019) Lung lobe torsion in 35 dogs and 4 cats. *Canadian Veterinary Journal* **60**, 60–66

Bennett AD, Lalor S, Schwarz T and Gunn-Moore DA (2011) Radiographic findings in cats with mycobacterial infections. *Journal of Feline Medicine and Surgery* **13**, 718–724

Berry C, Gallaway A, Thrall DE and Carlisle C (1993) Thoracic radiographic features of anticoagulant rodenticide toxicity in fourteen dogs. *Veterinary Radiology & Ultrasound* **34**, 391–396

Berry CR, Hawkins EC, Hurley KJ and Monce K (2000) Frequency of pulmonary mineralization and hypoxemia in 21 dogs with pituitary-dependent hyperadrenocorticism. *Journal of Veterinary Internal Medicine* **14**, 151–156

Berry CR, Moore PF, Thomas WP, Sisson D and Koblik PD (1990) Pulmonary lymphomatoid granulomatosis in seven dogs (1976–1987). *Journal of Veterinary Internal Medicine* **4**, 157–166

Bertolini G, Stefanello C and Caldin M (2009) Imaging diagnosis – pulmonary interstitial emphysema in a dog. *Veterinary Radiology & Ultrasound* **50**, 80–82

Boag AK, Lamb CR, Chapman PS and Boswood A (2004) Radiographic findings in 16 dogs infected with *Angiostrongylus vasorum*. *Veterinary Record* **154**, 426–430

Breheny C, Fox V, Tamborini A et al. (2017) Novel characteristics identified in two cases of feline pox virus infection. *Journal of Feline Medicine and Surgery Open Reports* **3**, 1–5

Brownlee L and Sellon RK (2001) Diagnosis of naturally occurring toxoplasmosis by bronchoalveolar lavage in a cat. *Journal of the American Animal Hospital Association* **37**, 251–255

Brummer DG, French TW and Cline JM (1989) Microlithiasis associated with chronic bronchopneumonia in a cat. *Journal of the American Veterinary Medical Association* **194**, 1061–1064

Burk RL, Joseph R and Baer K (1990) Systemic aspergillosis in a cat. *Veterinary Radiology & Ultrasound* **31**, 26–28

Cannon MS, Wisner ER, Johnson LR et al. (2009) Computed tomography bronchial lumen to pulmonary artery diameter ratio in dogs without clinical pulmonary disease. *Veterinary Radiology & Ultrasound* **50**, 622–624

Carpenter DH, Macintire DK and Tyler JW (2001) Acute lung injury and acute respiratory distress syndrome. *Compendium on Continuing Education for the Practicing Veterinarian* **23**, 712–725

Chandler JC and Lappin M (2002) Mycoplasmal respiratory infections in small animals: 17 cases (1988–1999). *Journal of the American Animal Hospital Association* **38**, 111–119

Clercx C, Peeters D, Snaps F et al. (2000) Eosinophilic bronchopneumopathy in dogs. *Journal of Veterinary Internal Medicine* **14**, 282–291

Clercx C, Reichler I, McEntee K et al. (2003) Rhinitis/bronchopneumonia syndrome in Irish Wolfhounds. *Journal of Veterinary Internal Medicine* **17**, 843–849

Cohn LA, Norris CR, Hawkins C et al. (2004) Identification and characterization of an idiopathic pulmonary fibrosis-like condition in cats. *Journal of Veterinary Internal Medicine* **18**, 632–641

Coia ME, Hammond G, Chan D et al. (2016) Retrospective evaluation of thoracic computed tomography findings in dogs naturally infected by *Angiostrongylus vasorum*. *Veterinary Radiology & Ultrasound* **58**, 524–534

Coleman MG, Warman CGA and Robson MC (2005) Dynamic cervical lung hernia in a dog with chronic airway disease. *Journal of Veterinary Internal Medicine* **19**, 103–105

Confer AW, Qualls CW Jr, MacWilliams PS and Root CR (1983) Four cases of pulmonary nodular eosinophilic granulomatosis in dogs. *Cornell Veterinarian* **73**, 141–151

Corcoran BM, Cobb M, Martin MWS et al. (1999) Chronic pulmonary disease in West Highland white terriers. *Veterinary Record* **144**, 611–616

Corcoran BM, King LG, Schwarz T, Hammond G and Sullivan M (2011) Further characterization of the clinical features of chronic pulmonary disease in West Highland white terriers. *Veterinary Record* **168**, 355.

D'Anjou MA, Tidwell AS and Hecht S (2005) Radiographic diagnosis of lung lobe torsion. *Veterinary Radiology & Ultrasound* **46**, 478–484

Dear JD (2014) Bacterial pneumonia in dogs and cats. *Veterinary Clinics of North America: Small Animal Practice* **44**, 143–159

Dear JD (2020) Bacterial pneumonia in dogs and cats: an update. *Veterinary Clinics of North America: Small Animal Practice* **50**, 447–465

Diana A, Guglielmini C, Pivetta M et al. (2009) Radiographic features of cardiogenic pulmonary edema in dogs with mitral regurgitation: 61 cases (1998–2007). *Journal of the American Veterinary Medical Association* **235**, 1058–1063

Drobatz KJ, Walker LM and Hendricks JC (1999) Smoke exposure in cats: 22 cases (1986–1997). *Journal of the American Veterinary Medical Association* **215**, 1312–1316

Drobatz KJ, Walker LM and Hendricks JC (1999) Smoke exposure in dogs: 27 cases (1988–1997). *Journal of the American Veterinary Medical Association* **215**, 1306–1311

Drolet R, Kenefick KB, Hakomaki MR and Ward GE (1986) Isolation of group eugonic fermenter-4 bacteria from a cat with multifocal suppurative pneumonia. *Journal of the American Veterinary Medical Association* **189**, 311–312

Egenvall A, Hansson K, Sateri H, Lord PF and Jonsson L (2003) Pulmonary oedema in Swedish hunting dogs. *Journal of Small Animal Practice* **44**, 209–217

El Kaddouri B, Strand MJ, Baraghoshi D et al. (2021) Fleischner Society visual emphysema CT patterns help predict progression of emphysema in current and former smokers: results from the COPDGene study. *Radiology* **298**, 441–449

Felson B (1979) A new look at pattern recognition of diffuse pulmonary disease. *American Journal of Roentgenology* **133**, 183–189

Fitzgerald SD, Wolf DC and Carlton WW (1991) Eight cases of canine lymphomatoid granulomatosis. *Veterinary Pathology* **28**, 241–145

Flückiger MA and Gomez JA (1984) Radiographic findings in dogs with spontaneous pulmonary thrombosis or embolism. *Veterinary Radiology* **25**, 124–131

Foster SF, Martin P, Allan GS, Barrs VR and Malik R (2004) Lower respiratory tract infections in cats: 21 cases (1995–2000). *Journal of Feline Medicine and Surgery* **6**, 167–180

Foster SF, Martin P, Davis W et al. (1999) Chronic pneumonia caused by *Mycobacterium thermoresistibile* in a cat. *Journal of Small Animal Practice* **40**, 453–464

Godshalk CP (1994) Common pitfalls in radiographic interpretation of the thorax. *Compendium on Continuing Education for the Practicing Veterinarian* **16**, 731–739

Gottfried SD, Popovitch CA, Goldschmidt MH and Schelling C (2000) Metastatic digital carcinoma in the cat: a retrospective study of 36 cats (1992–1998). *Journal of the American Animal Hospital Association* **36**, 501–509

Gunn-Moore D (2010) Mycobacterial infections in cats and dogs. In: *Textbook of Veterinary Internal Medicine, 7th edn*, ed S Ettinger and E Feldman, pp. 875–881. Saunders, Philadelphia

Gunn-Moore DA, McFarland SE, Brewer JI et al. (2011) Mycobacterial disease in cats in Great Britain: I. Culture results, geographical distribution and clinical presentation of 339 cases. *Journal of Feline Medicine and Surgery* **13**, 934–944

Hahn H, Specchi S, Masseau I et al. (2018) The computed tomographic "tree-in-bud" pattern: characterization and comparison with radiographic and clinical findings in 36 cats. *Veterinary Radiology & Ultrasound* **59**, 32–42

Hahn KA and McEntee MF (1997) Primary lung tumors in cats: 86 cases (1979–1994) *Journal of the American Veterinary Medical Association* **211**, 1257–1260

Hansell DM, Bankier AA, MacMahon H et al. (2008) Fleischner Society: glossary of terms for thoracic imaging. *Radiology* **246**, 697–722

Hayward NJ, Baines SJ, Baines EA and Herrtage ME (2004) The radiographic appearance of the pulmonary vasculature in the cat. *Veterinary Radiology & Ultrasound* **45**, 501–504

Hermanson JW, de Lahunta A and Evans HE (2020) *Miller and Evan's Anatomy of the Dog, 5th edn*. Elsevier Inc., St. Louis

Hoover JP, Henry GA and Panciera RJ (1992) Bronchial cartilage dysplasia with multifocal lobar bullous emphysema and lung lobe torsions. *Journal of the American Veterinary Medical Association* **201**, 599–602

Hornby NL and Lamb CR (2017) Does computed tomographic appearance of the lung differ between young and old dogs? *Veterinary Radiology & Ultrasound* **58**, 647–652

Hudson JA, Montgomery RD, Powers RD and Brawner WR (1994) Presumed mineral oil aspiration and cavitary lung lesion in a dog. *Veterinary Radiology & Ultrasound* **35**, 277–281

International Committee on Veterinary Gross Anatomical Nomenclature (2017) *Nomina Anatomica Veterinaria, 6th edn*. World Association of Veterinary Anatomists. Available at: www.wava-amav.org/downloads/nav_6_2017.zip

International Committee on Veterinary Histological Nomenclature (2017) *Nomina Histologica Veterinaria*. World Association of Veterinary Anatomists. Available at: www.wava-amav.org/downloads/NHV_2017.pdf

Jarvinen AK, Saario E, Andresen E et al. (1995) Lung injury leading to respiratory distress syndrome in young Dalmatian dogs. *Journal of Veterinary Internal Medicine* **9**, 162–168

Jefferies AR, Dunn JK and Dennis R (1987) Pulmonary alveolar proteinosis (phospholipoproteinosis) in a dog. *Journal of Small Animal Practice* **28**, 203–214

Jerram RM, Guyer CL, Braniecki A, Read WK and Hobson HP (1998) Endogenous lipid (cholesterol) pneumonia associated with bronchogenic carcinoma in a cat. *Journal of the American Animal Hospital Association* **34**, 275–280

Johnson VS, Corcoran BM, Wotton PR, Schwarz T and Sullivan M (2005) Thoracic high-resolution computed tomographic findings in dogs with canine idiopathic pulmonary fibrosis. *Journal of Small Animal Practice* **46**, 381–388

Johnson VS, Ramsey IK, Thompson H et al. (2004) Thoracic high-resolution computed tomography in the diagnosis of metastatic carcinoma. *Journal of Small Animal Practice* **45**, 134–143

Jones DJ, Norris CR, Samii VF and Griffey SM (2000) Endogenous lipid pneumonia in cats: 24 cases (1985–1998). *Journal of the American Veterinary Medical Association* **216**, 1437–1440

Kerr LY (1989) Pulmonary edema secondary to upper airway obstruction in the dog: a review of nine cases. *Journal of the American Animal Hospital Association* **25**, 207–212

Kirberger RM and Lobetti RG (1998) Radiographic aspects of *Pneumocystis carinii* pneumonia in the miniature Dachshund. *Veterinary Radiology & Ultrasound* **39**, 313–317

Kramek BA, Caywood DD and O'Brien TD (1985) Bullous emphysema and recurrent pneumothorax in the dog. *Journal of the American Veterinary Medical Association* **186**, 971–974

Lennon PF and Murray PA (1996) Attenuated hypoxic pulmonary vasoconstriction during isoflurane anesthesia is abolished by cyclooxygenase inhibition in chronically instrumented dogs. *Anesthesiology* **84**, 404–414

Lipscomb VJ, Hardie RJ and Dubielzig RR (2003) Spontaneous pneumothorax caused by pulmonary blebs and bullae in 12 dogs. *Journal of the American Animal Hospital Association* **39**, 435–444

Liu SK, Suter PF and Ettinger S (1969) Pulmonary alveolar microlithiasis with ruptured chordae tendineae in mitral and tricuspid valves in a dog. *Journal of the American Veterinary Medical Association* **155**, 1692–1703

Lo E, Schwarz T and Corcoran B (2021) Topographical distribution and radiographic pattern and lung lesions in canine eosinophilic bronchopneumopathy. *Journal of Small Animal Practice* **62**, 655–661

Lord PF (1975) Neurogenic pulmonary edema in the dog. *Journal of the American Animal Hospital Association* **11**, 778–783

Lord PF (1976) Alveolar lung diseases in small animals and their radiographic diagnosis. *Journal of Small Animal Practice* **17**, 283–303

Lord PF and Gomez JA (1985) Lung lobe collapse: pathophysiology and radiologic significance. *Veterinary Radiology* **26**, 187–195

Major A, Holmes A, Warren-Smith C et al. (2016) Computed tomographic findings in cats with mycobacterial infection. *Journal of Feline Medicine and Surgery* **17**, 510–517

Major A, O'Halloran C, Holmes A et al. (2018) Use of computed tomography imaging during long-term follow-up of nine feline tuberculosis cases. *Journal of Feline Medicine and Surgery* **20**, 189–199

Matros L, Riediesel EA and Myers RK (1994) Silicate pneumoconiosis in a dog: case report and current concepts of pathogenesis. *Journal of the American Animal Hospital Association* **30**, 375–381

McEntee MC, Page RL, Cline JM and Thrall DE (1992) Radiation pneumonitis in 3 dogs. *Veterinary Radiology & Ultrasound* **33**, 190–197

Mclaughlin R, Canada RO and Tyler WS (1961) A study of subgross pulmonary anatomy in various mammals. *American Journal of Anatomy* **108**, 149–165

Mesquita L, Lam R, Lamb C and McConnell F (2015) Computed tomographic findings in 15 dogs with eosinophilic bronchopneumopathy. *Veterinary Radiology & Ultrasound* **56**, 33–39

Moise NS, Wiedenkeller D, Yeager AE, Blue JT and Scarlett J (1989) Clinical, radiographic, and bronchial cytologic features of cats with bronchial disease: 65 cases (1980–1986). *Journal of the American Veterinary Medical Association* **194**, 1467–1473

Moon ML, Greenlee PG and Burk RL (1986) Uremic pneumonitis-like syndrome in ten dogs. *Journal of the American Animal Hospital Association* **22**, 687–691

Mortier JR, Fina CJ, Edery E and White CL (2018) Computed tomographic findings in three dogs naturally infected with *Crenosoma vulpis*. *Veterinary Radiology & Ultrasound* **59**, 27–31

Munden RF and Hess KR (2001) 'Ditzels' on chest CT: survey of the members of the Society of Thoracic Radiology. *American Journal of Roentgenology* **176**, 1363–1369

Murphy K and Brisson BA (2006) Evaluation of lung lobe torsion in Pugs: 7 cases (1991–2004). *Journal of the American Veterinary Medical Association* **228**, 86–90

Myer W (1980) Radiography review: the interstitial pattern of pulmonary disease. *Veterinary Radiology* **21**, 18–23

Neath PJ, Brockman DJ and King LG (2000) Lung lobe torsion in dogs: 22 cases (1981–1999). *Journal of the American Veterinary Medical Association* **217**, 1041–1044

Nemanic S, London CA and Wisner ER (2006) Comparison of thoracic radiographs and single breath-hold helical CT for detection of pulmonary nodules in dogs with metastatic neoplasia. *Journal of Veterinary Internal Medicine* **20**, 508–515

Nykamp SG, Scrivani PV and Dykes NL (2002) Radiographic signs of pulmonary disease: an alternative approach. *Compendium on Continuing Education for the Practicing Veterinarian* **24**, 25–35

O'Neill RG, Schwarz T, Thompson H, Sullivan M and Argyle DJ (2006) Pulmonary alveolar microlithiasis: undoubtedly underdiagnosed. *The Irish Veterinary Journal* **59**, 627–632

O'Sullivan SP (1989) Paraquat poisoning in the dog. *Journal of Small Animal Practice* **30**, 361–364

Olsson S-E (1957) On tuberculosis in the dog. A study with special reference to X-ray diagnosis. *Cornell Veterinarian* **47**, 193–219

Parent C, King LG, Walker LM and Van Winkle TJ (1996) Clinical and clinicopathologic findings in dogs with acute respiratory distress syndrome: 19 cases (1985–1993). *Journal of the American Veterinary Medical Association* **208**, 1419–1427

Park KM, Grimes JA, Wallace ML et al. (2018) Lung lobe torsion in dogs: 52 cases (2005–2017). *Veterinary Surgery* **47**, 1002–1008

Perez-Accino J, Liuti T, Pecceu E and Cazzini P (2020) Endogenous lipoid pneumonia associated with pulmonary neoplasia in three dogs. *Journal of Small Animal Practice* **62**, 223–228

Phillips S, Barr S, Dykes N et al. (2000) Bronchiolitis obliterans with organizing pneumonia in a dog. *Journal of Veterinary Internal Medicine* **14**, 204–207

Radlinsky MG, Homco LD and Blount WC (1998) Ultrasonographic diagnosis – radiolucent pulmonary foreign body. *Veterinary Radiology & Ultrasound* **39**, 150–153

Reed JC (1997) *Chest Radiology: Plain Film Patterns and Differential Diagnoses*, 4th ed. Mosby, St. Louis

Rooney MB, Lanz O and Monnet E (2001) Spontaneous lung lobe torsion in two pugs. *Journal of the American Animal Hospital Association* **37**, 128–130

Schultz RM, Peters J and Zwingenberger A (2009) Radiography, computed tomography and virtual bronchoscopy in four dogs and two cats with lung lobe torsion. *Journal of Small Animal Practice* **50**, 360–363

Schwarz T, Crawford PE, Owen MR, Störk CK and Thompson H (2001) Fatal pulmonary fat embolism during humeral fracture repair in a cat. *Journal of Small Animal Practice* **42**, 195–198

Schwarz T, Störk CK, Mellor D and Sullivan M (2000) Osteopenia and other radiographic signs in canine hyperadrenocorticism. *Journal of Small Animal Practice* **41**, 491–495

Scott-Moncrieff JG, Elliott GS, Radovsky A and Blevins WE (1989) Pulmonary squamous cell carcinoma with multiple digital metastases in a cat. *Journal of Small Animal Practice* **30**, 696–699

Scrivani PV (2009) Nontraditional interpretation of lung patterns. *Veterinary Clinics of North America: Small Animal Practice* **39**, 719–732

Scrivani PV and Percival A (2023) Anatomic study of the canine bronchial tree using silicone casts, radiography, and CT. *Veterinary Radiology & Ultrasound* **64**, 36–41

Scrivani PV, Thompson MS, Dykes NL et al. (2012) Relationships among subgross anatomy, computed tomography, and histologic findings in dogs with disease localized to the pulmonary acini. *Veterinary Radiology & Ultrasound* **53**, 1–10

Shimbo G and Takiguchi M (2021) CT morphology of anomalous systemic arterial supply to normal lungs in dogs. *Veterinary Radiology & Ultrasound* **62**, 657–665

Silverman S, Poulous PW and Suter PF (1976) Cavitary pulmonary lesions in animals. *Journal of the American Veterinary Radiological Society* **17**, 134–140

Silverstein D, Greene C, Gregory C, Lucas S and Quandt J (2000) Pulmonary alveolar proteinosis in a dog. *Journal of Veterinary Internal Medicine* **14**, 546–551

Stampley AR and Waldron DR (1993) Reexpansion pulmonary edema after surgery to repair a diaphragmatic hernia in a cat. *Journal of the American Veterinary Medical Association* **203**, 1699–1701

Starrak GS, Berry CR, Page RL, Johnson JL and Thrall DE (1997) Correlation between thoracic radiographic changes and remission/survival duration in 270 dogs with lymphosarcoma. *Veterinary Radiology & Ultrasound* **38**, 411–418

Staub NC, Nagano H and Pearce ML (1967) Pulmonary edema in dogs, especially the sequence of fluid accumulation in lungs. *Journal of Applied Physiology* **22**, 227–240

Suter PF and Chan KF (1968) Disseminated pulmonary diseases in small animals – a radiographic approach to diagnosis. *Journal of the American Veterinary Radiology Society* **9**, 67–79

Suter PF and Lord PF (1974) Radiographic differentiation of disseminated pulmonary parenchymal diseases in dogs and cats. *Veterinary Clinics of North America: Small Animal Practice* **4**, 687–710

Suter PF and Lord PF (1984) *Thoracic Radiography: A Text Atlas of Thoracic Diseases of the Dog and Cat.* Peter F Suter, Wettswil

Tamura A, Hebisawa A, Fukushima K, Yotsumoto H and Mori M (1998) Lipoid pneumonia in lung cancer: radiographic and pathological features. *Japanese Journal of Clinical Oncology* **28**, 492–496

Thierry F, Handel I, Hammond G et al. (2017) Further characterization of computed tomographic and clinical features for staging and prognosis of idiopathic pulmonary fibrosis in West Highland white terriers. *Veterinary Radiology & Ultrasound* **58**, 284–294

Thrall DE and Losonsky JM (1976) A method for evaluating canine pulmonary circulatory dynamics from survey radiographs. *Journal of the American Animal Hospital Association* **12**, 457–462

Tiemessen I (1989) Thoracic metastases of canine mammary gland tumors: a radiographic study. *Veterinary Radiology* **30**, 249–252

Tsai S, Sutherland-Smith J, Burgess K, Ruthazer R and Sato A (2012) Imaging characteristics of intrathoracic histiocytic sarcoma in dogs. *Veterinary Radiology & Ultrasound* **53**, 21–27

Warwick H, Guillem J, Batchelor D et al. (2021) Imaging findings in 14 dogs and 3 cats with lobar emphysema. *Journal of Veterinary Internal Medicine* **35**, 1935–1942

Winegardner K, Scrivani PV and Gleed RD (2008) Lung expansion in the diagnosis of lung disease. *Compendium on Continuing Education for the Practicing Veterinarian* **30**, 479–489

Wolf AM and Troy GC (1989) Deep mycotic diseases. In: *Textbook of Veterinary Internal Medicine – Diseases of the Dog And Cat. Volume 1, 3rd edn*, ed. SJ Ettinger, pp. 341–372. WB Saunders, Philadelphia

Woodring JH and Reed JC (1996) Types and mechanisms of pulmonary atelectasis. *Journal of Thoracic Imaging* **11**, 92–108

Index

Page numbers in *italic* refer to figures

Get the full picture with our imaging manuals...

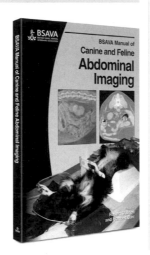
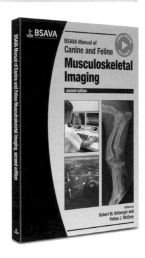
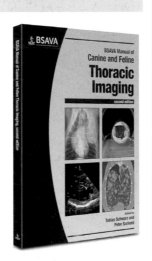
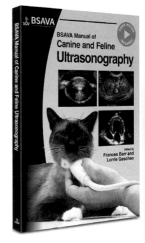